Pye's **Surgical Handicraft**

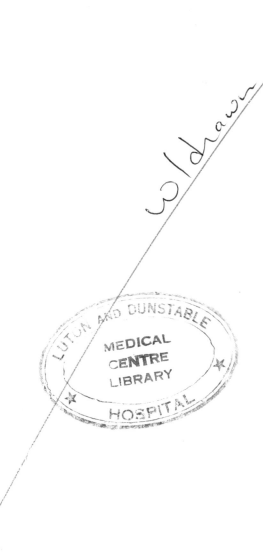

Pye's
Surgical Handicraft
Twenty-second edition

James Kyle CBE, DSc, MCh, FRCS, FRCS Ed, FRCSI
Consultant Surgeon, Aberdeen Royal Infirmary; Honorary Clinical Senior Lecturer in Surgery, University of Aberdeen

J. A. R. Smith PhD, FRCS, FRCS Ed
Consultant Surgeon, Northern General Hospital, Sheffield; Clinical Lecturer in Surgery, University of Sheffield

D. H. Johnston FRCS
Lecturer in Surgery, The Royal London Hospital, Whitechapel, London

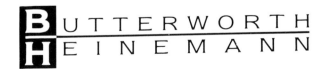

Butterworth-Heinemann Ltd
Linacre House, Jordan Hill, Oxford OX2 8DP

 PART OF REED INTERNATIONAL BOOKS

OXFORD   LONDON   BOSTON
MUNICH   NEW DELHI   SINGAPORE   SYDNEY
TOKYO   TORONTO   WELLINGTON

First published 1884
Twenty-second edition 1992

© Butterworth-Heinemann Ltd 1992

British Library Cataloguing in Publication Data
Kyle, James
  Pye's surgical handicraft. – 22nd ed.
  I. Title   II. Smith, J.A.R.   III. Johnston. D. H.
  617.001

ISBN 0 7506 1363 7

ISBN 0 7506 0623 1   Butterworth-Heinemann International Edition

Library of Congress Cataloguing in Publication Data
Pye's surgical handicraft. — 22nd ed./ [edited by] James Kyle, J.A.R.
  Smith, D. H. Johnston.
      p.   cm.
   Includes bibliographical references and index.
   ISBN 0 7506 1363 7
   1. Surgery, Operative.   I. Kyle, James.   II. Smith, John A. R.
III. Johnston, David H. (David Howard)   IV. Pye, Walter, 1853–1892.
Pye's surgical handicraft.   V. Title: Surgical handicraft.
   [DNLM: 1. Postoperative Care.   2. Preoperative Care.   3. Surgery,
Operative.   WO 178 P9951]
RD32.P94   1991
617.6'91–dc20
DNLM/DLC
for Library of Congress   91-19452
                                                              CIP

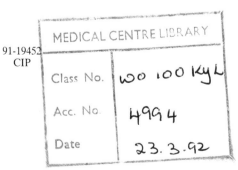
Composition by Genesis Typesetting, Rochester, Kent
Printed and bound by Courier International Limited, East Kilbride

Contents

Preface

It is almost exactly 30 years since I assumed the editorship of 'Pye' following the death of Hamilton Bailey early in 1962. During these three decades there have been great changes in medicine, and particularly in surgical practice. Many new and much more effective drugs are now available. Transplants have become commonplace, and minimally invasive surgery is expanding rapidly. Surgical oncology and vascular surgery have become recognized and separate specialties. The staffing patterns within British hospitals are changing. Surgical audit is of great importance, and now that patients have the right to see their own records, the young doctor must be particularly careful about what he writes in those records.

Markets for British textbooks have altered; the ships' doctors who used to roam the seven seas have now virtually disappeared; many countries in Africa and Asia now print their own books, or purchase them elsewhere. The advice given in this 22nd edition should be useful in any part of the world.

Nowhere have the changes of the last 30 years been more noticeable than in the publishing houses of Britain. For most of this century, 'Pye' was produced by John Wright & Sons, of Bristol. Then a few years ago the title passed to Butterworth Scientific and the typescripts for this edition had to be transferred to Guildford. The material's stay there was brief, because last year Butterworth joined Heinemann Medical, and operations moved to Oxford. Confusion and delay were inevitable. It is thanks to the untiring efforts of Jennifer Bew and June Fettes that the scattered parts at last have been assembled, and this new edition completed.

Amid all the swirling changes of recent years, the one steadfast rock has been my secretary, Mrs Jan Amonoo. Her tact and courtesy, her diligence and accuracy have been of inestimable value. Now entering her retirement, she has my most sincere gratitude and best wishes.

James Kyle
Aberdeen
October 1991

Contributors

D. F. Badenoch FRCS
Consultant Urologist, The London Hospital,
London

R. W. Blamey FRCS
Professor of Surgery and Consultant Surgeon,
Nottingham City Hospital, Nottingham

T. K. Choi FRCS
Queen Mary Hospital, Hong Kong

H. A. Crockard FRCS
Consultant Neurosurgeon, The National Hospital
for Nervous Diseases and University College
Hospital, London

T. Duckworth FRCS
Professor of Orthopaedic Surgery; Head, University
Department of Orthopaedics, University of
Sheffield; Consultant Orthopaedic Surgeon, Royal
Hallamshire Hospital, Sheffield

H. A. F. Dudley CBE, ChM, FRCS, FRCS Ed,
FRACS
Academic Surgical Unit, St Mary's Hospital,
London

J. R. Farndon FRCS
Professor of Surgery and Consultant Surgeon,
Bristol Royal Infirmary, Bristol

J. P. Gowar FRCS, FRCS Ed
Consultant Surgeon, Burns Unit, Birmingham
Accident Hospital, Birmingham

Graham Hill FRACS
Professor of Surgery, University of Auckland, New
Zealand

M. Horrocks FRCS
Consultant Surgeon, Bristol Royal Infirmary

Geoffrey Hooper MMSc, FRCS,
FRCS Ed (Orth)
Consultant Orthopaedic Surgeon, Princess
Margaret Rose Orthopaedic Hospital and the Royal
Infirmary, Edinburgh; Honorary Senior Lecturer in
Orthopaedic Surgery, University of Edinburgh

David A. Humberstone MB, ChB
Late Surgical Registrar. Dr Humberstone died very
shortly after the completion of his contribution to
this book

J. M. Imray FFARCS
Consultant Anaesthetist, Aberdeen Royal
Infirmary, Aberdeen

C. P. D. Isaac MEd, DipEdTech, RGN, RCT,
RNT
Clinical Teacher, Learning Resources, Foresterhill
College, Aberdeen

D. H. Johnston FRCS
Lecturer in Surgery, The Royal London Hospital,
London

James Kyle CBE, DSc, MCh, FRCS, FRCS Ed,
FRCSI
Consultant Surgeon, Aberdeen Royal Infirmary;
Honorary Clinical Senior Lecturer in Surgery,
University of Aberdeen, Aberdeen

Alasdair B. Matheson OBE, FRCS Ed
Consultant in Accident and Emergency Care,
Aberdeen Royal Infirmary; Clinical Senior Lecturer
(Surgery, Occupational and Environmental
Medicine) University of Aberdeen

R. J. Nicholls FRCS
Consultant Surgeon, St Marks Hospital, London

G. S. Robertson MD, FFARCS
Consultant Anaesthetist, Aberdeen Royal
Infirmary, Aberdeen

R. D. Rosin FRCS
Consultant Surgeon, St Mary's Hospital, London

G. H. Smith FRCS
Consultant Surgeon, Cardiothoracic Department,
Northern General Hospital, Sheffield

J. A. R. Smith PhD, FRCS, FRCS Ed
Consultant Surgeon, Northern General Hospital,
Sheffield; Clinical Lecturer in Surgery, University of
Sheffield

Louis Spitz FRCS, FRCS Ed
Nuffield Professor of Paediatric Surgery, Institute of
Child Health, London; Honorary Consultant
Paediatric Surgeon, Hospital for Sick Children,
Great Ormond Street, London

D. F. M. Thomas MRC, FRCS
Consultant Paediatric Surgeon/Urologist,
Department of Paediatric Surgery, St James's
University Hospital and the General Infirmary,
Leeds

D. A. Warrell MRCS, FRCP
Professor of Tropical Medicine, John Radcliffe
Hospital, University of Oxford, Oxford

D. C. White FFARCS
Consultant Anaesthetist, Northwick Park Hospital,
Harrow

J. Wong FRCS, FRACS
Professor of Surgery, Queen Mary Hospital, Hong
Kong

1

Duties of the house surgeon

James Kyle

The advice given in this chapter is based on more than 40 years' experience in hospital medicine. Careful perusal of this chapter by the house surgeon when he first takes up his appointment will provide him with this information that will enable him to perform his duties in a safe and satisfactory manner.

Good communications between all grades of staff are essential for the efficient and effective management of patients in hospital.

Obtaining information about his patients and communicating such information to appropriate persons are two of the main duties of a house surgeon. As the resident doctor on the spot, at times he will have to counsel and co-ordinate, initiate action and implement instructions. A modern hospital is a highly complex organization. When he takes up his appointment, the house surgeon should visit all the principal departments, and should find out from his predecessor, or other surgical colleagues, who are the most helpful members in the various departments.

The new house surgeon, if he wants to be treated as a doctor, should look and behave like one. Surgical wards should be clean and tidy, while in operating theatres an aseptic ritual is practised. Dirty, polo-necked sweaters and long, unkempt hair are not acceptable in either place. A clean white coat always looks professional. If it becomes soiled or contaminated it should be changed at once. It is safer to carry and use a notebook or clipboard than to rely on memory.

When talking to patients and relatives it is advisable to keep the conversation professional, but using simple words that are readily understood. Bad language and imputations against other doctors must always be avoided. Jokes are liable to be misconstrued; at the time of admission many patients are nervous, and not in the mood for jokes. As rapport is gradually built up, then a less formal attitude shows that the doctor is human. With some elderly patients it may be necessary to use a local dialect to obtain accurate information, but in general gimmicks are better avoided. Most patients are reasonable and sensible; they will be reassured if shortly after admission they are given an outline of the investigations that are proposed, of the options available, and of the form and duration of treatment.

Undue haste is rarely necessary. A doctor should not run except in a dire emergency such as cardiac arrest or total respiratory obstruction. Patients are not going to have much confidence in a doctor who always appears to be in a panic. Conversely, there is no place for haughty or high-handed behaviour. Arrogance is a sign of ignorance and immaturity. An experienced ward sister or secretary knows a great deal more about the running of a surgical ward than the most recent medical recruit. If he is wise, a house surgeon can learn a great deal from these permanent members of the surgical team, from the physiotherapist, pharmacist, head porter and other personnel who keep a modern hospital functioning smoothly.

Smoking

Smoking is dangerous to health, and doctors should set an example to the public by not smoking. A house surgeon should never smoke in front of patients, or in parts of the hospital where he may be seen by members of the public. Cigarettes should not be sold in hospital, and any patient who is going to have a general anaesthetic should be encouraged to stop smoking completely. A major operation

1

provides a good opportunity to give up the damaging habit permanently.

Time keeping

Patients in an acute surgical ward need to have a doctor readily available at all times. One of the first tasks of a new house surgeon is to check up in detail on the suggested duty or off-duty rota in his hospital. He has to make certain that there is continuous medical cover for his patients, 24 hours per day, 7 days per week. Consultation with other junior colleagues usually enables a safe and satisfactory rota to be worked out. Senior medical and nursing staff should be informed about and agree to the proposed rota.

When on duty the doctor should endeavour to be punctual. This usually means being in the ward 30 minutes before the consultant is expected, so that the latest state of the patients may be ascertained. Reliability and punctuality are major factors in a young doctor's chances of promotion. If for any reason he has to absent himself from his usual place of work while on duty, the house surgeon should tell the ward sister and hospital telephonist exactly where he can be quickly contacted in an emergency. Any sudden signal such as that provided by a 'bleeper' system should be answered at once. All emergency admissions must be seen without delay.

Responsibility and consultation

Assuming immediate responsibility for a ward full of sick patients for the first time is a daunting prospect. The consultant and other members of the team realize this, and will advise and support a new house surgeon. After a few weeks, when he knows all the patients thoroughly and has become accustomed to the ward routine and hospital procedures, the house surgeon becomes more confident and a valuable link-man in the team. If he is ever in doubt about a ward technique or how to proceed, the house surgeon should ask a more senior doctor for advice and help–that is how an apprenticeship system works. The young doctor should know his own limitations, without at the same time allowing himself to become a nuisance to others. It is not always easy to strike the right balance.

The consultant in charge will generally want to know at once of any unusual happening in his ward such as an accident, sudden death, unexpected complication, threatening relatives or anything that may lead to litigation later. Always inform the consultant of any late major changes in the plans made for the next day, for example cancellation of an operating list caused by illness, strikes or staff shortages.

Relations with staff and relatives

Relations with family doctors

The family doctor should always be treated courteously and his telephone calls answered promptly. He is in a unique position to provide vital information about a patient whom he may want to admit. Besides noting down the patient's history and personal particulars, the family doctor should be asked about previous episodes, drugs given, family history and social circumstances. There can rarely be any justification in refusing a request for an admission made by an outside doctor. When there is no other general hospital in the district, then the patient must be admitted, and somehow a bed be found for him in the hospital.

It is good practice for the surgeon to send the family doctor a letter at the time of any operation. If the practitioner wants to visit his patient in hospital he should be made welcome and given full information. When the patient goes home, the house surgeon should give him a note to hand to his doctor briefly indicating: (1) the diagnosis, (2) treatment, (3) dosage of any drugs suggested, (4) arrangements for follow-up or after-care. One of the more senior members of the team normally sends a detailed, typed letter as soon as possible after the patient's discharge.

Relations with nursing and other staff

Patients sometimes confide in nurses information which they have been afraid to tell the doctor. Nurses often gain considerable insight into home circumstances, and an experienced nurse may be almost as good as a medical social worker in sorting out the patient's domestic problems. The intelligent house surgeon can learn a lot from the nursing staff. He should always be considerate and polite towards them. Try to avoid interviewing patients in bed at times when nurses are known to be serving meals, dispensing drugs or giving out bed pans. Student nurses appreciate the doctor in the ward explaining a patient's symptoms and treatment to them when time permits.

A surgical ward which has a permanent physio-therapist and medical social worker attached to it is very fortunate. The house surgeon is responsible for telling them about foreseeable problems and cooperating with them in the management of complications and other difficulties. They should be alerted at an early stage, and be kept informed of progress. Verbal communications are always better than written messages. It is profitable for the house surgeon to build up a good personal relationship with other skilled technicians, such as biochemists, radiographers and electrocardiographers, as their services are frequently required in a surgical unit.

Relations with relatives

It is not uncommon for relatives to be even more worried than the patient who is admitted to hospital. Consequently they should be handled carefully and with sympathy. The doctor's first duty is always to his patient. First find out exactly what is the degree of kinship between relative and patient. If the relationship is close and there is no reason to suspect that the relative may take any action that would be against the patient's best interests, then the relative should be given a short, simple account of the medical condition and prognosis. Stick to the truth and do not pretend to be a prophet. A close relative should be notified of any sudden deterioration in the condition of a patient, and of course of a patient's death.

Sometimes relatives become unreasonable and make a nuisance of themselves. That is the time to be firm and to enlist the support of a senior doctor. A tired patient may need to be protected from excessive visiting by unthinking relatives.

Relations with the police

While the first duty of a doctor is to his patient, he also does have a civil responsibility to help the police when appropriate. Information should not be divulged to the police hastily; snap disclosures over the telephone should be avoided. Such information may be used in court proceedings. Ideally, witnessed consent should be obtained from an adult patient before medical information concerning him is given to the police. If the young doctor finds that there is a conflict between his obligations to preserve confidentiality on the one hand and to do his civil duty on the other, he should say nothing, but ask the police to contact the senior surgeon or hospital medical administrator next morning.

Autopsies

If a patient dies, the house surgeon should take time to say a few sympathetic words to bereaved relatives. It is desirable to get an autopsy in all cases, unless there has been histological confirmation of the diagnosis from a recent operation or other procedure. The relatives naturally wish to avoid delay and want to proceed with funeral arrangements. If it is explained to them that an autopsy may prevent some other patient dying from a similar condition, the relatives will mostly give consent to the examination. Reasoned argument rather than threats should be used.

When consent is refused and the cause of death is genuinely unknown, then the house surgeon must refuse to issue a death certificate and should notify his consultant at once. When the cause of death is unknown and the case needs to be notified to the Coroner (or the Procurator-fiscal), then an autopsy should not be performed unless the legal authority gives permission to proceed.

Note-taking

Good patient records are essential for correct diagnosis and management, and for follow-up and research purposes at a later date. They form a useful index of the standards maintained in a surgical unit, and some institutions for higher surgical training take ward records into account when deciding whether or not a hospital post should be recognized for training purposes. Good records are invaluable for the preparation of insurance reports and in any legal proceedings. They play an important role in surgical audit.

Notes about patients should be written legibly at once and not left until later. Several systems are in use. All should include simple statements: (1) of what the patient complained; (2) duration of complaint; (3) how it began.

It is advisable to record specific dates and times. There may be several different symptoms to be dealt with in sequence. Ask the patient about any industrial injury or hazard for which he may be able to claim compensation. Has he had any adverse reactions to drugs in the past? A provisional diagnosis or list of differential diagnoses should be suggested after the first round of questions and investigations. Make it clear that at that time the diagnosis is provisional, i.e. it may have to be altered at a later date. At the end of a ward admission the definitive diagnosis is written down, along with the arrangements for after-care.

Progress notes should be made during the patient's stay in hospital. It is particularly important to make contemporaneous notes should any serious emergency or complication develop. Brief, factual notes written at the time will prove invaluable in surgical audit, in dealing with complaints or rebutting a charge of medical negligence.

The problem-orientated medical record is frequently advocated but has not been widely adopted. Each patient has in his case notes a master problem list; this is a simple column of defined problems (with dates) and firm diagnoses. Problems can be secondary to other problems and may be active or passive. Investigation and diagnosis are conducted in a dynamic and logical manner.

Use and abuse of laboratories

It is the result of an investigation that is important, not the despatch of the specimen. When a patient's life depends on getting a result rapidly, then not only may the house surgeon have to take the specimen to the laboratory, but he may have to call back in person or telephone to get the result quickly.

During the past 30 years, the numbers of laboratory tests and of other special investigations being performed in hospitals have risen alarmingly. Many are totally unnecessary and constitute an unjustifiable waste of scarce health care resources. Before ordering any test the house surgeon should ask himself: 'On the clinical evidence available, is there any reasonable chance that in this patient this test is going to show an abnormal result?' If the answer is a clear 'yes', the test is performed forthwith, but if the answer is 'no', then the test is not requested at that time, although it may have to be performed later and after further consultation. The art is as important as the science in the practice of good medicine, and common sense is an essential component of both.

Writing on a request form to be sent to a laboratory should be legible. As well as particulars of the patient, the ward number, consultant and date, the form should quote any hospital unit number, mention any similar previous tests (with dates), and relevant drugs that the patient is taking. It should end with a clear statement of what information the ward or clinic doctor wants from the laboratory.

There can be no justification for endlessly repeating tests with normal results when the patient's clinical condition and therapy remain unchanged. Such behaviour indicates either that the young doctor has no understanding of the tests he is ordering or that the supervision by the senior doctor is gravely deficient, or both. A continuous intravenous infusion running for some days can, of course, lead to excessive accumulation of electrolytes, whose levels need to be checked. Another temptation which should be avoided is attempting to confirm an already proven diagnosis by half a dozen different techniques. It is very doubtful if a patient with a typical duodenal ulcer history, whose ulcer has been demonstrated by a competent radiologist, then needs to be subjected to gastroscopy/duodenoscopy.

Department of radiodiagnosis

The house surgeon is involved both in requesting radiological investigations and in the preparation of his patients for same. He must also ensure that the results of the investigations are made known to the senior member of the surgical team as quickly as possible.

When ordering a radiograph, the request form should (1) indicate the provisional diagnosis, (2) mention relevant clinical findings, such as a palpable mass or jaundice, (3) give details of any operation on the relevant part, (4) show the dates of any previous radiological studies, (5) mention factors which may be of practical importance in carrying out the investigation, e.g. a stiff hip or gross obesity before (6) stating clearly which particular investigation is required, if need be after consultation with the radiologist.

Avoidance of accidental irradiation of an early pregnancy

Female patients of childbearing age should be asked about the possibility of early pregnancy. If there is any doubt radiograph examination should be avoided (except in dire emergency) until pregnancy tests have been performed. Some hospitals confine irradiation of the lower abdomen in females to the 10 days following the first day of a menstrual period – The Ten Day Rule.

Types of radiological investigation

Imaging is a rapidly expanding speciality. It includes investigations by X-rays, ultrasound, computerized tomography (CT), positron emission and magnetic resonance imaging. New techniques are constantly being developed. The house surgeon is not expected to know the details of performing all the types of investigation and therapy which can now be practised in a modern radiology department. He should, however, possess an understanding of the role of imaging in the study of patients under his care, and of the relative merits of and place for the different types of investigation and of interventional radiology.

Straight radiograph

A straight radiograph is useful for fractures, in chest diseases, the acute abdomen, with opaque foreign bodies, etc.

Contrast studies

Contrast studies are useful for outlining hollow organs or channels with compounds containing opaque barium or iodine. In the alimentary tract they may be complementary to endoscopic studies. In some systems such as the biliary tract contrast studies have been largely superseded by ultrasonic (or CT) scans.

Ultrasonic scanning

This involves no irradiation and has now achieved a high degree of accuracy in detecting fetal abnormalities, cysts, abscesses, abdominal masses, biliary and pancreatic disease, congenital and valvular lesions of the heart, and in imaging major arteries.

Computerized tomography (CT scan)

This is expensive but valuable in intracranial lesions, mediastinal and abdominal masses (particularly in obese subjects), lymphomas and retroperitoneal tumours. CT scans should only be ordered after consultation with the radiologist.

Nuclear magnetic resonance (NMR)

There is no radiation hazard. Magnetic resonance imaging is helpful in detecting hepatic tumours and in central nervous system diseases. Tissue characterization may be possible.

Isotope imaging

Isotope imaging depicts changes of a functional nature. It is useful for demonstrating thyroid uptake, bone metastases, pulmonary emboli, myocardial ischaemia, intracardiac shunts and differential renal function.

Interventional radiology

The radiologist can now undertake therapeutic procedures under direct visual control, e.g. aspirating renal cysts, embolizing bleeding vessels, dilating arterial stenoses (transluminal angioplasty), percutaneous biopsies of bones or tumours and removal of renal or retained biliary calculi.

Digital radiography

The development of television enhancement systems using digital electronics and improved electronic recording enables an image to be stored (e.g. on video disc) and be handled by a computer.

Requesting another opinion

When the surgeon wants advice from a colleague in another ward or department, first ascertain if that person is available. If the matter is urgent, a personal visit is made to the other doctor and the nature and urgency of the situation explained to him. This is more courteous than an impersonal letter sent through the hospital mail. When the matter is less urgent, a tactful, factual letter can be delivered by hand to the unit where advice is being sought. It is unwise to rely on important letters reaching the correct specialist by entrusting them to impersonal delivery services. A telephone call can supplement a written communication.

Prescribing drugs

This is a task that has to be performed carefully and with attention to detail, particularly when dealing with controlled and other dangerous drugs. On the drug prescription card commence with: (1) the date, then insert (2) the pharmaceutical name of the drug, (3) the dose in metric units, (4) the route and (5) the times of administration, and finally (6) sign the entry. Usually it is inadvisable to mark drugs to be given 'as required', but an experienced ward nursing sister can be given some discretion with regard to mild laxatives and domestic types of analgesics. When a drug is discontinued, the date should be written down and signed. It is bad medical practice to administer drugs longer than is necessary, and furthermore they are costly. The house surgeon should frequently review the prescription card for each patient and know the cost of the drugs.

Any unusual reaction to a drug is noted on the prescription card and on the front of the patient's case notes.

Ward rounds

The resident doctor should go round all the patients under his care first thing each morning, checking not only on temperatures and intravenous infusions, but also on such mundane matters as urine output and bowel function. He should note the number of empty beds, particularly if his ward is to receive emergency cases that day.

The time of the nursing staff is just as valuable as that of the doctors. Rounds should not normally be started when meals are about to be served. If the registrar and senior registrar are available, they should go round with the house surgeon, and not expect the senior nurse to accompany each of them on separate peregrinations. When the consultant goes round, the house surgeon should have all the case notes and latest results available for inspection and discussion.

Nowadays many house surgeons will be off duty in the evening, but their ill patients still need careful supervision. Before he leaves the ward, the house surgeon must make a clear arrangement with another doctor in the surgical team, or with a colleague in an adjacent ward, to visit his ward in the late evening. It is important to tell the senior nurse whom to contact in case of difficulty, and leave a prominent note to this effect – nurses go off duty too.

Discharging a patient

When possible, a patient should be told a few days before it is likely that he will be able to leave hospital. He can then tell his relatives and make arrangements. It is very expensive to keep a patient in a hospital bed. The house surgeon should show intelligent anticipation in each case and try to ensure that every patient gets home to his family as soon as it is medically safe for him to do so. Before the patient leaves the ward, the doctor needs to check on the state of any incision and make sure that the patient is fit to make the journey. A patient should not be sent home to an empty house after an operation. If he has any doubts about the home circumstances, the house surgeon is advised to contact the patient's family doctor by telephone.

Patient taking his own discharge

A patient of sound mind has the right to decide what treatment he will accept and when he will leave hospital. If the doctor considers it medically unsafe for the patient to leave hospital, he should reason and explain to the patient in front of a witness. The consequences of his action having been explained, if the patient still insists on leaving, he should be asked to sign a form acknowledging that he is leaving contrary to medical advice. This form is duly witnessed. If the patient refuses to sign the form, then the doctor and witness sign it, noting down the patient's refusal to accept advice and to complete the form.

When the patient is considered to be of unsound mind the duty psychiatrist should be called at once.

Operating lists

Consent

Each patient having an operation has to sign a consent form after the nature of the operation has been explained to him – informed consent. The house surgeon must give this explanation in simple terms. It is most important that the patient understands what is involved, particularly if a limb or breast is to be removed, an external intestinal stoma established, or the patient rendered sterile.

It is now necessary to inform patients of the options available and the possible risks and complications of operations. But exercise discretion is so doing – do not destroy the peace of mind of the timorous or feed the appetite of the morbid.

The patient has to agree that the operative and anaesthetic techniques can be varied as considered necessary, and no undertaking is given that the procedure will be performed by any particular doctor.

Marking

With bilateral structures, limbs, etc. the side to be operated on must be clearly marked beforehand with a felt pen. Remember that a swelling may seemingly vanish once the patient is under a general anaesthetic.

Timing

The consultant (or operating surgeon) should always take the responsibility of compiling his operating list. On taking up the appointment, the house surgeon must find out from permanent members of the team approximately how long it takes the surgeon to perform different operations. Surgeons vary greatly; one may complete a straightforward gastric operation in 40 minutes, while another surgeon takes twice as long. The change-round time between cases for the anaesthetist involved also has to be taken into account. By adding these various times together, it should be possible to ensure that the complete elective operating list can be safely completed within the allotted duration of the operating session. Theatre nurses, orderlies and anaesthetists are entitled to their off-duty. Only for a genuine emergency should they be asked to stay on beyond the limit of their rostered duty time.

Notification of infectious diseases

It is not often that a disease which is liable to cause an epidemic is detected in a surgical ward. The regulations vary between different countries, but in many places it is necessary to formally notify the community health authorities. The main categories of disease of which notification may be required are:

1. Infections of childhood: exanthemas – diphtheria, measles, whooping cough, scarlet fever, erysipelas, meningitis.
2. Enteric infection – cholera, dysentery, typhoid and paratyphoid.
3. Adult infections – tuberculosis, poliomyelitis, anthrax, leptospiral and viral hepatitis.
4. Tropical fevers – malaria, plague, typhus and yellow fever, relapsing fever, smallpox, leprosy, lassa fever.

In some countries puerperal sepsis, ophthalmia neonatorum and food poisoning are also notifiable.

Confidentiality

Always remember that information gained about a patient is confidential and should only be divulged readily to professional personnel directly concerned with the patient's management.

Be on guard when inquiries are made by employers, lawyers and insurance companies. Ask the patient if he wishes them to be told about his medical condition, and where appropriate get his written consent. If in doubt, refer the request for information to the consultant in charge.

Protection against litigation

For their own protection all doctors are strongly advised to belong to a medical protection society. This is often a condition of employment. Litigation is becoming more common. Keep your society informed of any change of address.

In the UK it is still important for doctors to have their own medical protection even though employing authorities now provide indemnification for professional acts that have taken place within NHS hospitals. You may suddenly wish to render assistance at the site of a road traffic accident or at a sports meeting!

Death certificates

When the cause of a patient's death is known, the necessary certificate should be issued to the distressed relatives as soon as possible. They should not be kept waiting – the house surgeon should leave some less urgent task to complete the certificate.

The formalities for recording deaths with central government authorities vary in different parts of the world. The main purpose is to provide accurate information on the causes of deaths within the different countries. Health care resources and research can then be directed towards tackling the principal killing disease. Every 10 years the World Health Organization revises its classification of the causes of death.

The following details of death certification apply to Britain, but the principles are generally applicable. The certificate is in two parts: Part I lists the sequence of fatal events, while Part II records other conditions present which may have diminished the patient's chances of survival, but did not directly contribute to the patient's death. Incidental and completely unrelated pathological conditions do not need to be entered in Part II.

The immediate cause of death is inserted on the first line of Part I, e.g. bronchopneumonia, peritonitis or myocardial infarction. The second line shows the cause or reason for the first entry, e.g. hemicolectomy or perforation. A third entry may be made to complete the sequence, e.g. indicating that the reason for the hemicolectomy was carcinoma of sigmoid colon or that the perforation was of a chronic duodenal ulcer. For some patients only the first line needs to be completed, for example carcinoma of lung when the diagnosis had been confirmed earlier by biopsy and the patient's lungs and liver were clearly full of metastases. When possible, information should be provided on the primary site of a tumour, whether the condition was acute or chronic, or in the case of an earlier accident, whether it occurred at home or on a public road.

Part II might include generalized diseases such as chronic bronchitis, diabetes and hypertension. The house surgeon also records if an autopsy was performed, and whether or not he or another doctor saw the body. The Registrar of Deaths may later seek clarification or amplification. The house surgeon should sign the tear-off slip 'Notice to Informant' and give it to the informant. Usually the signing doctor should have seen the patient in his last 24 hours, and certainly within his last 14 days.

In some cases of death from natural causes it is not possible to complete the certificate in the detail outlined above. A patient may die from a widespread anaplastic neoplasm, the primary site being unknown. This is a natural death. In Britain it is only unnatural, unexplained or violent deaths that have to be reported to the Coroner (see below) or in Scotland to the Procurator-fiscal. In a doubtful or borderline case, the Coroner's officer or his Scottish counterpart is always willing to give advice.

Reference to the Coroner or Procurator-fiscal

A registered medical practitioner in attendance on a patient who dies has a statutory duty to complete a death certificate when he knows the cause of death and believes it to result from natural causes. On the other hand when the doctor does not have this certain knowledge there is no legislation to instruct him as to the action he should take. However, it is the generally accepted practice that when a doctor does not know the cause of death, or knows that unnatural factors played a role in causing the death, he will notify the Coroner in England and Northern Ireland, and the Procurator-fiscal in Scotland. Both these officials are charged with the responsibility of investigating and establishing the cause of death in the cases referred to them and they instruct police officers to inquire on their behalf. It is obvious that a medicolegal system cannot operate efficiently unless the appropriate cases are referred to it in the first place, and it must be appreciated that important medical information may be obtained by police officers in the course of their investigations. In many of these cases a medical practitioner will be required at a later date to give evidence at an inquest or public inquiry.

The circumstances in which a death should be reported to the Coroner or Procurator-fiscal are as follows:

1. When a death certificate cannot be completed on the grounds that:
   (a) The cause of death is not known, or
   (b) A doctor was not in attendance during the terminal illness or within 14 days of the death.
2. When a death is apparently due to an unnatural cause:
   (a) Accident, suicide or suspected homicide.
   (b) Any injury of any date including burning, neglect and starvation.
   (c) Poisoning from any source including therapeutic and occupational, alcoholism, drug addiction and food poisoning.
   (d) Abortion, other than natural.
3. When a death may be associated with medical treatment:
   (a) Death occurring under or attributable to general or local anaesthesia.
   (b) Death occurring during or attributable to a surgical operation.
   (c) Death apparently associated with medical mishap, diagnostic procedure, drug reaction or therapeutic hazard. (When negligence has been alleged or dissatisfaction is expressed by a relative every doctor concerned must inform his medical defence society immediately.)
4. When a death falls within a specified category, viz:
   (a) Foster children
   (b) Obscure infant deaths
   (c) Notifiable industrial diseases
   (d) Notifiable infectious diseases
   (e) Persons in legal custody
   (f) Persons receiving disability pensions.

The above list of reportable deaths is representative of the practice in the UK, combining the requirements of both the Procurator-fiscal and the Coroner. In other countries the jurisdiction will have similar, but not necessarily identical, provisions and if a doctor is in doubt as to whether a case warrants reporting he should discuss the matter with the appropriate legal official. While a case is being referred a certificate of death should not be issued and an autopsy should not be arranged until permission has been granted by the medicolegal authority.

Cremation

The regulations in the UK under the Cremation Acts are much more stringent than those for burial because of the irrevocable disposal of the body that cremation entails. The procedure obviously precludes the possibility of subsequently recovering medicolegal evidence by exhumation. The Acts also ensure that disposal by cremation is not against the wishes of the deceased or of the surviving relatives.

In the first place a certificate of death must be issued and the death registered in the ordinary manner as outlined above. The procedure requires that a cremation form, normally obtained from an undertaker, is completed and referred to the cremation authority, who appoint a medical referee to act on their behalf. This form consists of three parts:

Form A

The form of application which has to be completed and signed by the nearest relative or an executor. The applicant must confirm that the deceased had no objection to cremation and that there is no reason to believe that the death was due to any unnatural cause.

Form B

This medical certificate is completed by the doctor who attended during the last illness and who issued the death certificate. He must see and identify the body. He is obliged to disclose any relationship with the deceased or pecuniary interest he may have in the death.

Form C

This is a confirmatory medical certificate which has to be completed by a doctor of at least 5 years' standing. The 'second' doctor must not be a relative of the deceased nor a relative or partner of the doctor who completed Form B. In hospital practice the two doctors should not be members of the same clinical unit. The 'second' doctor is required to question the 'first' doctor and to examine his completed certificate. He must see and carefully examine the body. Thereafter he should make further inquiry by questioning other professional persons such as the ward sister involved in the case and relatives who were present at the death. If the 'second' doctor is a pathologist he may as an alternative to this inquiry give the cause of death from his autopsy findings.

When a death occurs in hospital where the deceased has been an inpatient, and a post-mortem has been performed and its result is known to the 'first' doctor signing Form B, then Form C may not be required.

Rarely a pathologist is requested to perform an autopsy by the medical referee, in which case he completes Form D, and this obviates the need for Forms B and C.

When Forms A, B and C are completed they are returned to the undertaker who then submits them to the medical referee, and if he is satisfied that all the legal requirements have been fulfilled, he grants authority to cremate. When a death has been reported to the Coroner or Procurator-fiscal then either authority on completion of his inquiry will give the considered cause of death on Form E. In this circumstance Forms B and C are unnecessary.

Removal of human tissues for transplantation

Before the parts are removed the law requires that a registered medical practitioner should satisfy himself that the patient is dead. In the case of a potential donor whose life is being maintained by a ventilator the determination of death may present considerable difficulty. In the UK the problem has been resolved by the Conference of the Royal Colleges which expressed the considered opinion that death can be diagnosed by the irreversible cessation of brainstem function, that is 'brain death'. In coming to this decision the criteria and tests laid down by the Colleges must be followed closely (see p. 454).

When death is to be determined on the basis of brain death, the diagnosis should be arrived at by the following combination of doctors.

1. A consultant who is in charge of the case or, in his absence, his deputy, who should have been registered for 5 years or more and have had adequate previous experience in the care of such cases, and
2. One other doctor, of comparable seniority.

Neither doctor should be a member of the transplant team and their findings, opinion and the time of death should be recorded in the case notes. The tests of brain death should be repeated at least once. Thereafter artificial ventilation and heart beat should be maintained until the removal of the organs is completed by the transplant surgeon; he also must have satisfied himself that the donor is dead.

Only the person who is legally in possession of the dead body can give consent to the removal of organs. In a National Health Service hospital, initially this means the hospital authority, until the body is claimed by whoever has legal right of possession – next of kin, executor or Coroner.

In a case where it is apparent that the Coroner or Procurator-fiscal has an interest no action should be taken until his approval is sought and obtained. Indeed, bearing in mind the surgical urgency of the situation, it is essential to make this approach before the death of the donor.

If a person wishes to donate his body for teaching purposes then this is provided for under the more complicated legislation of the Anatomy and Human Tissue Acts. He should be advised to contact the Head of a Department of Anatomy under whose guidance he can express his request in a formal document. When the patient is dying in hospital the doctor may have to help him make the necessary arrangements.

Stillbirth certificate

The definition of a stillborn child is a child which has been born after the 28th week of pregnancy and which did not, after having been completely expelled from its mother, breathe or show any other sign of life. The law of England requires that a medical practitioner or a certified midwife who was present at a stillbirth completes a stillbirth certificate on the prescribed form. Either is required to have been present at the birth or to have examined the body of the child before coming to an opinion. If the birth was unattended the legal authority should be informed, unless the fetus shows clear evidence of maceration or of a deformity incompatible with life.

When a fetus is delivered dead before the 28th week of pregnancy, it is presumed by law to be non-viable and therefore no legal certificate of any kind is required. On the other hand, should a child at any stage of pregnancy be born alive, then its birth will have to be registered and the usual certificate of death be completed by the ward doctor regardless of the time that it survived.

2

Resuscitation

H. A. F. Dudley

Cardiac arrest and resuscitation

General considerations

Cessation of the heart's action followed by fatal ischaemia of the brain is the sequence of events leading to death in most human beings. In many the heart's failure is the direct result of a progressive disease for which there is no cure. Consequently to interfere in the natural and inexorable progression of events is wrong. To do so is not really prolonging life, only prolonging the act of dying. Because in cardiac arrest it is necessary to act quickly, some hospitals have developed a policy of designating patients who have irremediable disease as 'not for resuscitation'. Though distasteful, this is necessary to avoid futile attempts by an incompletely informed 'arrest team' and subsequent distress both for staff and relatives. The matter has been made more complicated by the possibility of those who are destined to die being potential donors of organs. This is not common in surgical practice (except neurosurgery) where patients ending their lives are usually suffering from malignant disease and/or sepsis. Suffice it to say here that every member of the surgical team must be familiar with the local institutional guidelines about organ procurement.

However, cardiac arrest may occur in subjects believed to be otherwise healthy or in those with an expectation of life of many months. It is these patients who need urgent resuscitation.

Definition

Cardiac arrest means cessation of heart action in either asystole or ventricular fibrillation. Unless an ECG monitor is in position the distinction is hard to make clinically. However, the term is generally applied to a situation in which there is circulatory collapse or insufficiency to a degree which endangers the survival of the brain. With cerebral survival as the primary aim of management, precise diagnosis is not essential to the prompt institution of resuscitation though it aids appropriate treatment.

Causes of cardiac arrest

1. Myocardial infarction, which may precipitate ventricular fibrillation or so-called electromechanical dissociation.
2. Hypoxia: this is probably the single most common feature preceding cardiac arrest in surgical patients. It may be associated with airways obstruction, hypovolaemia, metabolic acidosis or a primary cardiac deficiency.
3. Acid–base upset, particularly metabolic acidosis.
4. Electrolyte imbalance, e.g. hyperkalaemia, gives diastolic arrest or ventricular fibrillation.
5. Drugs: accidental or intentional (suicidal) overdosage, e.g. with adrenaline, potassium salts, calcium salts and drugs used in the treatment of cardiac failure.

    The combination of adrenaline, hypercapnia and certain anaesthetic agents, e.g. halothane, is particularly hazardous.
6. Cardiac tamponade.
7. Hypothermia: accidental due to exposure, or intentional as part of the management of cardiac or neurosurgical operations.
8. Induced hypotension, especially the 'first dose phenomenon' in the use of agents such as angiotensin-converting enzyme inhibitors. though this is extremely rare.
9. Sudden fright and viscerocardiac reflexes.
10. Embolism: pulmonary or air embolism.
11. Haemorrhage and shock – from poor venous return.

12. Electrocution.
13. Drowning.
14. Anaphylaxis.
15. Investigations involving cardiac catheterization.

Diagnosis of circulatory arrest

1. Sudden loss of consciousness, occasionally with convulsions.
2. Appearance: combination of pallor, cyanosis and skin blotching; the patient looks dead and soon will be unless urgent action is taken.
3. Absence of respiration; there may occasionally be irregular gasps.

The diagnosis should be strongly suspected from the above factors in a few seconds, and should be confirmed in a further 10–15 s by finding:

4. Absence of femoral pulses (usually more easily ascertained than absence of carotid pulses).
5. Dilatation of the pupils (provided the patient is not on opiate drugs in large doses).

Note that sudden loss of consciousness occurs in fainting but there is bradycardia with usually an easily detectable pulse. Many examples of successful resuscitation by the 'kiss of life' are in patients who have merely fainted and would have recovered anyway provided their airway was kept clear and they could fall to the ground (see below). Nevertheless it is appropriate to *assume* that arrest has occurred until more information is available to disprove the assumption.

Initial treatment

1. Call for help, oxygen and resuscitation equipment. In hospitals this means alerting the cardiac resuscitation team using a special telephone number and the paging system. It is often referred to in North American hospitals as 'coding'. Note the time.
2. Lay patient flat, e.g. removing any pillows from the bed and make a quick check of the upper airways for any cause of respiratory obstruction which may have precipitated cardiac arrest, e.g. false teeth or a food bolus.
3. Thump the precordium hard with the ulnar border of the clenched fist (this may act as a stimulus to restart an arrest in asystole).
4. *Immediately* proceed to carry out external cardiac compression, applied over the lower third of the sternum (Figure 2.1).
5. If single-handed, interrupt cardiac compression after 10 s to apply expressed air resuscitation by mouth-to-nose (easier than mouth-to-mouth) respiration or by the use of an artificial airway, (Figure 2.2).
6. Provided there are sufficient assistants, the patient is best placed on a firm surface – the floor makes endotracheal intubation and the setting up of i.v. infusion difficult, and a bed with a firm base under the trunk is better.
7. Elevate the legs.
8. Pass an endotracheal tube (8 or 9 mm for an average adult) and inflate the cuff. Administer oxygen by means of a reservoir bag and valve, or a self-inflating bag such as the Ambu or the

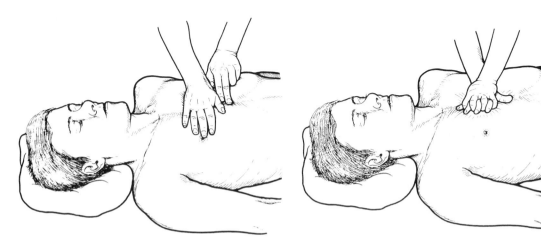

Figure 2.1 External cardiac massage. Having established an airway and after 2–3 breaths, check for a pulse. If it is absent, start external cardiac massage. Place the heel of the right hand over the sternum 8 cm above the xiphisternum and place the left hand on top. Keeping the arms straight, compress the sternum by 5 cm and then release; ensure that compression occupies at least a third of the cycle. Repeat the cycle 60–80 times per minute. If you are working single-handed, then 15 compressions to two lung inflations is the method to use. (From 'A guide to practical procedures in medicine and surgery' Butterworths, with permission.)

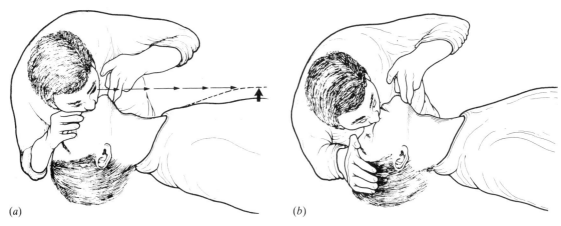

(a)   (b)

Figure 2.2 (a) Mouth-to-mouth resuscitation. Keeping the chin and neck in the same position as in Figure 2.1, and with the finger and thumb of the right hand pinching the nose, place your lips firmly over the mouth (having taken a large breath) and exhale. Look for the chest rising as you exhale. Next, release your seal and wait for the passive exhalation, again checking that the chest is moving. Repeat the process once exhalation is complete; this usually means 12–15 breaths/min; (b) oronasal resuscitation. Frequently it is more desirable to use the nose as the airway, particularly if you cannot get an airtight seal over the mouth or if the mouth contains blood or vomit. Use the left hand to hold the chin forwards and upwards and to keep the mouth shut. If this is not possible, use a pad over the mouth to seal it. Place your mouth over the entire nose and exhale. Then follow the same procedure as for mouth-to-mouth resuscitation. (From 'A guide to practical procedures in medicine and surgery' Butterworths, with permission.)

Laerdal type. If intubation is not possible, apply a face mask with the head fully extended, and give oxygen by intermittent positive pressure ventilation (this tends to be difficult for untrained personnel). One inflation of the lungs should be given for eight cardiac compressions. *Caution*: make sure endotracheal intubation has been achieved, otherwise oxygenation will be inadequate and gastric rupture may occur.

9. When external cardiac compression and ventilation with oxygen are under way, set up an i.v. infusion. Immediate cut-down at the elbow without aseptic technique may be more rapid than repeated attempts at percutaneous puncture of collapsed veins. Alternatively, if the skills are available a percutaneous puncture of the subclavian or internal jugular vein may be done. The bicarbonate may be given as 200 ml of a 4.2% solution.

10. Connect ECG monitor (this may be incorporated in the defibrillating equipment). Make a diagnosis of asystole or ventricular fibrillation or electromechanical dissociation (see below).

Technique of external cardiac massage

Press with the heel of the hand over the lower third of the patient's sternum. Rest the other hand on top of the first and keep the arms straight. With a sharp jerky movement press vertically backwards once per second, lifting the hands off the chest momentarily between compressions. The aim is to move the sternum backwards 4–5 cm with each compression. In an old person one or more ribs are frequently broken, but mechanical damage to the myocardium or liver must be avoided. Only one hand, and much less force, is needed in a young child. Get someone to check that the compressions produce a palpable carotid pulse.

If only one person is present, interrrupt cardiac massage every eight strokes to inflate the lungs.

Treatment once the initial emergency is over

Spontaneous recovery may occur as indicated by the return of heart beat and respiration, contraction of previously dilated pupils, spontaneous limb movements and restlessness. The ECG shows normal or near normal complexes.

Alternatively, asystole may persist with no detectable ECG complexes (flat tracing), there may be obvious ventricular fibrillation, or QRS complexes may be present but there is no cardiac output (electromechanical dissociation). The treatment of these three categories of 'cardiac arrest' is now standardized and is summarized in the flow diagrams designed by the Resuscitation Council (Figures 2.3, 2.4 and 2.5).

ASYSTOLE

Atropine 1 mg i.v.
↓
Check pulse
15 compressions
Read ECG
↓
Adrenaline 10 ml of 1:10 000
↓
Check pulse
15 compressions
Read ECG
↓
Sodium bicarbonate 50 ml 8.4%
↓
Check pulse
15 compressions
Read ECG
↓
Isoprenaline 100 μg
↓
Consider intracardiac adrenaline
Consider pacing

Figure 2.3 Flow diagram of management of asystole

VENTRICULAR FIBRILLATION

Defibrillate
200 joules (J)
↓
Check pulse
15 compressions
Read ECG
↓
Defibrillate
200 J
↓
Check pulse
15 compressions
Read ECG
↓
Defibrillate
400 J
↓
Check pulse
15 compressions
Read ECG
↓
Give lignocaine 100 mg
↓
Defibrillate
400 J
↓
Check pulse
15 compressions
Read ECG
↓
Give adrenaline 10 ml of
1:10 000
↓
Defibrillate
400 J
↓
Check pulse
15 compressions
Read ECG
↓
Give sodium bicarbonate 50 ml
8.4%
↓
Defibrillate
400 J
↓
Consider further lignocaine,
bretylium or other anti-arrhythmics
Consider changing the position of
the paddles and/or a change of
defibrillator

Figure 2.4 Flow diagram of management of ventricular
fibrillation

ELECTROMECHANICAL
DISSOCIATION

Consider causes: Drugs
Cardiac tamponade
Tension pneumothorax
Pulmonary embolus
↓
Adrenaline 10 ml 1:10 000
↓
Check pulse
15 compressions
Read ECG
↓
Isoprenaline 100 μg
↓
Check pulse
15 compressions
Read ECG
↓
Calcium chloride 10 ml 10%

Figure 2.5 Flow diagram of management of
electromechanical dissociation (defined as the presence of
QRS complexes in the absence of cardiac output)

(All 3 figures from 'A guide to practical procedures in medicine and surgery' Butterworths, with permission.)

Precautions in using a defibrillator

1. Disconnect ECG machine from patient.
2. Continue external cardiac compression and ventilate until the defibrillator is completely prepared for use.
3. Apply electrode jelly to the external electrodes to prevent skin burning.
4. Apply the electrodes to the chest, so that the electrical discharge passes through the largest bulk of heart tissue, i.e. one electrode at the base of the heart (to right of upper sternum) and the other over the estimated area of the apex of the heart, usually the sternal angle.
5. Make certain that nobody is in direct or indirect electrical contact with the patient before activating defibrillator.
6. Resume cardiac compression and ventilation *immediately* while awaiting the reappearance of the ECG pattern.

After spontaneous heartbeat has been restored following any type of dysrhythmic arrest careful supervision is needed:

1. Monitor patient's ECG.
2. Record blood pressure and temperature every 15 min.
3. Count respiratory rate; check adequacy of respiration.
4. Check acid–base status several times and correct metabolic acidosis.
5. Watch urinary output. Insert urethral catheter.
6. Be prepared for further episodes of cardiac arrest.
7. Transfer to an intensive or coronary care ward if possible.

When to stop attempts at resuscitation

Patients have returned to a normal life after an hour of cardiac massage. Recovery is unlikely, however, if spontaneous beating of the heart has not recommenced within 30 min of the start of resuscitative efforts. Certainly no junior doctor should cease his efforts in under 30 min. The decision to stop is best taken by the anaesthetist and senior clinician together. Frequent repetition of the steps outlined above for the treatment of ventricular fibrillation often brings success. Asystole carries a worse prognosis.

Other measures

Periods of anoxia cause cerebral oedema, which may interfere with the circulation to the brain and lead to permanent brain damage; they may also adversely affect renal function. To counteract these tendencies hypothermia and dehydration therapy may be used.

Hypothermia

The brain's oxygen requirements decrease sharply as the body temperature is lowered. If consciousness is not regained shortly after the heart is restarted, if there are other neurological changes or hyperpyrexia, then the patient should at once be cooled down 3–5°C to 32–35°C (89.6–95.0°F), by placing packs of broken ice around him at an early stage or if available by the use of a circulating blanket. Small doses of chlorpromazine (12·5 mg) i.v. may be used to help this process. Accurate monitoring of the core temperature is necessary and smaller doses of drugs are needed by the hypothermic patient.

Dehydration therapy

Urinary output can be increased by giving 500 ml of 10% mannitol intravenously. This loss of fluid from the body may reduce the tendency to cerebral oedema but the effect is temporary.

Dexamethasone

This agent is said to reduce the incidence and severity of cerebral oedema but there is continuing controversy about its efficacy. A dose of 4–6 mg may be given intramuscularly every 4 h for 24 h. Continued use beyond this time in the surgical patient may cause delays in wound healing.

Plasma expander

If the cardiac arrest was precipitated by hypovolaemia, a plasma expander, e.g. 500 ml of 6% dextran (Macrodex), may be infused intravenously.

Intracardiac injections

With effective cardiac massage and an intravenous line established, it should usually be unnecessary to inject drugs into the heart, a manoeuvre which is difficult and potentially dangerous because:

1. The average disposable hypodermic needle is almost always too short.
2. A needle may cause a pneumothorax.
3. There may be puncture of an anterior descending branch of one of the coronary arteries.
4. The injection may be placed into the pericardium and may cause haemopericardium and tamponade, or the injection may be given into the substance of the myocardium, forming a small 'infarct'.

Internal (open) cardiac message

This method of massaging the heart will be used when there is a cardiac arrest during an intrathoracic operation. It is also indicated when there is acute cardiac tamponade from a penetrating wound, air embolism or bilateral pneumothorax. In cardiac wounds with tamponade there are many examples of bold surgery in the Emergency Room being followed by success.

Technique of internal (open) cardiac message

When the thorax is not already open, without counting the ribs, a short, rather deep incision is made in what is believed to be the fourth or fifth left intercostal space. If there is no bleeding, the incision is enlarged so as to divide the intercostal muscles from the lateral border of the sternum to the posterior axillary fold (Figure 2.6). The pleura is

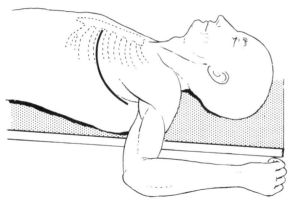

Figure 2.6 Incision for internal cardiac massage: it is made in the fourth or fifth left space and extends from sternum to posterior axilla

opened. By passing the left hand into the thoracic cavity the palm is insinuated beneath the heart and the intact pericardium, and the heart is compressed against the sternum. Rhythmical compression and complete relaxation (to allow the heart to fill) are continued at the rate of 1/s for about 25 s. In all probability by this time the wrist will become painful from constriction by the ribs, but sufficient blood to oxygenate the vital centres will have been delivered to enable the next step to be undertaken without endangering the viability of the cerebral cortex.

The hand is withdrawn, the costal cartilages above and below the incision are severed with a knife, and an assistant is instructed to hold the ribs apart or else a rib-spreader is inserted. Following the long axis of the heart, the pericardium is opened widely in front

of the phrenic nerve and cardiac massage is recommenced.

Ventricular fibrillation and asystole are treated as described above; the small electrodes of the defibrillator are applied directly to the front and back of the ventricular mass.

Cardiac tamponade

By far the commonest cause of this dangerous situation – which culminates with arrest – in modern surgical practice is a stab wound, particularly in communities where knives and sharpened screwdrivers are common weapons of aggression. Blood leaking from a cardiac chamber or from a coronary vessel often clots in the pericardial sac and there is thus little hope of effective relief by needle aspiration. The patient should, if hypotensive and hypoxic, be immediately moved to the operating room. While this is being done a needle (15–18 gauge) is inserted upwards and backwards from the left of the xiphoid because even the removal of 10 ml of blood or serum adds the same volume to stroke output. A median sternotomy is made as quickly as possible and the pericardium decompressed. A finger on the bleeding point will stem the loss until expert help can be summoned. It is better in desperate circumstances to operate with local anaesthesia or none at all than to risk further reduction in cardiac output by general agents. For the same reason a median sternotomy without opening the pleural cavity is the incision of choice. Once decompression has been achieved general anaesthesia with endotracheal anaesthesia can be instituted.

Air embolism

Air embolism is a rare accident; in most cases air has entered the venous side of the systemic circulation. In the old and frail surprisingly small quantities of air rapidly entering a vein may prove fatal.

Causes of venous air embolism

The application of positive pressure to a conventional intravenous infusion delivered from a bottle, e.g. with a Higginson's syringe, is always potentially dangerous and may cause air embolism. This method of administration should *never* be used. During an operation air may enter the large veins within the skull or neck; mismanagement of an open heart operation may cause the problem under anaesthesia; induction of a pneumothorax or pneumoperitoneum and vaginal douching may cause the emergency.

Clinical manifestations

Usually in the conscious patient the onset is abrupt, with deep inspirations, coughing expirations, cyanosis, then a few gasping breaths, succeeded by unconsciousness and cessation of respiration. The pulse becomes imperceptible and the blood pressure falls to an unrecordable level. A stethoscope applied to the precordium reveals the 'water-wheel' sound – a most unpleasant churning and splashing noise which masks the true heart sounds. In not a few instances, if the pulps of the fingers are placed over a jugular vein, bubbles of air can be felt moving beneath. Especially in cases where the patient was in a sitting position, or resumes an upright position after the entry of air into a vein, the state of unconsciousness is preceded by convulsions.

Treatment

To be successful, immediate action and sustained effort are imperative:

1. Tilt the patient so that the head is low. Large bubbles in the venous system then pass to the veins of the pelvis and the lower extremities, there to be absorbed slowly.
2. Turn the patient on to his left side, i.e. with the right side uppermost. By placing the patient on to the left side, air in the right ventricle rises towards the apex of the heart, breaks the air lock and permits the organ to pump whole blood into the pulmonary artery.
3. Ventilate the lungs, preferably with pure oxygen, at the earliest possible moment. Even if there is a slight improvement, persevere with postural treatment, if necessary for hours. Success has crowned 8 h of such treatment.

If these measures do not rapidly bring some evidence of improvement, the patient must be turned on to his back and the heart exposed via an incision through the fifth left interspace (see Figure 2.6). The right ventricle can then be aspirated under vision, and after discarding froth the blood is returned to the left ventricle. Massage the heart if necessary, but on no account commence cardiac massage until all the froth has been aspirated.

Shock and resuscitation

Patients presenting at the Accident and Emergency Department or to the surgeon on duty with the diagnosis of 'shock' may be suffering from a wide variety of clinical states, for shock is an imprecise but useful word. It does not describe a physiological single entity but rather a clinical appearance. Thus, its use in everyday practice is valuable in conveying information about what a patient looks like but is rarely helpful when it comes to deciding treatment. As with any other therapeutic manoeuvre, adequate treatment is dependent upon the understanding of mechanisms when these are capable of being elucidated. When summoned to a patient said to be in shock the first question that must be asked is, 'What is the cause?' Only by deciding this can a plan of treatment be arrived at. Though this is so and more harm can come from rushing about doing far too many things all at once because the diagnosis is not established in terms of cause, it is equally vital not to spend excessive time trying to reach too detailed a diagnosis while the patient is obviously deteriorating. Certain quick checks – on the airway, sites of possible continuing blood loss, for the presence of an external wound (for example, in the precordium, the abdomen and importantly the back) that might indicate an extremely urgent internal problem such as cardiac tamponade or the penetration of a large vessel – should take precedence. Survival for the patient admitted in 'shock' is predicated on quick decision-making by those who see him first.

Causes of the shock picture

In dissecting out the major aetiological agents in the causation of a state of shock the first premise is that our use of the term to describe a clinical state of affairs is a shorthand for the appearance of *reduced peripheral bloodflow*. Not only does this affect the easily visible skin and subcutaneous tissues but also the viscera, for example kidney and brain, accounting in this way for the oliguria and disorientation that may accompany a shock state. Most of the clinical manifestations of shock syndromes can be explained by peripheral tissue *hypoxia* based on the low blood flow. It is the method of production of the reduced perfusion that varies from instance to instance.

The principal aetiological agents responsible for the clinical picture of shock are:

1. Vasovagal overactivity, i.e. fainting.
2. Reduction in circulatory blood volume.
3. Massive sepsis.
4. Coronary occlusion.
5. Adrenocortical insufficiency.

Fainting and neural phenomena

In the past it has been customary to include bradycardia, hyperpnoea and the fainting of emotional stress under the heading of 'shock'. Certainly this is so to the layman who habitually describes as 'shocked' anyone who has had a fright. The term 'neurogenic shock' is best not used, although peripheral tissue hypoxia in the brain is characteristic of fainting which has a neurogenic basis. What is important for the doctor to remember is:

1. Other factors such as blood loss and pain can, if the patient is upright, contribute to the development of the physiological chain of events – adrenaline secretion, muscular vasodilatation, bradycardia and cerebral hypoxia – which leads to fainting. Thus, fainting may be a component of some particular circumstances of blood loss; perhaps the most frequently encountered in civilian practice is the patient who has a major gastrointestinal haemorrhage and then either defaecates or vomits. The Valsalva effect so produced reduces venous return to the heart and precipitates a faint so that he is picked up from beside the toilet or may sustain a head injury as he falls.
2. If, when a patient faints, he is prevented from falling, the cerebral hypoxia is self-perpetuating and may result in irreversible brain damage and/or a cardiac arrest. Death under light general anaesthesia in the dentist's chair (though most dentists now use the supine position) and possibly some fatalities in elderly patients propped upright in bed in hospital may be assigned to this cause.

Diagnosis

Sudden loss of consciousness has many causes. Fainting is usually easily recognized by the profound bradycardia that is always present, and the absence of any focal signs.

Management of fainting

The patient is placed flat and semiprone. Unconsciousness is rarely so deep that reflexes are lost but the airway should be checked and made safe. Usually consciousness is soon recovered and there is rarely, if ever, the need to administer vasopressor drugs. Unless the cause is obvious, the patient should be subsequently investigated for precipitating factors such as blood loss.

Shock caused by reduction in circulatory volume

Three major causes of volume reduction are known – loss of whole blood, loss of plasma as in a burn and loss of extracellular water. The clinical pictures produced by each have many points of similarity and some points of difference (Table 2.1).

Whole blood loss may be external (which includes by definition the gastrointestinal tract) or internal into damaged tissues (e.g. a fracture haematoma or an infarcted organ). The effects are the same, although the rate of loss may be slow and get progressively less in tissues where tension increases gradually.

Plasma loss occurs in burns (p. 79) as a consequence of leakage of protein and exudate through damaged capillaries. Dilute plasma is also lost into an area of inflammation or tissue damage (e.g. peritonitis and massive contusion), but the protein content of such loss is rarely important in considering fluid replacement.

Loss of extracellular fluid (ECF) is a consequence of three situations:

1. Deviation of normal exchange mechanisms. Extracellular fluid is in a constant state of exchange across the gastrointestinal tract and the nephron. Normally, although large quantities are moved every day in this manner, the net amount of extracellular water that is 'transcellular' (mainly in the lumen of the gut) at any instant is quite small. However, by interfering with reabsorption the extracellular fluid can be continuously drained from its normal site. Such losses occur in vomiting, diarrhoea, fistulae and failure of tubular reabsorption of urine. In each instance the fluid lost varies in composition, but basically it is rich in sodium ions. Big losses are accompanied by shrinkage of plasma volume and the onset of shock.
2. By increased loss of ECF along a normal pathway. The best single example of this situation is excessive sweating without replacement in a non-acclimatized individual. Sufficient dilute extracellular fluid may be leached out to produce a profound reduction in ECF and a

Table 2.1 Points of differentiation between whole blood, plasma and ECF loss

	Whole blood	Plasma	ECF
Haematocrit	Normal initially; falls over some hours	Rises	Rises
Skin colour	Pallor	Usually unchanged	Usually unchanged
Tongue	Moist	Moist	Dry

shock state but this is very rare in temperate climates.

3. The 'third-space phenomenon'. This concept is briefly summarized as follows. The ability of the cell to extrude sodium and so maintain both intracellular integrity and the volume of extracellular fluid is dependent upon active extrusion of the sodium ion by the expenditure of energy; a hypoxic or otherwise damaged cell is deprived of ability to expend such energy, thus permitting the ingress of sodium and draining such ions out of the extracellular fluid. The effective volume of the ECF is thus reduced and may aggravate the hypoxic insult. Third space must be taken into consideration whenever there has been more than a transient period of markedly reduced tissue perfusion, but it is not an important phenomenon in deliberate surgical injury without hypotension. However, in very big tissue dissection (e.g. total gastrectomy, hip replacement) considerable oedema formation occurs at the site of injury as a consequence of capillary damage (an anatomical third space) and should be replaced with normal saline.

Physiological adjustments to loss of circulatory volume

Two major physiological adjustments occur. First, there is peripheral vasoconstriction which adapts the volume of the vascular tree to the reduced volume of blood it contains (it must be noted that a phrase beloved of many writers on shock – discrepancy between volume of blood and the capacity of the vascular tree – is a physical impossibility). The vasoconstriction is widespread, affecting the capacitance vessels on the venous side of the circulation as well as arterioles. In both instances, as the vascular network shrinks the pressure tends to fall, but initially because of increased resistance to flow it is maintained on the arterial side, with or without a mild increase in heart rate. Measurements of intravascular pressure are thus usefully made both on the arterial and venous side of the circulation, particularly the latter (see Central venous pressure below). Secondly, there is, by virtue of the altered pressure relations in the arteriole–capillary–venule loop, an ingress of extracellular water into the circulation, producing haemodilution. Initially, this is quite a rapid process and after a haemorrhage of 1.5–2.0 litre three-quarters of the resulting haemodilution is over in 6–8 h; this is of importance in the management of patients with suspected continued bleeding into, say, the gastrointestinal tract. Repeated determinations over some hours indicating a progressively falling haemoglobin, haematocrit or red cell count (all rough indications of haemodilution) mean, more often than not, a continued haemorrhage.

Reduction in circulating volume: correlation with physical findings

Computation of blood volume deficits is difficult and even direct measurement of blood volume is only accurate to about 5% (±300 ml in an average man). No single parameter should be relied on, rather a summation as shown in Table 2.2.

In some circumstances it may be possible to correlate the clinical assessment with measured loss, for example, of blood during the course of an operation or ECF from a fistula. Even if the measurement lacks refinement (e.g. simple swab weighing), it gives more useful information than an ill-educated guess. Historical evidence may also be useful although lay people and members of the medical and nursing profession all tend to exagger-

Table 2.2 Parameters for computation of blood volume deficit

Clinical status	Vital signs	Existing introvascular deficit in adult
Patient well, not anxious	Pulse, 70–80 BP, 120 systolic CVP, 5–10 cmH$_2$O. Urine volume at least 40–50 ml/h	Less than 700 ml
Mild anxiety, restlessness, pallor, coldness, possibly sweating. Thirst. Fainting in upright position	Pulse, 90–100 BP, 90–100 systolic CVP, 0–5 cmH$_2$O. Urine volume less than 30 ml/h	1–2 litres
Great anxiety, disorientation. Air hunger, icy extremities, fall in body temperature. Severe thirst	Pulse, 130+ BP, 70 systolic CVP below atmospheric – 5 cmH$_2$O Urine volume, nil	2–3.5 litre

ate visible blood loss (except surgeons who always underestimate the amount of blood they spill). Finally, semi-objective assessment may be possible by seeing the extent of injury and referring to previously established figures.

When an assessment of whole blood loss has been made, a decision must be reached on the extent of third-space requirements. When blood loss exceeds 1 litre, a 2-litre deficit of extracellular fluid should be included for every additional 2 litres of lost blood.

Metabolic acidosis in low circulating blood volume

When a condition of low flow and hypoxia exists in an actively metabolizing tissue, oxidation is reduced and increased amounts of lactic acid are formed. This leads to the escape of hydrogen ions into the circulation and the development of metabolic acidosis. Increased hydrogen ion concentration depresses myocardial and smooth muscle contractility, thus interfering with the pumping action of the heart and with the ability of the vascular tree to exert pressure on the contained blood. Metabolic acidosis may complicate the picture of any low blood volume state and tends to be particularly severe when there is, in addition, a locally compromised area of circulation such as a strangulated loop of gut.

Management of reduced circulating volume

The object is to restore volume as rapidly as possible taking into consideration losses of ECF in addition to blood or plasma. Restoration is achieved by two means: (1) stopping the loss, and (2) replacing that which has occurred. In most, but not all, instances and by the adoption of the techniques to be described it is possible to replace volume faster than the loss is occurring, but sometimes it may be necessary to establish the conditions under which resuscitation can proceed by taking operative steps to control bleeding. Thus, a furiously bleeding spleen or ruptured ectopic gestation may need to be controlled before blood volume can be restored. Failure to respond, or a response that is temporary, indicates a hidden source of bleeding which must be diligently sought for and controlled.

Volume replacement should be undertaken once and for all, either as a preliminary to or after control of loss. It has often been observed that allowing the pendulum to swing from normovolaemia to hypovolaemia by repeatedly allowing losses to occur usually produces a crumbling physiological framework. Accordingly, it is extremely important to have a clear plan outlined by the surgical team which will allow a smooth progression from resuscitation to operation if this is necessary, or from operation to

resuscitation if the one must precede the other. When there are multiple casualties with a number in shock other than that occasioned by emotional disturbance, careful ordering of priorities is vital.

Replacement of circulating volume

The first essential is to withdraw blood for grouping and cross-matching. Thereafter the following principles should be observed.

Technique

A large-bore cannula or needle (No. 14 or bigger) *must* be used. Every young doctor seems to have to relearn the lesson that blood loss from the splenic artery or a ruptured aorta cannot be adequately replaced through a 22-gauge needle. Four alternatives are available:

1. Insert a standard No. 14 transfusion needle into a forearm vein.
2. Use a needle-cannula combination which, if it is plastic, may be inserted at the bend of the elbow.
3. Cut down on the veins of the elbow and insert a large-bore cannula.
4. For really massive blood loss cut the end off a sterile giving set and insert the tubing of this directly into an exposed vein after dilating the nick made in it with a pair of mosquito forceps.

These techniques will be found described in detail on pp. 38–40. Without exception the saphenous vein at the ankle should not be used as it is thick-walled and goes into spasm with monotonous regularity. Nor should time be wasted in futile attempts at needling collapsed veins. There are few patients who would not gladly endure a scar on the arm as a means of attaining increased longevity.

Initial infusion

Even if the cannula is the largest available, blood may initially flow only reluctantly through it. The patient's urgent need is for increased volume which will increase cardiac output and relax vasoconstriction. A healthy individual can maintain peripheral oxygenation with a haemoglobin concentration of 6 g/dl provided cardiac output (which is dependent on intravascular volume) is normal. Thus, it is good practice to administer initially a 'trailer dose' of crystalloid solution and for this purpose the fluid best suited to ECF replacement is ideal. One litre of Ringer-lactate (Hartmann's solution) is rapidly run in over a period of 5 min. This large infusion will be rapidly dissipated (within an hour or two) into the ECF, but for the moment it expands circulating volume more rapidly than any other technique, particularly because crystalloid fluids flow easily.

Later infusion

Subsequently blood and other appropriate fluids are transfused plus additional Ringer-lactate to provide for third-space losses (see above). Control of rate of transfusion is guided by continued assessment of: (1) pulse, (2) arterial blood pressure, (3) central venous pressure and (4) urine output. How many of these parameters will be used depends upon the severity and complexity of the situation, but it is a good rule to observe and record too much rather than too little. For this purpose it is essential to have a clear chart and to discipline oneself into meticulous entries at half-hour intervals.

Central venous pressure (CVP)

For reasons implicit in the outline of the physiology of volume reduction, CVP measured by the insertion of a cannula into the great veins is one of the most reliable guides to the adequacy or inadequacy of fluid replacement. Return of CVP to normal ($+5\,cmH_2O$) in the presence of presumed normal cardiac function is usually an indication that transfusion has been adequate. Because of peripheral vasoconstriction, arterial blood pressure (but not necessarily peripheral flow) may be normal when the deficit is incompletely replaced. A reduced CVP will more likely reveal this state of affairs and prevent the mistake of proceeding to anaesthetize a patient inadequately replaced when, if anaesthesia is prematurely begun, vasoconstriction is abolished and a decline in arterial pressure and flow is precipitated. The measurement of CVP is made after the insertion of a cannula into a great vein (pp. 39, 242).

In recent years there has been a tendency to move to 'high technology' devices which can measure pulmonary artery and wedge pressure (an indicator of left atrial pressure), and which also permit direct determination of cardiac output by thermal dilution. These devices certainly provide more information but exactly how to use the data in management is not always clear. Their most important use is probably where the heart muscle is damaged and at the same time something else has happened – hypovolaemia, a major operation or severe sepsis.

Urine output is a further satisfactory method of assessing a situation in which loss may be continuous as in a burn or a major operative procedure. A judicious reluctance to insert a urethral catheter in either sex should not be transformed into a doctrinaire refusal to exploit a useful technique which is certain to benefit patient management and, if properly controlled, is devoid of significant risk. In the complicated circumstances of shock when the patient is often restless, when many things may be done to him and when he may have to be moved from place to place, a No. 14 or No. 16 Foley catheter is the most reliable (see p. 342).

Restoration and maintenance of urinary volume should not be confused with 'more means better'. An hourly volume of 40–50 ml is adequate. Over-infusion of crystalloid is not usually a problem in the young and healthy. Care must, however, be taken not to drown an elderly person by the excessive use of Ringer-lactate solution. This may occur if attempts are made to increase urine output above, say, 50–60 ml/h by increasing the infusion rate. It is true that large infusions can achieve modest, though unnecessary, diuresis but not all the infused volume is excreted and a positive balance insidiously builds up.

Correction of acidosis

When acute volume loss has exceeded 2 litres or arterial hypotension below 100 mmHg systolic has existed for an hour, or when response to presumed adequate infusion has been incomplete, metabolic acidosis should be suspected. Confirmation should be sought by arterial blood analysis (see p. 38), but if this technique is not immediately available it is better to assume that acidosis is present and to administer sodium bicarbonate, 1 mmol/ml in 40 ml aliquots on the basis of 1 aliquot to each 3 units of blood required. This rule-of-thumb approach is moderately satisfactory, but control by pH studies is vitally necessary to intelligent therapy.

Management of ancillary features

Pain. In spite of the experience of World War II and subsequently, there is still a reluctance to use opiate drugs by the only route that will do any good, i.e. intravenously. Subcutaneous or intramuscular morphine is too slowly absorbed in the shocked patient to be useful. Once diagnosis is complete, the best technique is to dilute 15 mg of morphine in 10 ml of saline and to inject 1 ml every 30 s until relief is afforded. Precision of this kind is rewarded by the use of a relatively small dose correctly adjusted to the individual patient and sufficiently limited to avoid respiratory depression or masking of physical signs. The same technique is useful in the postoperative patient.

Immobilization of fractures. This not only limits blood loss into fracture haematomas, but also reduces pain. Any major long bone fracture should be temporarily splinted, pending definitive treatment. Similarly, unnecessary manipulation, transference from bed to stretcher, washing and fussy documentation should all be avoided. The patient in shock should be got out of it, not subjected to catechism or nursing ritual.

Warmth. The shocked patient complains of *cold* because his metabolic rate falls and/or because he is exposed to a large temperature gradient with the environment. The latter can be corrected by providing a high ambient temperature (21–24°C), but correction of the former is impossible until increased tissue perfusion raises oxygen consumption. Therefore, external warming is useless and may be harmful if it encourages peripheral vasodilatation. A space blanket made from aluminium foil conserves what little heat the patient produces.

Oxygen therapy

Opinion has ebbed and flowed about the value of oxygen in states of circulating blood volume reduction. Observation of desaturation of arterial blood and of experimental benefit suggests that it is not to be despised, and an intranasal catheter or venturi mask delivering 4–6 litre/min should be used until haemodynamics and urine output have returned to normal.

Plasma and plasma substitutes

When blood has been lost replacement is by lactated Ringer's solution and whole blood. However, in burns and peritonitis, plasma or plasma substitutes should be used. Whole plasma, usually made from a pool of outdated blood, has enjoyed an unsavoury reputation in the past because of the transmission of infective hepatitis. As now supplied, it is probably as safe or safer than whole blood, but because the major colloid of plasma is albumin, albumin solutions are also satisfactory volume expanders and a good substitute for unrefined plasma. The availability of albumin varies throughout the world. There is also a continuing debate about whether it has any virtues over lactated Ringer's solution in any circumstances. Indeed, there is a school of thought that suggests that it is harmful when the pulmonary capillary endothelium is damaged, which may occur in burns, severe sepsis and often profound hypotension. Alternatively, but far less satisfactory, is the use of dextran – a long-chain polysaccharide. Although many thousands of units of this substance have been used with success, mystery surrounds its effects on the microcirculation and on blood coagulability. While useful as a stop-gap and in some special circumstances, its use should be eschewed when adequate balanced salt solution and blood are available. Yet another currently popular choice is gelatin (Haemaccel). It is probably safe and is relatively cheap. If the resuscitation team prefers selective plasma volume expansion to less selective ECF expansion, then smaller volumes of gelatin may be used instead of Ringer-lactate.

Preparation for anaesthesia of the patient in shock

The need to have the patient's blood volume adequately replaced has already been mentioned. In addition, the stomach must, if possible, be empty. Gastrointestinal propulsion comes to a halt with a severe injury (and particularly when there is hypotension), so that the important interval is not the time between eating the last meal and the proposed anaesthetic, but the time between eating and injury. If this is less than 3 h residual gastric contents must be assumed. In some instances an oesophageal tube can be easily passed, but distressing efforts to persuade a patient to swallow a tube should not be persisted with. Furthermore, even a stomach tube will not effectively deal with semisolid or solid gastric content. In such circumstances, it is mandatory to practise an anaesthetic induction technique which does not permit regurgitation. Either the cricoid cartilage is firmly pressed directly posteriorly to occlude the oesophagus at its origin, or a No. 16 Foley catheter is passed into the oesophagus and gently inflated until the balloon just grips the oesophageal wall, so obstructing the lumen. Subsequent to the induction of anaesthesia and the passage of an endotracheal tube, an oesophageal or stomach tube can safely and easily be inserted to permit gastric aspiration.

Massive sepsis (septic shock; bacteraemia shock; bacterial shock; toxic shock)

Definition

The term 'massive sepsis' is preferred to septicaemia because the latter is, in fact, a bacteriological diagnosis which may be achieved only in retrospect, if at all. Furthermore, there is good evidence that an acute local process may throw off not so much organisms, but products of infection which cause the shock state. The organisms involved are usually intestinal – *Escherichia coli, Pseudomonas, Proteus* – but staphylococci can also be responsible as in 'toxic shock syndrome' caused by a retained infected vaginal tampon. The situation may also exist that their multiplication is favoured by some reduction in host resistance, e.g. severe illness, steroids, immunosuppressive drugs.

It is customary and desirable to distinguish two pathological forms of shock in massive sepsis – instances with and without a focus. In the latter the prognosis is worse than in the former and common portals of entry are the urinary tract, the portal tract and badly managed intravenous therapy. The pathophysiology of shock with sepsis is incompletely understood, but the current view is that it is predominantly the result of intense arteriolar and possibly venular vasoconstriction, produced by endotoxin causing the release of intermediaries such as tumour necrosis factor. In addition, there may be a 'third space' because of damage to the cell membrane. The arteriolar vasoconstriction reduces or abolishes peripheral blood flow and the venous effects reduce the blood available for venous return. Thus, cardiac output falls, further aggravating the peripheral hypoxia. There is little evidence of a direct effect of bacterial toxins on the heart, nor does selective hepatic vasoconstriction seem to have the same importance in man as it does in the dog and some other species.

Many other factors may contribute to the individual circumstances of a patient who presents with a presumed diagnosis of shock with sepsis. Acute ECF reduction, blood loss, metabolic acidosis and adrenocortical failure (see pp. 23, 324) may complicate the picture and call for treatment in their own right. Respiratory insufficiency (adult respiratory distress syndrome or ARDS) is a particularly common feature of severe sepsis even without significant haemodynamic disturbance (see p. 273).

Clinical features and diagnosis

Causes of blood volume reduction sufficient to account for the profound clinical disturbances are absent, but there may be a history of predisposing drug ingestion or of a febrile illness. In favourable circumstances the diagnosis is made easy by the presence of obvious sepsis or of a portal of entry. On examination, the patient is anxious, cyanosed, has an extremely sluggish capillary return, a cold periphery and tightly constricted veins. The core temperature may be high and a core-to-periphery gradient of 6–8°C is characteristic though not conclusive. Arterial blood pressure and CVP are both low.

Although blood cultures should be taken repeatedly, in instances of shock thought to be associated with sepsis they are of more use for retrospective evaluation and the refinement of a chemotherapeutic regimen than for urgent diagnosis. By far the most important investigation is a *peripheral blood smear*. With rare exceptions, this will show a leucocytosis and of much greater importance the neutrophils will usually contain toxic granulations and Döhle bodies. Both these are manifestations of severe infection and greatly strengthen the diagnosis. A Gram's stain should also be obtained; organisms are identified, though of course cannot necessarily be characterized, in about a third of cases.

Management

The outlook is poor in septic shock, particularly when there is no obvious focus. The management may be outlined as a series of steps:

1. Establish a fluid pathway preferably into a great vein so that CVP can be measured.
2. Insert a catheter into the bladder and check hourly urine output.
3. Draw blood for smear and blood culture.
4. Administer a massive dose of antibiotics chosen with regard to possible cause; unless staphylococcal sepsis is likely, 1 g of gentamicin and 1 g metronidazole is a good starting dose to be modified later in the light of bacteriological studies and blood levels.
5. If CVP is low, replace fluid losses with balanced salt solution.
6. If the patient now comes out of shock, renew the search for a focus and drain it if feasible.
7. If shock persists, it is worth while to give 1 g of hydrocortisone on the assumption that adrenocortical insufficiency exists. A non-specific effect of hydrocortisone has been described in some instances but is extremely rare in clinical practice.

If the patient remains in shock, often with oliguria, after these manoeuvres he is almost certainly going to die. It is usual then to administer an inotrope such as dopamine. This will usually raise blood pressure and also improve urine flow, so buying time to eradicate sepsis. When there is a high core temperature (as measured in the rectum or oesophagus) with severe peripheral vasoconstriction it is rational to attempt to promote blood flow by inducing vasodilatation. Small intravenous doses of chlorpromazine (10 mg) are given at 20-min intervals accompanied by blood volume expansion with blood or balanced salt solution. The importance of measuring core temperature in states of peripheral vasoconstriction cannot be overemphasized.

Oxygen therapy and the *relief of anxiety* or *pain* are as much indicated in this form of shock as in any other.

Coronary occlusion

Shock in myocardial infarction is more common in medical than in surgical wards, but it may occasionally complicate a surgical situation. Such association between an operation and a coronary occlusion is much rarer than many surgeons believe, and before assuming that the cause of a postoperative collapse is the consequence of myocardial infarction the doctor must carefully search for other causes and also seek positive confirmation of the diagnosis. Thus, in a recent series of 71 fatalities after gallbladder surgery – disease traditionally linked by many with the occurrence of cardiac disorders – not one was found to have been caused by coronary occlusion although many were so diagnosed.

Clinical features

The clinical features are not usually difficult to analyse, although pain may not be so severe. Shock, out of proportion to blood loss or the extent of other possible precipitating factors, combined with a raised CVP or one that becomes so after the infusion of a small (500-ml) challenge dose of colloid, are the diagnostic features confirmed by progressive ECG signs and ultimately by transaminase determinations. The aim in a surgical setting should be to correct any additional factor which will further embarrass the heart – a full stomach, the pain of an abdominal wound and the laboured breathing of a postoperative state. Expert cardiological advice should be sought in regard to monitoring, arrhythmias and the use of cardiac drugs such as digitalis, dopamine and β blockade.

Adrenocortical insufficiency

This syndrome is rare but perhaps not so rare as it used to be. *De novo* it may occur during the course of severe acute sepsis or after a severe head injury, but it is more common to encounter it after steroid drugs have been administered and endogenous cortical activity so reduced. Thus, it may be seen when surgery is called for in a patient with ulcerative colitis or rheumatoid arthritis. Adrenocortical suppression subsequent to steroid therapy may last up to 1 year, gradually declining in severity; but most instances of acute insufficiency have occurred within 9 months or take place while the patient is on a maintenance dose and is exposed to additional stress, e.g. an operation or infection.

Clinical features

The clinical features are non-specific; the diagnosis is made only by a high sense of suspicion and the therapeutic trial of a large (200 mg) intravenous dose of hydrocortisone. If adrenocortical insufficiency is present the response is dramatic, but it is fair to add that the suspicion is rarely confirmed, some other cause usually being confounded with the diagnosis of hypoadrenocorticalism.

Prophylaxis

Prophylaxis is more applicable to this form of shock than any other. Patients who have received steroids in therapeutic doses within 1 year should be regarded with suspicion if they have to undergo a major surgical procedure, but there is no indication to administer steroids unless they show signs of circulatory failure. Patients actually on therapy should have the operative procedure and postoperative period for the first 4–6 days covered by a dose of 300 mg daily of hydrocortisone in three divided intramuscular doses of 100 mg. Because of the slow effect of this drug intramuscularly the first dose on the day of operation should be given intravenously. Similarly, patients requiring emergency surgery should receive a large booster dose of 200 mg intravenously. After the fourth day, and *provided progress is satisfactory*, the dose is halved on successive days until the original maintenance dose is reached.

Disseminated intravascular coagulation

During the course of any episode of shock, and also in severe sepsis, a state of disseminated intravascular coagulation (DIC) may develop for reasons which are not clear. The condition manifests itself as a *consumptive coagulopathy* in which a fall in the concentration of a number of coagulation components – fibrinogen and platelets in particular – leads to spontaneous bleeding and increased loss from raw areas. The fibrin degradation products (FDPs) formed by lysis of the diffuse coagulum also act as anticoagulants, so worsening the situation. DIC also often leads to renal failure, presumably by coating the glomeruli with fibrin.

DIC carries a gloomy outlook unless detected early. Thus, in shock and severe sepsis, platelet counts should be done frequently if circumstances permit. If there is evidence of DIC then the vicious circle of consumption and feedback of FDPs into the coagulation cascade must be broken by preventing the initial coagulation sequence with heparin; 2000–4000 units are given intravenously and 1000 units thereafter by the same route every 1–2 h to maintain the clotting time in excess of 8 min. This will usually control the problem in sepsis and hypovolaemia provided the causative agent can be brought under control. When DIC occurs as it sometimes does in the course of malignant disease the outcome is usually fatal.

Prevention of renal insufficiency

When glomerular filtration rate is reduced by any of the mechanisms that are associated with shock, and particularly if at the same time nephrotoxins such as free haemoglobin, myoglobin or perhaps bacterial toxins enter the circulation, renal tubular damage is a possibility. Such circumstances occur in mismatched transfusion (pp. 24, 35), burns and severe sepsis although adequate conventional resuscitation by the energetic infusion of colloid and balanced salt solution (Hartmann's Ringer-lactate) should reduce their occurrence to a minimum. If urine output is falling below 30 ml/h in a patient who is in an unstable circulatory state, or if circulating nephro-toxin is suspected then either 100 ml of 15% mannitol should be rapidly infused over 10 min, or frusemide 60–80 mg should be given intravenously. Both these can produce a diuresis in spite of the antidiuresis that accompanies severe injury or shock. A lack of response is *not* an indication for repeating the dose. It must be assumed that irreversibility is present. In such circumstances the administration of massive doses of frusemide is said to improve the outcome, but their use is associated with a risk from cardiac arrhythmia and caution is therefore necessary.

The diagnostic administration of mannitol or frusemide is useful in dissecting reversibility from irreversibility.

Anaphylactic shock

This is a convenient term – although probably a gross oversimplification – for the acute circulatory collapse which is the consequence of hypersensitivity to a drug, toxin or serum.

Clinical features

The clinical features are acute hypotension, loss of consciousness, patchy mottling of the skin, urticaria and often, when consciousness is recovered, a persisting sense of anxiety – *the angor animi* of Ryle.

Treatment

Treatment is expectant and empirical: a large dose of hydrocortisone intravenously (200–300 mg) seems to give better results than adrenaline which was for long the main standby. If mismatched transfusion is suspected, 1 litre of balanced salt solution and 50 ml of 25% mannitol should be infused.

3

Fluids, nutrition and transfusion

David A. Humberstone and Graham L. Hill

As a consequence of the vast spectrum of diseases the modern surgeon encounters and as a result of the treatment modalities employed in dealing with them, a relative or absolute period with no oral input is frequently necessary. When this is combined with the metabolic disturbances associated with major surgery, the risk to the patient who does not receive careful perioperative care is enhanced. Finally, there may be accelerated rates of catabolism, dramatic changes in blood volume and substrate handling, all of which need to be taken into account.

For these reasons a firm grounding in fluid and electrolyte therapy, the use of nutritional support and blood transfusion are important aspects of all surgical disciplines. In this chapter normal body fluid distribution and some of the changes induced by surgical illness will be discussed, as will the fluid management of surgical patients. Furthermore, the importance of nutritional assessment and a discussion of available nutritional therapies will be undertaken. The chapter concludes with the role of blood and blood component therapy in current surgical practice.

Anatomy of body water and electrolytes

Body fat and lean

When considering the patient as a whole the total body mass can be subdivided into body fat and the fat-free mass. Fat is of undoubted importance as it is the major energy reservoir of the body. However, as it is anhydrous this has major implications as far as fluid therapy is concerned. For two patients of the same weight, the patient with the greater amount of fat will require less fluid as both the intracellular and extracellular fluid (ICF and ECF) volumes will be smaller.

In the state of health approximately 72% of the fat-free body is composed of water. In the presence of serious surgical illness, however, this may increase to 80% due to the erosion of the fat-free mass with relative preservation and therefore expansion of the extracellular fluid. A similar normal physiological expansion is seen with advancing years.

Extracellular and intracellular water

The total body water can be further subdivided into the extracellular and intracellular water (ECW and ICW). The interface between these two compartments is at the cell membrane. This partly explains the fluid shifts associated with serious illness as the function of the cell membrane is also known to undergo changes in these circumstances. All the enzymatic reactions and metabolic processes occur within the ICW, whereas the ECW bathes the cells and provides a constant milieu.

ECW compartmentalization

ECW can further be subdivided into five compartments, namely plasma, interstitial fluid/lymph, connective tissue and cartilage water, bone water and transcellular water. Problems may arise in fluid balance of the surgical patient when there is a failure to appreciate the interrelationships between these compartments, and fluid from one may become lost at the expense of others. Dramatic clinical examples of this include the patient with severe burns and the patient with intestinal obstruction.

Many surgical illnesses are associated with wasting due to changes in substrate handling, energy expenditure and accelerated rates of catabolism and this wasting is further accentuated by inanition. In this situation the ECW tends to be preserved whilst the cell mass is shrinking. The clinical message from this is that wasted patients without evidence of sodium or water depletion are likely to be both volume and sodium intolerant. In such patients cardiac failure may be easily precipitated if excessive quantities of saline are administered.

Sodium and potassium

Of the 4200 mmol of sodium in a healthy adult male, only 2.4% of this is intracellular and 70% of it is exchangeable. Up to 40% of total body sodium may be contained within the skeleton. In contrast, of the 3500 mmol of potassium within the body almost all is exchangeable and less than 2% is outside the cells. Thus it is apparent that sodium is the primary extracellular cation and potassium is primarily intracellular. This observation prompted the development of techniques to measure body cell mass based on measurements of total body potassium.

Unfortunately, in the presence of serious surgical illness changes in membrane potential are associated with changes in the intracellular potassium concentration making interpretation of results difficult. Changes in pH also induce changes in measured potassium, with hypokalaemia being associated with metabolic alkalosis (e.g. gastric outlet obstruction) and hyperkalaemia being associated with metabolic acidosis (e.g. renal failure).

Chloride

In the 70 kg healthy male there are approximately 2300 mmol of chloride. Of this, approximately 70% is contained within plasma, interstitial fluid and lymph. Hence chloride has been used as an index of ECF volume and most is exchangeable. Chloride also undergoes changes with acid–base disturbances with increases being seen in acidosis and decreases in alkalosis.

Magnesium, calcium and zinc

The healthy adult contains approximately 1000 mmol of magnesium with a distribution similar to that of potassium. Magnesium has an important role in the functioning of enzyme systems and depletion of magnesium which may be seen in starved hospitalized patients with serious illness manifests itself with signs of CNS and neuromuscular excitability similar to those seen with hypocalcaemia. The daily requirement is approximately 10 mmol.

The skeleton contains 99% of the 1200 g of bodily calcium. It is important to realize that the other 1% has major biological actions and is under the control of calcitonin, parathormone and vitamin D. Of the serum calcium, 50% is bound to proteins and the other half is responsible for the observed biological effects. The ratio of ionized to bound calcium is sensitive to acid–base changes, explaining the apparent symptomatic hypocalcaemia associated with overbreathing and respiratory alkalosis.

In the long-stay hosptial patient, especially those with enterocutaneous fistulae or wound problems such as dehiscence, there is an increased requirement for zinc and this zinc appears to have an important role in wound healing.

Surgical physiology

The body may be regarded as a finely balanced osmometer. When surgical illness is superimposed upon this system a series of alterations in the osmotic pressures between the intracellular and extracellular compartments results in a redistribution of fluid which may manifest itself in several different ways. One of the commonest observed changes will be the development of hypotonicity with hyponatraemia. This may be compounded by an excess of exogenous water, e.g. replacement of electrolyte-rich losses from a nasogastric tube with water as 5% dextrose. In this situation a decrease in the osmotic pressure of the ECF results in water diffusing into cells leading to swelling. When the swelling affects the brain this may have disastrous consequences, with fitting and loss of consciousness.

Conversely, if the extracellular compartment increases or decreases in volume without a change in the osmotic pressure, then no transfer of water occurs. In other words the ICF shares in changes of composition or concentration of the ECF, but not in those changes of volume alone.

Water balance

The average man takes in approximately 1500 ml of water/day in the form of fluids, the remainder being from the water content of food. Water is lost in the stool (100 ml/day), urine (1500 ml/day) and sweat (500 ml/day) with further insensible losses from the skin and the lungs. Water requirements will increase with fever, hyperventilation and hypermetabolism. Clearly, if the ambient temperature is higher or the subject very active, more will be lost from the skin. The requirements for water vary from 30 to 70 ml/kg body weight/day.

Sodium balance

The daily requirement for sodium is 80–120 mmol/day although the Western diet undoubtedly contains more than this. Regulation of sodium balance is primarily a function of the kidneys with approximately 100–150 mmol being lost in the urine each day. In the case of sodium depletion as seen in the patient with the high output ileostomy, the sodium content of urine, sweat and faeces can approximate zero. One consequence of this may be hypokalaemia as the subsequent hyperaldosteronism causes potassium loss to compensate for the sodium conservation.

Potassium balance

The daily requirement is 60–80 mmol/day with 60 mmol/day being lost in the urine and some in stool. Small intestinal fluid has a low potassium content (approximately 8 mmol/l) with somewhat more being seen in colonic content (approximately 50 mmol/l). Patients with mucus-secreting villous adenomas may present with hypokalaemia due to loss of mucus in the stool.

Abnormal gastrointestinal losses

Loss from the upper gastrointestinal tract should be replaced ml for ml with normal saline (0.9% NaCl). If this loss is from the stomach as in the patient with pyloric outlet obstruction, then 15 mmol/l of KCl should be added per litre of saline. Other gastrointestinal losses from lower down should be replaced ml for ml with Hartmann's solution.

Acid–base balance

Body cells and enzyme systems demonstrate extreme versatility in that they can function between a pH of 7.2 and 7.5 with acidosis being better tolerated than alkalosis. Due to the logarithmic nature of the pH scale, this range reflects a 400% alteration in the hydrogen ion concentration.

Acidosis

Acid is produced as a consequence of the metabolism of substrate, be it carbohydrate, fat or protein. Various surgical problems can generate increased quantities of acids. For example, hypoperfusion with consequent increased anaerobic metabolism in shock, increased lactate production in association with ischaemic gut and ketoacidosis in diabetes aggravated by surgical stress will all promote the development of acidosis.

The body removes acid with the aid of various buffering systems, the most quantitatively important one being the carbonic acid system, with acid being disposed of through the lungs in the form of carbon dioxide. Proteins and haemoglobin are other buffering systems with important roles.

Alkalosis

Alkalosis is less commonly seen than acidosis. The common situation in which metabolic alkalosis occurs is with pyloric obstruction with subsequent loss of acid from the stomach. A respiratory alkalosis is encountered in the anxious patient hyperventilating and hence blowing off an excess of acid in the form of carbon dioxide.

Compensatory mechanisms

When acid is added to a buffer system within a patient, whether endogenously or exogenously, the concentration of bicarbonate falls. The response is an increase in ventilation to blow off more carbon dioxide which tends to return the pH towards normal. This short-term rapid compensation is then succeeded by a slower but more thorough compensation involving the kidneys. This involves an increased excretion of acid salts and a tendency to retain bicarbonate. The converse occurs in a metabolic alkalosis.

Respiratory acidosis and alkalosis are produced by disturbances in alveolar ventilation, being excessive or insufficient. The kidneys once again are responsible for compensation, with retention of bicarbonate and excretion of acid in acidosis and the reverse process occurring in alkalosis.

Common body fluid changes seen in surgical patients

Extracellular fluid (ECF) depletion (surgical dehydration)

This is the commonest volume aberration confronting the surgeon, be it due to blood loss, vomiting due to bowel obstruction, diarrhoea, fistulae, burns, sepsis or shock. The diagnosis of ECF depletion must be clinical as in the short term there are no reliable laboratory changes to aid the clinician.

Mild deficit

In the presence of a mild deficit (less than 2 litres) there may be no clinical signs but the history is of great importance.

Moderate deficit

Once the deficit is of 2–4 litres in magnitude, cardiovascular signs become apparent with a tachycardia and a low central venous pressure. The patient may appear apathetic and have decreased tissue turgor and dry mucous membranes. Tissue turgor is not a reliable sign in the elderly and mucous membranes may appear dry if oxygen has been administered for prolonged periods without a humidifier.

Severe deficit

Once the ECF deficit becomes greater than 5 litres the patient may become pale, hypotensive and frankly comatose. His circulation will be shut down peripherally and the eyes will be markedly sunken.

Extracellular fluid (ECF) excess

With the exception of the patient in congestive cardiac failure which may be due to a perioperative myocardial infarction, the commonest cause of this overload is due to the administration of an excess of sodium-containing fluids during resuscitation for major injury or serious sepsis. ECF is also expanded in the oedematous patient with liver or kidney failure.

The plasma volume is increased as may be the interstitial fluid volume. There may be oedema present in dependent areas and the pulse, blood pressure and venous pressure may all be elevated. *The practical implications of this are most important in the elderly or those with impaired cardiac function.* Not only is an excessive strain placed on the heart, but tissues become oedematous which may impair healing. This is particularly important in the vicinity of an anastomosis.

Changes in electrolyte concentration

As tonicity tends to be a reflection of the sodium concentration, increases or decreases should be detected and the cause treated early before disastrous clinical sequelae supervene. Hyponatraemia and hypotonicity usually occur secondary to excessive water administration combined with the effects of increased levels of antidiuretic hormone (ADH) as part of the metabolic response to stress or trauma.

$$[Na_s] \propto \frac{Na(e) + K(e)}{TBW}$$

From this equation it can be seen that observed changes in serum sodium concentration Na_s are proportional to the total exchangeable cations in total body water (TBW). Thus, alterations in serum sodium are likely to reflect changes in water balance with hyponatraemia being the result of water excess and hypernatraemia being the result of water depletion.

Hyponatraemia

Once sodium becomes less than 130 mmol/l, signs of excess intracellular water may appear. If the level drops to less than 120 mmol/l, CNS signs including convulsions may occur due to brain swelling. This condition may usually be treated with water deprivation alone and it is exceptional for hypertonic salt solutions in combination with diuretics to be required.

Hypernatraemia

In contrast, hypernatraemia is usually the result of pure water depletion, i.e. dehydration. This is corrected by increasing the intake of free water which must be done cautiously to minimize the chances of cerebral oedema.

Hyperkalaemia

Hyperkalaemia is seen in response to severe injury culminating in extensive cell death where appreciable amounts of potassium leak into the ECF. It is also seen in renal failure and in metabolic acidosis, as well as in situations where there has been overzealous potassium supplementation. Providing the urine output and renal function are adequate, a dangerous level of hyperkalaemia is rarely encountered.

Clinically this may be silent but there may be evidence of gastrointestinal disturbances and if an ECG is performed there may be some characteristic abnormalities. These include high-peaked T waves, a widened QRS complex and depressed ST segments. These cardiac abnormalities may be sufficient to promote an arrest.

Hypokalaemia

Hypokalaemia may occur as a consequence of prolonged therapy with potassium-losing diuretics, alkalosis and replacement of gastric losses with saline without added potassium. It is important to remember that hypokalaemia may also be a manifestation of sodium depletion due to high levels of aldosterone secretion. The clinical signs that may be present include weakness and lethargy, decreased reflexes and ileus. Indeed, hypokalaemia is one of the causes of a pseudo-obstruction. These patients have a tendency to develop dangerous ventricular arrhythmias and this tendency is more pronounced if they are digitalized.

Treatment of electrolyte disturbances

Hyperkalaemia

The first aspect of treatment is to withhold any further potassium supplementation. If there are ECG changes a dextrose insulin infusion should be commenced to drive potassium back into the cells. Arterial blood gas should be checked and if there is evidence of a severe metabolic acidosis then bicarbonate should be administered. For less marked hyperkalaemia (<6 mmol/l), a dextrose insulin infusion may not be necessary and a cation exchange resin such as resonium should be administered.

Hypokalaemia

The therapy for this condition involves potassium replacement. It is essential to ensure a good urine output, particularly if high-dose potassium is being infused. The infusion rate should not exceed 20 mmol/h and at this rate urethral catheterization is helpful and cardiac monitoring should be considered. The level should be rechecked after several hours.

Routine fluid therapy

Three separate but overlapping aspects need to be considered:

1. Maintenance requirements.
2. Replacement of pathological losses.
3. Repair of deficits.

Maintenance requirements

The average man with no complicating factors requires approximately 2.5 litres of fluid/24 h. In addition there is also a requirement for 80–120 mmol Na/day and 60–80 mmol K/day. This can simply be met by prescribing 500 ml of 0.9% NaCl and 2 litres of 5% dextrose/day. To this should be added supplemental potassium at approximately 1 mmol/kg/day. Alternatively this could be given as 2500 ml of 0.18% NaCl and 4.2% dextrose with added potassium.

As well as dextrose being a convenient way of administering water, there is also a small protein-sparing effect of infused dextrose, due in part to the insulin response to the dextrose infused and in part to the inhibition of gluconeogenesis by infused glucose. Although this is a small effect it may be of importance in the protein-depleted postoperative surgical patient.

In the first 24 h after surgery potassium may not be required as the breakdown of cells induced by

surgical trauma will be releasing some potassium into the ECF.

Replacing ongoing pathological losses

Most of the losses from the gastrointestinal tract are isotonic and those losses due to vomiting, diarrhoea and fistulae can be replaced ml for ml with 0.9% NaCl with added potassium as KCl. Losses from other sites such as high ileostomy output can be adequately replaced ml for ml with Hartmann's solution (see Table 3.1). With ongoing losses that

Table 3.1 Composition of Plasmalyte and 0.9% NaCl (mmol/l)

	Hartmann's solution	0.9% NaCl
Na	130	150
K	4	
Ca	3	
Cl	109	150
Acetate	28	

are becoming unmanageable, pharmacological manipulation in an effort to modulate gut secretion may be worthwhile. In its simplest form this may involve the addition of an H_2 receptor antagonist and occasionally somatostatin may have a dramatic effect on reducing output.

With prolonged ongoing losses zinc and trace metal deficiency become real possibilities and may require supplementation. It is also important to realize that extra water will be lost in the presence of fever or tachypnoea and may require an extra 500 ml of 5% dextrose/day.

Sequestration occurs in several situations, e.g. in an established small intestinal obstruction 5–8 litres of fluid may be sequestered within the lumen of the gut. This phenomenon also occurs at the site of an operation and may be of particular import if a lengthy and extensive dissection has been carried out. Intraoperative fluid requirements in such situations may be up to 500 ml/h.

Repair of deficits

It is a useful exercise to be able to identify the compartment(s) involved in any deficit. Usually this will be the ECF compartment. Plasma volume should be restored rapidly as this will result in improved oxygen delivery to the tissues but interstitial fluid should be replaced at a slower rate. When large volumes are required, as is the case with severe pancreatitis, distal small intestinal obstruction or severe burns, it is important to monitor the patient during replacement.

This is crucial in the elderly with poor cardiac reserve and may necessitate frequent measurements of pulse, blood pressure, urine output, central venous pressure and, if in a critical care unit, a Swann–Ganz catheter may be useful. In all cases where large volumes are to be replaced, meticulous fluid balance records should be kept, monitoring input and output from all sources, including drains. A daily weight is also an important adjunct to management.

Nutritional care of surgical patients

Since the time of Studley it has been realized that poor nutritional state as evidenced by preoperative weight loss is associated with a higher postoperative morbidity and mortality. Recently the presence of weight loss occurring in association with evidence of physiological impairment has been identified as carrying a significantly worse prognosis in terms of infective sequelae postoperatively.

It was not until the late 1960s that the means of repleting starving patients intravenously became available. This has changed surgical practice to the extent that it is undoubtedly life-saving in certain situations, e.g. short gut, high output pancreatic fistula, although it is certainly not the panacea for all surgical illness.

Before any form of nutritional repletion can be undertaken – be it enteral or parenteral – it is important for the surgeon to be able to identify the nutritional deficiency syndromes he is likely to encounter. To this end it is also necessary to be familiar with basic techniques of nutritional assessment.

Nutritional assessment

Although there is a wide variety of tests recommended the best and most useful approach is clinical.

Dietary history and history of weight loss

As with the approach to evaluating any organ system, nutritional assessment involves both a history and an examination. Aspects of importance in the history relate to the dietary intake and the duration of any abnormality. This should be related to the history and duration of any weight loss. It is important to get the patient to relate the current weight to the weight when well. A useful guide is the fact that a patient who eats only half his normal food intake over a 1 month period will lose about 5 kg body weight.

Physical examination

Clinical examination is directed towards detecting objective evidence of weight loss and the assessment of protein and energy stores. Furthermore, signs of increased metabolic stress or increased energy expenditure are also important to detect.

The next aspect of the assessment involves the identification of any physiological impairment or organ dysfunction that may be occurring as a result of the altered nutritional status. Finally, at the completion of the assessment it should be possible to categorize the patient as belonging to a particular nutritional syndrome and appropriate recommendations for nutritional support should be given.

General appearance

The general appearance of the patient is important to note. He may be listless and apathetic, appearing haggard and emaciated. The face is thin with prominent cheekbones and may resemble the emerging skeleton. There may be marked wasting of the soft tissues, especially noticeable in the vicinity of the buttocks. However, malnourishment may not always be so easy to identify. One of the quirks of metabolism in the severely septic patient is the relative preservation of fat stores in the presence of severe erosion of protein due to accelerated rates of catabolism. Due to the preservation of fat stores and the relative expansion of ECF, dangerous protein depletion could be overlooked. A similar picture is seen in the patient on high-dose steroids, e.g. with active inflammatory bowel disease.

Assessment of body fat stores

Body fat stores may be grossly evaluated by the palpation of a number of predetermined skin folds. The principle behind this has led to the development of anthropometry. The skin folds examined are those over biceps and triceps as well as in the subscapular region. For ongoing evaluation it is important for the same person to continue measurements as there may be large interobserver variation.

If on palpation of skin folds the two layers of the dermis can be felt rubbing together, then the total fat stores of the patient comprise less than 10% body weight.

Assessment of protein stores

In a similar way it is possible to assess body protein stores, examining certain skeletal muscle bellies. This is based on the fact that the greatest proportion of body protein is located within skeletal muscle. The muscle groups examined are the temporales, the interossei, the supra and infraspinati, the biceps, deltoid and triceps. As well as the wasting of bellies of muscles being clinically important, when the tendons are prominent to palpation it is apparent that marked wasting has occurred.

Physiological function

Impairment of physiological function is determined both by history and examination. Poor wound healing, easy fatiguability and impaired exercise tolerance are all obtainable from the history and may suggest a serious nutritional deficiency state. The patient should be examined for signs of unhealed sores or indolent wounds. Skeletal muscle function can be assessed by estimating grip strength. This involves getting the patient to squeeze tightly upon middle and index fingers. Respiratory muscle function may be assessed by examining chest expansion and asking the patient to cough while a strip of paper is held 8 cm in front of the mouth. If the paper does not move forcefully there is marked impairment of the respiratory musculature.

Assessment of metabolic stress

It is also important to have an idea of any metabolic stress that the patient may be experiencing. This may be done with indirect calorimetry to determine resting energy expenditure. More simple parameters that may yield important information are temperature, white cell count, pulse rate, positive blood cultures or the presence of an abscess.

Nutritional syndromes

Moderate to severe nutritional depletion without stress

This is the situation seen in the patient with uncomplicated starvation due to insufficient food being ingested. Clinical examples of this include the patient with the benign stricture of the oesophagus or with pyloric stenosis due to peptic ulceration. Such a patient will have a weight loss of greater than 10% 'well weight' with clinical signs of malnutrition. The metabolic rate will be low as will be the rate of urinary nitrogen excretion. This demonstrates the protein-conserving response seen in uncomplicated starvation.

Mild depletion with added stress

This may be encountered in the patient with major sepsis following surgery, the young trauma victim with unstable fractures, the patient with the

pancreatic abscess, etc. Such a patient will initially have normal fat and protein stores but may have low serum albumin. These patients have vastly elevated catabolic rates, and if nothing is done will rapidly become seriously protein-depleted.

Moderate to severe nutritional depletion with stress

This is most commonly seen in the patient who comes to surgery nutritionally depleted, undergoes major surgery and has a serious complication such as an anastomotic leakage, e.g. post-gastrectomy or post-oesophagectomy.

Having identified the various nutritional syndromes, it is important to decide who will benefit from nutritional support and what form that support should take. It is unlikely that weight loss without physiological impairment is associated with increased postoperative complications, therefore weight loss alone is not sufficient reason for preoperative nutritional support. If there has been a weight loss of 10–20% in association with a decreased albumin and impaired skeletal and respiratory muscle function, the patient may benefit from 1 week of preoperative feeding if the clinical circumstances allow this.

After major surgery nutritional support is mandatory in the hypercatabolic septic patient losing weight and in the patient with enterocutaneous fistula. A softer indication exists in the patient with 15–20% weight loss with no immediate prospect of resuming normal intake postoperatively.

Nutritional support

Broadly speaking, nutritional support can be subdivided into that given by the enteral or by the parenteral route. Whichever mode is employed the daily requirements will be:

Water	30–70 ml/kg
Calories	30–50 kcal/kg
Protein	1.5–2.0 g/kg
Sodium	0.9–1.2 mmol/kg
Potassium	0.7–0.9 mmol/kg

In addition, magnesium, calcium, chloride, phosphate, trace elements and vitamins are also required.

Enteral nutrition

Enteral nutritional support may be administered through fine-bore nasogastric tubing, jejunostomy or gastrostomy and is the route of choice for patients with an intact and functional gastrointestinal tract, e.g. head injury patients. The current nasogastric

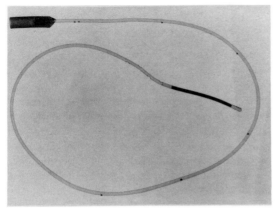

Figure 3.1 Nasogastric feeding tube. The tube is made of silicone rubber (no. 7 gauge) with a mercury weighted tip. (From Hill, G. L. (1988) Nutrition in surgical practice. In: Cuschieri, A., Giles, G. R., Moossa, A. R. *Essential Surgical Practice,* Bristol, John Wright and Sons Ltd.)

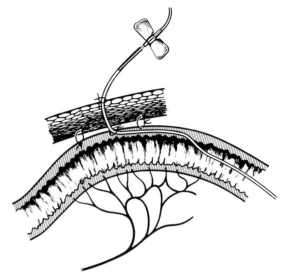

Figure 3.2 Fine needle catheter jejunostomy. (From Hill, G. L. (1988) Nutrition in surgical practice. In: Cuschieri, A., Giles, G. R., Moossa, A. R. *Essential Surgical Practice,* Bristol, John Wright and Sons Ltd.)

tubes are fine-bore silicone rubber and are comfortable for prolonged therapy (Figure 3.1). There are many defined formula diets available that are best delivered through an infusion pump as this minimizes the chances of blockage and results in smoother delivery to the gut compared with boluses several times per day.

When commencing therapy it is advisable to start at one-half or even one-quarter strength feeds to minimize the incidence of troublesome cramps and diarrhoea which sap both the confidence of the patient and the staff dealing with him. Before commencing feeding the tube position must be confirmed by a radiograph. If the patient is very hypoalbuminaemic it is likely that both gastric emptying and absorption will be impaired and it may be advantageous to replenish albumin parenterally with 100–200 ml of 25% albumin solution. Once feeding has commenced the patient should be weighed daily and both electrolytes and albumin should be monitored twice weekly.

Another technique of feeding a patient enterally involves the insertion of a needle jejunostomy at the time of an operation. This is particularly useful in the patient with a proximal obstruction, fistula or fragile anastomosis. The technical aspects involve the fashioning of a 10 cm submucosal tunnel some 30 cm from the duodenojejunal flexure through which a catheter is threaded into the jejunum and secured with a purse string suture (Figure 3.2). A contrast study is carried out on the operating table to ensure the catheter tip does lie within the lumen of the bowel.

The most recent development in enteral feeding in the 1990s involves the combined endoscopic/percutaneous placement of feeding gastrostomy or jejunostomy tubes. In future their use may avoid the need for an open operation.

Parenteral nutrition

This is now a practical therapy which can be administered safely in most hospitals, especially where a nutritional support service exists, and there are a considerable number of patients worldwide recieving home total parenteral nutrition (TPN), usually for short gut syndrome.

The nutrient solutions involved must be mixed in a hospital grade pharmacy using strict aseptic technique to minimize the potentially lethal complication of sepsis. The indication for TPN is usually in a seriously ill patient with a gastrointestinal tract that is blocked, short, fistulated or cannot cope (Table 3.2).

If the gut is blocked by oedema or a stricture following surgery which is expected to resolve, the parenteral route must be employed. Patients with the short gut syndrome usually require TPN for the

Table 3.2 Indications for TPN

Problem	Example
Gut short	Volvulus with infarction
Gut blocked	Anastomotic oedema
Gut unable to cope	Radiation enteritis
Gut fistulated	Crohn's disease

first 2 months while gut adaptation is occurring. As enteral feeding is necessary for optimal gut adaptation oral feeding should be instituted once faecal output and electrolyte problems have plateaued. If less than 1 metre of gut remains, permanent home TPN may be necessary for survival.

In the presence of a fistula proximal to the distal ileum the patient must be starved and commenced on TPN. If the fistula is of low output and distal to this, enteral feeding may be a realistic alternative. If the fistula does not close within 6 weeks, definitive surgery is required.

When the gut is inflamed and partially obstructed, as in Crohn's disease, some patients will experience a remission with the administration of gut rest, steroids and TPN. In the hypermetabolic trauma patient frequently seen in critical care departments, the demand for calories and nitrogen may exceed what can be delivered enterally. In such a situation additional parenteral nutrition may help to slow the ongoing protein losses. The responses of nutritional syndromes to TPN are shown in Figure 3.3.

Table 3.3 Typical TPN mixture for 55 kg patient

50% dextrose	550 ml
20% lipid solution	550 ml
Amino acid solution	1000 ml
Free water	400 ml
Total volume	2500 ml
Infusion rate	104 ml/h
Volume for electrolytes	2000 ml
Na (mmol/l)	50
K (mmol/l)	40
Mg (mmol/l)	4
Cl (mmol/l)	50
Acetate (mmol/l)	10
PO$_4$ (mmol/l)	15
Trace element solution	10 ml/day
Extra Zn	10 mg/day
Multivit infusion	10 ml/day
Folic acid	1 mg/day

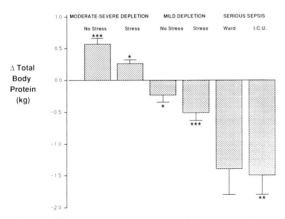

Nutritional Syndromes

Figure 3.3 Nutritional syndromes and their response to total parenteral nutrition

A typical TPN solution will consist of a solution of 8.5% amino acids and calories sufficient to provide 40 kcal/kg/day delivered as a 50:50 mixture of 20% lipid and 50% dextrose. To this is added water, albumin, sodium, potassium, magnesium, zinc, chloride, phosphate, acetate, trace metals and vitamins. One litre of this solution will provide approximately 1000 kcal and 42.5 g of protein. Table 3.3 lists the composition of a TPN mixture suitable for a 55 kg patient.

To achieve tissue growth the provision of protein and calories alone is not sufficient and potassium must be added at 40 mmol/1000 kcal and phosphate at 20 mEq/1000 kcal. One ampoule of MVI (multivitamin infusion) containing both fat- and water-soluble vitamins is added to the TPN solution each day. Additional folate and vitamin K are given weekly and vitamin B$_{12}$ once a week by intramuscular injection. Trace elements are given daily and extra zinc is important in the patient with problems related to the wound or fistulae.

Administration

Because of the hypertonic nature of the TPN solution it must be administered into a central vein with a high flow rate to minimize local complications. The subclavian approach using the Seldinger technique is preferred for in-hospital therapy, although for patients on home TPN a Hickman catheter may be more convenient. Line insertion is carried out using a strictly aseptic technique and the line is dedicated solely to TPN and is never to be used for additives, CVP recordings, etc. (Figure 3.4).

The dressings over the insertion site are changed three times per week as is the tubing. Following insertion of the line a chest radiograph is obtained to check the position of the line. The tip should lie in the superior vena cava, and complications of insertion such as pneumothorax should also be checked for. Other complications include malposition of the catheter, usually up the internal jugular, and arterial puncture and brachial plexus injury are not unheard of.

Until a patient is stabilized on TPN, blood is taken daily to check electrolytes and glucose. Once stable, blood is checked three times per week for electrolytes and zinc; magnesium and haemoglobin are checked once a week. The patient is weighed daily and a strict fluid balance record is kept.

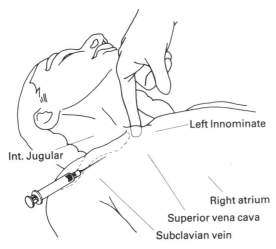

Figure 3.4 Central venous catheter placement. The needle is inserted lateral to the mid part of the clavicle and directed towards the suprasternal notch. Puncture of the subclavian vein is indicated by a flush of blood into the syringe. (From Dudrick, S. J. and Copeland, E. M. (1973) Parenteral hyperalimentation. In: Nyhus, L. M. (ed.), *Surgery Annual,* New York, Appleton-Century-Crofts)

Central line sepsis

If the patient on TPN has a temperature above 38.5°C and there is no obvious site for this, blood cultures are taken both peripherally and centrally. The TPN is taken down and a sample sent for microbiology. Antibiotic sensitivities of any bacteria cultured are requested. The central line insertion site is also cultured and the line changed over a guidewire, with the tip being sent for culture. Administration of 10% dextrose is commenced to avoid rebound hypoglycaemia. If the temperature has not started to come down after 4 h the line is removed and antibiotics started. If the catheter tip shows growth within 24 h and the blood cultures are positive, the line is removed whether or not the temperature has settled and 24 h later is inserted on the opposite side.

Blood transfusion

Any blood transfusion is a serious undertaking. If it is regarded as a form of transplantation of regenerative tissue from a donor being given to a recipient, its importance is not likely to be underestimated. The process of transfusion is not without hazard and it is therefore important for the surgeon to be familiar with the indications, risks and techniques involved.

Indications

In surgical practice blood may be transfused to correct anaemia of long standing or to combat acute blood loss. The anaemia of long standing may be due to chronic disease, e.g. Crohn's disease, or due to chronic bleeding and present as iron deficiency anaemia as in carcinoma of the caecum. Conversely blood may be required to sustain life in the presence of torrential haemorrhage due to preoperative problems such as trauma or a vascular emergency, or intraoperatively when heavy bleeding is encountered.

A further indication for blood transfusion may be in immune system modulation, e.g. renal transplantation. There is evidence that graft survival may be enhanced following blood transfusion preoperatively.

Preparation

All patients undergoing surgery where the potential exists for bleeding should at the very least have blood grouping carried out so that should the need arise blood can be crossmatched for them rapidly. For major operations where a transfusion is to be expected the operation should not proceed without blood being available in theatre. This requirement may vary from case to case with up to nine units being required routinely for ruptured aortic aneurysms and major trauma cases.

Rationale for transfusion

The reason for transfusion is to increase the red cell mass of the patient and hence optimize oxygen delivery to the tissues. The fate of transfused red cells depends somewhat on the time the blood has been stored for, but may undergo two routes. Dead or damaged cells will be completely removed from the circulation in under 24 h whereas the remainder will be removed in the normal fashion as they reach senescence. With modern storage techniques <20% of red cells are removed rapidly and with fresh blood this figure is <10%.

The increased oxygen carrying capacity resulting from a blood transfusion must not be attained at the expense of precipitating cardiac failure in the elderly by volume overloading or increasing haematocrit to the extent that viscosity increases to an unacceptable level. This is particularly important in vascular surgery and may jeopardize graft survival. In hypovolaemia, expansion of the blood volume may be more important than raising the haematocrit.

Who to transfuse

The most important issue regarding blood transfusion is that of who should be transfused. There are few hard and fast rules and it is dependent on the clinical situation. For example, patients with ischaemic heart disease tolerate worsening anaemia very poorly. The reason for this is that maximal oxygen extraction from blood is already occurring in the coronary system and the only way for oxygen delivery to be increased is for flow to increase. This may not be possible in very diseased coronary arteries and anaemia in such patients may precipitate angina. If there is a surgical cause for the worsening anaemia such a patient will need very careful transfusion preoperatively.

On the other hand, a fit young man recovering from surgery for multiple fractures can tolerate a low haematocrit very well and should be allowed to replace his own haemoglobin postoperatively. The key point is that there are very few absolute numbers at which all patients require transfusion and the decision should be individualized for each patient.

What to transfuse

Most transfusions are best undertaken with reconstituted packed red cells. This not only reduces the volume requirement but also minimizes exposure to potentially hazardous components in whole blood. In addition, with techniques available in modern blood banks, it means that platelets, white cells and cryoprecipitate can all be harvested from the whole blood and used in special circumstances.

Red cells are stored in a liquid state in a citrate-based anticoagulant. The citrate functions by binding calcium to prevent coagulation from occurring. Because of the effect of the citrate when multiple transfusions are being given over a short period of time, difficulties with low calcium may occasionally be encountered but only rarely require exogenous calcium administration.

Hazards of transfusion

Red cell antigen/antibody reactions

These are manifest clinically as haemolysis reactions and occur when either A or B red cells are transfused into a patient with either anti-A or anti-B antibodies in the plasma (group O with anti-A and anti-B antibodies, group A with anti-B antibodies or group B with anti-A antibodies) or by infusing plasma with anti-A or anti-B antibodies into a patient with either blood group A, B or AB. In its most dramatic form this reaction will manifest itself as haemoglobinaemia, haemoglobinuria, acute renal failure and disseminated intravascular coagulation (DIC).

A similar picture is seen if blood is administered through a line containing either 5% dextrose or water as red cells will haemolyse due to the osmotic gradient. Occasionally a delayed haemolytic reaction occurs due to an antibody/antigen reaction other than the ABO system. This will usually present as jaundice or anaemia and only very rarely as kidney failure.

Non-red cell antigen/antibody reactions

Approximately 1% of all patients undergoing transfusion will experience pruritus. This is thought to be related to plasma proteins. Similarly, many patients experience mild elevations in temperature whilst being transfused which is thought to be related to leukocyte factors. Occasionally a generalized anaphylactic reaction is seen and is thought to be related to IgA.

Miscellaneous

It is highly unusual for blood to be contaminated with bacteria or endotoxin but when it occurs the appearances are those of 'warm' or septic shock with elevated temperature and pulse, hypotension and vasodilatation. Overzealous transfusion, particularly in the elderly with impaired ventricular function, may result in circulatory overload, cardiac failure and pulmonary oedema. However, the practice of routinely prescribing diuretics following each unit of blood is also to be condemned. If the patient's state is that precarious, his volume status should be frequently reassessed over the course of the transfusion.

Viral infection

Both hepatitis B and the AIDS virus have been transmitted in the past and it is patients such as haemophiliacs and those on dialysis that have suffered. With screening tests, hopefully the incidence of transmission of both of these virus groups will be reduced, if not eliminated. Unfortunately, approximately 80% of transfusion-related hepatitis is non-A, non-B, and although generally less severe than B, it is still associated with a considerable morbidity and some mortality and cannot be screened for.

Immunological consequences of transfusion

There is some evidence accruing that the transfusion of whole blood in patients with colorectal cancer puts such patients in a higher risk category for recurrence than non-transfused controls. This may be related to the same immunological suppression that is beneficial in organ transplantation. Other workers have found a possible increase in septic sequelae following surgery involving blood transfusion. In both areas more work is needed before the true situation will become apparent.

Massive transfusion

Several problems are encountered when the transfusion given is greater than or equal to the patient's own blood volume.

Coagulopathy

Transfused blood is somewhat poor in clotting factors and platelets and this has been thought to be the reason for bleeding in massive transfusion. Some recent work has suggested that this is more likely to be a DIC-type phenomenon related to tissue hypoperfusion. However, it is still standard teaching in most centres to administer platelets and fibrin degradation products in the presence of ongoing massive transfusion.

Impaired oxygen delivery

There is impaired oxygen delivery due to a decreased level of 2,3-DPG in transfused red cells. This can be minimized by using blood as fresh as possible.

Hyperkalaemia

The theory is that potassium leaks out of cells due to the cold of storage. However, as the blood is warmed in the patient the potassium returns into the cells. The only potassium that permanently remains in banked blood is that from effete red cells, and if the blood used is fresh this should be <10%. Although often quoted, hyperkalaemia usually is not a problem in massive transfusion.

Hypocalcaemia

This may occur as a consequence of the citrate used as a preservative binding ionized calcium. Calcium should only be administered if there is evidence of failing cardiac function in the absence of hypovolaemia.

Hypothermia

Hypothermia may be severe enough to lower the patient's temperature to the point of producing cardiac arrest. Both the transfused fluids and the patient should be kept as warm as possible.

Specific blood products and their uses

Stable plasma protein solution (SPPS)

This is a 5% isotonic protein solution containing mainly albumin. It cannot transmit infective diseases and is a useful plasma volume expander where a sustained oncotic effect is required. It may be administered through the same line as blood.

Fresh dried plasma

This product may be used in the same circumstances as fresh frozen plasma and should only be given where there is an identified or potential loss of multiple coagulation factors. If used, at least 1–2 litres are necessary in a 70 kg adult to fully correct coagulation deficiencies. This product has the same risks as red cell transfusion as far as transmitting diseases is concerned.

Whole blood

Whole blood is only very occasionally required in massive blood loss and in some cardiac bypass procedures.

Resuspended red cells

Nearly all blood transfusion should be administered in this form. This product has a shelf life of 35 days and may transmit infective diseases.

Platelet concentrates

These may be required for massive transfusions, particularly once 8–10 units of blood have been used. Platelet concentrates may also be useful in DIC, haematological disorders and prolonged cardiac bypass procedures. The dose required is 0.08 platelet concentrates/kg body weight. These may also transmit infective diseases.

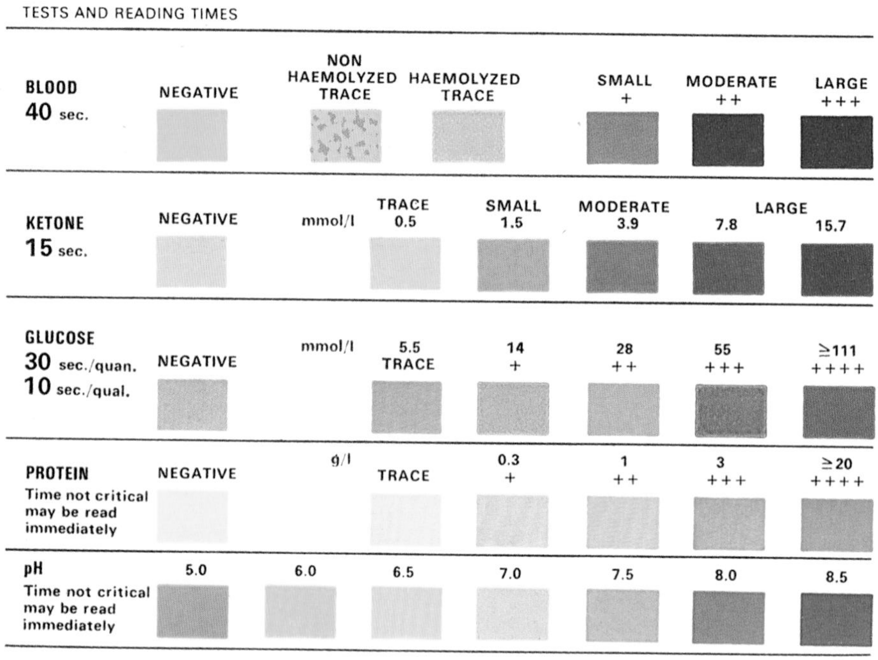

TESTS AND READING TIMES
BLOOD
40 sec.
NEGATIVE
NON HAEMOLYZED TRACE
HAEMOLYZED TRACE
SMALL +
MODERATE ++
LARGE +++
KETONE
15 sec.
NEGATIVE
mmol/l
TRACE 0.5
SMALL 1.5
MODERATE 3.9
LARGE
7.8
15.7
GLUCOSE
30 sec./quan.
10 sec./qual.
NEGATIVE
mmol/l
5.5 TRACE
14 +
28 ++
55 +++
≥111 ++++
PROTEIN
Time not critical may be read immediately
NEGATIVE
g/l
TRACE
0.3 +
1 ++
3 +++
≥20 ++++
pH
Time not critical may be read immediately
5.0
6.0
6.5
7.0
7.5
8.0
8.5

Plate 1 Ames Clinitest colour chart

4

Minor procedures

J. A. R. Smith

The word 'minor' is used somewhat erroneously to differentiate minor surgical operations from those more major procedures requiring special facilities or the use of an anaesthetic in theatre. However, it is vital that all such procedures are practised by all junior surgical staff in order to minimize patient discomfort, to avoid destruction of patient confidence and to save the practitioner time. Until each junior doctor is confident under supervision he should always ensure that experienced assistance is available.

Urine testing

Microscopy

Naked eye examination detects gross differences in colour and clarity, but microscopy is usually more valuable. A small sample, with or without centrifugation, allows examination for red or white blood cells, casts or the Brownian movement characteristic of bacterial infection. More specific information is obtained from a mid-stream specimen sent to the laboratory, but initial screening is valuable for emergencies.

Biochemical tests

Urine testing has been greatly simplified by the availability of standard 'strips' manufactured by Ames Co. With these it is possible to ascertain urine pH and the presence of any blood, protein, glucose, ketones, bilirubin and urobilinogen. Once the stick has been dipped fully into the specimen, time must be allowed for colour change to be detected, varying from immediately for pH to 60 s for urobilinogen. Standard colour charts are available for each substance (Plate 1).

Clinitest tablets allow quantification of any glucose present. Using a dropper provided with the kit, five drops of urine, followed by ten drops of water, are added to the test tube provided. One tablet is added and stimulates boiling. The tube is held steady for 15 s, shaken gently to ensure an even mix of colour, which is then compared with a standard chart provided (Plate 1).

Bence Jones Protein

To detect this abnormal protein in the urine, the specimen is divided in two test tubes. One is a control and the other is heated carefully over a Bunsen burner. If a cloud develops, it is due either to protein or to phosphates. Three to four drops of 5% acetic acid are then added, and if the cloud persists it is confirmed as due to excess protein in the urine. If continued heating disperses this cloud, then Bence Jones protein is present as it is seen as a cloud only between 45° and 55°C (113 and 131°F).

Blood tests

Venepuncture

Skill at obtaining venous blood samples can only be learned by practice. The skill is important as the more traumatic the venepuncture the less the confidence felt by the patient during future management.

Any suitable vein in the antecubital fossa or the dorsum of the hand may be selected – a Y-junction is usually best. A tourniquet is applied above the proposed site, but is left in place as short a time as possible and is not used at all if serum calcium is to be estimated. The skin injection site is thoroughly cleaned with spirit. The vacuum in the disposable syringe is released and the needle is rapidly inserted through the skin some 3–4 mm distal to the entry site on the vein. The needle is then passed proximally into the vein, at which point there is a characteristic feeling of 'give', and blood may be drawn back. The tourniquet is then released. Once the sample has been obtained, the needle is withdrawn and pressure applied for 2–3 min (Figure 4.1). The Vacutainer system allows several specimens to be obtained directly into the specimen bottles without using a syringe or any transfer of blood being required.

In obese patients, a distended vein may have to be palpated by the experienced finger. Occasionally *femoral vein stab* (Figure 4.2) is required, but leg veins should be avoided if possible both for venepuncture and for infusion purposes. To perform a stab, the femoral artery is palpated in the groin, the skin is cleaned and the needle is inserted just medial to the femoral pulse. If back pressure is applied as the syringe is depressed, both the feel and the obtaining of venous blood confirms entry into the vein.

Arterial puncture

To obtain arterial blood for blood gas analysis, strict local asepsis is essential. The femoral artery is the site of choice. The pulse is felt by two fingers of one hand lying longitudinally and the needle is then inserted between the fingers. One can feel the needle entering the artery and bright red arterial blood enters the syringe under arterial pressure. Once the needle is removed, the syringe must be sealed at once to prevent contamination with room air. Firm pressure is applied over the puncture site for 3 min.

Intravenous infusion

The principles involved in venepuncture are also applied to setting up a fluid infusion except:

1. It is kind to infiltrate some local anaesthetic at the skin puncture site and if the skin is at all tough to use a scalpel to nick the skin to facilitate entry of the cannula.
2. If at all possible, a site away from the antecubital fossa is preferable as elbow flexion may displace the cannula.
3. Firm fixation of the cannula and the giving set are essential to minimize night calls to attend to problems

Various cannulae are available and only by trial will personal preference be determined. It is vital to check infusion sites for: (1) thrombophlebitis, (2) tissue collection of fluid and to change the site if

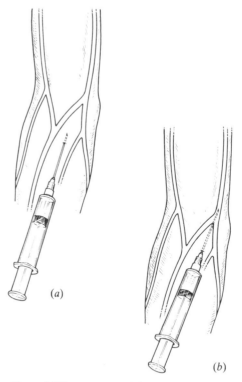

Figure 4.1 Venepuncture. (*a*) Needle inserted 1 cm distal to Y-junction in antecubital fossa. (*b*) Needle enters vein at confluence

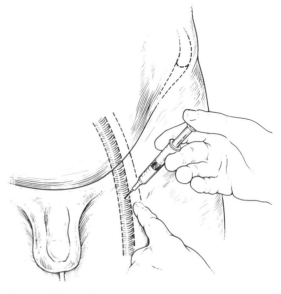

Figure 4.2 Femoral triangle venepuncture. A contralateral finger palpates the artery lateral to the femoral vein 1 cm distal to the inguinal ligament

either is found. Local symptomatic therapy may be required. Great care must be taken when changing infusion bottles to minimize the risk of bacterial contamination and to avoid air embolism.

Central venous cannulation (see also p. 241)

Whether required for central venous pressure monitoring or for total parenteral nutrition, strict asepsis using full theatre sterile techniques is essential if a central vein is to be cannulated.

Of the three most popular – subclavian puncture; internal jugular puncture; antecubital fossa puncture and cannula passage proximally – the first is the easiest to master, with least morbidity.

Technique

1. A sandbag is laid longitudinally between the shoulder blades (Figure 4.3).

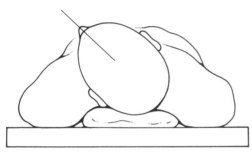

Figure 4.3 Central venous cannulation. A sandbag is placed between the shoulders and the patient's chin is turned to the left

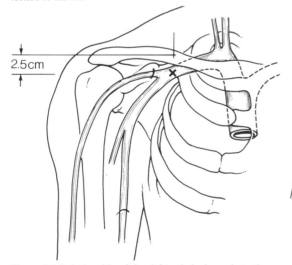

Figure 4.4 Relationship of the right subclavian vein to the clavicle and the first rib

2. The patient is placed in the supine head-down position to increase proximal venous pressure and landmarks are located (Figure 4.4).
3. The area around the right clavicle is thoroughly cleansed and draped.
4. Local anaesthetic is infiltrated in the skin about 2.5 cm below the midpoint of the right clavicle and the skin is nicked with a scalpel.
5. An 8 cm long cannula with syringe is inserted and passed upwards towards the suprasternal notch, keeping a line parallel to the medial one-third of the clavicle (Figure 4.5). If slight backward pressure on the syringe is maintained, the vein can be identified by the feel on entry plus the delivery of venous blood. A guide wire is directed through the cannula into the vein and a silicone catheter of 16 cm length is passed over the guide wire and into the vein. Whenever the syringe is disconnected the patient is asked to breathe out to minimize the risk of respiratory air embolus. The catheter is advanced into the superior vena cava, the patient's head being turned to the left to discourage passage upwards into the neck veins. An intravenous fluid infusion is then connected, but before commencing flow, the bottle should be lowered below the level of the head and flow of blood back into the catheter visualized to confirm patency and the presence of the cannula in a vein. Where central venous access is required for nutritional support, it is advisable to (a) cut down on the right cephalic vein; (b) cannulate the vein and pass the cannula into the superior vena cava; and (c) create a subcutaneous tunnel between a site on the anterior chest wall and the cephalic vein site. This makes managing the cannula more straightforward and reduces the incidence of infection. Chest X-ray to confirm the site of the catheter in the superior vena cava is essential before total parenteral nutrition (TPN) is commenced or before monitoring starts.

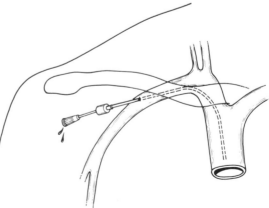

Figure 4.5 Cannula inserted parallel to the medial one-third of the right clavicle

Central venous pressure (CVP) monitoring

Clear fluids only should be infused if CVP monitoring is required. A reference point marking the position of the right atrium is used to measure zero and CVP can be read in cmH$_2$O from a simple side arm manometer (Figure 4.6). It is important:

1. To alter reference point as the patient's position changes.
2. To make allowance for the effect of assisted ventilation which tends to increase CVP.
3. To remember that CVP is *not* an absolute measurement, but is only valuable as a method of assessing response to fluid infusion. Whenever a central venous cannula is removed, the tip should be sent for bacteriological investigation.

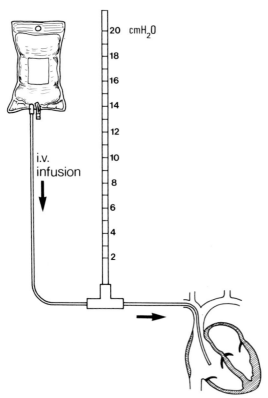

Figure 4.6 Schematic diagram of the infusion pack and side-arm manometer and their relationship to the right atrium

Venous cutdown (Figure 4.7)

Very occasionally in a shocked patient neither peripheral nor central venous cannulation is possible. If so, it is possible to identify a vein in a standard anatomical site by cutdown.

Under aseptic conditions, the area is cleaned and locally anaesthetized. A transverse incision is made in the skin and is deepened until a reasonably sized vein is identified. The vein is dissected free and two linen ties passed around it. The distal is firmly tied: only one throw is made in the proximal. The vein is opened using a fine scalpel or scissors and a venous cannula inserted carefully. The proximal thread is then tied firmly and a fluid infusion commenced. Standard skin closure is performed.

Blood culture

Using strict aseptic conditions, a venepuncture specimen of 20 ml is obtained. Taking a fresh needle, an aliquot of blood is injected into culture medium bottles for aerobic and anaerobic culture and the bottles are placed in an incubator at 37°C (98.6° F).

Samples are obtained from each bottle for plating and for microscopy as appropriate. The sensitivity to antibiotics of any bacteria is determined.

The best time to obtain positive blood cultures is at the peak of a pyrexia, and cultures should be repeated with each subsequent spike of temperature.

Biochemical testing of blood

The only standard test essential in the house surgeon's expertise is the measurement of blood sugar using Dextrostix. The colour change obtained when the stick is inserted into a sample is compared with a standard and the level read off. It is important that laboratory confirmation of the result is obtained.

Other tests are done in the laboratory, but it must be ensured that the correct tube is used for the estimation required. The number of venepunctures should be kept to the minimum possible. The needle must be removed before blood is transferred from the syringe to the tube in order to minimize trauma to red cells.

Risks of hepatitis (For Aids etc. see Chapter 10)

Where there is any possibility of category III or IV risk, it is essential that the doctor wears gloves and pays particular attention to the avoidance of spillage or contamination. All tubes must be identified and placed in a polythene bag. The laboratory forms should make the fact of possible category III/IV risk very clear.

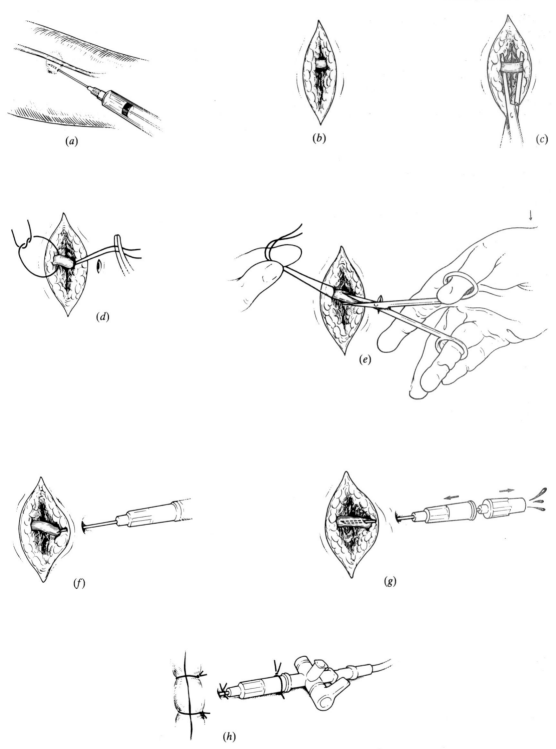

Figure 4.7 Venous cutdown. (*a*) Infiltrating local anaesthetic in forearm. (*b*) Incision at right-angles to vein. (*c*) Clearing vein. (*d*) Sling stitches around vein. (*e*) Making nick in vein for large cannula. (*f*) Inserting cannula. (*g*) Removing stilette. (*h*) Three-way tap and infusion line attached to cannula. Main incision sutured, and two sutures securing cannula in position

Cyst aspiration and cytology

The most common site for aspiration is the breast. The area is cleaned, the cyst localized with the left fingers and a needle is inserted into the cyst cavity. The fluid is aspirated to dryness. If no fluid is obtained, it is worthwhile to continue aspiration as the needle is withdrawn as a specimen can be obtained for cytology. On removal, the syringe is detached from the needle; air is aspirated; needle and syringe are reconnected and any cells in the needle can be expelled onto a clean slide by emptying the syringe of air. The specimen is dried and sent to the cytology laboratory for staining and microscopy. Alternatively, the aspirate may be placed into a transport medium to be processed later in the cytology laboratory. If the cyst does not resolve on aspiration, if it recurs or if it contains blood, cytological examination by an expert is essential, followed by formal biopsy. If the breast cyst is emptied completely, the patient should none the less be checked clinically in 4 weeks. Recurrence indicates the need for biopsy.

Faecal occult blood

An ideal method to detect occult blood in the faeces which is sensitive, but not too sensitive, has still to be devised. The simplest test presently available is the Haemoccult test which involves:

1. Smearing a specimen of faeces on one side of a paper in a prepacked kit;
2. The dropping of a standard reagent on the opposite side once the faeces have dried;
3. Reading any blue discoloration – indicative of occult blood;
4. Repeating the test three times to avoid false negative results in suspicious clinical circumstances;
5. Repeating the test on a meat-free diet to minimize false positives.

Lumbar puncture

Before embarking on lumbar puncture it is essential to ensure that there are no clinical signs of raised intracranial pressure nor any fundal signs, such as papilloedema. As in all procedures, the steps involved are explained carefully to the patient, who then lies on the left side with hips and neck flexed (Figure 4.8). An aseptic technique is essential. After carefully washing and gloving the hands, thoroughly clean the skin overlying the lumbar spine and towel the area. Identify the posterior superior iliac crest and palpate the space between two lumbar spines just distal to this level. Infiltrate about 2 ml of 1%

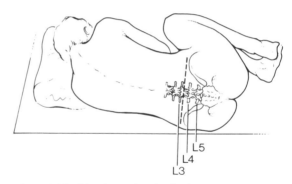

Figure 4.8 Position for performing lumbar puncture

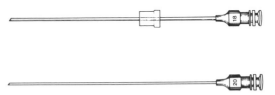

Figure 4.9 Lumbar puncture needles; the larger with a marker

plain lignocaine. The lumbar puncture needle and trocar (Figure 4.9) are inserted and passed in the midline upwards and then straight to enter the spinal canal. The sensation of 'give' is characteristic both as ligamentum flavum and outer dura are penetrated. If leg pain is complained of, withdraw the needle a little and reinsert it more centrally. Fluid is obtained on removing the trocar. Cerebrospinal pressure can be measured using a simple manometer and fluid sent to the laboratory for biochemical (sugar and protein) and bacteriological investigation. The needle is removed: a firm dressing is applied and the patient is kept supine in bed for 24 h.

Abdominal paracentesis

Abdominal paracentesis is used in the following circumstances:

1. To obtain a specimen of ascitic fluid for diagnostic purposes.
2. To allow drainage of such fluid causing symptoms.
3. To assist in the diagnosis of intra-abdominal trauma, or more recently, of acute pancreatitis.

The procedure is explained to the patient and the abdominal wall cleaned thoroughly with antiseptic solution. The entry site of choice is midway between anterior superior spine and umbilicus (Figure 4.10) but particular care is required where there are scars

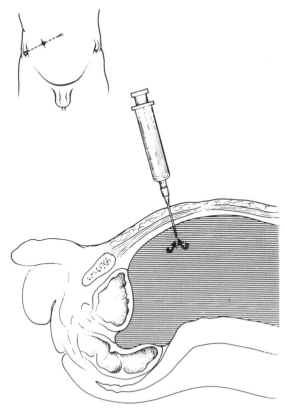

Figure 4.10 Abdominal paracentesis

from previous surgery. The site chosen is infiltrated with local anaesthetic down to the peritoneum. A needle attached to a syringe, or a special peritoneal dialysis catheter is inserted along the line used to infiltrate with local analgesia, to enter the peritoneal cavity. Specimens of fluid are sent for biochemical, bacteriological and cytological examination. Care must be taken not to remove too much fluid too quickly lest hypovolaemia results.

Where there is minimal fluid and either trauma or pancreatitis are suspected, lavage of the cavity is performed using a fixed volume of warmed normal saline and the effluent is examined for blood and/or amylase.

Examination of pus

In most centres pus is sent to the laboratory for examination and for both aerobic and anaerobic culture. Both the naked eye appearance and the smell of pus may be characteristic, e.g. greenish pus indicates *Pseudomonas*; watery, golden pus suggests *Staphylococcus*; and sulphur-granular pus, actinomycosis. However, these features are unreliable and further investigation is essential.

It is important to send either a sterile container of pus or a fresh swab in transport medium as swabs tend to dry out in transit and prove worthless

Gram stain

If no laboratory is available, some information may be obtained by Gram staining:

1. Smear specimen of pus on slide.
2. Dry in air and fix by heat.
3. Add ammonium oxalate crystal violet for a few seconds.
4. Wash off excess stain with water.
5. Cover with Gram's iodine and leave for 10 s.
6. Wash off iodine with acetone for 2–5 s and immediately wash with water.
7. Counterstain with dilute carbon fuchsin for 10–20 s.
8. Wash and dry.
9. Examine under microscope.

This will distinguish Gram positive (purple staining) from Gram negative (pink staining) and cocci in clumps (staphylococci) or chains (streptococci) from bacilli.

5

Wounds and minor surgery

A. B. Matheson

Many wounds and minor surgical procedures may be managed by junior medical staff or in a doctor's surgery, but the inexperienced or occasional operator should be wary of embarking on any operation which might prove to be beyond his ability. Full discussion with a senior colleague before starting an operation is much to be preferred to a call for help during it. Some wounds will require the skills of a specialist surgeon and should be referred appropriately.

No matter how wounds are caused, be they deliberate as part of a surgical procedure, accidental or even self-inflicted, the aims of management remain the same: to restore as much function as is possible to the affected part, to achieve the best possible cosmetic result and to avoid as far as possible both early and late complications. In practice this usually means creating the best conditions under which primary healing can take place and protection against infection.

Soft tissue wounds

Wounds are common injuries, occurring in a wide variety of situations – in road traffic accidents, accidents in the home or at work, as a result of the activities of terrorists or criminal assault, or they may be self-inflicted. The doctor's approach must be methodical and thorough. Criminal and civil court actions are often raised following wounding incidents; they are most commonly pursued against the person allegedly causing the wound, but sometimes civil litigation is directed towards the doctor for alleged negligence, such as failure to detect a retained foreign body or damage to an important deep structure. Although the doctor's actions should not be unduly influenced by the fear of litigation, he should be alert to possible medicolegal implications.

The Accident and Emergency department should have an established policy for the management of wounds which the staff should follow closely. The adoption of methodical, careful and thorough techniques of examination and treatment and the keeping of good written records may save much anguish later.

Records

The records, which should be made at the time, should note:

1. The history;
2. The findings on examination (where a sketch can be useful) including the interpretation of radiographs;
3. The procedures carried out and drugs or antibiotics prescribed; and
4. The arrangements for aftercare.

First aid

In all injured patients the ABC of basic life support, i.e. attention to the airway, breathing and circulation, must take precedence over all other measures. In wounding, first aid is directed at the control of bleeding and the prevention of further contamination. If hospital treatment is thought necessary, an ambulance should be called. It is seldom a good idea to convey a badly injured or semiconscious patient to hospital in a private car if proper ambulance transport is reasonably available. The waiting time can be spent usefully in preparing the patient for the journey and reassuring him. In severe injury, or where distances are great or road congestion is a problem, the use of a helicopter should be considered.

Venous bleeding may be reduced by elevating the wounded part but arterial haemorrhage is best controlled by digital or manual pressure over a suitable pad. Open wounds should be covered with sterile gauze pressure dressings secured with bandages. If proper dressings are not available clean household linen may be used. Fluffy materials such as cotton wool should *not* be applied directly to open wounds. If a fracture is suspected some form of splintage will be necessary. Analgesics are very seldom indicated for wounds, and are contra-indicated in the presence of significant head injury. If the doctor is not accompanying the patient to hospital he should make a written note of what has been done and send it with the patient.

History

If possible a detailed history of the incident should be taken from the patient. Sometimes valuable additional information is available from eye witnesses or from persons called to the scene of the accident such as police or ambulance crew. A good understanding of the mechanism of injury will prepare the doctor as to the type of wound he is likely to encounter and assist him greatly in his examination.

Examination

In all but the most trivial of cases the examination should be carried out with the patient recumbent in an area out of public view. It is reassuring for a child or a mentally handicapped patient to have a friend or relative present, but otherwise they should be excluded from the examination room. With foreign or deaf patients, an interpreter may have to be present.

Viral hepatitis and AIDS

Full aseptic precautions using gown, mask and gloves are not necessary for the examination of wounds and indeed these arrangements may be impossible to achieve in some Accident and Emergency departments or surgeries, but the risk of staff being contaminated with hepatitis virus or the human immunodeficiency virus (HIV), the causative agent of acquired immune deficiency syndrome (AIDS), should be well understood and at a very minimum plastic aprons and surgical gloves should be worn.

Some Accident and Emergency departments post notices requesting patients to inform the staff if they are carriers of the hepatitis virus or HIV. When a positive response occurs, some members of staff may wish to take additional precautions such as wearing a mask, two pairs of gloves and even goggles, but the sensitivities of the carrier must be treated with the greatest respect.

The question of testing patients for the hepatitis virus, and particularly HIV, raises difficult ethical considerations. This type of screening should only be carried out with the express permission of the consultant in charge of the case. Blood should always be regarded as potentially infectious for these conditions, and the doctor should take care not to place himself or his colleagues at risk, either through injury by pricks from sharp instruments or contamination of the mouth or eyes with splashes of blood. A pricked finger should be squeezed to encourage free bleeding and contaminated skin swabbed with Hibiscrub (chlorhexidine) or Betadine (povidone-iodine). Eyes should be washed out with water or saline. Should a member of staff be exposed to significant risk, the viral status of the patient should be established as soon as is convenient. If found to be HBsAg positive, the staff member should be offered immunization with a deep intramuscular injection of 500 mg high titre hepatitis B immunoglobulin (HIGB) as soon as practicable and preferably within 48 h of exposure. Better protection against hepatitis B can, of course, be offered by previous active immunization. At present there are no comparable measures which can be taken to protect staff against HIV, but it must be recognized that the risks are very small, and with good techniques vanishingly small.

General examination

The examination begins with inspection, both before and after clothing is removed. Adequate exposure is essential. When the history suggests multiple injury it is important to exclude wounds in other parts of the body; the back of a patient is just as vulnerable to wounds as the front half which is traditionally presented to the doctor.

Preliminary cleansing may be necessary at this stage to locate all wounds; for example, in a face which has been damaged by windscreen glass it may be necessary to swab it over with gauze soaked in warm water in order to decide what is wound and what is merely dried blood. Superficial pieces of clothing or foreign material can be lifted off the wound at this stage.

Local examination

If the character of the wound suggests that important deep structures might be damaged, they should be tested before any local or other anaesthetic is administered – sensory nerves by pinprick sensibility distally, motor nerves and tendons by appropriate motor function. It is best to regard all deep structures as being damaged until proved otherwise. X-ray examination is necessary when bony injury is suspected or if a radio-opaque foreign body might be retained in the tissues.

Types of wound

Contusion

A contusion is the familiar bump or swelling which arises often quite quickly following a blow. The skin surface remains intact but small blood vessels may be injured or torn and bleeding may discolour the skin producing a bruise. The bruise is at first red, turning to blue, which darkens to almost black before fading through greenish-yellow then yellow and so to the normal skin colour. The complete process takes several days. Generally a contusion requires no treatment.

Haematoma

This results from rather more severe injury, particularly to the vessels, allowing the escape of larger volumes of blood which collect in the tissues or tissue planes. Most commonly the blood is quickly reabsorbed and the haematoma resolves, but complications can occur. If the bleeding takes place into the tissues contained within the fascial compartment of a limb, pressure can be built up which will interfere with circulation and release of the pressure by fasciotomy may be necessary.

A subcutaneous haematoma may become infected, particularly if the overlying skin is damaged, and the resulting abscess will require incision. A haematoma may persist and if it remains fluid, aspiration through a wide-bore needle can be attempted. More commonly, the liquid blood will clot after a very few days and formal evacuation through an incision will be necessary. In the absence of infection the incision may be closed by suturing.

A persistent haematoma may organize, i.e. the original clot is replaced by fibrous tissue resulting in a very firm swelling. At incision an organized haematoma is often whitish, all the blood pigment having been removed, and frequently has a layered structure like an onion. A complication occurring specifically in haematomas of muscle is myositis ossificans where the blood clot is replaced by calcifying osteoid tissue rather than fibrosis. Typically this occurs in the quadriceps muscles following a haematoma of the thigh. A patient with such an injury should remain under review for at least a month and a radiograph of the thigh should be taken at about 3 weeks to exclude calcification.

Haematomas of the limbs are treated by rest, elevation and pressure bandaging with alternate layers of wool and crepe bandages encircling the limb. Once the acute pain and swelling have subsided, gradual mobilization can begin.

Abrasion

The mechanism producing an abrasion is readily understood – a rough surface, such as on a road, tears and scours superficial layers from the skin as the body or limb skids across it. Bleeding points and sensitive nerve endings are exposed and at the same time dirt and grit may be embedded in the tissues. Deep abrasions should be regarded and treated as lacerations, but superficial ones will heal readily by epithelialization.

Treatment consists largely of preventing infection. Contaminating grit should be removed – the larger pieces being picked out with forceps and the remainder by scrubbing with a sterile brush and a mild antiseptic solution, the scrubbing action following the line of the injury. If such ingrained dirt is not removed the skin will heal over it leaving a permanent tattoo which can be most disfiguring, particularly on the face, and which is very difficult to remove subsequently. All facial abrasions should be meticulously cleaned, small areas being dealt with under local anaesthesia, but for larger areas general anaesthetic is justified. On the face, no dressings are required and elsewhere a dry dressing can be placed for 2–3 days until the wound itself is dry. Thereafter no further dressing is required.

Degloving injuries

The term is self-explanatory. At the time of injury, shearing forces are set up which detach the skin from the underlying structures which may be left relatively undamaged. The area of skin may be lost entirely, it may remain attached by one edge in the form of a flap, or the skin can remain intact but separated from the deeper structures – the so-called physiological degloving. Areas of complete skin loss may require grafting and should be referred to the appropriate specialist.

A particular degloving injury is often seen affecting the thin atrophic skin on the front of the shin of elderly women. After a blunt injury, such as knocking the shin against a step, a triangular flap is raised. Sometimes, particularly if the flap is proximally based, it is possible to replace it with excellent results. The wound should be carefully cleansed with sterile saline, any contaminating material, non-viable fat and adherent blood clot removed from both surfaces, and then the flap gently spread out to cover the defect. It can be held in position with a few sutures or with paper adhesive closures. Over the dressing a firm supportive bandage from the toes to below the knee is applied and if possible left undisturbed for about 10 days. Not all shin injuries will lend themselves to this treatment and where the flap is obviously devitalized it should be excised and immediate or early grafting performed by a competent surgeon.

In physiological degloving, when the skin is not disrupted, the diagnosis may be difficult. It should be suspected when the tissues have been drawn into the rollers of a machine or under the tyre of a road vehicle. The affected area will be insensitive to pinprick, will lack a capillary circulation and may be pale, but these last two features may be obscured by abrasion or friction burning. Such cases should be referred to a plastic surgeon, whose management will be aimed first at minimizing the area of skin necrosis and secondly at early covering of any area which cannot be saved.

Incised wounds

These are wounds caused by sharp cutting edges such as a knife, glass or metal, or even the edge of a sheet of paper. The wound itself is neat although the subcutaneous tissues may tend to pout through it. It bleeds profusely initially because of the cleanly cut vessels and may be painful due to the many cut nerve endings. Deep structures such as nerves and tendons may well be divided. Contamination is uncommon because the causative cutting edge is likely to be relatively clean and the initial brisk haemorrhage has a cleansing action on the wound. Infection therefore is less likely than with other wounds and healing is usually quick with little scarring. Treatment consists of thorough cleansing and suturing.

Lacerations

Lacerated wounds are untidy and irregular, being caused by crushing or tearing forces. The area of tissue disruption – the actual laceration – may be surrounded by an area of other damage, contusion or abrasion. Similarly, the tissues deep to the laceration may be bruised and contused. The surrounding torn skin edges are irregular and may be pale or blue denoting devitalization. In the depths of the wound nerves and blood vessels may be mangled or stretched rather than cleanly divided so that brisk bleeding may not be a feature, but this is not always the case. Damaged muscle may be dusky in colour, again indicating doubtful viability.

Frequently these wounds are grossly contaminated by clothing material or dirt forced into the tissues at the time of injury. Inevitably there is accompanying bacterial contamination. The bacteria are protected from the natural body defences by the zone of devitalized tissue and by the presence of foreign material, and multiply rapidly so that infection is soon established and is likely to persist. Without adequate treatment, these wounds heal slowly and with much scar tissue.

Treatment is directed at removing foreign material and dead tissue leaving healthy tissue with a good blood supply which can effectively eliminate bacteria. Dead spaces in which blood clot or serum could collect, offering a culture medium for bacteria, must be obliterated. Compromise of the circulation by swelling in fascial compartments should be avoided. If these surgical aims are achieved the body's natural defences will destroy bacteria and allow sound healing. Antibiotics and antiseptics may have a part to play in management but they cannot be expected to replace good surgical practice.

Puncture wounds

These are wounds which are deeper than they are long. They may be caused by a stabbing action with a long thin weapon, instrument or object, or by a missile such as a bullet or flying fragment from an explosion. The dangers are the possibility of damage to deep structures and organs, and the risk of infection from contamination along the track of the wound.

Penetrating and perforating wounds are variations of puncture wounds. A penetrating wound has an entry wound only, while a perforating wound has both entry and exit wounds, the object causing the injury passing through the tissues.

In stab wounds the possible depth can be judged if the causative weapon or a description of it can be obtained, but probing a wound to ascertain its depth is quite useless and should not be attempted. All puncture wounds to the neck and to the trunk should be regarded as having caused deep damage and should be referred to an appropriate specialist surgeon. The abdominal organs are vulnerable to injury from wounds to the back, and wounds to the buttocks may involve the pelvic organs or the gluteal vessels. Often the patient's clinical condition will immediately suggest internal injury, but no stab wound in these areas should be dismissed. Puncture wounds to the hands may result in serious infection and even the seemingly most trivial ones demand meticulous treatment (see Chapter 26).

In missile injuries the degree of damage relates to the speed of the projectile and its path through the tissues. A low velocity bullet such as an airgun slug will leave a relatively straight track with little surrounding damage, but deeper structures may be injured. A flying fragment from an explosion may spiral through the air and continue to do so through the tissues producing much damage. High velocity bullets, as they pass through tissues, create shock waves and cavitation with widespread gross destruction of tissues. The entry wound may be small but the exit wound enormous, indicating the degree of deep damage. Such wounds, even in limbs, can threaten life and the junior doctor's task will be the resuscitation of the patient before referring him to an appropriate unit.

Hydraulic injection injuries

In these cases liquid under high pressure in some sort of hydraulic system escapes in the form of a fine jet and, on striking the skin, is injected into the tissues. Water, oil, hydraulic fluid, grease and paint may be involved and considerable volumes of liquid can be injected. The entry wound may be insignificant and even difficult to detect, but these injuries demand careful treatment. In regions where possible expansion of the tissue spaces is limited, such as the hand, the build-up of pressure is considerable and in many cases the injected material is highly irritant. Even with meticulous and vigorous management, loss of part or whole of a digit may be inevitable. Referral to a skilled surgeon is therefore advisable. The affected tissue should be incised and widely laid open, the tracks of the liquid followed and as much as possible of the foreign material removed. The wound should be left open and secondary closure only performed when it is clear that all the injected material has been expelled.

Bites

Infection is the major risk with bites due to mixed mouth organisms being deeply implanted into the tissues. Whatever the animal inflicting the bite, tetanus is always a possibility and prophylaxis essential. A common type of human bite is where the teeth damage the metacarpophalangeal joints in a fist fight. Suppurative arthritis can result from organisms which are often insensitive to phenoxymethylpenicillin. In these circumstances a compound of broad-spectrum antibiotics such as Augmentin (amoxycillin and clavulanic acid) is useful.

Cats have thin, sharp, needle-like teeth which can innoculate organisms into deep structures such as the joints and tendon sheaths. Mixed infections are common but often *Pasteurella multocida* is encountered which also responds to Augmentin.

Dog bites can result in lacerated wounds, sometimes of considerable extent. Thorough surgical management can allow primary closure.

Snake bites are dealt with in Chapter 28.

Rabies

Many animals can transmit rabies, but cats and dogs are most likely to transmit it to humans. In endemic areas contact with an animal suspected as rabid, i.e. a bite or even a lick on an area of broken skin, should be treated seriously. The patient must be started on a course of human diploid rabies vaccine and the animal observed in quarantine for 10 days. If the animal remains healthy for 5 days treatment is stopped. If the animal develops rabies, human antirabies immunoglobulin should be added to the treatment and the course of vaccine completed. If the animal is known to be rabid at the time of contact or is unavailable for observation, the patient should be given a complete course of vaccine and immunoglobulin. This should also be the line of treatment when a patient travels from an endemic area to a non-endemic area after contact.

Principles of the treatment of wounds and minor surgery

Before embarking on the definitive treatment of a wound or a minor operation, the junior doctor should consider carefully if he has the necessary resources in terms of anaesthesia, assistance, experience, skill and time to perform the task. If he has any doubts he should not be diffident about calling the help of a senior colleague or offering the case to a specialist surgeon. There is no disgrace in referring to a textbook to refresh one's memory of the anatomy before entering unfamiliar territory.

Anaesthesia

Careful consideration should be given to the type of anaesthesia to be employed – general, regional or local – and this too can usefully be discussed with a senior surgical or anaesthetic colleague. The techniques of local and regional anaesthesia are fully described in Chapter 8.

If intravenous regional anaesthesia (Bier's block) is selected it is essential to have another doctor, preferably an anaesthetist, present to apply and supervise it, thus leaving the operator free to concentrate on the surgery.

Tourniquet

Bloodless fields can be obtained in the limbs and digits by the use of tourniquets. A pneumatic tourniquet, which should be regularly maintained and calibrated, is appropriate for the limbs and the doctor should apply it himself to minimize any risk of failure or injury to the patient. It should be placed around the upper arm or upper thigh over a thin layer of orthopaedic wool and all connections should be checked before it is inflated to a safe correct pressure, e.g. 200 mmHg for an arm, 300 mmHg for a leg. The tourniquet should *not* be left inflated for longer than 45 min and after release the doctor should confirm that distal circulation has been re-established. For a digit fine rubber tubing can be used as a tourniquet, but it should not be tied in a knot. It is much preferable to hold it in position with stout artery forceps. This simplifies release and elminates the possibility of the tourniquet being concealed by dressings and so left *in situ* at the end of the procedure.

Skin preparation

In wounding the surrounding skin may be cleaned first using a proprietary degreasing agent or soap or detergent and water. The wound itself can then be thoroughly washed out using aqueous Savlon or similar preparation and obvious contaminating material removed. The operative field should be shaved with a safety razor, again using soap and water as lubricant, and care should be taken not to nick the skin. In the scalp, an area of 2–3 cm around the wound or lesion will be sufficient, but on the chest or abdomen a wider surrounding area should be prepared. Eyebrows should never be shaved off, firstly because it is unnecessary and, secondly, because they take an inordinate time to regrow.

A wide variety of proprietary and other skin antiseptics is available. They are all effective but some may have disadvantages in certain situations. Before surgery it is important to establish that the patient is not allergic or sensitive to the material to be used. Some materials act as a dye on the skin, staining it for several days. This is useful to the surgeon during application as he can readily see if an area of skin has been missed, but it may be an embarrassment to the patient in the days following surgery and these solutions are probably best avoided in exposed regions such as the face.

Tincture of iodine 2% is a highly effective and widely used skin antiseptic, but if left in contact with the skin for long periods it can cause irritation. It should not be used for open wounds or on sensitive areas such as the scrotum and vulva and at the end of any procedure it should be washed off using 70% alcohol.

Hexachlorophane should probably not be used as a skin preparation in babies and small children as there is a theoretical risk that it might be absorbed through the skin.

Other useful skin antiseptics for minor surgery are povidone-iodine (Betadine) and Savlon Hospital Concentrate which contains chlorhexidine and cetrimide.

The techniques of draping an operation site are best learned from an experienced surgeon or theatre nurse and this is particularly true of difficult areas such as the head and neck. The important principle is that the towel should be laid directly onto the operating field and not subsequently moved about so as to avoid the risk of the contaminated part of the undersurface of the towel making contact with the operative field. For minor surgery a towel with a small aperture in its centre is useful as are the modern non-permeable film materials which adhere to the skin.

Instruments and materials
Scalpel blade

Skin incisions should be made with a blade which has a curved belly. The belly of the knife is drawn gently across the skin and with experience the depth of the incision can be very accurately controlled. For most minor surgical work, a No. 10 blade will be ideal, but for finer work the small No. 15 blade may be used. Straight spear-shaped blades such as the No. 11 are designed for a slicing action and should not be used to incise the skin in a stabbing manner.

Materials for wound closure

When deeper layers require to be approximated, absorbable materials such as catgut or a synthetic alternative on a round-bodied curved needle of suitable size should be used.

For skin closure non-absorbable suture materials are usually used, and these fall into two broad categories: (1) braided materials such as silk and nylon, and (2) monofilaments such as nylon and polypropamide. They each have advantages and disadvantages. Braided materials are easier to handle and knot, the tension of the stitch can be adjusted very accurately. They suffer from producing a degree of drag through the tissues, and by their capillary action may cause tissue reaction at the stitch site which can lead on to stitch abscess. Monofilaments, while causing less drag and less tissue reaction, are rather difficult to knot and so it is difficult to adjust the stitch tension with them. The junior doctor will probably find braided materials easier to use while he is gaining experience.

Regarding needles, only the cutting types should be used on the skin. Fine, so-called slim-line needles should be used for facial work. A 3/0 gauge suture material on a stout cutting needle will be found suitable for most minor surgical procedures, but on the face a 4/0 suture on a slim cutting needle should be used by the inexperienced doctor. As skill increases finer sutures and needles can be employed.

Manufacturers now produce ranges of skin staples in disposable applicators in varying sizes and numbers. The technique of using them is readily mastered and with them skin closure is simple and swift. They are best avoided on the face and on the hand only the dorsum lends itself to their use.

Proprietary adhesive paper strips are also effective skin closures. They are comparatively painless to apply so that when used for wound closure, anaesthesia is sometimes omitted. Unfortunately this can lead to skimping of other aspects of the wound management, a fault of the operator and not the material.

Instruments

A needle holder of appropriate size will be required, except on the few occasions when hand needles are used. The Gillies' pattern of combined needle holder and scissors is a very useful instrument, but it does require a little experience to be used properly. Small retractors of the catspaw type and fine skin hooks can be of great value. Fine mosquito forceps and small curved Mayo scissors are essential. When dealing with abscesses, sinus forceps and a Volkmann spoon are useful additions.

Drains

Drainage is not very often required in this type of surgery, but when it is corrugated natural or synthetic rubber material has wide application.

Suction drains consisting of fine perforated plastic tubes of 3 mm and 6 mm outside diameter can be used to prevent deep collections of blood or serum. Suction is applied by attaching a disposable light plastic collapsible container or an evacuated glass jar.

Surgical management of wounds

There are three distinct aspects to the surgical treatment of a wound – exploration, toilet and repair – but the emphasis placed on each will vary with the wound. In superficial incised wounds, for example, it may be evident that no deep structure has been damaged; after cleaning only repair by suturing is necessary. In a heavily contaminated laceration exploration and toilet may be the only procedures carried out at the initial operation, repair being delayed to a later date.

In exploration, the extent of the damage is assessed. Sometimes, particularly in puncture wounds, proper exposure will require extension of the wound by incision (Figure 5.1). Such incision should be carefully planned so as to avoid further

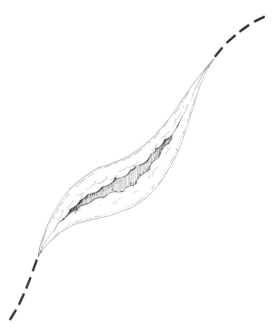

Figure 5.1 Extension of wound

damage and with due regard to subsequent closure. Adequate exposure having been obtained, the depths of the wound can be examined. Further dissection may be required but the unnecessary opening up of tissue planes should be avoided.

During exploration, any contaminating foreign material encountered should be removed. The next step is surgical toilet. The aim is to remove all remaining foreign material and devitalized tissue, leaving healthy tissue which can resist infection and heal rapidly. Irregular devitalized skin edges are cut back to leave healthy straight or smoothly curved margins which will come together neatly. Only the minimum amount of tissue should be removed and care should be exercised in the hands and face to avoid removing too much. Skin excision should be carried out with a scalpel as scissors tend to have crushing action. Subcutaneous tissue, fat and muscle may be cut back with scissors. The wound should again be thoroughly washed out with aqueous Savlon. Any important deep structures identified

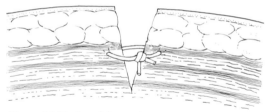

Figure 5.2 Placing of deep suture

are examined again for damage and if all is well repair can begin.

Deeper tissue layers should be approximated with absorbable material, either catgut or polyglycolic acid (Figure 5.2). It is important to avoid undue tension, but dead spaces should be obliterated if at all possible. The skin edges may then be approximated as accurately and as neatly as possible without inversion of one side or any puckering. One of a variety of techniques can be used.

Skin closure techniques

Simple suture is the most widely adopted technique (Figure 5.3a). The point of the needle is driven into one skin edge a little distance from the margin and perpendicularly to the surface. Using the curve of the needle the point is taken across the wound at depth and then directed through the subcutaneous tissues of the other edge aiming a little beyond the intended spot of penetration. The point is then drawn back to its intended position and taken out through the other skin surface, again perpendicularly. A reef or square knot is then tied, adjusting the tension on the first throw. In this way the skin edges are a little everted so counteracting any tendency to invert. In certain situations the tendency to invert is so marked that positive steps must be taken to evert the skin edge. Interrupted mattress sutures do this. In the vertical mattress suture (Figure 5.3b) the first step is the same as a simple suture, but then the needle is passed back taking tiny bites of both skin edges in the same vertical plane and tied. In the horizontal mattress suture, after placing what is essentially a simple suture, another one is placed in the opposite direction a few millimetres along and the ends are again tied (Figure 5.3c). Neither of these sutures should be used on the face.

Continuous subcuticular suture (Figure 5.3d) is an excellent technique when it has been mastered; either monofilament or absorbable material may be used. Starting at one end of the wound, the thread is first fixed by placing a simple suture or by tying it over a bead. Working inside the wound, small equal bites of tissue are taken alternately at each skin edge just below the surface. When the end of the wound is reached, the suture is taken back onto the surface through a single puncture, the tension carefully adjusted along the length of the wound and then tied, again with a simple suture or bead.

Continuous over and over suture is quick to insert but sometimes does not give a very satisfactory cosmetic result and should certainly be avoided on the face.

Skin staples are quick and easy to use but an assistant is usually required to hold the skin edges together accurately with forceps or skin hooks. The applicator is then aligned on the wound, and often there is an arrow or mark to assist in this, and the trigger pulled. In one action the staple is driven into the tissues and closed. For removal a special extractor is required which bends the staple back into its original configuration, whereupon it can be withdrawn (Figure 5.4).

Adhesive paper strips can be rather awkward to apply, especially when wearing surgical gloves and without assistance. Ideally, the skin edges should be prepared using Compound Benzoin Tincture (Tinct. Benz. Co.) which should be allowed to dry thoroughly. The assistant then approximates the

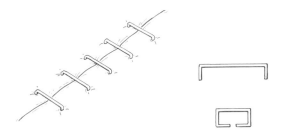

Figure 5.4 Skin staples

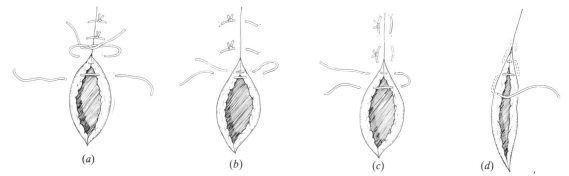

Figure 5.3 (*a*) Simple suture; (*b*) vertical mattress suture; (*c*) horizontal mattress suture; (*d*) continuous subcuticular suture

wound edges and the strips are placed squarely across the wound. The strip itself should not be used to achieve approximation as this can lead to puckering. If necessary additional strips can be placed diagonally. They can be left *in situ* until they no longer adhere and there is some evidence that their use reduces the incidence of wound infection.

Dressings

Just as much care should be taken over dressings and bandaging as the rest of the operative procedure. A bewildering array of dressings is now available, many of which are highly effective in their specific applications. Dry gauze remains the most versatile dressing, however, and is quite suitable for sutured wounds. Liberal wool should then be applied and held in place by crepe or other conforming bandages (see Chapter 6). The proper application of dressings can do much to control haematoma formation and so lessen the risk of infection. In limbs elevation can reduce swelling, and splintage, with the limb rested in the position best suited to subsequent function, will assist later rehabilitation.

Frequent redressing of a sutured wound is unnecessary, but the wound should certainly be inspected if the patient complains of pain or throbbing at the site or if the general condition suggests that infection may be occurring.

For small surgical wounds proprietary adhesive vapour-permeable dressings can be perfectly adequate.

Timing of wound treatment

The timing of wound treatment is important. Arguably wounds should be treated surgically within the first 6 h. In clean wounds with no extensive muscle damage definitive treatment may be undertaken at any time thereafter up to 24 h. Sometimes a contaminated wound is not seen for some days, by which time it is grossly infected. In this case a swab is taken for bacteriological culture. The wound should be explored, surgical toilet performed, but the wound should not be closed. It should be dressed with non-adherent material, appropriate antibiotics given, and closed by delayed suture or grafting when all infection has been eradicated.

Late infection

Despite all precautions and with good surgical care, occasionally sutured wounds do subsequently become infected. The patient complains of throbbing pain at the site of injury and on examination the wound is tense and inflamed. Under these circum-

stances all the skin closures should be removed and the wound laid open to establish continuing drainage. A swab of the pus should be sent for culture and the wound gently cleansed. Frequent redressing and cleaning and an appropriate antibiotic will be necessary to bring the infection under control. Close liaison with the microbiologist is advisable. When all signs of inflammation have gone secondary suturing may be performed.

Tetanus

The organism causing tetanus (*Clostridium tetani*) is found in animal and human faeces. When conditions are unfavourable for its multiplication it forms spores and these are plentiful in soil, road dirt and house dust. These spores are difficult to destroy and may resist prolonged boiling. Germination of the spores into the vegetative form requires anaerobic conditions and these are not found in healthy tissues which have a good blood supply, but wounds containing devitalized tissue due to trauma, ischaemia or infection with other organisms, can provide ideal conditions for germination.

Deep puncture wounds involving muscle are the most liable to give rise to tetanus but any wound in which there has been contamination of deeper tissues poses a risk. The wound need not be large and those sustained on farms or gardens, playing fields and roads, in garages and sewers are most likely to be contaminated.

Cl. tetani releases a neurotoxin which is absorbed by the motor nerve endings and passes along the nerves to the anterior cells where it interferes with the transmission of impulses and so stimulates contractions.

Protection against tetanus
General measures

The rigid application of the principles of surgical treatment in all wounds is the cornerstone of tetanus prevention. The aims of these measures are to remove contamination which may contain spores and the anaerobic conditions in which they develop. Thorough cleansing must be carried out and all foreign material removed. All devitalized tissue at all levels must be excised and the wound should be closed without tension.

Specific measures

These are directed at conferring immunity to the toxin on the individual either actively or passively and at destroying the vegetative forms of *Cl. tetani* with antibiotics before toxin is released into the tissues.

Active immunity

To be effective, active immunity must be conferred before exposure. Tetanus toxoid (TT) adsorbed on to aluminium hydroxide is injected intramuscularly in two doses of 0.5 ml with an interval of 6–8 weeks between injections. This gives some degree of protection, but a third injection 6–12 months later produces a high level of immunity which can be maintained by the injection of a booster dose every 10 years. A booster dose given any time after an adequate primary course will produce a high level of response and this is useful after wounding, but in a non-immune patient tetanus toxoid given after exposure offers no immediate protection. Tetanus toxoid is safe and reactions to it are uncommon. Local reactions in the form of redness and induration at the injection site can occur. Allergic reactions are very uncommon and are most likely to occur in over-immunized adults. For this reason, the indiscriminate use of tetanus toxoid must be avoided.

Passive immunity

Passive immunity can be immediately conferred by the injection of human tetanus immunoglobulin (HTIG). This material is prepared from the blood of human donors who have been actively immunized with tetanus toxoid. A dose of 250 units injected intramuscularly gives protection which lasts for about 6 weeks. Adverse reactions are very uncommon. Its use is particularly indicated in a patient not known to have received active immunization, and in this case the first dose of a course of tetanus toxoid should also be given. The two materials must not be mixed in the same syringe and they must be injected at different sites.

Antibiotics

Antibiotics may protect against tetanus in two ways, firstly by destroying *Cl. tetani* in the vegetative form and, secondly, by destroying other bacteria which could consume the meagre supply of oxygen so creating the anaerobic conditions within the wound for *Cl. tetani* to develop. Useful drugs are penicillin and erythromycin. They have no power to neutralize toxin and therefore must be given soon after injury. Treatment should be continued for 5 days.

Procedure

A guide to the use of tetanus toxoid and immunoglobulin is given in Table 5.1. It should be remembered that tetanus toxoid and HTIG offer no protection against organisms other than *Cl. tetani* and the doctor may wish to add an antibiotic to provide wider cover.

Table 5.1 Guide to the use of tetanus toxoid (TT) and human antitetanus immunoglobulin (HTIG)

Patient's immunity status	Type of wound	
	Recent, clean wound	Wound >6 h old or contaminated or deeply penetrating
Immunized, booster within 1 year	Nil	Nil
Immunized, booster within 10 years	Nil	TT booster
Immunized, no booster within 10 years	TT booster	HTIG + TT booster
Not immunized or status unknown	TT full course	HTIG + TT full course

Established tetanus

The management of extablished tetanus is beyond the scope of this book. The presenting symptoms are very often trismus and dysphagia (hence the archaic name lockjaw) because the toxin first reaches the spinal cord cells of the muscles with the shortest motor nerves.

For successful treatment an intensive care facility is essential. The patient is paralysed and ventilated mechanically and given large doses of penicillin. The treatment may require to be continued for several weeks until all the toxin has been eliminated and the contractions cease.

Gas gangrene

This is another clostridial infection occurring in wounds. The three main organisms are *Cl. welchii (perfringens)*, *Cl. oedematiens* and *Cl. septicum*, again found in the soil. Conditions of low oxygen tension are necessary for their development, and wounds where there has been extensive muscle damage, particularly in the lower limbs of patients with compromised circulation, are at risk. The organisms release toxins which destroy muscle and also have a more general effect leading to circulatory failure. Gas is released into the tissues so giving the condition its name.

Bursting or throbbing pain at the wound site is often the first indication that all is not well. The patient may be toxic with a rising pulse and a falling blood pressure. Examination of the wound will show it to be tense and indurated and the skin red and shiny. Gas in the tissues, which can be detected by crepitation on palpation or by X-ray, is a late sign. The wound may have a characteristic sickly sweet smell. Antisera are of doubtful value in the prevention of gas gangrene and general surgical measures as described for the prevention of tetanus must be relied on. All these clostridia in the vegetative form are sensitive to penicillin and it, or an equivalent preparation, should be given for 5 days in all wounds where clostridial contamination is a possibility.

Treatment

A swab of pus or discharge should be obtained for laboratory confirmation of the diagnosis and the patient then given massive doses of penicillin. Antiserum is of doubtful therapeutic value. The basis of treatment is aggressive and even sacrificial surgery. The wound should be laid open widely and all necrotic and doubtful muscle excised. The loss of some function in a limb may be the price to be paid for survival. The wound should be thoroughly washed out at the end of the procedure and then left open, being lightly packed with fluffed up gauze. Rarely, amputation of the limb may be necessary. Intravenous fluids including blood may be indicated to combat circulatory failure. Hyperbaric oxygen, by increasing the oxygen tension in the tissues, can be a valuable adjunct to surgery, but this facility is available in only a few centres.

Retained foreign bodies

Three problems confront the junior doctor when the possibility of a retained foreign body arises:

1. Is there a foreign body in the tissues?
2. Does it require to be removed?
3. Does the doctor have the skill and resources to remove it safely?

The first question may be difficult to answer. A scout radiograph will quickly settle the matter when the foreign body is radio-opaque, but wood and other vegetable material may not show up even with the softest of radiographs. In these circumstances, ultrasonography in the hands of a skilled operator can be most valuable. It is wise to believe a patient who thinks there is something in the tissues.

Not all foreign bodies need to be removed and sometimes removal can do more harm than good, but vegetable material such as wood or clothing fabric and animal matter such as bone or tooth will cause trouble in the form of tissue reaction and must be eliminated. Metallic alloys such as brass may corrode in the tissues by electrolytic action but glass, lead and steel usually remain inert. Small objects like flakes off a hammer head are difficult to find and even quite large objects may be left in the large muscle masses of the thigh or buttock. An inert foreign body should only be removed if it is causing trouble or is lying close to a structure, e.g. a joint, tendon or nerve which may be irritated by it in the future.

Having decided to remove the foreign body, it must be located accurately. If it is palpable this is no great problem, but generally radiographs or ultra-sonographs will be required. Radiographs in two planes should be taken immediately prior to surgery and some form of reference or marker placed on the skin surface is essential. Much better than the often recommended paper clip is a little grid like the framework for the game of noughts and crosses made out of four pieces of fuse wire, held in place by adhesive tape. It should be left there until the operation begins. With ultrasonography a printout of the image is useful, but the operator may mark the skin overlying the object and give some indication of its depth.

The operation itself should be properly planned. There is hardly ever any need to do this type of surgery at night. General anaesthesia is often indicated as the surgery may be quite lengthy and the foreign body may be found some distance from where it was thought to be lying. A bloodless field is a great advantage if it can be achieved. The incision should be carefully thought out. At right angles to a linear object for instance, sometimes it is useful to raise a flap. Commercially available metal detectors have their greatest value during surgery, although they can be used to confirm the presence of both ferrous and non-ferrous metal objects. Using the smallest probe and with the sensitivity turned down, the surgeon can define precisely where in a wound a tiny object is lying. If a junior doctor fails to locate a foreign body he should immediately call assistance or abandon the operation rather than to continue fruitlessly doing more harm than good.

Facial wounds

These injuries are common after road traffic accidents and assaults. Frequently achieving a good cosmetic result will be a major aim of treatment, but it should not be forgotten that important structures may be damaged in facial wounds. The face is a well vascularized area and, while this aids healing, it also means that often a facial wound will bleed profusely. Usually digital pressure will control this, but any artery in the face may be tied off without fear of compromising the circulation. Careful clinical ex-amination is necessary to exclude damage to deep structures such as the facial nerve or parotid duct. Examination of the inside of the mouth should not be overlooked. X-ray examination may be indicated where bony damage or retained foreign bodies are suspected.

Injuries to the eye should be referred to an ophthalmic surgeon and so too should wounds involving the margins of an eyelid or the inner canthus where the cannaliculi may be damaged. Facial wounds where there is appreciable loss of tissue are best dealt with by a plastic surgeon from the outset. Management of damage to the bony skeleton of the face is the province of the maxillofacial surgeon.

Surgical treatment of facial wounds follows the principles described, but rarely is extensive excision of tissue necessary. More usually after cleaning a facial laceration all that is necessary is to trim any ragged skin edges, removing only the minimum. It may be necessary to place a few deep absorbable sutures after which the skin is accurately approximated with several fine non-absorbable sutures. Wounds crossing linear features of the face must be accurately aligned to avoid healing with a 'step' deformity. In the eyebrows, which should never be shaved off, a stitch should be placed at the upper and lower borders to ensure alignment, and in the lips the first external stitch should be placed to locate accurately the red margin. Any suturing inside the mouth should be done before repairing external wounds. If done in reverse order, retraction on the lips may tear out the external sutures.

Because of its excellent blood supply, wounds to the face heal rapidly and skin sutures may be removed at an early date. If left longer than 4 days there is a risk that the result may be marred by marks of the stitches themselves.

Wounds to the neck

Wounds to the neck may damage major blood vessels, the air passages or the oesophagus, and the patient's life may be at risk from haemorrhage or airway obstruction (Figure 5.5). The junior doctor's primary tasks will be to establish and maintain a clear airway, to control haemorrhage and to restore blood volume.

The airway may be obstructed by aspiration of blood through an opening or by external pressure due to emphysema, haematoma or oedema, and endotracheal intubation or tracheostomy may be required (see Chapter 11). Bleeding is best controlled by direct digital pressure, compressing the vessels against the vertebral column. Blood clots or foreign bodies should not be disturbed at this stage as doing so may increase the bleeding. Blood loss may be considerable and the volume should be restored promptly using crystalloid or colloid solutions initially.

While superficial neck wounds involving not more than the platysma may be repaired by a competent

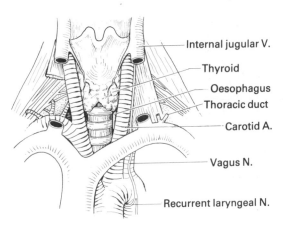

Figure 5.5 Anterior neck structures

junior doctor, deep wounds will require the skills of an experienced surgeon and should be appropriately referred.

Minor surgery

Pathological and bacteriological specimens

Most specimens excised should be sent for histological examination. Even the most ordinary and innocent-looking lesions sometimes provide surprises. Pus or caseous material should be submitted for culture and determination of the antibiotic sensitivities of organisms present. It is important to make sure that the results of these tests are received, are entered in the patients' records, and any appropriate action taken, including informing the family doctor.

Excision biopsy

Many small superficial skin lesions can be excised by this method, either for cosmetic or diagnostic purposes. Local infiltration is usual. An elliptical incision is made centred on the lesion with the axis along Langer's lines. If sinister pathology is suspected, a margin of at least 3 mm should be left in all directions. Using a blade or fine scissors, the skin ellipse, including the lesion, is dissected away ensuring an adequate depth deep to the lesion. Larger bleeders are tied off with fine absorbable material and the smaller ones crushed in the points of fine artery forceps. The skin is closed with simple sutures. Undue tension can be avoided by undercutting both skin edges.

Sebaceous cyst

Local infiltration anaesthesia is employed or general anaesthesia if multiple cysts are to be removed. An elliptical incision is made as above, centred on the punctum, rather longer than the cyst and about a third of its diameter in width. The ellipse is dissected away, care being taken not to rupture the cyst, and the line of cleavage sought. If the cyst has never been infected it can be shelled out readily. Should rupture occur it is important to dissect away all the so-called epithelium. Haemostasis is attended to and, if necessary, the dead space obliterated with absorbable stitches and the skin closed.

Implantation dermoid

The hands and feet are common sites for this lesion. In some, previous wound epidermis is driven under the surface of the skin where it remains viable and sequesters and continues to grow, forming a little nest of keratin. Left untreated these cysts will sometimes rupture through the skin surface and in that way be self-limiting. Occasionally there is indication for excision. Local infiltration or digital block are satisfactory; a bloodless field is useful. The incision is made over the cyst in the line of a skin crease and enucleated. Skin closure may not be necessary.

Lipoma

Some lipomata can prove to be much more extensive than their superficial appearances would suggest. This is true for example in the axilla and supraclavicular areas. Local infiltration or general anaesthesia may be indicated, depending on the size and number of lesions to be removed. A solitary rounded lipoma can be approached by the tissues being squeezed to make it bulge forward and the incision is then made down to it when it can be enucleated. With large and multilocular types, an approach similar to that described for sebaceous cysts can be adopted, the line of cleavage established, and the swelling removed with a mixture of blunt and sharp dissection. Haemostasis should be meticulous and the dead space closed off, or a small suction drain inserted where dissection has been extensive or oozing persists.

Ganglion

A ganglion is a diverticular swelling related to a joint or tendon containing synovial fluid. A common site is the wrist, particularly the dorsum. Sometimes the cyst may be ruptured by trauma and the ganglion then disappears, but permanent cure is unlikely. Even after excision the condition sometimes recurs.
  General anaesthesia or regional block are to be preferred, as is a bloodless field. The incision should be in the line of a skin crease. The sac is then identified and followed down to its neck. Sometimes the neck can be transfixed with a fine absorbable suture before division. If solid tissue is encountered, a biopsy specimen should be sent for histological examination to exclude synovioma.

Management of ingrowing toenails

Ingrowing of the nail of the great toe results from tight footwear. The condition is troublesome when infection supervenes caused by injudicious trimming and lack of personal hygiene. It is seen most commonly during adolescence and early adulthood, and the junior doctor should beware of operating on the toes of any elderly or diabetic patient as the diagnosis may be incorrect and digital block may prove disastrous.

Conservative management

Tight shoes and socks should be avoided. The latter should be changed frequently and the feet washed regularly, at least once a day. Mild infection can be controlled by lightly packing a little pledget of cotton wool soaked in antiseptic along the sulcus and beneath the sharp corner of the nail where it cuts into the soft tissue. With several applications, infection can be brought under control and further trouble avoided by cutting the toenail squarely so that the incurled edge projects beyond the skin.

Surgical management

Few surgical conditions have as many procedures attached to them as ingrowing toenail. Of the dozen or so, three will be described. Digital block (with the above caveat) or general anaesthesia may be employed. The latter allows the use of a pneumatic tourniquet which gives more operative freedom than the rubber tube type.

Avulsion of the nail plate

Avulsion of the nail plate is indicated in heavy infection where there is exuberant granulation tissue along the sulcus and at the corner of the nail. One jaw of a stout straight artery forceps is inserted beneath one edge of the toenail and advanced to the nail fold. The jaws are then closed and the nail is rolled off in an action similar to opening a can of sardines. The granulation tissue is removed using a Volkmann spoon. The raw area is dressed with non-adherent material like tulle gras and will be dry in a few days. Antibiotics are seldom indicated. As soon as the new nail appears, the patient may be referred to a chiropodist so that the ingrowing nail may be 'trained'.

Wedge resection

Wedge resection is indicated in recurrent cases where one sulcus only is involved. It is best performed when infection is quiescent. The aim is to remove a narrow wedge of tissue containing one-third of the nail, the sulcus, the nail bed and the matrix on the affected side (Figure 5.6). A stout

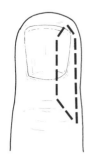

Figure 5.6 Incision for wedge resection

blade is required to make a vertical incision through the nail and nail bed down to bone. A second parallel incision is made through the skin just beyond the sulcus and angled slightly so as to nearly meet the first in the depth of the wound. The intervening block of tissue is dissected out. Nail matrix cannot be identified on sight, and at the proximal end the dissection should be carried to within a few millimetres of the level of the interphalangeal joint and beyond the line of the nail sulcus to ensure that all germinal material is removed. Raising a little skin flap here may assist. The narrow trough-like wound may be left to granulate or can be loosely approximated with one or two monofilament sutures.

Nail bed ablation

Nail bed ablation is indicated in recurrent cases where both sulci are involved; it may also be used in onychogryphosis. The quiescent phase is preferable. The patient must understand that the cosmetic deformity of permanent loss of the nail will result. The nail plate is first avulsed, taking care not to damage the nail bed. Both sulci are excised as for wedge excision but with very much narrower wedges. Again, these are curved outwards proximally. The very edge of the nail fold is trimmed off and a thin skin flap between the two incisions reflected back almost to the level of the joint. The

nail bed is divided with a horizontal incision at the same level as the nail fold and the block of tissue contained within the three incisions underlying the flap is dissected away down to periosteum (Figure 5.7). Care should be taken not to damage the extensor tendon nor enter the interphalangeal joint. Again, particular attention should be paid to the proximal corners of the tissue block being excised to ensure removal of all matrix. After haemostasis the flap is replaced and may be held with a few monofilament sutures; it is usually unnecessary to close the narrow wedges.

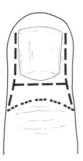

Figure 5.7 Incision for nail bed ablation

Warning note

Variations of the above two procedures are described where the nail matrix is destroyed using powerful corrosive chemicals such as 80% phenol or 20% sodium hydroxide. These substances are *dangerous* and represent hazards to the patient and theatre staff as well as the surgeon. On no account should an inexperienced operator attempt these procedures unsupervised without first having the techniques fully demonstrated to him by a competent surgeon.

Management of abscesses

Soft tissue infection may proceed to abscess formation, i.e. the collection of pus in the tissues. Correct surgical management is incision and drainage. The presence of pus may sometimes be difficult to detect clinically, but fluctuation is generally a late sign and should not necessarily be awaited. A continuing fever, failure of the site to show signs of resolution, and pain sufficient to disturb the patient's sleep are all indicative of abscess formation. The aims of surgical management are:

1. To decompress the abscess;
2. To remove as much pus and necrotic material as possible; and
3. To establish free and continuing drainage.

Antibiotic treatment is not always necessary. Many superficial abscesses can be treated by surgery alone, but whenever pus is encountered, a swab of it should be sent for culture and sensitivity tests so that an appropriate antibiotic can be given if indicated.

Axillary abscess

Axillary abscesses are common in young women who shave the axillary hair. Not infrequently multiple or bilateral abscesses are present. They should be treated vigorously to avoid the risk of chronic infection of the apocrine glands (hidradenitis suppurativa).

General anaesthesia is used. The arm is abducted and can be held in position by placing the hand under the patient's head. Incision is made directly over the abscess and usually pus is released immediately. The abscess cavity is rubbed out with dry gauze and any infected glands encountered can be curetted away or excised with scissors. Small ellipses of skin are cut from both skin edges to ensure free drainage and suitable dressings applied.

Breast abscess

Although common in the lactating breast, abscesses are occasionally seen in the non-lactating phase. Small abscesses near the nipple may be associated with duct ectasia, and if this is suspected and the patient is to be referred to a specialist surgeon for this, it is preferable that he deal with the abscess also.

Superficial breast abscesses can be managed exactly as an abscess elsewhere, a radial incision being employed for those near the nipple or areola so as to minimize damage to ducts, but the incision following the Langer lines elsewhere.

A lactating patient may present when infection is at the stage of mastitis and conservative treatment should be attempted. Breast feeding should be discontinued from the affected side, but may be resumed later. The breast itself should be supported by a firm bandage and the patient given a broad-spectrum antibiotic. Milk can be sent for culture, but if delivery has taken place in hospital the organism is likely to be a penicillin-resistant *Staphylococcus*. In many cases the mastitis will resolve without proceeding to abscess formation.

If an abscess is not drained but antibiotic treatment continued, the pus may be sterilized and a so-called antibioma or sterile abscess formed. This is palpable in the breast as a discrete hard mass, very similar to a carcinoma. The diagnosis is made by finding pus with an exploratory needle which produces no growth on culture. The antibioma may be evacuated by aspiration or formally drained.

Operation for breast abscess is indicated when a tense induration can be palpated in the breast after it has been emptied of milk. General anaesthetic is necessary and the skin incision is as above. The abscess cavity, which may be lying at some depth, is entered with scissors and a swab of the pus taken. Loculi are broken down digitally to form one large cavity and necrotic material curetted or dissected out before rubbing out with dry gauze (Figure 5.8).

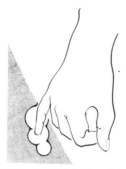

Figure 5.8 Digital breakdown of loculi in breast abscess

If drainage is problematical, dependent drainage should be established. A counter-incision is made in a lower part of the breast and a soft rubber drain drawn into the cavity (Figure 5.9). Dry dressings with liberal wool and a comfortable supporting bandage are applied. An antibiotic is given and the wound dressed frequently until healing is complete.

Frequently, it is possible to excise and obliterate an abscess cavity. Once all necrotic tissue has been removed, the cavity wall is excised by sharp

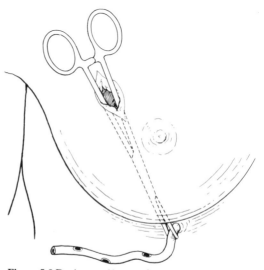

Figure 5.9 Drainage of breast abscess

dissection. The dead space is then obliterated using large stitches of monofilament material which are tied on the surface over gauze to prevent skin marking. This technique greatly shortens the time for complete healing.

Whatever technique is adopted it is always worthwhile sending a biopsy of the cavity wall for histological examination.

Acute suppurative parotitis

Dehydration is a predisposing factor of this condition which in the past was seen as a postoperative complication of elderly debilitated patients denied oral fluids. Improved pre- and postoperative care, particularly with respect to fluid and electrolyte balance, has reduced its incidence.

It presents as a painful swelling of the parotid gland and conservative management should be tried at first. Dehydration should be corrected, a specimen of saliva, obtained by milking the gland gently, sent for culture, and an antibiotic given. Oral hygiene should be attended to and a silagogue such as chewing gum or citrus fruit may be useful.

If there is no resolution within 24 h, incision and drainage should be performed. Fluctuation is a late sign and should not be awaited. General anaesthesia is preferable, but if the patient's condition does not allow this the procedure can be performed under local infiltration. A vertical incision is made from the zygomatic arch to the angle of the jaw, about 1 cm in front of the ear, taking care to incise only the skin. The parotid fascia is approached by blunt dissection and incised transversely in two or three places, avoiding the main divisions of the facial nerve. Pus is sought with sinus forceps, cavities dealt with in the usual manner and the skin edges loosely approximated over a corrugated rubber drain brought out inferiorly.

Collar stud abscess

Such an abscess has two components, a deep one and a superficial one. Suppuration commences at depth, sometimes in association with a lymph node. At some point the fascia is breached and a superficial collection forms which may be the presenting feature. If only the superficial abscess is dealt with the pathological process continues and a sinus may form. Such abscesses may be encountered in the neck resulting from either pyogenic or tuberculous infection.

For operation general anaesthesia is preferred. The incision should be made along a skin crease and the superficial cavity drained and rubbed out. Pus may be seen welling up from the deeper collection. The fascia should be incised in the same line and the deep collection or granulation tissue dissected or curetted away. Swabs of pus or caseous material should be taken and any clearly involved lymph node excised for histological examination. The skin should be lightly approximated with a few stitches about a corrugated rubber drain. A primary focus of infection, such as carious teeth, septic tonsils or very occasionally, spinal tuberculosis, must be sought and treated.

Bed sores

Without adequate precautions bed sores may develop with great rapidity in paralysed, debilitated or elderly patients who are bedridden and unable to move freely in bed. The skin over the heels, sacrum and the greater trochanters is particularly at risk. Pressure on these areas compromises the skin circulation and necrosis eventually occurs. Matters may be compounded by the skin and bed linen being sodden or soiled due to urinary or faecal incontinence, and by roughness or wrinkles of the undersheets.

Prevention

Prevention is much better than attempted cure. Prophylaxis of bed sores is dependent on good nursing care. To avoid prolonged pressure over susceptible areas the patient's position should be changed every 2 h. This routine allows the pressure areas to be inspected and soiled bed linen changed immediately. Paralysed patients may be nursed alternately prone and supine on a rotating bed such as a Stryker frame. Ripple beds, which rhythmically inflate and deflate ridges in the mattress pneumatically, are useful in spreading the pressure of the patient's weight more evenly. Sheepskin or similar man-made fibre under-blankets play a similar role and allow better ventilation to the skin. Physiotherapy can help by exercising the patient in bed and assisting in mobilization.

Where the skin remains intact it can be protected by the application of various proprietary creams and rubs, but alcohol rub remains useful. The spirit keeps the skin surface dry and the rubbing action stimulates the circulation. If the skin does break down no effort should be spared to promote healing. The sore should be frequently dressed with saline soaks, avoiding antiseptics which might irritate the skin. Infrared radiation can assist healing by drying the sore and eliminating moisture-loving organisms.

The patient's general condition may be improved by ensuring good calorie and protein intake. The haemoglobin should be maintained at an acceptable level with oral iron or blood transfusion and vitamin supplements may be indicated. Measures must be taken to control incontinence. Temporary urinary incontinence in the male may be managed by applying Pauls tubing or a similar appliance to the penis and connecting it to a closed urinary collecting system. Permanent male incontinence and urinary incontinence in the female are best controlled with an indwelling Foley catheter. Meticulous catheter care is always necessary. Any urinary infection should be vigorously treated and a good fluid intake maintained. Faecal incontinence is rather more difficult to control. A common cause is faecal impaction which, if found by rectal examination, should be treated by enema or manual evacuation. Lubricant laxatives should be avoided, but some measure of control may be re-established by bulking up the stool with added dietary fibre.

Surgical treatment

A large established bed sore with slough and necrotic bone at its base requires surgical treatment. The operation should be carried out when the patient's general condition allows it, under general anaesthesia. The sore is widely excised and the diseased bone at the base removed. A broad based rotational flap is then fashioned in an area not at risk to pressure and swung into position to cover the raw area. The remaining defect is covered with a split skin graft.

6

Application of bandages

C. P. D. Isaac

A bandage is defined as a piece of material used to cover, support, immobilize, or exert pressure to a part of the body. Good and effective bandaging can be learned only by frequent practice. It is worth mastering, for a well-applied bandage is greatly appreciated by the patient.

Bandages are used for many purposes: as a first-aid measure in the treatment of the injured, particularly to control bleeding; to immobilize a part or restrict its movement; to afford support; to hold splints securely; and to prevent or reduce swelling. They are also used to protect a surgical wound against infection, to hold surgical dressings or other local applications in place, and to assist in the correction of a deformity.

Before applying a bandage the following considerations must be kept in mind:

1. The type and purpose of the bandage.
2. The comfort of the patient.
3. The most natural position of the part to be bandaged.
4. The neatness and the economy of the bandage.

Roller bandages

There are many new proprietary bandages available which are proving effective and easy to apply. However, some roller bandages still have a place in hospital and general medical practice, and for this reason are included in this chapter. A roller bandage is defined as a length of material wound into a compact firm roll.

Size

Various lengths and widths are used according to the part to which the bandage is to be applied and the need (Table 6.1).

Material

A roller bandage may be improvised from any material but those available commercially utilize a

Table 6.1 Guide to approximate dimensions of bandages used for various parts of the body

Part of body	Length		Width	
	Yards	Centimetres (approx.)	Inches	Centimetres (approx.)
Toe or finger	1–3	90–270	0.75–1	1.8–2.5
Head	6	540	2–4	5–10
Arm	6	540	2–2.5	5–6.25
Leg	6–9	540–810	2.5–3	6.25–7.5
Trunk	6–9	540–810	4–6	10–15

variety of materials, natural and synthetic. Special bandages will be described later in the chapter.

Although the open-weave cotton bandage is still available, it has largely been superseded by an open mesh conforming bandage, frequently incorporating materials such as nylon, polyester and viscose. Equally, the cotton crêpe bandage, light and woven in such a way as to allow considerable elasticity, tends to be replaced by the crêpe knit bandage made of 60% nylon and 40% viscose. Both can be applied easily so that uniform pressure is maintained over the area covered.

Application

Before starting to apply a roller bandage the patient should be placed in a comfortable position and the part to be bandaged should be in the natural position if permitted. The person applying the bandage should stand in front of the patient and the part to be bandaged. A tightly rolled bandage should be used and only a short length, not more than 5–7.5 cm (2–3 in), unrolled at a time so that full control of the bandage is maintained.

Starting just below the part to be covered, the outer surface of the bandage is placed next to the skin, and two turns initially will firmly anchor the bandage. The bandage should be applied in an upward direction whenever possible and from within outwards for a limb. Absorbent material ought to be placed between two skin surfaces to absorb perspiration and to avoid friction. All prominences should be well padded. Particular care should be taken that the bandage is applied with even tension over the whole area. It should be borne in mind that the degree of pressure required will vary according to the purpose for which the bandage is used. One-third of each turn of the bandage should be left uncovered.

The bandage should be finished with a complete turn and fixed securely with a strip of inexpensive adhesive strapping or Sellotape; with the end of the bandage, which is split and tied; with a safety-pin, taking care that it will not cause harm; or by sewing the end with needle and cotton.

Mistakes

When applying a bandage every effort should be made to avoid the following:

1. A wet bandage, as it will shrink when dry.
2. Uneven tension of the bandage as it is being applied – a very tight bandage will interfere with the circulation of blood and cause death of tissue – a loose bandage will become displaced.
3. Reverse turns over a prominence or wound as they will not 'give' at all and can cause the patient discomfort and pain.

4. Use of too much bandage which will cause discomfort and is expensive.
5. Incorrect securing of the end of the bandage, which may do harm.

Basic turns

There are five turns commonly used in roller bandaging:

1. *Circular.* When the bandage is carried horizontally around the part. It is used mainly for securing a bandage at the beginning and end. It should not be used around a limb as it could interfere with the circulation of blood.
2. *Spiral.* When the bandage is carried spirally up the limb. It is applied over parts that are of uniform thickness as for the finger and the upper arm.
3. *Reverse spiral.* When a spiral bandage has a reverse turn. It is used for parts of varying dimensions, e.g. the forearm (Figure 6.1).

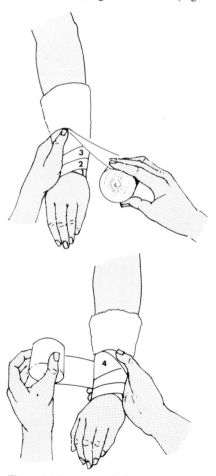

Figure 6.1 A reverse spiral turn

4. *Figure-of-eight.* When each complete turn of the bandage forms a figure-of- eight. It consists of overlapping turns, each of which crosses at a mid-point and ascends or descends alternately. It is used over joints and as an alternative to the reverse spiral. A spica is a modification of the figure-of-eight turn when one loop is much larger than the other. It is so named because the appearance of the pattern of the completed bandage suggests an ear of barley.

5. *Recurrent.* When a series of alternating turns are made. After one or two spiral turns the initial turn is made across the middle of the area to be covered and the succeeding turns pass to and fro over the end on first one side, then the other, of the initial turn until the entire area is covered. Finally, the bandage is completed with one or two spiral turns. This pattern is useful when applying a bandage to the stump of an amputated limb, or to the head (Figure 6.2).

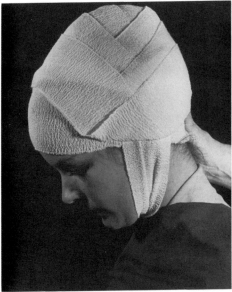

Figure 6.2 Recurrent turns when applying bandage to the head

Removal

If a roller bandage is to be used again it is unfastened and taken off by gathering it loosely together and passing it from one hand to the other whilst unwinding. It is then washed, rewound, sterilized and stored under cover until required. Alternatively, a bandage which cannot be used again is removed by cutting along its entire length on the side away from the injury or wound. A special scissors, one blade of which is probe pointed, should be used to avoid injury to the skin. The ends of the bandage are then carefully gathered and the bandage destroyed.

Head bandage

A 5–10 cm (2–4 in) cotton or crêpe bandage is required. An assistant will be needed to support the head and hold in place the recurrent turns unless the patient is fit to co-operate fully. Ensure that the dressings are in position and insert cottonwool behind the ears.

Commence with a horizontal turn around the head, beginning at the right ear, carry it backwards low on the occiput and forward over the left ear, across the forehead to the starting point. Repeat. Over the starting point make a reverse turn and guide the bandage over the centre of the head to the left ear. (Sometimes the central bandage is continued down the left side of the head under the chin and up the right side of the head over the right ear, up over the head to one side of the first turn to the left ear and then continued as already described.) Here reverse the bandage again and guide it back over the head to one side of the central bandage to the right ear. Pass the succeeding turns to and fro over the head on first one side, then the other of central bandage until the head is covered. Finish with two horizontal turns round the head and fix in front with a safety-pin or adhesive strapping (Figure 6.2).

This bandage is frequently used in neurosurgical units, but in some instances it has been superseded by the appropriate application of either cotton/rayon or elastic net tubular bandage.

Eye bandage

A 5 cm (2 in) woven edged bandage is used. The 'Kling' bandage is suitable for children. Place the bandage against the forehead above the affected eye, pass it horizontally around the head towards the sound eye and above the ears, bringing it low on the occiput and forward to the starting point. Here, take it over the back of the head under the ear on the affected side and up over the inner edge of the dressing to the centre of the forehead. Care is needed to keep the edge of the bandage clear of the sound eye. Take the bandage obliquely across the side and down the back of the head and again up over the eye. Finally, after two or three such turns make one horizontal turn around the head and secure the end of the bandage on the forehead. Crêpe bandages are used when pressure is needed (Figure 6.3).

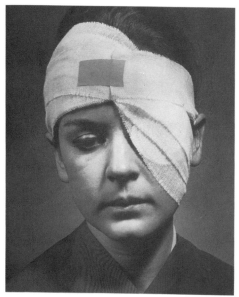

Figure 6.3 Bandage to left eye

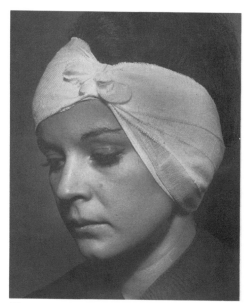

Figure 6.4 Bandage to left ear

Ear bandage

Take a 5 cm (2 in) bandage; cut off a length of approximately 22.5 cm (9 in) and lay it vertically across the patient's forehead. Fix by placing the free end of the bandage over the dressing and taking one and a half turns around the head; then carry the bandage from a point above the ear on the sound side obliquely downwards low on the occiput and forwards to cover the lower edge of the dressing on the affected side. Continue to carry the bandage forwards and upwards across the horizontal turn and over the front and side of the head. Repeat the complete turn, bringing the first part a little higher each time over the dressing, and the second part a little nearer the forehead over the head. Finish with a complete horizontal turn around the head. The strip is then tied tightly to fix the end of the bandage and to prevent any slipping (Figure 6.4).

The application of the single ear bandage to each side in turn is most practical when both ears require dressings.

If used for a mastoidectomy a crêpe bandage may be applied for the first 24 hours when it can be replaced by an open-weave cotton bandage for a few days.

Barrel bandage for fractured jaw

A barrel bandage may be used for a fractured jaw. Take approximately 150 cm (60 in) of a 7.5 cm (3 in) bandage and place the centre under the chin, carry

the ends to the top of the head and tie with the first loop of a reef knot; loosen and separate the loop bringing one-half over the forehead and the other low on the occiput. The ends are now taken to the top of the head and tied securely with a reef knot (Figure 6.5).

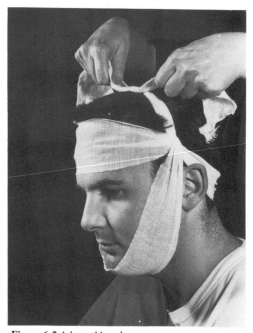

Figure 6.5 A barrel bandage

Shoulder bandages

There are two ways of applying a spica to the shoulder. If the dressing is low over the joint the ascending spica is used; conversely, if the dressing is high on the shoulder a descending spica should be used.

Ascending spica

Insert a pad of absorbent cotton wool in each axilla. A 7.5 cm (3 in) bandage is used. Commence by taking a spiral turn around the upper part of the arm on the affected side, follow with two reverse spirals and carry the bandage across the back and under the opposite arm well below the axilla, across the front of the chest and over the shoulder. Then take the bandage under the arm from behind forwards, up over the shoulder and across the back again. Repeat these turns until the dressing is covered and secure in front. If the dressing is not extensive the reverse spiral turns on the arm can be omitted (Figure 6.6).

Descending spica

The bandage is similar to that already described for an ascending spica but the figure-of-eight turns work downwards to cover the entire dressing and it is secured on the arm.

Bandage for fracture of the clavicle

Use a 10 cm (4 in) domette (i.e. cotton and wool weft) bandage. The patient sits with shoulders braced back, arms flexed and hands resting on hips. The person who is applying the bandage stands behind the patient. Place large pads of wool over the shoulders and under the axillae. Start in front of the sound shoulder. Take the bandage across the back, under the axilla, and up in front of the affected shoulder. Continue across the back under the axilla and up in front of the sound shoulder to complete a figure-of-eight. Repeat these turns until a firm bandage, which draws the shoulders well up and back, has been applied. Secure in front. Support on the affected side in a sling. Reapply bandage every few days over a 3–4 week period.

Although this technique is still used, it is more common to achieve clavicle bracing using a simpler form of figure-of-eight bandage. One method is to use the Seton Collar 'n' Cuff which is made of polyurethane foam covered with stockinette, therefore combining strength with padding. The technique involves taking about 1.5 m of the bandage and, standing behind the patient, laying the Collar 'n' Cuff round the back of the patient's neck, bringing

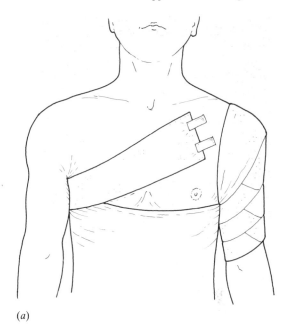
(a)

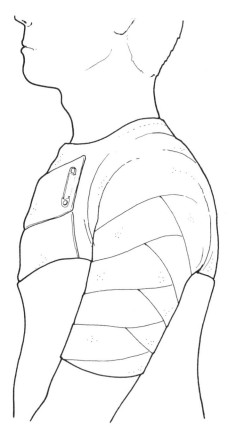
(b)

Figure 6.6 (a) & (b) Bandage of left shoulder – ascending spica

an end back under each axilla. A single knot is tied and one end is brought up and under the piece around the back of the neck and then pulled firmly down so that the shoulders are pulled back putting the clavicles into traction (Figure 6.7). The ends of

the bandage are firmly secured using either the fasteners provided or by tying a knot, first removing the foam from the two tails. In this way a flatter more comfortable knot will be achieved.

Bandage for the breast

For the left breast the patient's left arm is flexed and supported. Use a 10–150 cm (4–6 in) bandage. A 'Kling' conforming bandage is suitable for this purpose, but a cotton crêpe or crêpe knit bandage is more commonly used when it is important to ensure good wound support. Particularly appropriate is the Elset 'S' type, being of adequate width and length to provide single bandage application for the majority of patients. Begin by placing the bandage over the lower edge of the dressing and carrying it towards the left side. Make a complete turn around the body and then continue with three further turns in an upward direction, ensuring adequate support in the axilla of the affected side. Next, with the head of the bandage again on the right side, carry it obliquely over the left shoulder, and then continue in the same direction with a further three turns around the body from below upwards. Finish with a complete turn round and secure the bandage away from the

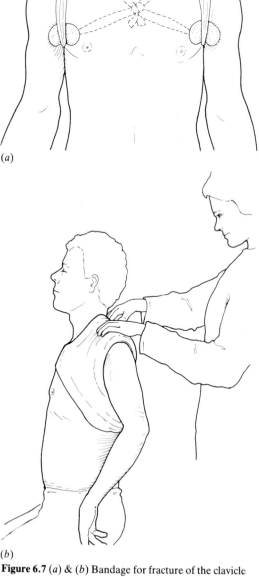

(a)

(b)

Figure 6.7 (a) & (b) Bandage for fracture of the clavicle

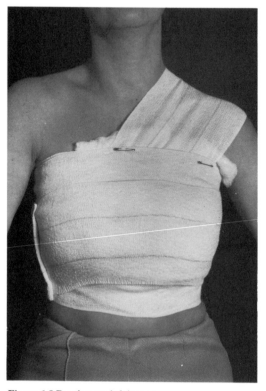

Figure 6.8 Bandage to left breast

affected side. The shoulder 'strap' assists in retaining the dressing well into the axilla, and it is secured with safety pins as illustrated, both at the front and at the back. This bandage is occasionally used following a mastectomy (Figure 6.8).

Bandages for the upper limb

Whole arm

A 6.25 cm (2.5 in) bandage is used. Turn the hand palm downwards and bend the elbow. Start with a spiral turn around the wrist, from within outwards. Then fix the bandage by taking one turn around the hand followed by a figure-of-eight turn, one loop being around the knuckles and the other around the wrist. Now make one spiral turn around the wrist and begin to reverse. Continue up as far as the elbow, keeping the turns near the centre of the arm to avoid pressure on the bone (alternatively, figure-of-eight turns can be used). Change to

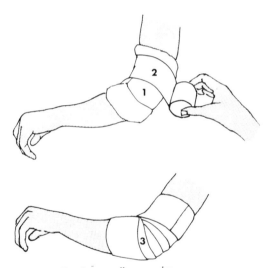

Figure 6.9 Bandage to elbow – spica

figure-of-eight turns over the elbow. Either continue these turns to the top of the arm or reverse again after the elbow is passed. Finish with a spiral turn and secure.

Spica of elbow

Use a 6.25 cm (2.5 in) bandage. Start with two spiral turns around the elbow so that the point of the elbow rests in the middle of it. Continue the bandage with figure-of-eight turns, working above and below the point of the elbow until the dressing is covered. Finish above the elbow with a spiral turn and secure (Figure 6.9).

Spica of thumb

Where there has been a thumb or thenar muscle injury it is usual to use Elastoplast strapping 2.5 cm 1 in) in order to achieve support. Commencing below the distal interphalangeal joint, two turns around the thumb are applied in an anti-clockwise direction on the left thumb and clockwise on the right thumb. The strapping is carried straight across the palm, around the hand and over the base of the thumb, around the thumb itself and back across the palm. These turns are repeated three or four times, overlapping each other by at least half, working down the thumb and palm towards the wrist (Figure 6.10).

Bandages for the lower limb

Whole leg and spica of knee and heel

A 7.5 cm (3 in) bandage is used. A similar technique is employed as described for the upper limb.

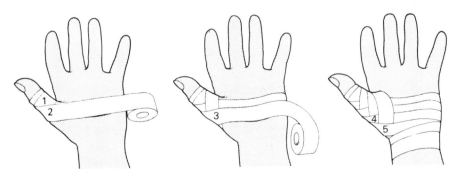

Figure 6.10 Bandage to thumb of left hand – spica

Knee pressure bandage

A 7.5 cm (3 in) domette or crêpe knit bandage is used. The patient lies in the dorsal recumbent position with knee extended and his heel resting on a wedge. Wrap a thick layer of wool around the knee. Apply two or three firm circular turns of the bandage around the knee, add another layer of wool, then two or three more firm circular turns of bandage. Repeat until a firm unyielding bandage has been applied. This bandage is used to control and reduce swelling, for immobilization of the knee following injury, and as a postoperative measure. Elasticated surgical tubular stockinette, e.g. 'Tubigrip' is often used in these instances. It is important that the limb is measured accurately using the Tubigrip Tension Guide, so that the correct size is applied.

Sprained ankle

As a temporary measure only, a crêpe knit bandage may be applied, and the method of application is similar to that described for the more effective adhesive strapping bandage.

Bandaging an amputation stump

This bandage is applied to condition the stump for limb wearing, the aims being:

1. To prevent terminal oedema of the stump.
2. To encourage healthy venous return.
3. To tone up 'flabby' tissue.
4. To prevent the formation of an adductor roll of flesh which would cause great discomfort when wearing an artificial limb.

This is effected by using a rayon and elastic bandage, the size depending upon the site of the stump. The degree of pressure exerted by the bandage depends upon the patient's ability to tolerate the pressure but it must be applied from the time of amputation.

Below-knee stump

Figure-of-eight turns are used commencing above the lateral tibial condyle, then bandaging diagonally across the front of the stump to the medial distal corner. The bandage is then taken firmly up along the posterior aspect of the stump, care being taken to place fixing turns around the limb only above the joint, leaving the patella exposed.

Above-knee or through-knee stump bandaging

This may be carried out as shown in Figure 6.11 and described by Seton Products Ltd, who recommend

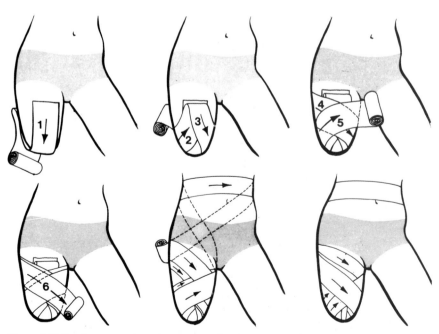

Figure 6.11 Bandage to an above-knee stump of an amputated limb

the use of the Elset 'S' bandage. Further information and literature may be obtained from their head office at Tubiton House, Medlock Street, Oldham OL1 3HS, UK.

Incorrect stump bandaging is one of the major causes of delayed rehabilitation following amputations and it may be necessary to obtain the advice of the Limb Fitting Service on this matter.

Special bandages
The T-bandage

This bandage may have one tail (single) or two tails (double) attached to a belt. The belt is passed around the waist and secured. The single or double tails are passed between the legs, which are extended, and tied or pinned to the belt. T-binders are used for fixing dressings on the perineum and in the groin, e.g. after haemorrhoidectomy or abdominoperineal excision of the rectum (Figure 6.12).

Tubular gauze

Tubegauz is a seamless tubular gauze available in rolls of standard size: the bandages are supplied with specially designed applicators (Figure 6.13). Table 6.2 sets out the sizes of the range of applicators with indications for their use. Each applicator is clearly marked both with its size and the size of the bandage with which to load it.

* Tubegauz (The Scholl Manufacturing Co. Ltd, 182–204 St John's Street, London EC1P 1DH, UK).

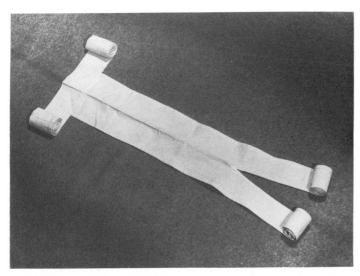

Figure 6.12 A T-bandage

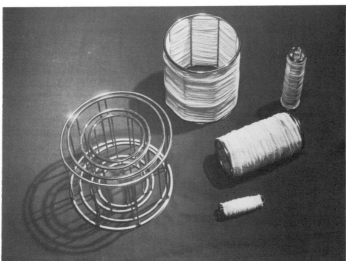

Figure 6.13 Loaded and unloaded Tubegauz applicators

Table 6.2 Applicators for tubular gauze

Bandage	Applicator	Uses
00	00* F/A†	Very small fingers, toes
01	{ 0* = 00 F/A† C (2.5 cm)	Adult fingers, toes
12	D (4 cm) (F/A)	Bulky finger, toe dressings
34	E (9 cm)	Small hands, limbs
56	{ F (12 cm) G (17 cm)	Adult hands, arms, legs
78	{ G (17 cm) H (19.5 cm)	Child's head, adult thigh
T.1	–	Adult head, small trunk
T.2	–	Adult trunks

* Sugar tong type.
† Shuttlecock type.

Since Tubegauz can be used quickly and effectively with or without applicators and the bandage can be adapted to fit any part of the body, it is commonly used in hospital practice, particularly in Accident and Emergency departments, fracture clinics and dermatological units, as well as in domiciliary practice and in industry.

Technique

The required amount of Tubegauz is cut from the roll and eased on to the applicator of suitable size; the bandage is drawn over the rim of the applicator and held lightly on the dressing. The applicator is then rolled and at the same time carried down the limb. The simple rolling movement is continued whilst the applicator is carried upwards and downwards over the area to be covered according to the number of layers required. The method of finishing is to cut the Tubegauz around the channelled rim of the applicator, split the edge of the bandage, and tie (Figure 6.14).

If pressure is required it can be applied effectively by adopting a method similar to that which has been described, the only difference being in the degree of control over the discharge of Tubegauz from the applicator and the amount of rotation used. A constant tension on the bandage and on every continuous rotary movement will produce pressure that is uniform throughout. As for roller bandages, the application of tubular gauze can be learned only by frequent practice. It is extremely important that the person applying tubular gauze bandages masters the technique of rolling the applicator correctly so that an overtight bandage which will interfere with the circulation of blood is avoided. Some other examples of tubular bandages are illustrated (Figures 6.15–6.18).

Further details of the purpose and techniques of application of ranges of tubular bandages are seen in a 16 mm colour film with sound entitled 'It's Quicker by Tube', available on request to Guild Sound & Vision Ltd, 85–129 Oundle Road, Peterborough, PE2 9PY. Information with regard to other new bandages is available on request from the manufacturers.

Bandages impregnated with medicaments

An increasing number of impregnated bandages are now available. They are made of cotton which may be impregnated with one of the following:

1. Zinc paste BPC.
2. Zinc oxide and ichthammol BPC 2%.
3. Zinc oxide, ichthammol and urethane 2%.
4. Zinc oxide, calamine 5.75% and urethane 2%.
5. Prepared coal tar 3% in zinc paste.
6. Iodochlorohydroxyquinoline 1% in zinc paste.
7. Zinc oxide and calamine 5.75%.

These bandages are used to protect and soothe the skin and to promote healing of wounds, in particular eczemas, dermatitis and gravitational ulcers. They also act as a buffer between a compression bandage (when used) and the skin and thus prevent skin damage. Detailed instructions are supplied with the bandages.

Cotton crêpe (elastocrêpe)

This is a smooth-surface cotton crêpe bandage which provides greater compression and support than the ordinary crêpe bandage. It stretches to nearly twice its length but regains its original length readily. This elasticity gives firm but controlled compression, and is particularly useful for this purpose when applied in conjunction with the impregnated bandages already described.

Cotton incorporated with rubber threads

This is a bandage incorporating strong rubber threads which provides even greater compression and support than the cotton crêpe (elastocrêpe) bandage. Blue line webbing is available in rolls of various lengths, while the individual varico leg bandage, of similar material, has a fashioned foot loop. This is designed to assist the patient to start the bandaging process correctly from the base of the toes. The 'blue line' woven into the centre of the bandage, and running throughout, provides a visual

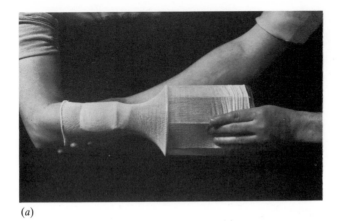

(a)

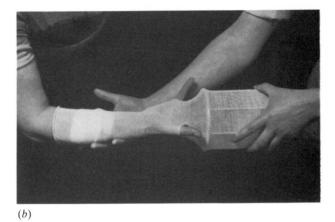

(b)

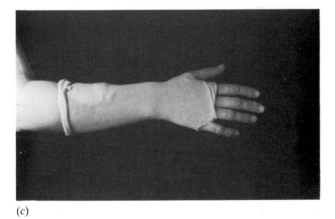

(c)

Figure 6.14 (a)–(c) The application of Tubegauz bandage to forearm

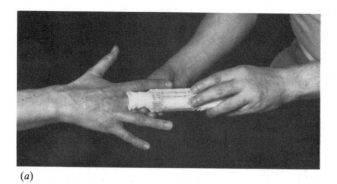

(a)

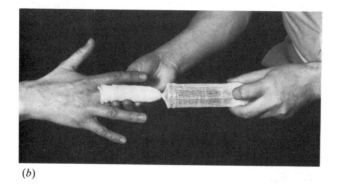

(b)

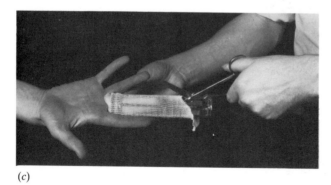

(c)

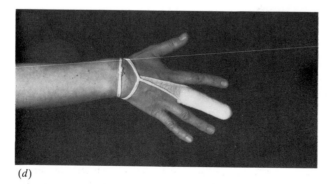

(d)

Figure 6.15 Application of Tubegauz to finger

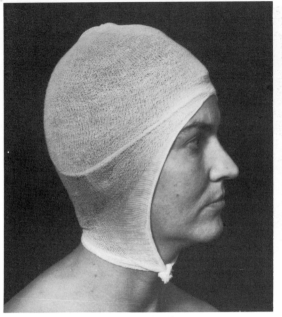

Figure 6.16 Tubegauz applied to head

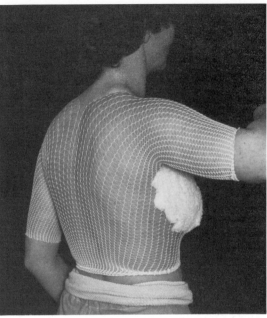

Figure 6.18 Setonet 'ready to wear' garment

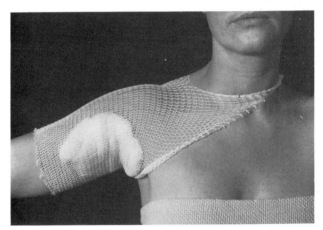

Figure 6.17 Setonet – tubular elastic net bandage applied to axilla

guide to the amount of overlap that should be allowed in the application of the bandage.

Method of application of this bandage for varicose veins of the leg

The patient is seated and an assistant supports the foot at right-angles to the leg. Place the loop over the foot with the edge level with the base of the big toe. Pull the bandage well out during application, especially when covering the lower third of the leg. Ensuring that the heel is incorporated, the bandage is applied using spiral turns, so that there is a consistent thickness of bandage throughout. It is finished just below the knee (Figure 6.19).

Adhesive bandages

An adhesive bandage is usually made of cotton and it may or may not be extensible. The bandage is usually rolled, wrapped and supplied in a sealed tin or other suitable container; it should be stored in a cool place.

Purpose

Adhesive strapping is used for almost all the conditions given in the previous paragraphs for a roller bandage and is tending to replace the latter. It is, however, particularly effective in providing:

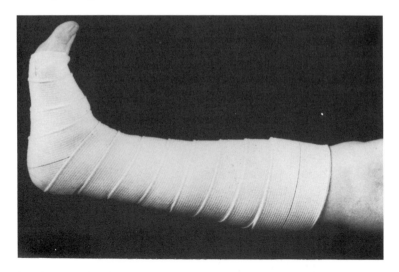

Figure 6.19 The application of a blue line bandage to the leg

1. Pressure and support for chronic conditions of the legs, e.g. varicose veins and ulcers.
2. Support for sprains and strains.
3. Immobilization of fractures.
4. Skin traction in the treatment of fractures and diseased joints.
5. Protection of wounds.

Types

The three types in common use are:

1. *Waterproof*. This is made from a thin, pliable plastic film spread with adhesive plaster. It is ideal as a temporary protection of wounds or of normal skin, for example, when the bandage is placed over the surfaces and edges of plaster-of-Paris casts.
2. *Porous*. This type of bandage is spread with an adhesive in such a way that it permits free circulation of air, evaporation of sweat from the skin and avoidance of skin irritation without loss of efficiency (Figure 6.20).
3. *Extension*. This is similar to the porous bandage, but the material is made so that it is rigid lengthways and extensible crossways (Figure 6.21). It is used for the application of skin traction.

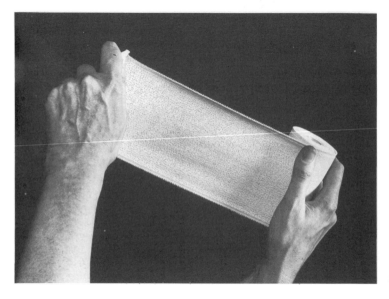

Figure 6.20 Porous adhesive strapping

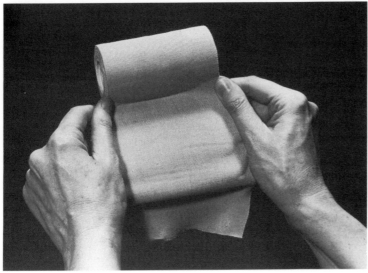

Figure 6.21 Extension adhesive strapping

Application

Adhesive bandages have many advantages if they are applied correctly. They are prepared for immediate use, are quickly and easily applied, effective, neat, and patients find them comfortable. Adhesive strapping should adhere to the skin, be free of creases, and not be so tight as to cause discomfort, pain or impairment of function. The bandage is applied more effectively if it is split at each end.

Precautions

Irritation of the skin is one potential hazard which can be minimized if the person who applies the bandages takes heed of the following directions:

1. The area to be covered should be clean and dry.
2. Sensitive skin may be protected by being painted with compound tincture of benzoin before application of the bandage, but with the new hypo-allergic strapping this is contraindicated.
3. The bandage should remain untouched unless the patient complains of discomfort or pain.

Technique

When strapping is applied to protect a wound, split the free end as required and unroll and cut the appropriate length of strapping. Apply the split end some distance from the dressing and smooth in place with the palm of the hand. Draw the strapping firmly over the dressing and split the opposite end before smoothing on to the skin. Light pressure may be required until the ends are stuck securely. Further lengths of strapping are applied as required.

Removal

The strapping should be removed with care by: (a) Peeling it off gently and slowly with ether or a special commercial non-inflammable plaster solvent (Zoff); (b) using special scissors as previously described (Figure 6.22).

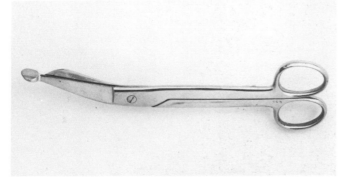

Figure 6.22 Lister's scissors for cutting adhesive strapping

Ankle strapping

Use a 7.5 cm (3 in) bandage. The patient is seated and an assistant supports the foot in an elevated position and at right angles to the leg. Cut and apply sufficient stockinette to cover the area from ankle to knee. Using the adhesive bandage and working from without inwards, start at the web of the toes and take two turns around the foot. Using moderate tension on the bandage, proceed by completing three or four figure-of-eight turns, as illustrated in Figure 6.23. Continue upwards using spiral turns, overlapping each by about half, to finish below the knee. This provides a firm support for a sprained ankle. It is greatly appreciated by patients as it is comfortable and they can walk with no danger of stretching the injured ligament.

Further information on the application of strapping for a variety of conditions is found in a booklet *Techniques with Elastoplast Bandages,* published by Smith & Nephew Medical Ltd, Woodlands Road, Birmingham B8 3AG.

Individual adhesive strapping bandages

Extensible adhesive strapping is used for the following bandages unless otherwise indicated.

Neck

A strip 7.3–10 cm (3–4 in) wide is required. Cover with gauze the adhesive surface of the part of the strip that will be placed around the back of the neck. Place the centre of the strip at the back of the neck and bring the ends (which may be split) forwards so that they cross over the dressing in front of the neck. This is a simple and effective method for fixing a dressing over a thyroidectomy wound (Figure 6.24).

Breast

Several lengths 10 cm (4 in) wide are required. Flex the arm on the affected side and support. Place the end of the strapping well back under the axilla. Apply overlapping strips exposing one-third of the width either horizontally or obliquely over the chest on the affected side so that the dressings are covered. The strips can be adjusted for a radical mastectomy, when they should pass around and beyond the opposite breast. If used to support the breast or to fix a dressing over a wound after removal of a fibroadenoma, the nipple should be protected with a light pad of gauze. The bandage should not interfere with normal breathing.

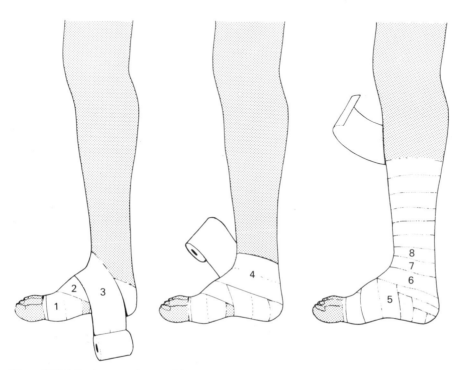

Figure 6.23 Adhesive strapping to ankle

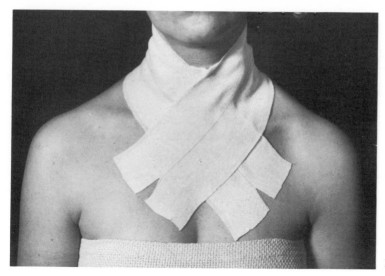

Figure 6.24 Adhesive strapping to neck

Ribs

Use either extension crosswise strapping or adhesive non-extensible plaster 5–10 cm (2–4 in) wide. Sit the patient in an upright position with the arm raised and the hand resting upon his head, giving assistance if necessary. Apply the end of the first strip approximately 5 cm (2 in) below the nipple on the unaffected side. Instruct the patient to breathe out

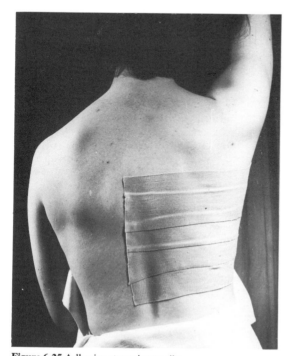

Figure 6.25 Adhesive strapping to ribs

to the fullest degree and carry the strip towards the affected side around the trunk, and fix at a point beyond the vertebral column so as to encircle three-quarters of the trunk. Apply further strips during expiration in a similar way so that each one overlaps the preceding one by a third of its width, to a level 5 cm (2 in) approximately above the injured area. This bandage is now only rarely used for fractured ribs when the patient complains of severe pain and discomfort (Figure 6.25).

Abdomen

Lengths varying according to the purpose for which they are to be used, each 10 cm (4 in) wide, are needed. Split the ends. Apply overlapping strips horizontally, obliquely, or vertically over the abdomen as required. These bandages are commonly used after abdominal surgery. The bandage should be applied with only moderate stretch if discomfort is to be avoided.

The following varieties of bandages are recommended as an abdominal support in patients who have had abdominal surgery and who have a persistent cough or weak abdominal muscles. They may also be used for approximating the edges of abdominal wounds.

Tongue and slot

Two strips, each long enough when stretched to encircle two-thirds of the body, and 10 cm (4 in) wide, are required. Apply the strips against the patient's back and bring forwards on either side. Make a transverse slit so that when in position the slit lies near the edge of the wound. Turn in the

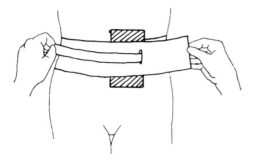

Figure 6.26 Tongue and slot adhesive strapping for abdomen

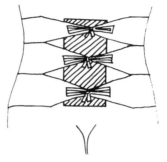

Figure 6.28 Abdominal corset using adhesive strapping

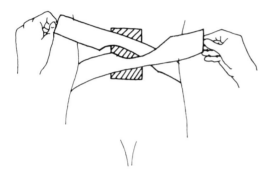

Figure 6.27 Interlocking cut-outs in adhesive strapping on abdomen

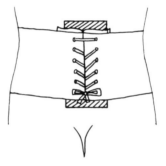

Figure 6.29 Many-tailed abdominal binder

lateral edges of the free end of the other strip and manoeuvre it through the slit. Then pull the ends across in opposite directions, having instructed the patient to take a deep breath, and securing the adhesive surfaces of the free ends while still taut to the strapping beneath (Figure 6.26). This type of strapping may be used for small umbilical hernias in infants.

Interlocking cutouts

Use two strips 45 cm (18 in) long and 7.5 cm (3 in) wide. Cut out a semicircle half the width of the bandage 15 cm (6 in) from the end of each strip. Place a prepared strip against either side of the patient's trunk and draw together so that the

semicircles face and fit into each other. Secure both ends while the bandage is still taut (Figure 6.27).

Abdominal corset

Two or more strips 10 cm (4 in) wide are required. Fold back one end of each strip and cut holes 1.5 cm (0.5 in) from the folded edge. Secure the strips to the skin on each side of the wound and lace up with tape. This forms a corset which can be adjusted to any part of the body (Figure 6.28).

A very effective abdominal support which does not ride up is a many-tailed binder. It is made by taking six 30 cm (12 in) lengths of 7.5 cm (3 in) wide bandage and attaching tapes at the end of each length. The three lengths are applied to the body from each side and the tapes are tied over the abdominal dressing (Figure 6.29).

7

Treatment of burns

J. P. Gowar

A burn may be defined as a dissolution in tissue continuity consequent on thermal damage. The tissue necrosis usually follows the application of heat; however, freezing may cause a very similar injury. Burns also result from the application of chemicals and electricity but in these cases the mechanism of injury is more complex and not completely understood. Heat is transferred to the tissues by physical means, i.e. conduction from contact with hot solids and liquids, convection of hot gases over the skin, e.g. flame, radiation, e.g. from a coal fire or the sun, or from a sudden release of great energy as in an electric arc or explosion.

Everyone has suffered a minor burn at some time and witnessed the spontaneous healing of skin. More serious burns requiring medical attention are a frequent cause of traumatic injury throughout the world. In England and Wales approximately 170 000 patients per annum attend accident and emergency departments for outpatient treatment of burns and a further 12 000 need inpatient care. Approximately 80–85% of such injuries occur in the home: most vulnerable are the very young who, through ignorance of the dangers and natural inquisitiveness, put themselves at risk. Those rendered unconscious by illness or drugs or who have skin insensitive to heat due to disease (peripheral neuropathy, e.g. leprosy, diabetes mellitus) or injury (severed sensory nerves, e.g. brachial plexus lesions) are also at particular risk from deep burns.

In the home the heat sources usually involved are those associated with cooking, heating and lighting, and with the habit of cigarette smoking. Some 15–20% of burn injuries are sustained by the working population, certain industrial processes such as iron and steel manufacture and processes involving high energy inputs being particularly risky for severe burns. There are many agents of thermal injury which may be grouped as shown in Table 7.1.

Table 7.1 Causes of burning injury

Common	Uncommon	Rare
Dry heat	Electric contact	Friction
Flame	Thermoelectric	Ionizing radiation
Scald	Chemical	Frostbite

The skin is the organ most often affected, but the lining of the respiratory and alimentary tracts can also be involved. Very deep burns affecting all tissues may be sustained by those who are unconscious or trapped.

Dupuytren was the first to classify burns by depth; his classification described six degrees of burning and this has led to confusion in modern times as people have altered the classification, defining the degrees differently. It is therefore best to use a classification which is descriptive in character. The key to spontaneous regeneration of injured skin is the germinal epithelium. Skin regenerates from surface epithelium, hair follicles and sebaceous and sweat glands and their associated ducts. Three main levels of injury are recognized. The intermediate level is often divided into two, superficial and deep dermal, for important clinical reasons.

Burn classification by depth

1. Superficial: epidermis partly destroyed.
2. Dermal: some dermal elements have survived.
3. Full thickness: deeper structures may be involved.

Shallow burns which heal spontaneously in less than about 10 days tend not to scar although there may be a permanent mark, visible on close inspection of the healed skin. Intermediate depth burns healing in less than 3 weeks will scar to some extent, but the appearance of the mature scar is usually acceptable (Figure 7.1). Those burns taking longer than this are deep dermal or full thickness in depth and heal with unacceptable scarring. It is in this latter group that surgical intervention is appropriate to improve the quality of healing.

In a full-thickness burn germinal epithelium only survives at the margins of the wound (Figure 7.2).

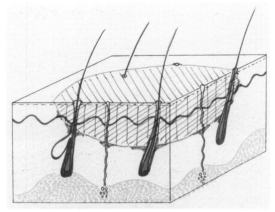

Figure 7.1 A dermal burn (partial thickness): epidermis regenerates from remaining viable germinal epithelium

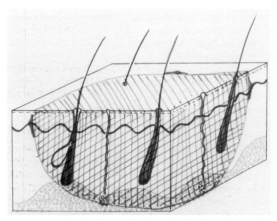

Figure 7.2 A full-thickness burn: epithelium is only regenerated from the margins

Healing is by the formation of granulation tissue, wound contraction and the growth of epidermis from the margins of the wound. This process is slow. A full-thickness wound 3 cm in diameter will take 3 months to heal if the only treatment is with dressings: the result will be a scar. Burns involving subcutaneous tissue, muscle, tendon, cartilage, bone, joints and viscera contained in body cavities have their own special problems.

Recognition of depth of burn

An accurate history is important in determining the temperature of the burning agent and the time during which it operates. When a burn is sustained from heat of very low intensity applied for a long time, circulation in the burnt skin will carry some of the heat away. Such burns tend to be patchy as the flow of blood through the skin is uneven. These three factors, together with skin thickness, determine the depth of injury.

$$\text{Depth of injury} = \frac{\text{Temperature} \times \text{duration}}{\text{Blood flow}}$$

In general, most scalds are partial thickness in depth whereas most flame burns due to clothes catching fire will destroy the full thickness of the skin.

Wound appearance

Superficial burns are characterized by initial exquisite pain and redness, and once the initial pain has settled, hyperaesthesia. A good example is sunburn sustained in fair-skinned individuals. There may be a lag phase during which the patient is unconscious of injury; there will then be reddening and pain, and if the skin surface is touched it feels hot due to the increased circulation (the inflammatory response) and is exquisitely tender. Even once the initial pain has subsided light touch induces a marked withdrawal reaction.

Dermal burns are divided, for important clinical reasons concerned with management, into superficial partial-thickness burns and deep partial or deep dermal burns. There is usually blistering of the skin but not always so. When blisters are opened by peeling away the dead epidermis the underlying dermis may be red, mottled red and white, or dead white in colour. Short exposure to high heat intensity may sear the skin surface making it brown or black, and blistering may be slow to occur, e.g. electric flash burns.

Full-thickness burns tend to be white, yellow or brown in colour, and blistering may occur at the margins where the burn is less deep. The skin tends to shrink below the general surface of the surrounding undamaged skin: this is due to the action of the heat on dermal collagen fibres.

It is important to the understanding of the burn wound to realize that at no time is one dealing with a static entity. If a burn is caused by heat of great intensity the tissues are damaged immediately, but gentle heating takes time to burn and the body's response also tends to be slow so that the full effect of the injury may not be apparent for many hours. This is particularly so in superficial partial-thickness injuries where the patient may only have redness of the skin when first seen but, over the course of the succeeding day, blisters may appear. Thus, what was initially thought to be a superficial injury is then recognized as a dermal injury. Such slow evolution of a burn indicates a very shallow injury and one can make a confident prognosis that healing will be fairly rapid and without scarring.

The final factor in determining depth of injury, apart from history and appearance, is the sensibility to pin prick. In cooperative patients the wound can be tested by pricking with a sterile hypodermic needle. If sensibility to pin prick is retained because the pain nerve endings are viable, the diagnosis is a superficial dermal injury (otherwise known as a superficial partial-thickness burn). If the burn is insensitive to pin prick, it may be deep dermal or full thickness in depth. This test is particularly useful as it distinguishes those burns which will heal with acceptable scarring in less than 3–4 weeks (superficial partial-thickness injury) and those which will not (deep dermal or worse).

The diagnosis of the depth of injury from a burn is shown diagrammatically in Figure 7.3.

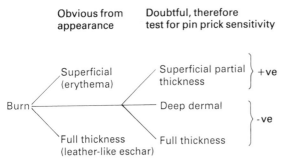

Figure 7.3 Diagnosis of burn depth

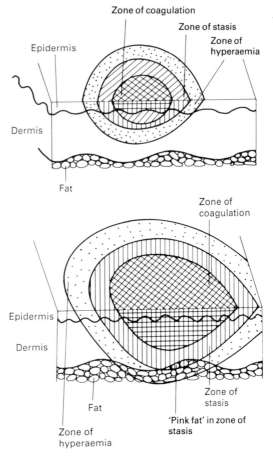

Figure 7.4 Three zones of tissue injury: central zone of coagulation, outer zone of hyperaemia and intermediate zone where initially there is a circulation which later ceases (zone of stasis)

Pathology

The severity of tissue injury is uneven and three zones of the burn wound have been described (Figure 7.4). Characteristically there is a central zone of coagulation, an outer zone of hyperaemia and a zone intermediate between these where initially there is a circulation which later ceases; this is the zone of stasis.

It is important to recognize the changes in the vascular system due to heating. Mild heat produces a dilatation of arterioles and capillaries, a hyperaemic phase giving the appearance of erythema. Higher temperatures damage the capillary wall and increase its permeability. A plasma-like exudate forms, either as blisters on the surface of the wound or as a subcutaneous oedema. This loss of plasma from the circulation causes haemoconcentration; the blood eventually becomes so viscous that circulation

ceases. Surrounding tissues then die of ischaemia. The red cells will autolyse and the leaked haemoglobin pigment stains the ischaemic tissues a pink colour. Thus after a couple of days the zone of stasis is readily defined clinically if the wound is explored surgically. The loss of plasma from damaged capillaries occurs rapidly in the first few hours after burning and gradually diminishes over the first 2–3 days, depending on the severity of the burn. This loss of liquid from the circulation is predictable and the likely loss can be determined by assessing the extent of the injury.

Extent

The extent of a burn is expressed as a percentage of the body surface area. The entire body surface must be examined front and back, top and bottom. The

CHART FOR ESTIMATING SEVERITY OF BURN WOUND

NAME_____WARD_____ NUMBER_____DATE_____
AGE_____   ADMISSION WEIGHT_____

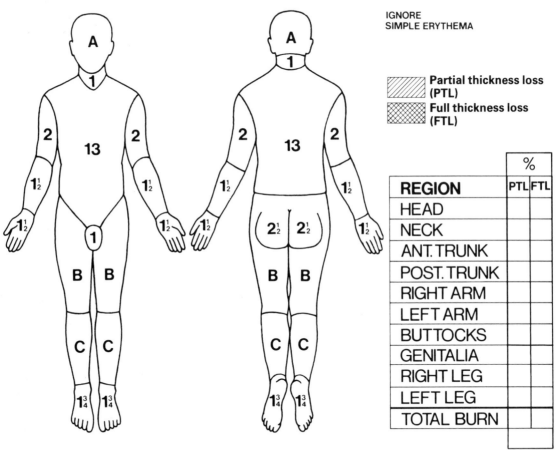

IGNORE
SIMPLE ERYTHEMA

Partial thickness loss
(PTL)
Full thickness loss
(FTL)

REGION	%	
	PTL	FTL
HEAD		
NECK		
ANT. TRUNK		
POST. TRUNK		
RIGHT ARM		
LEFT ARM		
BUTTOCKS		
GENITALIA		
RIGHT LEG		
LEFT LEG		
TOTAL BURN		

RELATIVE PERCENTAGE OF BODY SURFACE AREA AFFECTED BY GROWTH

AREA	AGE 0	1	5	10	15	ADULT
A = ½ OF HEAD	9½	8½	6½	5½	4½	3½
B = ½ OF ONE THIGH	2¾	3¼	4	4½	4½	4¾
C = ½ OF ONE LEG	2½	2½	2¾	3	3¼	3½

Figure 7.5 Lund and Browder chart for calculating body surface areas

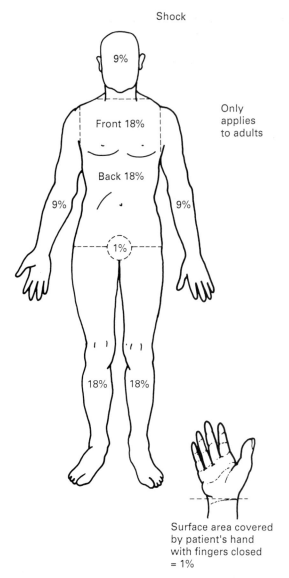

Shock

9%

Front 18%

Only
applies
to adults

Back 18%

9%

9%

1%

18%   18%

Surface area covered
by patient's hand
with fingers closed
= 1%

Figure 7.6 'Rule of Nines' for quick calculation of area

use of a Lund and Browder chart (Figure 7.5) is necessary for accuracy. Alternatively, a quick assessment may be made in the adult using Wallace's 'Rule of Nines' (Figure 7.6). It is important to stress that this only applies to adults and *not to children*. The values given for different body parts in the adult on the Lund and Browder chart have to be modified when used in children. In the newborn, 20% of the body surface area is occupied by the head and neck, and this shrinks to 9% in the adult. Failure to recognize this fact is a frequent cause of misjudging the size of a burn in a child.

Burns shock

Burns shock is the hypovolaemia which follows the more extensive body surface area burns. Shock is predictable if an accurate assessment of the surface area involved is made. Burns of more than 10% of body surface area in a child and of more than 15% in an adult are likely to lead to hypovolaemic shock. If this is recognized early it is possible to prevent the hypovolaemia by administering a plasma-like substance at the predicted rate of loss from the circulation. The leak of plasma from the circulation lasts between 1 and 3 days depending on the severity of injury, being most rapid in the first few hours after injury and gradually diminishing. This is shown diagrammatically in Figure 7.7(a).

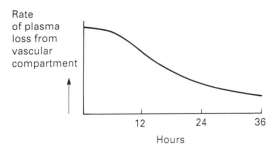

Rate
of plasma
loss from
vascular
compartment

12   24   36

Hours

Figure 7.7 (*a*) Rate of plasma loss from circulation. After Muir and Barclay (1963)

This predictable behaviour of burn wounds has led various authorities to put forward formulae to assist in the resuscitation of the patient. From the outset it must be recognized that these are only a *rough guide* and clinical and laboratory means should be used to judge the adequacy of the infusion. In the UK, most burns units use colloids to replace the liquid loss from the circulation, the most commonly used colloid being human purified protein fraction or human albumin solution, but some units use dextran 110 in normal saline (i.e. average molecular weight of dextrans is 110 000) when it is available. Ideally the colloid used should be plasma and some burns units do have access to fresh frozen plasma. However, large volumes of this substance are difficult to infuse owing to the need to defrost the bags. The ideal and most practical solution was made up from a freeze-dried small pool plasma but this is no longer available. The oncotic pressure of a solution depends on the number of molecules of solute per unit volume. With a leaking container (the injured vascular system) the rate of loss (and therefore the final amount of leakage) from the container will be less, the larger the individual molecules of solute. Colloid solutions are more effective than crystalloid solutions in maintaining the intravascular oncotic pressure because they contain larger molecules. This is why they are more effective when used to treat the hypovolaemia of burns.

The vascular leak of liquid diminishes over 2–3 days. When colloids are used the total volume infused to maintain adequate peripheral perfusion and also the severity of burn oedema are both less than when crystalloid resuscitation is employed.

Resuscitation of the shock case

Any formula used to guide the colloid infusion should take into account the gradually diminishing rate of loss of liquid from the vascular compartment. The Mount Vernon formula does just this by dividing the resuscitation phase into six periods of successively 4, 4, 4, 6, 6 and 12 h respectively. The formula suggests a volume in millilitres of plasma to be infused during each period. The response to the infusion is assessed at regular intervals (at least at the end of each period but more often than this in extensive burns) and the infusion rate is adjusted if necessary.

$$\frac{\begin{array}{c}\text{Area of burn}\\\text{(as \% total body}\\\text{surface area)}\end{array} \times \begin{array}{c}\text{Body weight}\\\text{(in kg)}\end{array}}{2} = \text{ml of plasma}$$

This ration of plasma is the amount to be infused during each period.

The shock phase commences at the moment of injury. Any delay in commencing treatment has to be made up by giving the calculated ration of plasma in a shorter time than 4 h (Figure 7.7(b)).

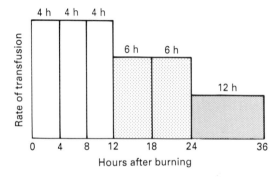

Figure 7.7 (*b*) Transfusion plan: blocks represent equal volumes of fluid to be given in periods shown

Assessment of response to infusion

This is done primarily by clinical methods, e.g. observation of the mental state (restlessness is often a sign of anoxia), peripheral perfusion as evidenced by skin temperature and colour (pallor, cyanosis), filling of peripheral veins, and the rapidity of capillary return after blanching the skin by finger pressure.

The vital signs are monitored at regular intervals; not only the rate but the volume of the pulse should be noted especially if it is difficult to measure blood pressure. (Sometimes there is not an unburned limb available upon which to apply a cuff.) In extensive burns, if it is felt blood pressure readings must be obtained, the only alternative is by means of an intra-arterial cannula and pressure transducer.

As well as heart rate the measurements should include respiratory rate, rectal (core) and skin (peripheral) temperatures and hourly urine volumes. This is very valuable.

The rate of loss of plasma from the circulation can be estimated using the haematocrit, estimations being made at intervals and the plasma deficit calculated as follows:

Plasma deficit =

$$\text{Blood volume} - \frac{(\text{Blood volume} \times \text{normal haematocrit})}{\text{Observed haematocrit}}$$

In order to apply this it is necessary to have tables of normal values at different ages (Figure 7.8).

In full-thickness burns red cells are both destroyed and damaged, and these are removed from the circulation. Thus, a patient will become anaemic as a result of the burn and this will confuse the picture if plasma deficit is relied upon to indicate the need for infusion of colloid solution. In very deep burns, particularly electrical injury, not only is there damage to red cells but also to muscle cells which release myoglobin pigment into the circulation. These two pigments, in conditions of hypovolaemia, may cause acute tubular necrosis, and it is to prevent this cause of acute renal failure that resuscitation is so important in the more extensive burns. Renal failure may go unrecognized and it is important to monitor renal function. The simplest way to do this is to catheterize the patient and measure hourly volumes of urine. The normal output is 0.5–1.0 ml/kg body weight per hour. Urine volume by itself is an inadequate indicator of renal function.

The quality of the urine should be assessed by estimating its osmolality. The measurements on the hourly urine samples can give early warning of the onset of renal failure. A low urine volume with a high osmolality is indicative of good renal function but small volumes of low osmolality may indicate failing kidneys. About half the cases of renal failure

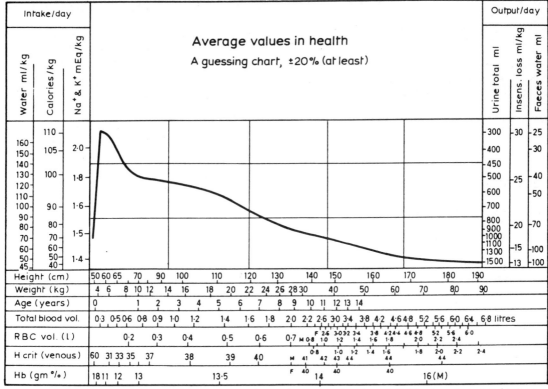

Figure 7.8 Guessing chart to help calculate plasma deficit (see text)

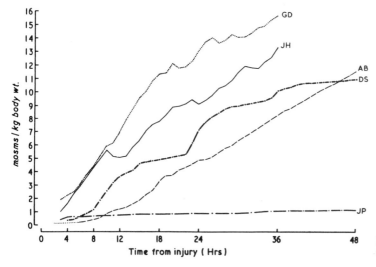

Figure 7.9 Diagram showing cumulative free osmolal output in four patients

due to burns are of the 'high output' or 'non-oliguric' type. Such apparently adequate volumes of urine may lull one into a false sense of security. A measure of effective renal work is required and this is measured as the free osmolal output. Plasma osmolality is normally 285 ± 10 mosm/kg. Urine with this osmolality has been produced without any renal 'work' as it is just a filtrate of the plasma. One may plot the cumulative free osmolal output as mosm/kg body weight against time since injury (Figure 7.9). This is the sum of the number of osmols being excreted per hour over and above that in an isotonic urine. GD and JH show good concentrating ability stimulated by antidiuretic hormone secretion evidenced by the steep slope; the dips represent periods of water diuresis. AB's trace shows poor early function (flat curve) which later improved. DS's trace shows good early function which then declined later (plateaus). JP had clinically obvious acute renal failure and virtually no work was done by his kidneys.

When treating the hypovolaemia of burns it is best to keep the calculations for the treatment of the hypovolaemia separate from calculation of other liquid requirements. The patient's metabolic needs should be met (Figure 7.8). In very large burns the waterproofing effect of the skin has been lost and there will be an evaporative loss of water from the wound. This occurs at the same rate as it would from an open bowl of water. The latent heat of vaporization of water is supplied by the patient. It is this heat loss which puts a severe metabolic stress on the patient, in addition to the stress of injury. The loss of water from the wound is 0.3 ml/cm²/24 h.

Metabolic response to injury

Cuthbertson in the 1930s described the changes in metabolic rate following injury (Figure 7.10). At first there is a fall in oxygen consumption and if the patient is not resuscitated this continues to death.

With successful resuscitation there is a turn and then a flow phase in which the metabolic rate and oxygen consumption are increased. For instance following a gastrectomy the metabolic response lasts about 5 days; following a fractured femur it lasts about 2 weeks, but in a major burn it may last for months. If sepsis is super-added the rate becomes even higher, and a severely ill septic burns case may have a metabolic rate which is twice the normal. Energy is required to sustain this high metabolic rate, and if the patient is unable to eat enough he will waste away.

Characteristic of this metabolic response to injury is sodium and water retention and potassium and protein loss. These may be readily monitored by recording fluid balance daily and estimating the content of sodium, potassium and urea in a sample of the 24-h urine collection. The metabolic response is mediated by corticosteroids and catecholamines. The patient in the early stages is relatively resistant to insulin and may exhibit a diabetic-like state with glycosuria, the so-called 'pseudodiabetes of burns'. Under the influence of these hormones, protein is broken down to form glucose (gluconeogenesis) and there is wasting of body muscle: fat stores are used to fuel this process. It has been realized that excessive weight loss predisposes to a fatal outcome and in recent years great efforts have been made to improve the nutrition of the patient, both by intravenous and nasogastric feeding. It is now recognized that there is a danger of over-feeding the patient and causing a respiratory acidosis, the reason being that excessive administration of carbohydrates causes the body to store them as fat. This is particularly the case when intravenous nutrition is used. This storage occurs primarily in the liver leading to enlargement. While carbohydrates are being converted into fat, for every three oxygen molecules inspired, 29 CO_2 molecules have to be expired. The elimination of the carbon dioxide may cause hyperventilation and, despite this, there will be a respiratory acidosis.

Immunosuppression and control of sepsis

Extensively burned patients have a large wound which is readily colonized, both with the patient's own organisms and with organisms from the environment. Great care must therefore be taken to prevent cross-infection from one patient to another in a burns unit. Initially patients are isolated and the staff attending them are fully gowned and gloved until a dressing is applied to cover the wound adequately. This is designed to prevent acquisition of organisms from the environment. In between patients, the staff should change their gowns, gloves

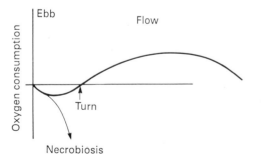

Figure 7.10 Oxygen consumption changes with time after injury

and aprons, and wash their hands. In general, patients acquire organisms about the fifth or sixth day after the burn, but invasive infection can occur much sooner or much later.

The large burn wound excites an inflammatory response. Many substances elaborated in this response have widespread effects. One of these is thought to be the re-setting of the temperature-controlling mechanism at a higher level. This fever is thought to be beneficial, but fever is also an indicator of invasive infection and to help distinguish whether this is occurring it is worth monitoring substances which indicate the level of the inflammatory response, such as C-reactive protein (CRP).

The microbiological flora of patients should be regularly and routinely monitored from admission onwards. At admission culture swabs are taken from nose, throat and wound. The nose and throat swabs are repeated weekly or preoperatively. Exposed wounds such as the face or perineum should have daily swabs cultured. Other wound swabs are taken at dressing changes or twice weekly from each main area of burn. Cultures from the wound in the early stages tend to be of Gram-negative organisms; it is only in the later stages that these are replaced by Gram-positive ones. When septicaemia is suspected and whenever there is fever of more than 39.5°C (103°F) blood cultures should be taken. The recovery of organisms when septicaemia is clinically diagnosed is difficult. In a good laboratory blood cultures are positive on about 10% of occasions when septicaemia is suspected clinically. Where possible cultures should be taken on at least three occasions before starting antibiotic therapy.

General effects

The synthesis of immunoglobulins is expensive for the body economy, especially when stressed by an extensive burn. Because of this immunosuppression, homografts may be applied to excised wounds and may not be rejected for several weeks when generally, in a fit patient, homografts are rejected at about 10–14 days. The progressive fall in serum proteins leads to a decrease in the colloid osmotic pressure; there tends to be a relative shrinking of the intravascular volume and monitoring of the urinary urea and electrolytes may show a gradual fall in the excretion of sodium and a rise in the excretion of potassium and urea. This is evidence of the 'sick cell syndrome' when there is a failure of the sodium pump which normally keeps sodium out of the cells. Potassium leaks from the cells, sodium leaks into the cells and there may be a fall in the serum sodium. This is not corrected by giving twice normal saline. One way to correct these effects is to transfuse blood, even in the presence of a normal haemoglo-

bin. A similar result may be obtained by giving glucose, potassium and insulin intravenously.

There is a progressive anaemia in burn cases which is due to primary red cell destruction at the time of injury, a decreased haemopoiesis and loss of red cells at dressing changes and operations. Invasive infection compounds all these effects, i.e. the metabolic response, the immunosuppression and the decreased haemopoiesis. Further effects which should be borne in mind are the malaise and anorexia which go with the fever. Sepsis may contribute to ileus diagnosed by a decrease in bowel sounds, nausea and vomiting. Occasionally attempts to increase the food intake result in diarrhoea due to intolerance of the feeds given. Constipation must be avoided. In children there may be a decrease in absorption of nutrients and lactose intolerance may contribute to a relative malabsorption. It may be necessary to change to lactose-free feeds to avoid this problem. Severely septic patients may develop respiratory failure, renal failure, liver failure, i.e. multiorgan system failure. All the resources of an intensive care unit will be needed to support such patients.

The burn wound

Once the epidermis has been destroyed there is an evaporative water loss from the wound. If the wound is left exposed, drying occurs. This extends to the dermis and, although the growth of micro-organisms is inhibited in a cool, dry wound, so also is the epithelial regeneration (Figure 7.11).

Where possible it is best to treat wounds occlusively, i.e. by means of a dressing which incorporates an antiseptic, a layer which prevents adhesion of the dressing to the wound, and the ability to absorb exudate and prevent strike-through. Traditionally this has been achieved with a tulle dressing incorporating the antiseptic such as 0.5% chlorhexidine, over which is laid first of all cotton gauze, and then at least 1 in (2.5 cm) thickness of cotton wool, secured by a bandage and sometimes additionally a splint. The dressing should extend for 4 in (10 cm) beyond the margins of the wound. The reasons for changing a dressing should be explained to patients, particularly those who are outpatients as they should return to have the dressing changed if any of the following occur. For this reason they are given dressing instructions which state:

Keep the dressing dry. If the dressing should become: (1) hot producing a fever; (2) wet; (3) loose uncovering the wound; (4) painful preventing sleep (throbbing); (5) too tight; or (6) smelly, return to the hospital to have it changed.

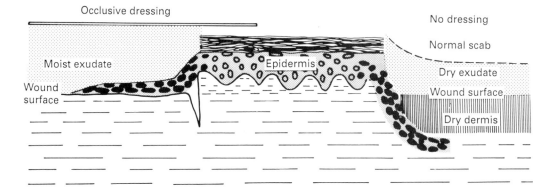

Figure 7.11 Comparison of the mode of epidermal regeneration in shallow skin wounds in a moist and a dry environment

A further medical reason for change of dressing is to inspect the progress of healing. In shallow burns the ideal is to apply a dressing which will remain in place until it is no longer needed, possibly 10 days or 2 weeks. For deeper wounds it may be necessary to change the dressing more frequently. Any but the smallest wounds which are not healed in 3 weeks should be grafted with split skin.

Steps to follow with a new burn emergency

1. Is the airway clear and the patient able to breathe? Indications for intubation include an unconscious patient, one with deep burns involving face and neck, and evidence of burns inside the mouth and throat and with stridor or hoarseness.
2. Obtain a history from the patient or his attendants. Establish *what* happened and *when* and whether the incident could have caused other traumatic injuries apart from the burn (e.g. explosions may blow someone from the upper storey of a house or the patient may jump to escape; they may sustain fractures of long bones or crush fractures of vertebrae; explosions may also cause penetrating injuries of the eye).
3. Corrosive chemical burns should be flooded with water. Advice about specific treatment is available from the National Poisons Advice Centre, Guy's Hospital, London, telephone no. 071 635 9191.
4. Make a short general examination. Estimate the size of the burn (percentage body surface area) using a quick method (Rule of Nines) and decide whether an intravenous drip is needed (>10% body surface area in a child; >15% body surface area in an adult).

5. Estimate colloid requirement using the Mount Vernon formula:

$$\frac{\text{Area of burn (\%)} \times \text{body weight (kg)}}{2} = \text{ml of plasma}$$

This is to be given in first 4 h from time of injury.

6. Cannulate a large vein away from a joint. In a severely vasoconstricted patient it may be necessary to cut down through intact or burned skin. A good place to start is the radial side of the forearm at the junction of the middle and lower thirds to discover the cephalic vein. (When matters are desperate remember the rectum will absorb liquid; a nurse can give warm Hartmann's solution as an enema).
7. Before connecting the drip set take 10 ml of *blood* for packed cell volume, haemoglobin, urea and electrolytes, group and cross-match. Then establish the drip initially with saline if colloid is not immediately available.
8. Relieve pain using:
   (a) cold water or by fanning a wet burn;
   (b) nitrous oxide and oxygen inhalation, or well diluted morphine given *intravenously* and titrated against the patient's response. The dose of morphine is 0.1–0.2 mg per kg body weight.
9. Catheterize the bladder in cases of burns of more than 25% body surface area. The catheter should be self-retaining and connected to a closed drainage system. Note the time, measure the volume and save a specimen. This first specimen may have forensic significance and a portion should be frozen in case it is needed for analysis for poisonous substances.
10. Establish whether the casualty has been trapped, burned in a confined space or inhaled smoke. Suspect lung damage; take *arterial*

blood and measure Pao_2 $Paco_2$ and carboxy-haemoglobin.

11. Make a systematic clinical examination and assess the patient's general condition as to whether the measures taken to support airway, breathing and circulation are effective and producing improvement. Check whether occult blood loss is occurring and whether vital functions are embarrassed by thoracic injury.

12. With every child consider whether the burn could be a non-accidental injury. In adult cases check whether there are any unexplained or suspicious circumstances. Consider whether to take urine and blood for forensic examination (e.g. common poisons).

13. Examine the depth of the burn more closely. Is it full thickness and circumferential on neck, trunk or a limb? Consider the need for incising the eschar (escharotomy).

14. Chart the extent accurately on a Lund and Browder chart and indicate the depth. N.B. *Do not* include simple erythema.

15. Take stock of events – has anything been missed? Recalculate colloid requirements. Reassess patient and write instructions for nurses. Complete the clinical record.

Special types of burn injury
Smoke inhalation

Smoke inhalation may occur as a single entity or combined with burns of any degree of severity. The individual may have inhaled smoke which contains irritants and poisons. If the atmosphere is very hot they may also have inhaled steam. The hotter the gases and the more irritant the smoke, the more is the injury confined to the upper airway; this is usually associated with burns of the face, singed nasal vibrissae and perhaps blistering seen on the palate with deposits of soot. Cooler smoke may not cause burns of the upper airway but inhalation of irritants and poisons can cause severe damage to the lower airway as well as causing asphyxia and loss of consciousness from carbon monoxide poisoning.

In a patient with minor burns with obvious deposits of soot on the skin one should beware of a slow onset of symptoms which may yet prove fatal. Any patient who gives a history of smoke inhalation or who has received burns in an enclosed space should automatically be assumed to have suffered inhalation injury and should be admitted for observation. The unconscious may require intubation and ventilation immediately. Initially 100% oxygen should be used. If the carboxyhaemoglobin (COHb) concentration is more than 10%, administration of 100% oxygen should continue for at least 4 h or until the carboxyhaemoglobin concentration has declined to a safe level. Apart from facial burns,

symptoms associated with smoke inhalation include hoarseness or even loss of the voice, stridor, wheeze and a cough producing carbonaceous sputum.

Investigations should include carboxyhaemoglobin level, blood gas estimations and a chest radiograph as a minimum. If there is any suspicion that the airway is compromised, an anaesthetic opinion should be obtained. It is better to intubate early and be safe rather than leave it until it is too late; emergency tracheostomy should then not be necessary.

Beware of the confusion and restlessness due to anoxia. This should never be treated by sedation with opiates. The treatment is adequate ventilation and oxygenation. Inspired gases should be humidified. If there is bronchospasm this should be treated with a suitable bronchodilator delivered by nebulizer, e.g. salbutamol, 0.5 ml of respirator solution (5 mg/ml) diluted with 2 ml of physiological saline in a nebulizer connected in the oxygen delivery circuit clipped onto the oxygen mask. This should be repeated 2–4-hourly as necessary at first. Later this may be reduced to a regular dosage four times a day. If there is no response to bronchodilators on their own, steroids may be given in addition. There is no place for steroids as a prophylactic measure. If respirations become increasingly shallow and rapid, respiratory failure is imminent.

Artificial ventilation should be instituted, if necessary with added post end expiratory pressure (PEEP) or continuous positive airway pressure (CPAP). The airways should be kept clear as necessary by regular suction using an aseptic technique (at least 2-hourly to begin with). Antibiotics are only indicated if there is pulmonary infection. In severe cases of smoke inhalation the maximum effect of the injury may not be seen for 2–3 days.

Occasionally artificial ventilation has to be carried out for so long that it is necessary to perform a tracheostomy electively. With careful management this should only be necessary after about 2 weeks of endotracheal intubation.

Chemical burns

The injury to the tissues depends upon the specific chemical involved. The mode of action may be, as with strong acids and alkalis, the vigorous combination with water to produce heat. Certain acids and alkalis may penetrate deeply owing to their chemical action and this applies especially to hydrofluoric acid and sodium hydroxide, potassium hydroxide and lime (beware of cement, this contains strong alkalis and can burn the unwary). If large areas have been involved with a chemical, the first aid is to flood the area with water and continue copious washing for at least 20 min. When such a case is received in a casualty department, further washing with water should occur before phosphate buffer solution is applied. The phosphate buffer solution is made up of: (1) potassium acid phosphate (monobasic) KH_2PO_4, 30 g; (2) sodium phosphate (dibasic) Na_2HPO_4, 220 g; and (3) water to 1 litre; dissolved with the aid of heat, filtered and checked for pH 6.8–7. This solution is safe to use in the eye and is equally effective in buffering the action of strong acids and alkalis.

If it is suspected that the chemical is continuing to penetrate deeply, excision of the wound as an emergency procedure may be necessary. This is most often the case in extensive hydrofluoric acid burns where the fluride iron precipitates body calcium, immobilizing it and leading to hypocalcaemia and tetany. The patient may require infusions of calcium gluconate to maintain the serum calcium. Poisons such as phenol are readily absorbed through the skin, particularly if excessively diluted with water. It is necesary to fix the chemical in some way and the specific treatment should be mopping the skin with polyethylene glycol, soap or olive oil. If extensive areas are involved by contact with phenol, penetration and systemic effects can only be prevented by excising the affected area while supportive measures are applied to maintain the life of the patient.

Where a chemical is known to affect organs such as the kidneys, the function should be carefully monitored. A prime example of this situation follows contact with chromium salts. Relatively minor burns may still lead to renal failure requiring dialysis. Information on the effects of chemicals, the necessary treatment measures and specific antidotes can be obtained from the National Poisons Information Centre at Guy's Hospital, telephone no. 071 635 9191.

The treatment measures for chemical burns can be summarized as follows:

1. Wash from the surface.
2. Neutralize where possible.
3. Remove tissue reservoir.
4. Facilitate detoxification or excretion.
5. General supportive measures.

Electrical burns

Contact with electric current may have very minor effects or may be immediately fatal. Burning is due to the heat produced by the resistance to the passage of current by the tissues (the Joule effect). The effects of the current are related to its strength measured in amperes. The passage of a current of 1 mA is just perceptible. Pain is experienced at 5 mA and tetany of voluntary muscles at about 15 mA.

Tetany of respiratory muscles occurs at 30 mA and ventricular fibrillation may occur between 60 and 5000 mA.

A patient who has received an electric shock may appear to be dead. The first action should be to isolate the victim from the current either by switching off or dislodging the conductor from the patient with some non-conducting object such as a wooden pole. Once the victim has been made safe, the rescuer can start resuscitation using external cardiac massage and mouth-to-mouth ventilation (see pp. 11–14). This should be continued until signs of life are seen or until a full assessment can be made in hospital. Quite often patients are not found until spontaneous recovery has occurred but the sign that there has been a cessation of respiration will be petechial haemorrhages caused by anoxia. These are best seen in the whites of the eyes and in the thin skin of the eyelids and behind the ears. Once in hospital the casualty should be investigated by means of an electrocardiogram and arrhythmias should be treated appropriately.

Electrical burns caused by low-tension (generally defined as voltages below 1000 V) tend to cause fairly small burns but these may penetrate deeply and involve joints and other deep structures. Excision and immediate repair are indicated in such cases, either with skin grafts or flaps. The patient should be inspected carefully all over the body, particularly looking within the hair for unsuspected burns. They may be found over bony prominences, sometimes as very small spark burns. Usually there is at least one fairly large and obvious wound but there may be other much smaller ones that are equally deep. These are due to earthing of the current. Because of the heat generated by resistance to the passage of current as it enters the body, the skin burn may be indented or even charred.

High-tension injuries are defined as contact with electricity over 1000 V. This is often many thousands of volts, e.g. from high-tension conductors over railway lines (25 000 V) or even higher tensions. The effects are quite devastating, leading to severe deep tissue injury. The deep injury may in fact be more severe than that of the skin as the current tends to follow the axis of limbs and much heat is produced as resistance to the current by bone is high. Surrounding muscles may be cooked when the external skin appears more or less intact. In such cases release of tight fascial compartments by fasciotomy may be necessary. Dead tissue should be excised (debridement) following the principles of war surgery where muscle which is blue and does not twitch when cut is excised. Successive excisions of dead tissue may be necessary over several days until the wound is safe. During this time it is advisable to give antibiotics to prevent anaerobic infection. The ideal combination is metronidazole and penicillin. Salvage surgery for these cases is the province of the expert, whose opinion should be sought. Frequently, amputation of parts becomes inevitable.

Treatment of the major burn wound

When faced with a large wound it is easy to forget that medical treatment is necessary. One should ensure that the patient is immunized against tetanus. During the shock phase of burns the large infusions of fluid so dilute the antitetanus immunoglobulin that it is wise to protect the patient with penicillin or erythromycin for the first 5–7 days. Besides being prophylactic against tetanus, there is the additional benefit of prophylaxis against *Streptococcus pyogenes*. It is important to judge the depth of the burn wound as the management depends on this. Wounds which are full thickness and for which early excision is planned may be treated with an oily dressing so that they remain relatively dry, as some surgeons feel that this type of slough is easier to excise. Others prefer to use a cream dressing such as silver sulphadiazine, feeling that the antibacterial efficacy is greater than a tulle dressing.

Early excision and grafting

Early excision of the burn wound may be defined as that occurring within the first 7–10 days of injury. It was first shown in 1960 that very aggressive early surgery, i.e. during the shock phase, does not improve the mortality rate in major burns, although the length of hospital stay may be shortened. This has been confirmed more recently by Herndon (1986) who treated two groups of children: those who underwent very early aggressive surgery had half the length of stay in hospital of those treated conservatively, but again the mortality rate was not improved. The difficulties experienced in attempting the more aggressive approach can be very great and are not suitable for most burns units in the UK. Such activities cause great dislocation of the general running of a burns unit, particularly if it is part of a plastic surgery department.

Before the operation it is important to have sufficient blood cross-matched and to perform a coagulation screen to ensure there are sufficient platelets and fibrinogen for effective blood coagulation. A safe practice is to excise an area which does not put the patient's general condition too much at risk. If there is undue blood loss the surgery should be curtailed. It should be the anaesthetist's duty to monitor blood loss and call a halt well before half the blood volume has to be replaced. Great problems with haemostasis should not be encountered provided no more than half a blood volume is lost during and after the procedure. This means the excision should stop when about one-third of the blood volume has been lost as there tends to be continued ooze from donor sites and the wound.

Deep dermal burns may be tangentially excised. This requires careful judgement. Using a skin graft knife the wound is shaved in layers down to punctate bleeding from the dermis. The correct level is that at which there is punctate bleeding on shaving which ceases over the course of several minutes. It is tempting to re-excise this area but this should not be done. It is important to cover the whole tangentially excised area with thin split skin grafts as any areas left uncovered will dessicate and die, thus increasing the wound depth at that site. Wounds that have been tangentially excised are more at risk of loss of grafts from Gram-negative infection and such areas should be dressed with a gauze soaked in 0.5% solution of silver nitrate as this is inhibitory to Gram-negative organisms. Tangential excision should be performed between the third and fifth days after the burn. If this opportunity is missed, deep dermal areas should be treated conventionally.

During surgery every effort is made to minimize blood loss. The areas which are to undergo excision or provide skin grafts are infiltrated subcutaneously with a solution made up in 500 ml physiological saline for injection of 1 ml 1:1000 adrenaline and 1500 units hyaluronidase. This 1:500 000 adrenaline has proved safe to inject using a spinal needle attached to a drip set which is under pressure. The method is time consuming but very effective in reducing bleeding. Alternatively, swabs soaked in 1:100 000 adrenaline may be applied topically to excised areas which continue to ooze after all the more major vessels have been ligated or coagulated.

Where possible inflatable tourniquets are used and excision is carried out on a limb lightly exsanguinated using the 'pillow' exsanguinator. The wound must be protected from contamination while this is done. As excision proceeds obvious vessels are picked up in haemostatic forceps and diathermized or coagulated using a bipolar coagulator. For large burn excisions diathermy is quicker and more effective. Once excision is complete the tourniquet may be deflated to facilitate further coagulation of bleeding points. It is re-inflated to allow careful application of skin grafts which should be dressed in place before final release of the tourniquet. The object of skin grafting a major burn is to achieve healing of the largest possible area in the shortest possible time. This means autografts should be as thin as possible consistent with easy handling and rapid application. The advantage of thin grafts is that they take well even in the presence of infection. The disadvantages are that the cosmetic appearance is poor and the subsequent contracture may be severe. Grafts cut with a thicker layer of dermis 'take' less well but contract less.

In very extensive burns autologous skin may have to be used very sparingly. Several different methods have been used to achieve this:

1. Postage stamps. The skin is cut into small pieces
   and spread over the wound surface leaving gaps
   around each piece of up to 1.5 cm. The wound
   epithelializes by outgrowth from the margins of
   the islands of skin once they have become
   established.
2. Jackson Mowlem alternate strip method. The
   wound is covered completely but most of the skin
   used is homograft. Viable human split skin grafts
   2 cm wide, from a live or dead donor are
   interspersed with 0.5 cm strips of autograft skin.
3. The Chinese described a method in which large
   sheets of viable homograft were applied to
   excised areas. When the large homograft had
   become established, individual holes were cut
   out and autograft inserted.
4. Method (3) has been automated to provide
   sheets of homograft on an adhesive backing strip
   from which square holes have been cut and
   autograft placed exactly into each hole (Hettich).
5. Subsequently the Chinese have modified method
   (3) to become the microskin grafting technique.
   Autograft is chopped very finely and dispersed
   on the inner surface of the homograft sheet so
   that it is sandwiched between the wound and the
   homograft. The autograft forms islets which grow
   and coalesce under the protection of the homograft which is eventually rejected.

Methods (2), (3) and (4) have an added advantage in
that the homograft dermis may be retained and the
foreign epidermis be replaced by a creeping
substitution process. If the homograft is poorly
antigenic or the patient severely immunodepressed,
the homografted areas may not even ulcerate as the
creeping substitution of homologous epidermis with
autologous epidermis occurs. This preservation of
homologous dermis has been claimed for method (5)
also, although it is difficult to see how this may
occur.

Meshed skin grafts

By cutting a series of parallel, staggered overlapping
slots in a sheet of skin it may be opened out like a
concertina to form a net. Depending on the length
of the cuts the skin net may be used to cover an area
several times the size of the original piece of skin.
Various devices exist to cut these slots quickly. The
Tanner Vanderput machine is able to cut mesh of
several different ratios depending on the grooving in
a flexible plastic backing sheet (dermacarrier).

A 3:1 ratio may be used on autograft covered with
a standard dressing. The interstices of the mesh heal
across in 7–10 days but the mesh pattern is retained
permanently. If the autograft is expanded much
more than 3:1 it is best protected by homograft
which itself may be meshed, for instance, 6:1
autograft mesh overlaid by 3:1 or 1.5:1 homograft
mesh.

Meshing, besides extending the area covered, has
the advantage of allowing wound exudate to escape
from under the graft. Frank bleeding will still give
rise to clots which will separate the meshed skin
from its bed and prevent successful graft take.

Later grafting

Where wounds are less extensive and the depth is
uncertain, it is permissible to await the formation of
granulation tissue as the slough separates. In
countries where blood is difficult to obtain this is the
best way to treat extensive burns, as the only reason
for blood transfusion should be to replace blood loss
from the donor sites. Once a clean granulating
wound has been achieved the application of skin
grafts is a simple matter. Again techniques may be
used to spread the skin over a larger area such as
using 'postage stamps' scattered over the wound or a
meshing method.

On limbs, grafts are fairly readily secured by
careful application of dressings upon which splints
are superimposed to prevent shearing forces on the
grafts. On areas of constant movement the exposed
technique may be used; this is particularly valuable
on the chest or back if the patient can cooperate.
Even in children immobilization may allow grafting
on the back or front; this requires that both legs are
splinted with plaster cylinders and a bar placed
between the feet so that they are spreadeagled, as
this prevents the child from turning over. A child's
elbow may be fixed with splints made of rolled
cardboard padded with cotton wool to prevent the
child disturbing the grafts on the trunk. The exposed
method also allows nursing staff to clean the wound
daily with saline and to express seroma and
haematoma from under the grafts.

If there is a shortage of operating time, it is
possible to excise wounds and harvest autografts
under general anaesthesia. A suitable dressing is
applied to protect the wound until the next day.
Nursing staff may then change the dressing at their
leisure, removing the temporary dressing and
applying the grafts. This is the delayed grafting
technique and is particularly valuable when troublesome bleeding at the time of surgery makes it likely
that graft take will be poor. Delayed grafting
minimizes the loss of grafts from seroma and
haematoma and is used extensively in some plastic
surgery units.

Special areas

Important functional areas should be given priority
for skin grafting. These include the face, particularly
the eyelids and around the mouth. The flexor
aspects of joints should have priority over the

extensor aspects and, where possible, sheet grafts should be used in these situations. A judgement has to be made between the need for saving life, i.e. closing as great an area of the wound as possible which usually means grafting large areas on the trunk or limbs, at the expense of devoting a lot of time to areas such as the hands and eyes. Very often time is spent on important functional areas when the patient is not particularly ill. Later on they may become severely ill and septic, even developing multisystem organ failure. This might have been prevented had more of the wound been closed in the early stages by devoting one's attention to area rather than function.

8

Local and regional anaesthesia

G. S. Robertson

Local or infiltration anaesthesia is produced by the injection of a local anaesthetic drug into the immediate area upon which an operation is to be performed. Regional anaesthesia is produced by blockage of sensory conduction in nerves before they enter the operation field; this may be produced by the precise placement of local anaesthetic solution into or near specific nerves, or by the infiltration of the region around the nerves by the use of larger volumes of solution. Specialized techniques such as spinal, epidural and caudal blocks should be carried out only by trained staff or under suitable supervision, and they will not be described here.

Although the effectiveness of a local anaesthetic technique is clearly important the prime consideration of the operator should be safety. Many local and regional techniques have specific dangers but the commonest cause of serious complications is the injection of a local anaesthetic drug in excessive dosage.

Local anaesthetic drugs

Only those local anaesthetic drugs of applied importance to local and regional use will be described.

Lignocaine (Lidothesin, Xylocaine, Xylotox, Lidocaine)

The most popular drug for local anaesthesia, lignocaine is also the drug responsible for the highest incidence of serious or fatal reactions. Such reactions are virtually never due to allergy or anaphylaxis but are caused by overdosage. The principal advantages of lignocaine are its rapid onset

of action and ready diffusion through tissues. It has little or no effect on small vessel tone.

Dosage

For a fit adult of about 70 kg the maximum safe total dose of lignocaine is 200 mg; when used with adrenaline the safe dose can be increased to 500 mg because the local vasoconstriction produced by adrenaline greatly reduces the rate of absorption of lignocaine (Table 8.1).

Table 8.1 Lignocaine dosage

Concentration	Maximum volume
Plain lignocaine (without adrenaline):	
0.5% (5 mg/ml)	40 ml
1% (10 mg/ml)	20 ml
2% (20 mg/ml)	10 ml
4% (40 mg/ml)	5 ml (for topical use only)
Lignocaine with adrenaline 1:200 000:	
0.5%	100 ml
1%	50 ml
2%	25 ml

Caution

The maximum safe total dose will be reduced in the following conditions: low body weight (including children), debility, old age, hepatic disease, renal impairment, epilepsy and heart block.

Which concentration to use?

For infiltration of wide areas where there is no risk of inadvertent intra-arterial injection it is generally safer to use lignocaine 0.5% with adrenaline

1:100 000 or 1:200 000. The weaker concentration of adrenaline is safer when large volumes are likely to be required; the use of 1:100 000 adrenaline limits the safe volume of solution to 40 ml maximum because of the risk of adrenaline toxicity. If the aim is to obtain a dry operating field by the use of vasoconstriction, adrenaline 1:200 000 is always effective provided the operator waits at least 5 min before making the skin incision.

For regional block a solution of 0.5% or 1% lignocaine should be used, depending upon the volume required, and for the regional blocks described in this chapter there is never any need to exceed a concentration of 1% lignocaine.

Topical anaesthesia for bronchoscopy requires 4% lignocaine but it is inappropriate to use it with adrenaline. This effectively limits the dose to 5 ml. For nasal surgery, 4% lignocaine may be applied to the nasal mucosa along with up to 1 ml of 1:1000 adrenaline. More effective vasoconstriction of the nasal mucosa is produced by 10% cocaine (up to 4 ml) and adrenaline 1:1000 (up to 1 ml). For gastroscopy topical anaesthesia may be obtained using 2% lignocaine (Xylocaine Viscous) in a maximum dose of 15 ml. Anaesthesia of the urethra is produced by the use of lignocaine in a lubricant, water-miscible base (Lidothesin Gel, Xylocaine Gel, Xylotox Gel) in a maximum dose of 10 ml, best given as two increments of 5 ml separated by an interval of 2 or 3 min.

Toxic effects of lignocaine

These are liable to occur when the recommended dosage is exceeded or when a substantial proportion is given by inadvertent intravenous or intra-arterial injection. Cerebral toxicity produces anxiety, excitement, drowsiness, coma, convulsions, cessation of respiration, areflexia. Cardiac toxicity causes hypotension, bradycardia, heart block.

Treatment of lignocaine toxicity

Excitability or drowsiness alone requires no specific treatment but it may give early warning of serious toxic effects and it is prudent to administer oxygen at an early stage and prepare for the possibility of convulsions or respiratory arrest. An intravenous catheter should be inserted. If convulsions develop, continue the administration of oxygen and give either diazepam (Valium, Diazemuls) slowly intravenously in increments of 5 mg or 2.5% thiopentone (Pentothal, Intraval) in increments of 50 mg (2 ml) intravenously until convulsions cease. Only the minimum dose of diazepam or thiopentone should be used as they may aggravate any separate toxic effects on the myocardium. If respiratory arrest occurs, administer oxygen by artificial ventilation using a bag (e.g. Ambu or Laerdal) connected to a tight-fitting face mask or a cuffed endotracheal tube. Respiratory depression or arrest associated with the administration of lignocaine must *never* be treated with a respiratory stimulant. Hypotension, if apparently due to bradycardia and myocardial depression, should be treated by the slow intravenous administration of atropine 0.6 mg. In the presence of persistent cardiovascular collapse, particularly with peripheral vasodilatation, a combined vasopressor and cardiac stimulant, such as ephedrine (15–20 mg) should be given intravenously. The patient should be placed flat, with the legs elevated, and a saline infusion should be given.

Note: In local anaesthetic procedures where it is evident that large total doses of local anaesthetic drug will be necessary, it is wise to insert a cannula in a vein before starting to inject the drug.

Prilocaine (Citanest)

This is pharmacologically similar to lignocaine and it is generally considered to be less toxic. However, it diffuses less readily and so its effects on nerves are more delayed. Slower absorption of prilocaine makes it less necessary to use it along with vasoconstrictor drugs. Its main application is in situations where large volumes of local anaesthetic solution are required, e.g. widespread infiltration in the head and neck and in intravenous regional analgesia. The maximum safe dose of prilocaine for an average adult is 400 mg (40 ml of 1% solution) and this may be increased to 600 mg by the addition of a vasoconstrictor. As well as having toxic effects on the central nervous and cardiovascular systems similar to those of lignocaine, prilocaine in excessive dosage will also cause methaemoglobinaemia.

Bupivacaine (Marcain, Marcaine)

This drug has a considerably slower rate of onset than lignocaine and a much longer duration of action (4–6 h compared with 1.5 h for lignocaine). It is of value in more prolonged surgery and for providing postoperative pain relief. The addition of adrenaline 1:200 000 will provide local vasoconstriction but it does not greatly increase the duration of action of bupivacaine. Maximum recommended dosages of bupivacaine are given in the section on 'Local anaesthetic techniques for postoperative pain relief' on p. 102.

Emla (Emla cream 5%)

This is a eutectic mixture of local anaesthetics consisting of lignocaine and prilocaine in the form of a cream. It is applied liberally to the skin at least 1 h and preferably 2 h before an injection, and an occlusive dressing is then applied over the cream. The cream should be applied as a thick layer and should not be rubbed into the skin.

Upper limb surgery

Intravenous regional analgesia (IVRA; Bier's block)

This is one of the commonest forms of local anaesthesia in current use for upper limb surgery.

Advantages

1. Simplicity.
2. Relative safety.

Disadvantages

1. Toxic reaction due to excessive dosage on cuff deflation or inadvertent premature deflation of the cuff.
2. Incomplete analgesia, especially in surgery of the digits – this can usually be avoided by careful technique.
3. Ischaemic pain in the area of the occluding cuff – this can be largely avoided by the use of a double occlusion cuff or two separate cuffs and by limiting the cuff inflation time to about 1.25 h maximum.
4. Oozing of local anaesthetic solution from veins and venules during surgery. This is rarely troublesome.

Choice of drug

Although lignocaine was favoured in IVRA for many years, there have been several reports of severe systemic reactions after deflation of the cuff. Such reactions may be minimized but not avoided completely by using lignocaine 0.5% rather than 1%. Bupivacaine (Marcain, Marcaine) in 0.2% solution may be safer because of its greater tendency to become tissue-bound, but as with lignocaine, toxic reactions have been reported. To make up 0.2% bupivacaine dilute 20 ml of the 0.5% solution to 50 ml with normal saline.

Probably the safest option at present is prilocaine (Citanest) which may be used in 0.5% or 1% solution, but the 0.5% strength may be insufficient to guarantee satisfactory analgesia for extensive sharp dissection. However, regardless of the choice of drug, IVRA involves the use of large doses of local anaesthetic and it should not be undertaken in circumstances where resuscitation facilities and expertise are not available.

Note: It is recommended that a venous cannula should be inserted in the unaffected arm or hand before IVRA is commenced.

Technique of IVRA

1. Apply a double tourniquet on the affected arm above the elbow. Alternatively, two blood-pressure cuffs may be used, one being applied distal to the other.
2. Check the systolic blood pressure.
3. Insert a flexible indwelling cannula (18 G or 19 G Venflon, Medicut or equivalent) in the dorsum of the hand on the affected side. If the dorsum of the hand is unsuitable or unavailable any vein in the forearm or antecubital fossa may be used, but the results may be less satisfactory. A metal indwelling needle is unsuitable unless the use of an Esmarch bandage is inappropriate (see 4 below).
4. Exsanguinate the affected arm using a firmly-applied Esmarch bandage, from the finger tips to the edge of the distal cuff. If the nature of the operation or injury (e.g. Colles' fracture) precludes the use of an Esmarch bandage the arm should be elevated fully for at least 2 min after which manual pressure should be applied over the accessible parts of the arm to aid exsanguination
5. Inflate the proximal cuff to about 100 mmHg above the systolic blood pressure.
6. Remove the Esmarch bandage, check that the cuff remains inflated and that there is no arterial inflow.
7. Inject local anaesthetic solution through the indwelling cannula. Prilocaine (Citanest) 0.5% or 1% is recommended; the stronger concentration being more suitable for extensive procedures or surgery involving fingers. The volume should be 30–40 ml depending upon the size of the limb. An average adult requires 38 ml. In elderly patients or where the dose is uncertain, a small dose, e.g. 30 or 32 ml should be used initially and if, after a wait of 10 min, there is inadequate analgesia a further 4–6 ml may be injected.
8. After a delay of 5 min, inflate the distal cuff (underneath which the arm should be analgesic) and after checking the operation of the distal cuff deflate the proximal cuff.
9. Surgery should not be commenced until at least a further 5 min (i.e. 10 min after injection of the local anaesthetic), and in some cases requiring sharp dissection, particularly involving the fingers, the interval should be extended to a total of 15 min from injection.
10. At the end of surgery the cuff should be deflated for a few seconds and immediately re-inflated once per minute for 5 min to avoid systemic

reactions to the local anaesthetic. In cases where the occlusion time has been longer than 30 min it is probably safe to re-inflate and deflate the cuff only once after the initial release.

11. Even with the use of a double tourniquet, a proportion of patients may develop severe pain in the area underneath the cuff after 30–60 min. If tourniquet release at this time is inconvenient, the pain can usually be relieved by infiltrating 20 ml of 0.5% lignocaine or prilocaine in adrenaline subcutaneously in a ring around the arm proximal to the cuff.

Causes of failed or incomplete block with IVRA

1. Inadequate exsanguination This leads to excessive dilution of local anaesthetic by blood remaining in the limb.
2. Arterial blood flow into the arm. This may be caused by leakage of air from the tourniquet or by a rise in blood pressure to a level above the tourniquet pressure The commonest times at which inadvertent cuff deflation may occur are during the change from proximal to distal cuff inflation and during transfer of the patient from an anaesthetic room into the operating theatre.

   If cuff deflation is incomplete, rapid re-inflation will minimize limb congestion and it is usually possible to proceed with surgery, particularly if the limb has already become analgesic. If cuff deflation is complete, venous outflow will carry a large proportion of the dose of local anaesthetic into the general circulation and the risk of a systemic reaction is greater after such early deflation. The cuff should be re-inflated immediately in order to delay the return of local anaesthetic to the circulation. The limb should be allowed to empty of anaesthetic in increments by successive deflation and re-inflation of the cuff over a period of 10 min. If no systemic reaction occurs it is usually safe to repeat the IVRA technique as described above but extra care must be taken to ensure that early release of local anaesthetic into the circulation is not repeated.
3. Incomplete analgesia may be found in surgery of the fingers, particularly the finger-tips. This may be due to inadequate dosage of local anaesthetic in an unusually large arm, and it may be possible to prevent it by reducing the venous capacity of the arm by applying firm manual pressure round the upper forearm during and for 5 min after the injection of local anaesthetic, thereby promoting selective distribution to the hand. For surgery confined to the distal phalanges of the fingers it may be better to employ a digital block.
4. A common cause of inadequate analgesia is failure to allow sufficient time for the block to take place. IVRA depends entirely upon diffusion from small vessels to sensory nerve endings, and this requires a lapse of at least 10 min. The testing of pin-prick sensation routinely is not recommended because some patients may misinterpret the feeling of incomplete analgesia, and in many procedures, particularly manipulations, surgery may be virtually painless even when pin-prick sensation is not completely lost.

As with any local anaesthetic technique, incomplete block may be largely corrected by the administration of a potent analgesic i.m. or i.v. in suitable dosage. Similarly, where conditions permit, better results from local anaesthetic techniques are obtained in patients premedicated with an analgesic or sedative drug.

Bilateral IVRA for upper limb surgery

The use of IVRA on both arms simultaneously is *not* recommended because of the risk of severe toxic reaction if the local anaesthetic drug from both arms is allowed to enter the general circulation within a short period of time. Surgery on one arm should be completed, the cuff deflated and absence of toxic reaction confirmed before IVRA on the second arm is commenced. The interval between cuff deflation on the first and second arms should be not less than 30 min.

Brachial plexus block

This may be carried out using either a supraclavicular or an axillary approach.

Supraclavicular brachial plexus block
(Figure 8.1)

Classically, this block is carried out at the point where the plexus crosses the first rib. This technique carries a high risk of pleural puncture. It is unsuitable for administration by the occasional user and will not be described here. An acceptable alternative which is much simpler and safer, but slightly less certain is as follows:

1. With the patient's head in the mid position (not rotated to one side) apply sustained traction to the affected arm abducted to about 45°. The object is to overcome tension in the neck muscles and allow direct palpation of the brachial plexus.
2. After a few minutes of traction it is possible to palpate the plexus some 2 cm above the clavicle in all but the most muscular or obese patients.
3. Using 1% lignocaine or prilocaine with adrenaline 1:200 000 inject through a 25 G or 23 G hypodermic needle placed into the middle of the largest mass of the brachial plexus. Up to 30 ml of

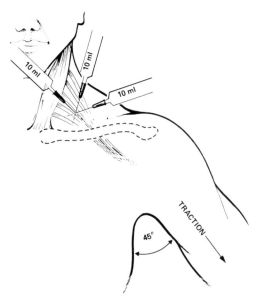

Figure 8.1 Brachial plexus block – supraclavicular approach

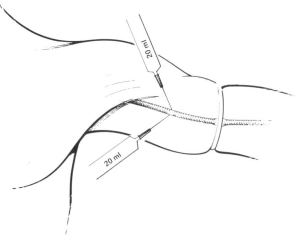

Figure 8.2 Axillary block of the brachial plexus

solution may be used in three increments of 10 ml injected in a fan-shaped distribution within the plexus. The injection commonly elicits paraesthesiae in the arm or hand. Allow an interval of 10–15 min before assessing the presence of analgesia. The length of needle used should allow adequate injection of the plexus without the risk of pleural puncture.

Axillary block of the brachial plexus

Although the axillary approach is safer than the supraclavicular approach, it does not produce analgesia of the shoulder region and lateral part of the upper arm. Also the lateral cutaneous nerve of forearm (musculocutaneous nerve) which supplies the radial aspect of the forearm may not be blocked. The technique is as follows:

Abduct the arm to an angle of 90°. Apply a rubber tourniquet (e.g. Sterivac tubing) tightly 2–3 cm distal to the insertion of pectoralis major in order to limit the distal spread of local anaesthetic within the axillary sheath (Figure 8.2). Palpate the axillary artery pulse as it emerges from the edge of pectoralis major and direct a small (25 G or 23 G) needle immediately above the arterial pulse to enter the axillary sheath. In an adult of average build, this does not lie deeper than 1–2 cm. When the needle point lies within the sheath the needle will show marked movement with the pulse. Aspirate the needle to test for arterial puncture and when this is negative inject 20 ml of lignocaine or prilocaine 1% in 1:100 000 or 1:200 000 adrenaline. Withdraw the

needle and re-insert it immediately below the axillary pulse to enter the medial part of the axillary sheath. Check for arterial puncture and inject a further 20 ml of the same anaesthetic solution. After some 15 min remove the rubber tourniquet and wait a further 5–10 min before commencing surgery.

Nerve block at the elbow

In view of the limited area of analgesia produced by ulnar nerve block at the elbow and the clear danger of nerve damage by direct injection into the ulnar nerve, nerve block at the wrist is preferred for hand surgery.

Nerve block at the wrist (Figure 8.3)
Ulnar nerve

At the level of the distal end of the ulna and about 1 cm proximal to the distal skin crease between wrist

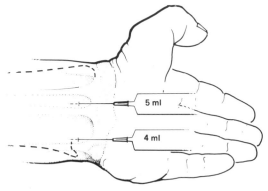

Figure 8.3 Wrist block (front)

and hand insert a 25 G needle to a depth of 1 cm immediately to the radial side of the flexor carpi ulnaris. Inject 4 ml of 1% lignocaine. The dorsal branch of the ulnar nerve is blocked by the subcutaneous injection of lignocaine between the proximal edge of the pisiform bone and the middle of the dorsum of the wrist.

Median nerve

At the same level and to the same depth as for ulnar nerve block insert a 25 G needle between the tendons of palmaris longus and flexor carpi radialis or 3 mm to the ulnar side of the flexor carpi radialis. This point is almost exactly in the middle of the anterior surface of the wrist or a few millimetres to the radial side of the midline. Inject 5 ml of 1% lignocaine.

Radial nerve

In view of the anatomical variations in the division of the radial nerve near the wrist joint, the simplest technique is to inject up to 10 ml of 1% lignocaine subcutaneously round the radial border of the wrist at the level of the ulnar and median nerve blocks. The injection should extend from the middle of the dorsum of the wrist, round the radial side to the middle of the palmar surface of the wrist (Figure 8.4).

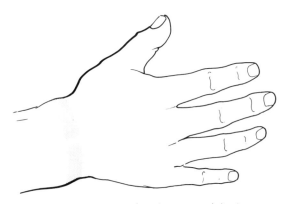

Figure 8.4 Wrist block (back). Subcutaneous injections

This triple block should provide analgesia of all digits and the whole hand except for the proximal 1–2 cm of the palmar aspect of the hand immediately distal to the wrist joint.

Digital nerve block

This is a simple block which is also safe provided that: (1) not more than 4 ml solution are injected into each finger, and (2) solutions containing adrenaline are strictly avoided. All injections should be made through the dorsal surface of the finger using a small-bore (27 G or 25 G) needle. Inject 1 ml of 1% lignocaine subcutaneously over each side of the dorsal aspect of the proximal phalanx at the level of the finger web. Insert the needle past each side of the phalanx until it is palpable on the palmar surface of the digit and inject a further 1 ml of lignocaine.

Lower limb surgery

The most suitable form of regional block for major surgery of the lower limb is usually unilateral spinal anaesthesia or epidural anaesthesia which are outwith the scope of this chapter. However, useful analgesia can be obtained by specific nerve blocks or by IVRA.

Intravenous regional analgesia (IVRA)

This is less satisfactory in the lower limb than the arm because: (1) venepuncture in the foot is more difficult and more painful; (2) good exsanguination is more difficult; and (3) often very large volumes (60–80 ml) of local anaesthetic solution are necessary. This increases the likelihood of toxic systemic reactions on cuff deflation.

The technique is as for IVRA in the upper limb with prilocaine (Citanest), 0.5% being the local anaesthetic of choice; the cuff around the thigh should be inflated to about 450 mmHg or 60–80 mmHg above the level at which the dorsalis pedis pulse disappears.

Local anaesthesia for long saphenous vein ligation and stripping

The area of the leg involved in ligation and stripping of the long saphenous vein is supplied by the femoral nerve and its superficial and deep branches. Femoral nerve block alone is usually adequate but separate injection of the proximal incision line is recommended as a routine procedure (Figure 8.5).

Technique of femoral nerve block

Palpate for the femoral arterial pulse 2 cm below the inguinal ligament and raise a skin weal 1 cm lateral to the artery using 1% lignocaine or 1% prilocaine in 1:200 000 adrenaline. Insert a needle perpendicular to the skin surface to a depth of 3–4 cm and lying lateral to the femoral pulse. Detection of accidental femoral artery puncture is best obtained

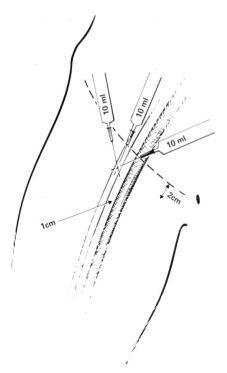

Figure 8.5 Femoral nerve block and subcutaneous infiltration for varicose veins surgery

by using the needle without a syringe attached. Inject 10 ml of the same solution as used for the skin weal. Withdraw the needle to a depth of 0.5 cm and re-insert at an angle of 15° medial and lateral to the initial position. Extra care should be taken to ensure the absence of arterial puncture in the medial position. Thus a total of 30 ml of local anaesthetic solution is injected in the region of the femoral nerve. A further 8–10 ml should be used to infiltrate the line of the groin incision.

Nerve block at the ankle

Anterior tibial nerve

Raise a skin weal midway between the lateral and medial malleoli about 1 cm proximal to a line joining the tips of the malleoli. Through the skin weal insert a needle immediately lateral to the tendon of extensor hallucis longus and direct it towards the medial surface of the medial malleolus. At a depth of 3–4 cm inject 5 ml of 1% lignocaine or prilocaine in adrenaline and a further 5 ml as the needle is withdrawn.

Saphenous nerve

Inject 7 ml of solution around the long saphenous vein on the anterior surface of the medial malleolus at a level approximately 2 cm proximal to the tip of the malleolus.

Musculocutaneous nerve

This nerve supplies the greatest area of the dorsum of the foot and runs between the tibia and fibula above the ankle joint. It divides at a variable distance above the ankle and is most effectively blocked by injecting about 10 ml of solution subcutaneously between the fronts of the tibia and fibula some 3–4 cm proximal to the tips of the malleoli.

Sural nerve

Through a skin weal 1 cm behind and proximal to the tip of the lateral malleolus inject 7 ml of solution between the malleolar surface and the skin.

Posterior tibial nerve

This is located near the posterior tibial artery pulse on the posterior border of the medial malleolus between it and the Achilles tendon. At a depth which is almost down to the posterior surface of the tibia inject 10 ml of solution while moving the needle in and out over a distance of 2 cm.

The total volume of solution for complete foot block at the ankle is 45–50 ml and thus the local anaesthetic should be used in combination with a vasoconstrictor.

Local anaesthesia for inguinal and femoral herniorrhaphy

This block involves the use of large volumes of local anaesthetic solution. It is therefore important to select either lignocaine 0.5% with adrenaline or prilocaine 0.5% with or without adrenaline and to keep note of the dose of local anaesthetic being injected. The use of a vasoconstrictor, apart from allowing a larger dose of local anaesthetic to be given safely also helps to delineate the field of analgesia by virtue of the skin blanching produced after subcutaneous infiltration.

The object is to block the iliohypogastric, ilio-inguinal and genitofemoral nerves together with cutaneous fibres from the opposite side. Separate injections are also required to obtain analgesia in the region of the pubic tubercle and the deep inguinal ring (Figure 8.6).

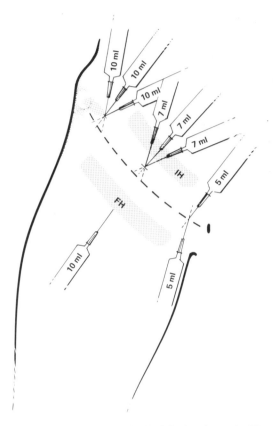

Figure 8.6 Local anaesthetic block for hernia repair: IH, injection of inguinal incision line; FH, subinguinal approach for femoral hernia

Technique

1. Using a small needle raise three skin weals as follows:
   (a) Two cm medial to the anterior superior iliac spine;
   (b) Directly over the pubic tubercle; and
   (c) Over the deep inguinal ring, 1–2 cm above the midpoint of the inguinal ligament.
2. Using a longer needle, preferably with a short bevel, inject 5 ml of solution subcutaneously between weal (a) and the anterior superior iliac spine. Inject three doses of 10 ml of solution in a fan-shape in the transverse plane, ensuring that each injection is deposited deep to the external oblique aponeurosis which is penetrated with a distinct click. The most lateral injection should be started with the needle in contact with the iliac bone below the iliac spine and the most medial injection should be vertically downwards through weal (a) to a depth of about 3 cm. (Total injected so far: 35 ml, including 5 ml for skin weals.)

3. Through weal (b) inject 5 ml of solution directly on to the pubic tubercle, a further 5 ml lateral to the tubercle at a depth of 2–3 cm and a further 10 ml subcutaneously towards the umbilicus for a distance of about 8 cm. (Total volume of solution: 35 + 20 = 55 ml.)
4. Through weal (c) pass the needle perpendicularly backwards to penetrate the external oblique aponeurosis. Inject 20 ml of solution in a fan-shape in the line of the inguinal ligament. This will block the genitofemoral nerve and possibly also the neck of the hernial (inguinal) sac. (Total: 55 + 20 = 75 ml.)
5. Inject 10 ml of solution subcutaneously in the line of the skin incision. (Total: 75 + 10 = 85 ml.)
6. During dissection of the hernial sac pain may be produced by peritoneal traction and this should be treated by injecting 10 ml of solution into the neck of the sac. A larger volume (up to 20 ml) may be necessary when dealing with a wide-necked or obstructed hernial sac. (Total: 85 + 10 to 20 = 95 to 105 ml.)

Local anaesthetic techniques for postoperative pain relief

In recent years there has been increasing interest in the use of local anaesthetic drugs for providing partial or complete relief of pain after surgery. This has arisen largely because of greater experience with the long-acting local anaesthetic bupivacaine, which acts for up to 6 h.

There are several important advantages in using local anaesthetic techniques for pain relief:

1. The avoidance of powerful narcotic analgesics (mainly of the opiate group) with their attendant side effects including nausea, vomiting, respiratory depression, and delayed mobilization.
2. The ability to avoid exacerbating the respiratory problems in patients with obstructive airways disease (asthma, emphysema, chronic bronchitis). Even in the absence of significant preoperative respiratory disease, simple local anaesthetic techniques can reduce postoperative complications, particularly after upper abdominal surgery.
3. The maintenance of the alert state, which allows earlier cooperation with postoperative instructions and physiotherapy.
4. The capacity to relieve pain completely or almost completely, if necessary using repeat injections of local anaesthetic. This improves patient morale and reduces fear, especially in patients who require a series of surgical procedures. Local anaesthetic methods of postoperative pain relief are particularly helpful and rewarding in relation to surgery in children.

5. The reduction or omission of systemic analgesic drugs in patients with impaired ability to metabolize or eliminate these drugs. This is particularly valuable in patients with significant liver or kidney impairment, although the ability to clear local anaesthetic drugs may also be reduced.

Techniques for pain relief

More complex methods of pain relief (such as continuous epidural block and caudal block) are used by many anaesthetists. However, experience of such techniques and the management of the potentially serious complications do not normally form part of surgical training, and so they are not described here.

Although any of the techniques already described for intraoperative local analgesia can also be used for postoperative analgesia, it is usually possible to employ simpler methods and lower doses of local anaesthetic for purely postoperative pain relief. In general, while intraoperative analgesia needs to be complete, valuable degrees of pain relief can be achieved even with limited or incomplete blocks in the postoperative period.

Upper abdominal surgery

Useful pain relief and improved lung function can be obtained by irrigation with a local anaesthetic of wounds which are closed in layers (as distinct from mass closure). After closure of the peritoneum, a perforated catheter (10 Fg Drevac) is placed for the length of the wound between the peritoneum and the muscles of the abdominal wall. The catheter is exteriorized through a separate stab skin incision (or using a sharp-pointed 10 Fg trocar) and sutured in place at the medial or superior end of the incision. The catheter is connected to a bacterial filter (Millex-GS, Millipore) using a short cannula (20 G or 18 G Medicut). A three-way tap is then connected and 10–15 ml bupivacaine 0.5% is injected. The tap is then turned off towards the patient. The same dose of bupivacaine is repeated at intervals of 4–6 h as required for about 48 h, after which the catheter is removed.

This technique has not caused detectable wound infection in a series of cholecystectomies, but it should not be used in the presence of intra-abdominal sepsis.

Inguinal herniorrhaphy

Adequate postoperative pain relief may be obtained by a simplification of the technique described for intraoperative local anaesthesia. The objective is to block the iliohypogastric and ilio-inguinal nerves in their course between the internal and external oblique muscles.

Through a point 2 cm medial to the anterior superior iliac spine insert a short-bevel needle deep to the external oblique aponeurosis and inject 10 ml bupivacaine 0.5%. Using an in-and-out vertical movement of 1–2 cm deep to the external oblique inject a further 10 ml of solution. This block will provide pain relief for up to 6 h after which it may be repeated. It is rarely necessary to repeat the block more than once.

The same technique may be used after herniotomy in children, but bupivacaine 0.25% should be used in volumes appropriate to the child's body weight. In order to avoid causing distress to children, Emla cream under an occlusive dressing should be applied to the site of injection at least 1 h beforehand and the injection should be made very slowly. Valuable pain relief can be obtained in children by injecting bupivacaine subcutaneously and deep to the external oblique at the lateral end of the wound during surgical exposure, and in adults direct injection of the ilio-inguinal nerve may provide satisfactory analgesia.

Penile block

This is valuable in adults after circumcision and in children after circumcision or urethroplasty. Place an index finger on the pubic symphysis and direct the needle past the finger tip at about 15° from the midline to lie just below the inferior margin of the pubis. After negative aspiration for blood inject 5 ml bupivacaine 0.5% on each side of the midline, moving the depth of the needle by 1 cm during injection (adult), or 0.5–2.5 ml bupivacaine 0.25% on each side (child).

In penile block adrenaline should never be used. Ring block of the penis is unnecessary since the nerve supply enters only along the dorsum.

Digital block

This simple block is useful during and after surgery of the toes, such as treatment of ingrowing toenails. For analgesia of the great toe in an adult inject 0.5% bupivacaine 0.5–1 ml in each of four areas as follows: two on the dorsal surface subcutaneously near the base of the proximal phalanx, injecting at points midway between the extensor tendons and the margins of the toe; two by inserting the needle beyond the two dorsal injections and past the phalanx to lie subcutaneously on the plantar surface. The needle depth is easily felt and controlled by an index finger placed on the plantar surface of the toe.

Subcutaneous bupivacaine

Although the above techniques may provide almost complete pain relief, useful degrees of analgesia can be obtained by the simple method of injecting bupivacaine subcutaneously into surgical wounds before closure of the skin. This may be used in virtually any wound which is surgically clean, including incisions for abdominal surgery, herniorrhaphy, nephrectomy, thoracotomy and breast lumps.

Dosage of bupivacaine

For postoperative pain relief the dose of bupi-vacaine in any 4 h period should not exceed the levels shown in Table 8.2.

Table 8.2

Body weight (kg)	Maximum volume 0.25% (ml)	Maximum volume 0.5% (ml)
10	8	Not recommended
20	16	Not recommended
30	24	Not recommended
40	32	16
50	40	20
60	48	24
70 and over	56	28

9

Preparation for operation

J. A. R. Smith

In the early days of surgical practice success depended on operative skill and speed. Anaesthetic advances have reduced the need for speed, and while operative skill remains important, there is little doubt that the improvements seen in surgical results over the past few decades have been due to the realization of the importance of careful pre-operative and postoperative management. Greater understanding of the physiological and metabolic consequences of disease and of surgery has been applied to patients' care with satisfying results but there is no room for complacency. The preoperative period not only allows time for careful assessment of the patient, but also permits him to develop a relationship with medical, nursing and ancillary staff which allays anxieties and helps postoperative management.

History

In surgical practice, the patient's problem is often more straightforward than in other specialties and the general health is otherwise excellent. However, the importance of a careful history cannot be over-emphasized and with care and experience will provide over 70% of the information required to reach the correct diagnosis.

Presenting complaint

Whether the presenting complaint is simple, such as the development of a groin swelling, or more vague, such as abdominal discomfort and weight loss, the same general principles apply. Thus, the duration of the presenting complaint, associated features and both precipitating and relieving factors, must be recorded. With continuing experience, the impor-

tant associated features can be recognized and more specific enquiry made to narrow the differential diagnosis.

Systematic enquiry

This is of great importance in the assessment of the patient and to establish any additional associated features which may have been overlooked. In a non-specific way it provides an assessment of the patient's general wellbeing: it may be possible to identify any features which are of greater import-ance than the presenting complaint, e.g. to discover symptoms of bronchial neoplasm in the patient who presents simply with a hernia or with piles. Finally, it is essential to make a specific assessment, particularly as regards the cardiorespiratory systems, as to the patient's fitness for anaesthesia. It is in this section of the history that one begins to be able to make a balanced judgement between the patient's need for a surgical procedure for his presenting complaint and his ability in terms of general health to tolerate the treatment that might be required. The most important adage of all is 'above all else, to do no harm'.

Past medical history

This is of importance to identify any episodes similar to the presenting complaint in the past. It may identify any previous surgical procedures which may or may not be related to the presenting complaint. To identify any illnesses which might interfere with general wellbeing is as important as it is to recognize any disease which would be a positive contraindi-cation to extensive investigation and treatment. Except in the direst emergencies, it is undesirable for a patient who has had a myocardial infarction to have a general anaesthetic prior to operation within 3–6 months of the infarct. The risk of further infarction is 75% with a mortality rate of 25%. It is necessary to record any history of bleeding disorders, or of such specific diseases as tuberculosis, diabetes mellitus or rheumatic fever.

Social history

This is important to identify first the work requirements of the patient, and secondly any possible precipitating factor in the work environment. Furthermore, the patient's smoking and drinking habits and his spare-time occupation, such as his enjoyment of exercise, are important to record.

The patients domestic situation should be investigated as this will influence the time of discharge from hospital and the need for convalescent facilities.

Family history

This may provide pointers to the diagnosis for illnesses with a familial disposition, e.g. gallstones or duodenal ulceration. In addition, in those situations where, for example, gastroenteritis masquerades as acute appendicitis, the history within the family unit may be of vital importance. As in the past medical history, it is necessary specifically to exclude diabetes mellitus, tuberculosis or rheumatic fever.

Drug history

Any medicament being taken by the patient must be recorded, not only because certain agents may precipitate surgical illness, e.g. haematemesis resulting from aspirin ingestion, but also because certain drugs will interfere with surgical management, e.g. treatment with anticoagulants. In female patients, the taking of the oral contraceptive pill should also be recorded in view of the increased incidence of deep vein thrombosis after surgery in this particular group. It must also be recorded whether or not the patient has any allergies to particular agents and whether, in the past, the patient has had any blood transfusion and for what reason.

The importance of drug interaction must be remembered, especially when a new agent is prescribed and results in an adverse reaction. It is not uncommon for a patient to deny symptoms, e.g. of cardiorespiratory disease, only for the doctor to find out he is on drugs which have clearly treated such disease effectively!

Industrial history

Could the disease or lesion result from some industrial hazard? Did a hernia appear during heavy work? Was the patient exposed to aniline dyes or asbestos many years ago?

Physical examination

A thorough physical examination is mandatory and although this may concentrate initially on the system suggested by the presenting complaint, a full examination of all the systems is essential if associated features are to be identified, if an accurate assessment of the patient's general health is to be obtained and, in particular, if conditions which might make treatment more difficult or impossible are to be identified and where possible, treated. For example, if it is thought that the primary diagnosis is some neoplasm, it is clearly important to identify any possible metastatic spread in the sites appropriate for the primary growth, e.g. lungs, liver, bone, etc.

It cannot be over-emphasized that all data obtained must be recorded accurately, with particular reference to clear description of the side of any unilateral problem. Certain features which are often overlooked are the presence of lymphadenopathy and the findings of digital rectal examination. Pulse and blood pressure, temperature and a general assessment of the patient's health are also recorded and although difficult to define in precise scientific terms, with experience it is usually possible to reach some conclusions about the patient's general mental state and his likely tolerance of any surgical treatment. This assessment can be particularly important where the initial presenting complaint is somewhat vague and does not fall clearly into a particular category.

Investigations

If an accurate history and careful physical examination are performed, then there is a greater than 85% chance either of having reached a definitive diagnosis or having identified a particular treatment plan. Thus, in general terms, any investigation should serve either to confirm or refute a particular diagnosis or to add information about the general assessment of the patient concerned. *The fewer investigations done the better.* The argument that hospital admission provides an opportunity to screen all patients can easily be refuted by the low incidences of unexpected diseases that are diagnosed. However, certain preliminary investigations are obligatory and others will clearly be dictated by the likely differential diagnosis.

Urine specimen

A urine specimen must be obtained and tested for the presence of sugar, albumin and ketone bodies. Any obvious abnormality of colour or content can readily be identified.

Full blood count

A full blood count, which includes assessment of haemoglobin, packed cell volume, total and differential white cell count, blood film and erythrocyte sedimentation rate, must be undertaken.

In any patient undergoing surgery, a critical assessment must be made of his likely need for blood transfusion. Certain operations will have such minimal blood loss that even cross-matching is not required. The tendency at present is to cross-match fewer and fewer patients. In patients undergoing ulcer surgery, cholecystectomy and even small bowel resection, transfusion is seldom required. For more major procedures, grouping the patient's blood and saving the patient's serum for matching should transfusion be required is an acceptable practice. Only for procedures such as oesophageal, hepatic, total gastric or colorectal resections is formal grouping and matching required.

In patients who are jaundiced or who have specific haematological defects, fresh blood, fresh frozen plasma or preparation of specific clotting factors may be required and need to be arranged well in advance of surgery.

Of the other investigations available, the ones which are most common to arrange in surgical practice are as follows.

Urea and electrolytes

Certainly in any patient who has had gastrointestinal pathology or who will be having an operation which will involve intravenous infusion with or without nasogastric suction, it is valuable to know what the baseline measurements of urea and electrolytes are. Where these are found to be abnormal, it is essential that these are corrected as far as possible before undertaking any surgery. This is particularly relevant to emergency surgery.

Chest X-ray

Even the majority of anaesthetists have now come to recognize that not all patients undergoing operation under general anaesthesia require a 'routine' chest X-ray. However, for patients over the age of 45 undergoing major surgery, or patients with a history suggestive of chronic obstructive airways disease, and most important of all, in patients who have primary malignant disease elsewhere, chest X-ray is essential.

Electrocardiogram

This is required in any patient with a history suggestive of ischaemic heart disease and in all patients over the age of 45.

Faecal occult blood tests

This is important in any patient with anaemia and patients suspected of having peptic ulceration or gastrointestinal neoplasia. However, at the present time the commercially available tests, although very convenient for side-room use, are either too insensitive or are over-sensitive. Thus the majority of such specimens must be sent to the biochemistry laboratory and, for obvious reasons, a degree of selectivity is required if laboratory services are not to be overworked. Of the side-room tests available, Haemoccult II is the most widely used and the most reliable.

Blood sugar tests

In any patient who is shown to have glycosuria, a random and/or fasting blood sugar test is required. It must be remembered that a proportion of some previously undiagnosed diabetics will be admitted to hospital. If undetected, anaesthetic and perioperative problems are more likely to occur. Any patient with preoperative glycosuria must be investigated further, involving a specialist in diabetes mellitus where possible.

Liver function tests

These tests will be important in the differentiation of the various causes of jaundice and will also be measured in any patient who has palpable hepatomegaly at the time of physical examination. It must be remembered that about 75% of the liver must be diseased before there is any serious impairment in liver function as measured by blood tests, and thus the presence of normal liver function tests does not necessarily mean that the liver is functioning normally. An elevated alkaline phosphatase in the absence of jaundice may be the first biochemical hint of liver metastases or of a bile duct stone in an elderly patient.

Platelet count

In patients who are jaundiced or have any history of it, it is important to arrange a platelet count and to have a haematological screen of any clotting abnormality.

In most cases, any abnormality detected during these investigations will require accurate evaluation and will merit further investigation before treatment and surgery are commenced.

Ultrasound

Perhaps the most reliable way of assessing the liver, if liver function tests have demonstrated abnormality, is to perform an ultrasound examination and this is shown to be more accurate than radio-isotope scanning in the detection of metastatic deposits. Ultrasound is also an effective method of detecting bile duct dilatation in the investigation of jaundice and has also a part to play in the investigation of abnormal masses, abscesses, abdominal aortic aneurysms, heart valve lesions, etc.

Computed tomographic (CT) scan

Computer-aided whole body tomography is now more widely available. It is of particular relevance in the management of head injury, differentiating between intracranial haemorrhage and oedema. It has also proved of value in the investigation of the liver, biliary system and pancreas, and of retroperitoneal or mediastinal structures.

Nuclear magnetic resonance (NMR)

Nuclear magnetic resonance is developing rapidly and carries the advantage of not involving ionizing radiation. This form of imaging is most valuable in neurology but can be used to test function of organs as well as to provide pictures. It is likely that the application of NMR will continue to increase.

Special problems
Obesity

Obesity is an increasing problem in surgical practice and while patients presenting for emergency surgery may have to take their chance, supported by any prophylactic measures available, it is inadvisable to perform elective surgery on the grossly obese patient without controlled attempts at weight loss by supervised dieting. The patient who is obese is at risk because:

1. Any procedure is technically more difficult as exposure is impaired and thus errors are more likely to occur.
2. In the postoperative period there is an increased risk of infection in wound, in deep structures and in the chest and therefore prophylactic antibiotics must be used.
3. Obesity carries an increased risk of venous thromboembolic disease.
4. With the difficulties of haemostasis and the increased risk of wound infection, obesity also has a higher risk of wound dehiscence and incisional herniation.

However, it is important to emphasize that sudden crash dieting should not be encouraged as this itself may complicate surgery which follows rapidly on weight reduction. It is in this field that a dietitian has a particularly important part to play in ensuring that not only is weight lost but that a suitably balanced diet is ingested during this time.

Malnutrition

Malnutrition occurs in varying degrees but the significance of minor degrees is difficult to define. However, in any patient who has lost more than 15% of his ideal body weight in the course of the illness which has precipitated surgery, there is an increased morbidity and mortality following operation. Similar figures for increased morbidity result if the plasma albumin is less than 30 g/l. In practice, malnutrition is seldom simply that of starvation, and the contribution of the disease process acting either as an obstruction or by itself interfering with normal body metabolism, is very important.

The evidence in favour of correcting malnutrition prior to surgery is not convincing where weight loss of less than 15% has taken place and it is probably sufficient to ensure that such patients have a high calorie, high protein intake during preparation for surgery, using the oral route wherever possible. The active cooperation of a dietitian in providing support and, if necessary, a liquidized diet or one of the commercially available preparations, is vital. Any form of nutritional support needs to provide carbohydrate, protein, fat, electrolytes, trace elements and vitamins. In surgical practice the importance of zinc and vitamin C in ensuring wound healing must be remembered.

Parenteral nutritional support is increasingly popular as all these requirements can be met, but this form of therapy is not without risk and the evidence in favour of its routine use in the malnourished surgical patient has not yet been reported.

Of greater importance is to ensure that any hypoalbuminaemia and any fluid and electrolyte imbalance consequent upon malnutrition are corrected prior to surgery.

Anaemia

The anaemic patient falls into two main categories in the preoperative period:

1. The patient who is anaemic because of some gastrointestinal pathology which is unlikely to respond prior to surgery, e.g. bleeding chronic duodenal ulcer; ulcerating gastrointestinal tumour. In this type of patient a balanced judgement is required, aiming to restore blood volume and haemoglobin as far as possible and then proceeding to early surgery to prevent further loss.
2. A more difficult problem is the patient who is chronically anaemic either because of the disease process or because of malnutrition. Current evidence would now suggest that provided the haemoglobin is 10 g/dl or above, and provided the patient does not have myocardial disease, then the ability of the myocardium to increase cardiac output will ensure that even at this level of haemoglobin, oxygen delivery to the tissues is adequate. Thus, in this group of patients, any requirements for blood transfusion can be deferred to the postoperative period.

Where the anaemia is more severe than the above, the treatment will depend on the urgency of the procedure. It may be sufficient to correct anaemia by iron supplements, or if surgery is more urgent, correction may be by blood transfusion alone. However, it must be remembered that transfusing stored blood has certain risks and that stored red cells are poor transporters of oxygen so that transfusion may restore blood volume but will not immediately restore oxygen delivery potential. Furthermore there is some evidence that in bowel surgery, blood transfusion increases the risk of wound infection and impairs prognosis.

Where blood loss has been acute, it may be helpful to optimize the time of surgery by the use of central venous pressure monitoring, particularly in the older age group of patients in whom myocardial disease is more likely to be present and for whom the risks of congestive failure are greatest.

Diabetic patients

Diabetic patients are at increased risk in surgery, partly because of the problems of wound infection and impaired healing, and partly because of alterations in the catabolic response to surgery. Furthermore there is an increased risk of cardiac and of renal disease, and this must be assessed carefully before elective surgery.

The main aims are to avoid both hypoglycaemia and ketoacidosis. In insulin-dependent diabetics the following routine should be carried out:

1. On the day before surgery obtain a blood glucose profile.
2. Plan surgery for as early on a *morning* list as possible.
3. When oral intake stops, start infusing each 5 h 500 ml of 5% dextrose in water, each containing 5 mmol KCl and 8 units Actrapid insulin.
4. Hourly, do Dextrostix tests and 2 h postoperatively arrange formal blood sugar, urea and electrolyte estimations.
5. Aim to maintain blood sugar between 5 and 10 mmol by adjusting insulin by ±2 units per 500 ml 5% dextrose.
6. Adjust potassium to keep at upper end of normal range (3.3–5.5 mmol/l).
7. Replace requirements for sodium, plasma or blood, in addition to 5% dextrose regimen.
8. Daily blood sugar profiles are needed while regimen in progress.

In non-insulin-dependent diabetics, observe urine tests using BM sticks. Avoid long-acting oral hypoglycaemic agents, and omit short-acting agents on the morning of surgery. Therapy is resumed with the first postoperative day. Remember, too, that the stress of major surgery may result in insulin being required for the first time in non-dependent patients, at least in the short term.

The elderly patient

Elderly patients are usually grouped together as a 'poor risk group'. In the absence of any coexisting medical condition, the very fact of survival to old age usually means that they respond remarkably well, even to major surgical procedures. However, it must be remembered that the reserves available are more limited and that considerable care must be taken as regards fluid replacement, chest infection, etc.

Elderly patients are much more likely to be taking certain medicaments and this is particularly important where the cardiovascular and respiratory systems are concerned. An additional feature to note in the elderly patient is that a moderate degree of hypertension may be for them normal, and may be essential to ensure adequate cerebral perfusion. Thus, fairly modest reductions in blood pressure during and after surgery may be more catastrophic to the elderly patient than to a younger counterpart.

The elderly patients are more sensitive to the effects of certain analgesic or narcotic agents and as over-sedation will further increase the risk of bronchopneumonia, smaller dosage will be required. Partly because of frailty and general immobility, elderly patients are more likely to develop venous thromboembolic disease and because of skin fragility, are more likely to develop bed sores in the postoperative period. Preoperative physiotherapy and fuller explanation than usual of these problems may help to minimize the risk in the postoperative period.

Jaundice

Patients who have jaundice due either to obstruction or to hepatocellular disease are a high risk group of patients. Because obstructed bile is infected in more than 95% of these cases, such patients are at risk from infection both in the wound and in other sites. Thus, prophylactic antibiotics are indicated.

For reasons which are not absolutely clear jaundiced patients have a higher incidence of renal failure in the postoperative period – the hepatorenal syndrome. This may be due to something as simple as abnormal fluid shifts occurring in such patients in response to surgery, or to the endotoxinaemia which may complicate surgery to the obstructed infected biliary system. Alternatively, it may be due to the deposition of bilirubin in the renal tubules, or to impaired handling by the obstructed liver of the various hormones responsible for normal renal function. It is important that all jaundiced patients have an adequate fluid load throughout the operation and in the postoperative period. It is customary for such patients to have an osmotic diuretic such as an infusion of 10% mannitol intraoperatively. In this group of patients, urinary output must be monitored by a urethral catheter and maintained at over 40 ml/hr.

Patients with jaundice and impaired liver function have a higher incidence of clotting abnormalities. This may be because of the disruption of liver function or because of the failure of absorption of vitamin K due to the relative absence of bile for fat absorption in the intestine. Thus the prothrombin time must be measured and vitamin K given i.m. prophylactically to minimize the risk of bleeding during and after surgery.

Patients with jaundice, especially those where the jaundice is secondary to malignant disease, have a poor record of wound healing and in order to minimize the risk of wound dehiscence, careful mass closure with non-absorbable sutures ought to be used.

Because of the impairment of liver function, there is a greater risk of such patients becoming hypoalbuminaemic and any deficits of plasma or blood volume must be corrected. Finally, patients with liver disease tend to retain salt and thus excessive use of saline solutions must be avoided.

Endocrine abnormalities

(see Chapter 22)

Hyperthyroid patients tolerate surgery badly and thus toxicity must be controlled therapeutically prior to any surgical procedure. This may be achieved by any of the antithyroid preparations, such as carbimazole, but it is customary now for those patients in whom early surgery is required for beta-blockers, such as propranolol, to be used to protect the heart against the effects of surgery in the hyperthyroid state.

Patients undergoing operation for phaeochromocytoma of the adrenal medulla are a particularly difficult problem. Very close cooperation between clinician and anaesthetist is essential before, during and after surgery, if such patients are to survive. Control of blood pressure may require the judicious use of both α- and β-antagonists. It is clear that such patients should be dealt with in specialist centres.

The most important endocrine abnormality of all concerns the *adrenal cortical hormones*. Any patient who has received steroid therapy in the 6 months prior to surgery requires parenteral steroids to cover the period of operation as their own reserves in response to the stress of surgery may be inadequate. It is usual to give 100 mg of hydrocortisone at the time of induction of anaesthetic; to give 100 mg q.i.d. for the first 24–48 h and gradually to diminish the dosage in the postoperative period.

Impaired renal function

The commonest problem in the urinary system after surgery is acute retention and thus a history of prostatism should put the surgeon on his guard. More insidious, however, is the chronic renal failure secondary to chronic retention of urine, so that any electrolyte disturbance detected before or after surgery must be thoroughly investigated and corrected.

Remediable causes of impaired renal function, such as obstruction, hypertension or congestive cardiac failure, must be recognized and treated preoperatively.

The contribution to impaired renal function of urinary tract infection must be remembered and any such infection treated. Instrumentation of the infected urinary tract, e.g. by catheterization or cystoscopy, carries a high risk of septicaemia and septic shock.

Where renal failure results in hyperkalaemia, potassium exchange resin, such as Resonium administered rectally, may be effective as an emergency treatment. Alternatively, the combination of infusion of 50% dextrose, together with intravenous insulin, will be sufficient to force potassium into the cells and thus reduce the risk of cardiac arrhythmia.

This must be seen as a 'first-aid measure' and steps taken thereafter to correct the underlying cause.

Where the patient is in established renal failure, collaboration with the renal physician may mean that a combination of dialysis, either peritoneal or haemodialysis, may be used to prepare the patient sufficiently well for surgery to be permissible.

It is important to remember that patients with impaired renal function are more susceptible to developing abnormalities of electrolytes but also that their clearance of drugs, including antibiotics, will be impaired and this is particularly important in those agents whose toxicity is related to blood levels, e.g. gentamicin.

Oral hygiene

Improved dental care in the UK has meant that the problem of dental sepsis and carious teeth is much reduced. However, there is little doubt that dental sepsis may contribute to postoperative infection and where oral hygiene is particularly bad, dental treatment may be required before elective surgery is carried out.

Anticipation of complications

Cardiac disease

Emergency treatment

Patients who have had a recent myocardial infarction, i.e. within 3–6 months, should not have a general anaesthetic unless the risks of not operating outweigh the increased risk of mortality which would occur. Where surgery is thought to be obligatory, some form of local or regional anaesthesia is to be preferred,

Where the cardiac problem is one of angina secondary to ischaemic heart disease, it is important to liaise with the anaesthetist and a cardiologist about the preoperative use of digitalis or beta-blockers. It is also necessary to be extremely careful in the postoperative period as regards the prescription of intravenous fluids.

When the patient is in frank congestive cardiac failure, the risks of operation and the risks of not operating must again be judged for the individual patient. If it is decided that surgery is unavoidable, then treatment with digitalis and with diuretic drugs must be part of the preoperative preparation. Treatment should contine after surgery, where the necessity for monitoring carefully any fluid infusion cannot be over-emphasized.

Elective surgery

In this situation in particular, cooperation with an expert in cardiological medicine is of great value.

Patients should not have elective surgery under general anaesthetic within 6 months of myocardial infarction. Otherwise it is important that such conditions as cardiac arrhythmias, congestive cardiac failure and hypertension are under medical control before any elective procedure is carried out. However, the introduction of more effective methods of controlling hypertension has made it unnecessary for such agents to be withdrawn prior to surgery. It is clearly important that in the postoperative period accurate control of electrolytes, particularly potassium, takes place.

General

Any patient who has congenital or rheumatic heart disease or who has had open heart surgery with valve replacement must be covered during and after the operative period with prophylactic antibiotics, the present favoured drug being cefuroxime.

Respiratory disease

One of the most important respiratory considerations of all is to ensure that all patients who smoke are warned prior to their name being put on the waiting list of the benefits of their stopping smoking prior to surgery

The history and physical examination will give some indication of the existence and severity of any obstructive airways disease. The degree of dyspnoea and the amount of exertion required to precipitate dyspnoea are important points to establish. Where there is any doubt about respiratory reserve, more sophisticated tests of respiratory function are now available and of these, the vital capacity, the forced expiratory volume and the forced expiratory volume in the first second are probably the most important parameters to assess. In the more severe cases, assessment of arterial blood gases is important, both to estimate the severity of the airways disease and also to give some indication of the methods of management in the postoperative period, i.e. the likelihood of artificial ventilation being required.

Any sputum must be cultured preoperatively and as would happen in the postoperative period, antibiotic sensitivity should be assessed. Where the sputum is purulent, elective surgery should not take place until the infection has been cleared by a combination of physiotherapy and antibiotic therapy. Various sprays and bronchial dilators are now available but should only be used under careful supervision. In this regard, the benefits of preoperative physiotherapy are well established.

As for cardiac disease, the decision to proceed or not with surgery will depend on the indications for that surgical procedure, but there has been a tendency towards elective ventilatory support in the postoperative period where there is any doubt about the patient's respiratory reserve and where major surgery is believed to be absolutely necessary.

Thromboembolic disease

It is now possible to categorize certain patients who are at high risk of developing vein thrombosis, e.g. those having pelvic surgery, patients who are obese and patients with peripheral vascular disease. The risk is greater in older age groups, in patients with neoplastic disorders and those who are obese. A past history of varicose veins or of throboembolism must be sought.

Managing patients on the oral contraceptive pill can be difficult. There is an increased risk of deep vein thrombosis, and ideally the pill should be stopped 6 weeks before surgery. Where the risk of pregnancy is unacceptable to the patient concerned, the risk of deep vein thrmobosis must be discussed with the patients and prophylaxis advised.

Prophylaxis

Patients over the age of 45 undergoing major surgery or surgery involving the hip or pelvis should have specific prophylaxis using calcium heparin, 5000 units subcutaneously, 2 h prior to surgery, continuing two or three times a day until the patient is fully mobilized. In addition, early mobilization is recommended. The use of specific graduated compression stockings, in conjunction with subcutaneous heparin, is recommended for high-risk patients.

Impaired wound healing

A number of conditions predisposing to impairment of wound healing have been identified. Not all are avoidable or preventable, but it is vital either to prevent them if possible or to alter surgical techniques to minimize the risk of wound failure.

Serious malnutrition (weight loss of greater than 20% of ideal body weight; serum albumin less than 30 g/l) interferes with wound healing as does jaundice secondary to malignant disease. Steroid therapy, irradiation and wound infection are important as are obesity or poorly controlled diabetes mellitus.

However, the most important is to recognize the various risk factors before, not after, surgery.

Wound infection

Infection after 'clean' abdominal procedures is uncommon and usually reflects either poor technique or cross-infection.

Most infections are caused by organisms endogenous to the patient. Infection rates are highest where an intestinal organ is breached, e.g. in colorectal surgery, or where there is pre-existing infection, e.g. biliary obstruction, achlorhydric stomach. It is in this group of patients that prophylactic antibiotics are required, an appropriate agent being given intramuscularly with premedication or intravenously at induction to ensure adequate tissue levels at the time of surgery.

Cefuroxime (750 mg) is the agent of choice supplemented with metronidazole (1 g rectally 2 h before surgery or 500 mg intravenously at induction) for colorectal procedures.

Preparation for surgery

The preoperative patient

At the latest on the day before operation, the wound area and its surroundings are shaved thoroughly and the patient bathed. Specific preparation of the bowel for colorectal surgery is considered in Chapter 20 but it remains sensible to prescribe an aperient before any major surgery.

Up-to-date blood results, a chest X-ray and ECG, if indicated, and blood grouping or cross-matching must all be arranged.

Before any medication is given the procedure should be explained to the patient and his written consent witnessed. The evening before surgery may be particularly stressful and a mild hypnotic may be helpful to avoid insomnia.

Where general anaesthesia is to be used or may be used, the patient is fasted for 6 h before operation. In the elderly or diabetic patient, this may necessitate the use of intravenous fluids.

The prophylactic use of antibiotics and heparin has been discussed. Where major surgery or a pelvic procedure is planned, a urethral catheter should be passed. In the male it is often kinder to wait until the patient is anaesthetized.

There is a movement away from the routine use of nasogastric tubes in abdominal surgery. Where there is pyloric or intestinal obstruction, tubes are obligatory but it is more sensible to leave other decisions to the intra-operative period and have a tube passed by the anaesthetist, if indicated.

Frozen section examination may be required when a breast lump, or other potential neoplasm, is to be operated upon; the pathologist should be alerted beforehand.

10

Assisting at operations

J. A. R. Smith

The operating theatre

Advances in surgical technique, in anaesthetic practice, in theatre design and the abilities both of the nursing staff and the operating department assistants, have all served to increase the sophistication and complexity of the modern operating theatre. While this has meant a significant contribution to the improvement in results of surgery, it has also served to emphasize the need for a closely coordinated surgical team, consisting of the surgeon, the theatre sister or scrub nurse, and the anaesthetist and their respective assistants. The precise responsibilities for each individual member of this team varies from establishment to establishment, but the overall responsibility rests with the surgeon performing the operation. While his delegation of duties is a matter for his personal decision, this chapter serves to describe the duties to be performed, certain items of important equipment and to give some indication of how the theatre suite works. Such organization is vital if any surgical procedure is to be performed in such a way that the surgeon and his team can concentrate on the operation in hand and not have to spend considerable time giving repetitious instructions. There is no doubt that the efficiency of the surgical team relates to practice together and to each individual having a feeling of confidence in the other members within that team.

Whether the theatre is a single unit or part of a complex suite, certain areas can be identified. It is important that the particular use of each area is not violated in order that the risk of contamination is kept to a minimum.

The entrance
Personnel

For any person entering the theatre complex, the minimum requirement is the use of overshoes. However, in most modern establishments it is necessary to change completely from outdoor to theatre clothing and in all cases this must be done before entering the theatre itself. Theatre clothing consists of either a dress for nursing staff, or a shirt and trousers for staff of both sexes. The material used should be of cotton and be reasonably cool and freshly laundered for each wearer. The use of modern synthetic materials may be associated with the generation of an electric spark and this is potentially hazardous in the theatre itself. Nowadays, disposable caps and masks are used to minimize the risk of contamination from hair, nose and mouth. In orthopaedic practice, an all-enveloping hood tends to be used. The masks are less permeable than the older cotton masks but it must be remembered that even they become permeable with time and should be changed after long surgical procedures. A malleable rim is now incorporated into most masks at the upper margin to allow the safer wearing of spectacles without the risk of fogging. More recently, it has been suggested that masks are unnecessary because the majority of infecting organisms come from the patient himself. However, even one staphylococcal or streptococcal infection from a member of staff is potentially lethal and ought to be avoided, if the small cost to pay is merely the wearing of a mask. It is usual also to wear antistatic boots or shoes, but these should be restricted to theatre use only. Both the theatre itself and, in some cases, the entire theatre complex, is positively ventilated and thus it is very important that all doors of entry to the theatre and exit from the theatre are kept closed.

Equipment

All members of staff need to know where their own particular equipment is stored and as this is the age of presterilized, prepacked, disposable equipment, the risks of cross-infection are minimal. However, in most hospitals instruments are no longer cleaned and sterilized by the theatre staff themselves, and thus it is important that all trays of instruments returning from the central sterile supply department are checked both for cleanliness and completeness as well as for sterility prior to use. The standard methods now used are change of colour of a vial of fluid contained within the pack itself, combined with change of colour of tape used to bind instrument packs prior to them being placed in the autoclave.

The patient

The patient is brought to the theatre either in his bed or on a trolley, but neither of these should enter the theatre area itself. The patient is transferred onto the theatre trolley or table and is then conveyed into the anaesthetic room and thence into theatre.

Movement into the operating room

Personnel

All staff enter theatre, usually through double doors, into the entry zone which is used for scrubbing, gowning and for storing equipment likely to be required for the procedures to be undertaken in that particular session. The amount of movement in and around the operating room and table itself should be kept to a minimum. There should be doors clearly marked for entry and exit as one-way traffic will minimize the risk of contamination.

Equipment

There should be a separate exit not used by personnel, for the passage of dirty instruments and waste swabs etc, to leave theatre after they have been checked. Clearly this will also minimize the risk of clean equipment becoming contaminated.

The patient

The patient leaves theatre by a special exit door and is conveyed to the recovery room. This allows for the next patient on the list to be accommodated in the anaesthetic room before the end of the first procedure.

Leaving the theatre complex

Personnel and patients leave the theatre complex in a reverse order to that of their entry. However, equipment and soiled goods tend to be passed out of the theatre complex as quickly as possible and many theatres now have a 'dirty corridor' surrounding the theatre complex which can be used to collect waste matter and convey it to disposal units.

Important equipment within the theatre

Various types of operating theatre table are available allowing for different positions of the patient and for rapid elevation of the table as a whole, or the foot or head ends of it. The importance of adequate theatre lighting need not be over-emphasized but, in addition, the operating department assistants need to develop some expertise in directing the light where the surgeon would like it to go. Where access of light is particularly difficult the use of a head lamp is recommended. Facilities within the theatre (usually by providing a hook rack) are essential to allow accurate counting of swabs and packs and there should be facilities for these to be weighed so that by subtracting dry from wet weight, some indication of measured blood loss can be obtained. Within the theatre, the book to record all operations done and by whom, and the fact that the swab count has been correct (see below) is gradually being replaced by computer-worked forms of the Korner type. In addition to any suture material required, it is important to have a supply of pathological specimen jars containing formalin in saline and a supply of pathology forms so that specimens can be conveyed to the laboratory with minimal risk of specimens being mixed up.

Responsibilities of the surgical team

The overall responsibility for the patient's safety and the correct performance of the operation rests with the surgeon. However, in order that he may concentrate his attention entirely on performing the procedure, it is important that he delegates certain responsibilities to his colleagues. Such delegation will vary from team to team and thus the different requirements will be described and some indication given of the likely member of staff on whom these responsibilities will rest.

Before the patient is anaesthetized, it is important that he/she is identified, that the nature of the operation to be performed is confirmed, that dentures are removed and any rings taped. The side of the operation and the particular extremity or digit requiring the operation are all identified. In most units, the responsibility for identifying the side and site of operation is two-fold:

1. That the assistant should mark the side with indelible pen prior to surgery, warning the patient not to wash it off.
2. That the surgeon himself should check with the patient both that the mark is present and that the side marked is correct.

At this stage, it is important to check that the consent form has been signed and that such medicaments as premedication, prophylactic anti-biotics and subcutaneous heparin have, in fact, been given.

It is sensible before commencing the procedure to know that any blood for transfusion is readily available and that the blood provided matches with the patient's name, blood group and hospital number.

It is essential that the various members of the surgical team are fully aware of the procedure that is planned and that any likely complications are discussed prior to commencing the operation. Thus, it is valuable for both the sister and anaesthetist to know if there is any likelihood of the thoracic cavity being entered or whether any major vascular structure is at risk, so that the appropriate clamps can be made available. It is important to check with the anaesthetist about any particular medical problems the patient has. Although he will probably have seen the patient prior to surgery, some cross-check before induction of anaesthesia is important so that any requirements for platelets, antihaemophilic fraction, etc. should be confirmed and the availability of each ensured.

It is particularly important to ensure that the supporting services have been warned the previous day if they are likely to be required, e.g. a pathologist for frozen section histology or a radiographer if any operative cholangiography is to be undertaken.

If the patient has a pacemaker *in situ*, the use of diathermy coagulation must be used with caution, if at all.

The problems of monitoring central venous or arterial pressures are the responsibility of the anaesthetist but where one has been requested, it is necessary that the assistant ensures that an intra-venous infusion has been set up and that a urethral catheter has been passed.

When the patient is brought into theatre, it is the responsibility of the operating department assistant, the surgeon and his assistant to ensure that the patient's position on the table is correct. Thus, no part of the skin surface should be in contact with anything metal if diathermy is to be used. There should be a pad underneath the heels and the arms should be positioned in such a way that they will not interfere with the functions of any member of the operating team. Care should be taken to avoid excessive abduction of the upper limbs or pressure over bony prominences to avoid neuropraxia or skin damage.

Opinions vary, but the responsibility for ensuring an accurate position of the patient and the table is that of the surgeon and the operating department assistants. However, the general principles are that any movement is gentle and not hurried, and that excessive pressure on skin surfaces, and particularly on areas where arteries and nerves are superficial, is minimized. It must be remembered that in patients who have been given intravenous muscular relaxant, the risk of bone and joint injury is increased because of the absence of protective muscle tone. The judicious use of sandbags, bridges on the operating table, mechanical supports and plenty of padding means that virtually any area can be adequately exposed. Thus, where it is likely that the patient will have a sympathectomy or where a retroperitoneal approach to the kidney, etc. is likely, the lateral position is used (Figure 10.1). Where the perineum or rectum is the area to be exposed, the lithotomy (Figure 10.2) or modified Lloyd-Davis positions (Figure 10.3) are used. When elevating the lower limbs by flexing both knees and ankles and abducting the limbs to put them into position, it is essential that these movements are performed simultaneously by separate assistants on either side. Where an operation is to be conducted in the pelvis

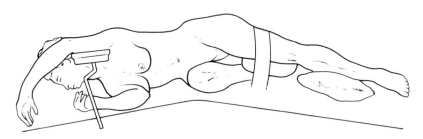

Figure 10.1 Patient in the lateral position. The lower knee is flexed, the upper knee and calf are cushioned, the upper arm is supported and the operating table can be 'broken' in the centre

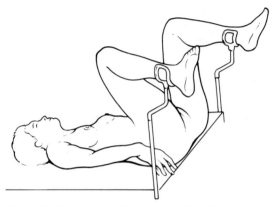

Figure 10.2 Patient in the lithotomy position. Be very careful with elderly patients, particularly if there is any abnormality of the hip joints. Protect the hands from the posts

and exposure may be difficult, or in varicose vein surgery, the head-down Trendelenburg position is used (Figure 10.4). However, in all cases it is the responsibility of the surgeon himself to ensure that the position is satisfactory prior to commencing any surgery.

Preparation for the operation itself
The surgical team

Any member of the team who is actually involved in the operation, i.e. surgeon, sister and one or two medical assistants, will be required to scrub thoroughly as a preliminary to gowning. Special sinks are designed for this purpose to allow an adequate flow of warm to hot water, the flow being

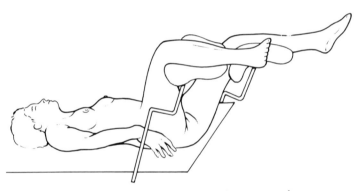

Figure 10.3 Lloyd-Davis position. Avoid localized pressure on the arms

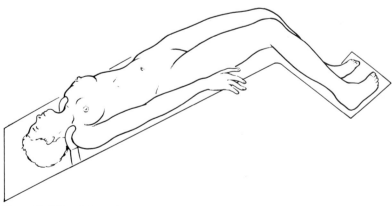

Figure 10.4 Trendelenburg position. The patient's shoulders must be adequately padded and supported

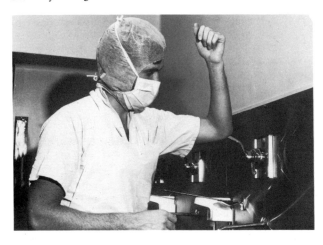

Figure 10.5 Regulating elbow taps. Wet scrubbed hands should be kept pointing upwards

controlled by elbow taps (Figure 10.5). An antiseptic solution, such as Hibiscrub or Betadine, is used and can again be obtained without the use of a hand. Other elbow-operated dispensers are available to obtain a sterile nailbrush.

Neither Hibiscrub nor Betadine actually sterilizes skin but they are effective in dealing with pathogens. During the course of an operation, bacteria will rise out of the skin crypts, but these are not usually of significance in causing surgical infection.

Following the initial scrub, the hands and forearms are washed and scrubbed thoroughly for about 3 min, particular attention being taken to cleaning under the nails. At the end of this scrub, the hands and forearms are rinsed and the hands are thereafter held up above the level of the elbows so that any water will run downwards and drop off at the elbows. Water is turned off and the hands, and then forearms, are dried. Once an area of towel is used, it should not again be used to dry any other

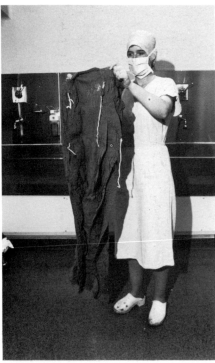

Figure 10.6 Gowning: holding gown by inner, top edge while gown unrolls

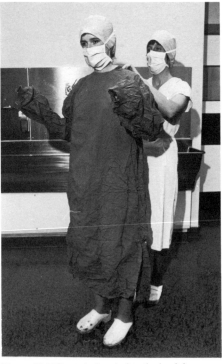

Figure 10.7 Gown being tied at the back by an assistant. Hands are kept pointing upwards

area. It should be said that when a second scrub follows immediately after one procedure before any particular contamination of the hands has taken place, a scrub of 1–2 min is usually considered adequate. This is again based on the principle that the majority of abdominal surgical infections are caused by the endogenous bacteria of the patient himself.

Once the hands are scrubbed and dried, it is important that both gown and gloves are put on before anything else is touched. It is now more common for each individual to put on his gown himself. The upper end of the gown is identified, as are the outer and inner surfaces, and holding the gown by its upper or neck margin, with the inner surface towards the individual, the gown is allowed to unroll and drop freely (Figure 10.6). Hands are inserted into each of the armholes and the back is tied by an assistant (Figure 10.7). Sterile, disposable gloves are then put on, carefully applying the gloves in order to avoid any contact between skin and the outer surface of the glove. Gloves are now available which do not require the prior application of powder. These are particularly recommended for abdominal surgery, to minimize the risk of adhesion formation stimulated by starch or talc. The inner forward surface of the right hand glove is grasped in the left hand and the right hand glove applied first. It is then possible with the glove's right hand to hold the inside forward edge of the left glove and, similarly, for this to be put on. The cuffs of the gloves can then be drawn up over the cuffs of the gown (Figure 10.8). Finally, the outer tie of the theatre gown is tied in combination with the scrubbed and gloved members of the team. Where talcum powder is used, it has become advisable to wash the outer surface of the glove in a solution of cetrimide or of chlorhexidine in water, 1:10000.

It is possible for a circulating nurse to assist in putting on gown and gloves but this has become less popular in recent years.

Where there is any suspicion of category III or IV risk double gloving is essential, combined with the other precautions described below.

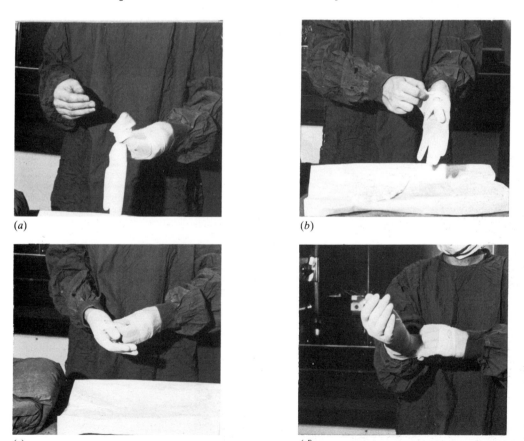

(a)

(b)

(c)

(d)

Figure 10.8 Gloving. (*a*) Pulling on left glove which is held by the upper edge of inner surface. (*b*) Holding right glove by inserting gloved left fingers under everted top edge. (*c*) Drawing glove up, holding outer surface. (*d*) Pulling glove up over cuff or gown

The patient intraoperatively

The patient is now suitably positioned, with any anaesthetic monitoring devices in place and infusions running. Precautions should also be taken that no limb is under any particular stretch as it is possible to damage nerve and nerve plexuses by traction neuropraxia. The patient's skin is then washed with an antiseptic solution such as chlorhexidine or povidone-iodine. The actual area covered will be the area of the incision and the immediate surrounding portion of the body, together with any other area that may be incised should the wound need to be enlarged. Thus, for abdominal procedures, the skin between the nipple and the upper thigh is washed, (Figure 10.9). If there is any possibility of an abdominal incision extending into the chest the appropriate part of the chest wall is

cleaned in continuity. It is usual to perform two washes, on each occasion starting with the area of the wound planned and then spreading radially round this, so that there is minimum contamination of the area of the incision itself. Particular attention must be paid to the umbilicus for even if a patient has been advised to clean that thoroughly in the bath, it is quite common to uncover unwanted debris in theatre.

Sterile drapes are then placed to cover all the body except that part to be used for the incision. The minimal amount of skin should be left exposed (Figure 10.10). The towels should be clipped in place, using towel clips, but the clips should be passed through the material of the drapes only, not into the skin. The drapes are usually of a distinctive colour, e.g. green, thus identifying the sterile field. Some surgeons recommend the application of an

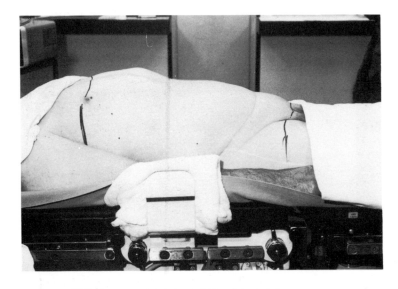

Figure 10.9 Skin area to be prepared for an abdominal operation. Note padding between arm guard and patient's elbow

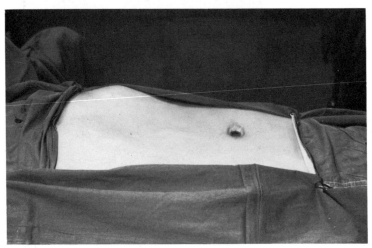

Figure 10.10 Skin drapes applied, clipped in position and exposing only the minimum amount of skin

adhesive transparent plastic sheet, either before or after application of the drapes. There is no evidence that this reduces wound infection and, in fact, because of skin sweating, may increase the amount of bacterial contamination.

The surgeon then positions himself where he will be most comfortable while performing the procedure and this usually means standing on the side of the organ or lesion to be approached. The first assistant stands opposite, on the same side as the theatre sister or scrub nurse and any additional assistant stands on the left or right of the surgeon, depending on whether an upper or lower body structure is being operated upon. The position and height of the table are dictated by the organ to be exposed and the surgeon's comfort. If the position is not suitable for the assistants or nurse, then they may be able to elevate themselves on a small foot stool but otherwise they have to be tolerant.

The surgeon then checks with the scrub nurse that the instruments are correct, as are swabs and packs, and with the anaesthetist that he is happy for the surgeon to proceed. Diathermy is connected and the operation commences.

Function of the surgical team

The scrub nurse

It is the responsibility of the scrub nurse to ensure that all the instruments which are likely to be required are available, either on the operating trolley or close at hand. In most theatres now, books are kept of the particular requirements of individual surgeons so that these can be made readily available. The instruments and the number of instruments are checked by the circulating nurse. The number of swabs and packs on the trolley are counted and noted, as are the suture materials and needles being used. She then prepares sponge-holding forceps and swabs for preparation of the skin and obtains any radio-opaque material which may be required for intraoperative X-ray. It is her responsibility to provide the surgeon with any instrument he requires; to ensure that any specially dangerous or contaminated instruments are kept away from the immediate operating field; that the instruments are kept in some semblance of order and that any suture/ligature materials and packs are readily available. Where it is possible that there will be contamination by gastrointestinal contents and traditionally where such operations as thyroidectomy or thoracotomy are performed, towels of separate colours may be used to minimize the risk of contamination and to identify areas where contamination has taken place. There is no real evidence that the benefit is anything other than aesthetic.

Where there is any possibility of the patient being infected with the virus of either hepatitis B or HIV, it is particularly important for the scrub nurse and surgeon to work in close harmony to avoid needle stick injury.

In addition to being an important and active member of the team, the scrub nurse is also responsible for keeping a check on swabs and packs and to check that all swabs and packs are accounted for before the end of the procedure. However, it is the responsibility of the surgeon if any foreign body is left in the operating field, and therefore the scrub nurse must report to the surgeon either the fact that the count is correct or that there is a discrepancy.

The medical staff

The role of the surgeon is to perform the procedure as safely, skilfully and expeditiously as possible. It is no longer necessary to concentrate on speed as anaesthetic technique has improved, but the longer the operation the greater is the risk of hypothermia, fluid and electrolyte imbalance and wound infection. Tissues are delicate and adequate haemostasis and delicate handling of the tissues must be the rule throughout the procedure.

The role of the first assistant is to ensure adequate exposure of the operating field for the surgeon and to assist him at all times to secure haemostasis and, in general terms, to make the operation as easy for him as possible. He must be able to anticipate the requirements of the surgeon and to respond instantly to any requests or instructions. The balance between excessive interference and inadequate assistance can only be learned by sometimes bitter experience. The cornerstone of surgical dissection is to provide exposure of tissues under reasonable tension by retraction, and thus correct application of such traction by hand or by metal retractor is essential. It is vital that all members of the surgical team maintain vigilance throughout the procedure in order that unforced errors are avoided. For this reason, only a minimal number of observers should be allowed. They should be warned about the need to stay clear of the sterile field and not to talk or otherwise distract the attention of the team. It is also vital both for the team and observers to ensure that if they feel in any way unwell, they should retire from the area before they fall into the operating field itself.

Any breach of sterile technique or any unwanted contamination of glove or instrument must be immediately recognized and either the instrument rejected or the glove changed. Recent evidence would suggest that glove puncture is a very common problem and should be detected as soon as possible, for the sake of both the patient and the surgeon.

Specific functions of the assistants

Retraction

Many surgeons may use self-retaining retractors or specific fixed retractors, e.g. Rochard (Figure 10.11) or Omintract, but in addition to these, the assistants, and particularly the second assistant, are responsible for ensuring adequate exposure of the operating field by retraction. This usually means holding a structure to one side under the direct control and supervision of the surgeon himself, but it must be remembered that injudicious retraction

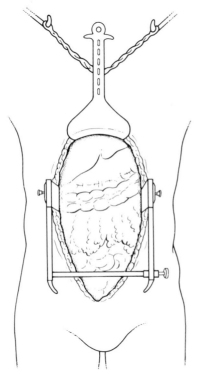

Figure 10.11 Self-retaining retractor, with Rochard retractor at top

may by itself cause damage. The assistants, too, must be aware that tissues are to be handled carefully and to recognize that aggressive retraction, whether by hand or by instrument, may tear tissues, including small blood vessels, and obscure the operating field by unwanted haemorrhage. In order to minimize the risk of dangerous retraction, it is often valuable for the surgeon actually to show his assistants what he is doing and why the particular exposure is required. Furthermore, it is seldom necessary to maintain a strong pull on the retractor or the tissues, but rather to hold the retractor gently in the position indicated by the surgeon. If a metal retractor is turned in too far, it may by itself produce tears of such relatively soft structures as liver or spleen. The assistant must not lean on the patient's chest or arm. It is important for the assistant to make it clear to the surgeon when he becomes fatigued or when the retractor begins to slip because of the effect of fat or body fluids.

Mopping

By careful use of pledgets, swabs or packs, the assistant must attempt to keep the operating field dry and free of blood and body fluid. This should be done as a dab rather than a rub, as excessive rubbing will remove any blood clot which has formed at the end of bleeding vessels and thereby induce further haemorrhage. Sudden haemorrhage should *not* be dealt with by the sudden application of large forceps into the depth of the wound. This is seldom effective and may damage associated vital structures. The bleeding is dealt with rather by the application of pressure on top of a pack until all the facilities are available to produce adequate control of haemorrhage.

The field may also be kept clear by careful use of a surgical suction device. Various types are now available but more general suction through multiple orifices or pinpoint suction through fine orifices are both available. However, it is important to avoid sucking viscera, e.g. part of the small bowel wall, into the sucker.

Haemostasis

Any bleeding points must be controlled except where minimal capillary oozing has taken place. Larger vessels should be clipped with an appropriate artery forceps, making strenuous attempts to take only the vessel and not the surrounding tissue. This may then be dealt with either by coagulation diathermy or by ligation. Where problems persist and where the end of a vessel cannot be readily identified, it is occasionally justified to undersew the bleeding point and then to ligate the vessel. For the majority of ligatures, a non-absorbable material is satisfactory, although the newer absorbable materials such as Vicryl are very effective.

Diathermy

Vessel coagulation is achieved by passing an intermittent oscillating current from a point electrode to the metal forceps holding the specific vessel which is bleeding. A diathermy plate will have been applied to the patient to provide earthing but it is important that no other part of the patient should be touched by metal.

The area surrounding the point to be treated by diathermy coagulation must be dry and there should be a minimal amount of fat in the controlling forceps. Diathermy should not be applied to skin or to skin flaps as this may produce a skin burn.

Ligation

When it is proposed to apply a ligature, it is important that the point of the forceps extends beyond the level of the vessel (Figure 10.12). It is then possible to pass a ligature round the point and

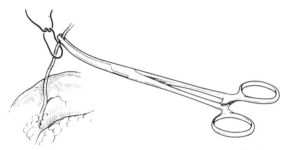

Figure 10.12 Ligating a vessel held in a haemostat. The tip of the forceps should extend beyond the vessel and its point should if possible be upwards when the ligature is being tied

the vessel, either by hand or using an instrument, and to tie-off the vessel using a square (reef) knot (Figure 10.13). This can only be achieved by adequate practice and may, in the early stages, produce particular problems deep down in a cavity. It is vital at all times, and particularly in a cavity where exposure is difficult, that the index finger of the hand being used to tie the knot is pushed well down to avoid undue traction on the vessel as this will increase the risk of the ligature being pulled off and bleeding recommencing. In addition, in areas where it is desirable to be meticulous in the placing of the ligature so that it does not encroach on surrounding structures, an aneurysm needle may be used to avoid the use of artery forceps.

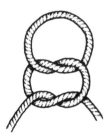

Figure 10.13 Square (reef) knot

A variety of is are available to assist haemostasis. Careful application is essential as most are relatively easy to dislodge. The development of clips made from biological materials which are biodegradable is awaited with interest.

A particular problem may arise in vascular tumours and, in this regard, early ligation of the proximal vessel may be of importance along with ligation of the vein, so that the risk of blood-borne spread of neoplastic cells is minimized.

Haemostatic agents

Such agents as Sterispon and Surgicel have been recommended for use in those situations where no solitary bleeding point can be identified but where oozing is troublesome, e.g. in the liver. In general terms they have little to recommend them, except as a last resort. However, bone wax is particularly important in controlling oozing from bone edges. Pieces of temporalis muscle may be of value in neurosurgery as muscle is a rich source of tissue thromboplastin. In controlling haemorrhage from the cut surface of the liver, the use of through-and-through catgut stitches with liver buttresses has been a significant improvement in recent years (Figure 10.14). More recently alginate materials have been shown to be effective haemostatic agents.

Ligatures and sutures

Recent years have seen remarkable innovations in the suture materials available. Non-absorbable materials have been made less and less irritant by various chemical methods, while absorbable sutures have been made in such a way that their absorption can be predicted in a much more accurate manner than previously.

Absorbable sutures

Catgut, particularly impregnated with chromic acid, remains the mainstay of the absorbable sutures in the world market. Its use in the UK continues to decrease. Contrary to the suggestion made by the name, this material is obtained from the connective tissue of sheep intestinal mucosa. This lasts in the tissue for 2–3 weeks and is used only for approximation of tissue rather than for tensile strength. There is now no place for its use in closing abdominal wounds.

Polyglycolic acid sutures are also absorbable but have been much criticized because of the difficulty in pulling smoothly through the tissues and in securing a square (reef) knot.

Vicryl (polyglactin 910) sutures and ligatures have a wide application in general surgery. Absorption

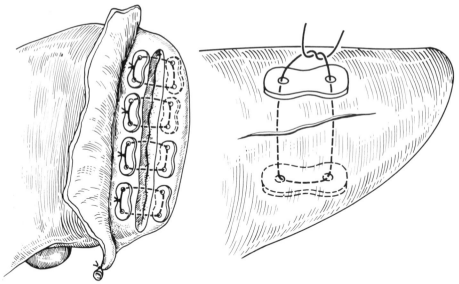

Figure 10.14 Suturing the liver. Through-and-through catgut stitches and buttress strips

takes place over 40–90 days so that this material is excellent for intestinal anastomoses and soft tissues where great tensile strength is not required.

Polydioxanone (PDS) is one of the newest absorbable materials. It is unusual in retaining its tensile strength over some weeks (50% at 4 weeks) with absorption commencing at 3 months and continuing until the sixth month. It is applicable for gastrointestinal anastomoses, but is used too for fascial closure and subcuticular wound closure.

Non-absorbable sutures

Braided silk remains the most popular of the non-absorbable sutures, especially for skin closure. However, attempts have been made to reduce its irritant qualities and coated silk (Nurolon) is a very

effective alternative, particularly for gastrointestinal anastomoses. For wound closure, the stronger nylon or Prolene sutures are increasingly popular and, as they have been shown to be effective methods of ensuring wound closure, such substances as stainless steel and wire have become less and less popular. Subcuticular closure using either polydioxanone (PDS) or Prolene produces a very satisfactory wound with minimal problems of suture removal. Tension sutures of non-absorbable material tied loosely in the abdominal wound have been widely used to minimize the risk of wound dehiscence, but are usually reserved for high-risk patients because of the somewhat unsightly scar which is produced (Figure 10.15) and because there is no scientific evidence that they are of value.

The size of the suture material is dictated by a standard gauge. The finer the suture, the larger the

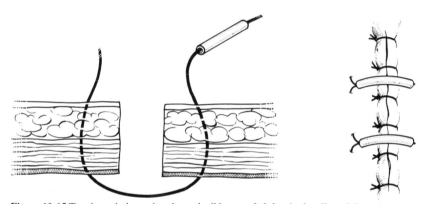

Figure 10.15 Tension stitch passing through all layers of abdominal wall, and threaded through 2 cm length of plastic tubing

number of zeros from 0 to 00 to 000, etc. The heavier sutures go from 0 to 1 or rarely 2, the larger sizes of suture materials no longer being commonly used.

Once the sutures are tied using a square (reef) knot, the method of cutting is very important. Skin sutures of non-absorbable material are cut with an end of some 1 cm in order that they may be easily identified and removed at a later date. Within the body cavities, silk may be cut shorter, but as catgut tends to swell once tied, a longer margin must be left to prevent the knot becoming undone.

Needles are available in two main forms: (1) Cutting: which is used for passing through such tissues as skin, fascia or scar tissue; and (2) Round bodied: which is used for softer tissues where it is necessary to ensure the smallest residual hole possible, e.g. in bowel anastomosis. The shapes of other needles are too various to mention and may be held by hand or by needle-holder, depending on the particular preference of the surgeon.

Although for many years it has been possible to approximate the skin edges using either sutures or clips, the use of automatic stapling or clipping devices for bowel anastomosis, for dissection and for skin closure, has become more popular of late. At the present time, the cost effectiveness of these is debatable except for low anterior resection of the rectum and for oesophageal surgery. Multicentre studies have shown a shorter time for anastomosis but no other benefit. However, stapling devices are of particular value for reversing a Hartmann's procedure or for oesophageal transection for varices.

Surgery in high-risk patients

The patients concerned fall into two main categories: those carrying hepatitis B antigen and those who are HIV positive. Hepatitis B is more infective than HIV, but HIV infection is permanent; 30% will develop AIDS and virtually all of these will die as a result of the disease.

It is important to recognize patients at risk (Table 10.1) and to advise medical, nursing, laboratory and theatre staff accordingly.

Table 10.1 Patients at risk of carrying hepatitis B and HIV antigens

Hepatitis B	HIV
Blood transfusion	Male homosexuals
Tattoos	Drug addicts
Jaundice	Haemophiliacs
	Patients from sub-Sahara Africa
	Opportunistic infection
	Anorectal pathology

Hepatitis B has been transmitted from surgeon to patient and vice versa. It is likely the risk for the surgeon from a patient who is HIV positive is small and to date no patient has been infected by a surgeon. However, the risks of transmission of the disease are so devastating that formal precautions are essential whenever the risk is perceived. A major problem is that failure to detect the HIV virus does not indicate freedom from infection – precautions should be taken on suspicion of risk alone.

Ward precautions

Only where there is a discharge of body fluids, or an open wound, is there a significant problem. Standard barrier nursing precautions are required, including the use of double gloves and goggles. Isolation of the patient should be kept to a minimum.

Operating theatre precautions

Only essential personnel and equipment should be in theatre. Any member of staff possibly coming into contact with the patient should have a plastic apron, visor and double gloves. Disposable gowns and drapes are essential.

Use of sharp instruments should be minimized, e.g. scissors or diathermy for cutting rather than scalpel. Stapling devices are particularly helpful to avoid the use of needles. Passage of sharp instruments should not be hand to hand, but via a dish.

At the end of the procedure disposable items are gathered into labelled sacks and discarded. The floor is cleaned with dilute hypochlorite.

Any accidental injury should be thoroughly cleaned and dressed. The injury is recorded and reported. Blood is taken and stored lest there be any later confirmation of HIV positive status in the patient.

Before the patient returns to the ward any blood-stained dressings are removed and replaced taking the same precautions as described above.

All specimens from a patient believed to be 'at risk' must be clearly labelled for the information and protection of all staff.

Completion of the operation

Prior to the wound being closed, it is important that the surgeon and scrub nurse are agreed that the count of swabs and instruments is correct. Areas of operation, particularly where large vessels have been ligated, are checked to ensure that haemostasis is adequate and the position of any drain is checked, both to ensure that it has remained in the correct place and that it has not become compressed in passing through the surface stab incision. It is important that the drain is stitched in position at an early stage to avoid dislodgement. Where a nasogastric tube has been used, its position should be checked, particularly if it is wished to pass this through any anastomosis: its position at the nose can then be checked and marked.

Method of closure

There are no hard and fast rules about closure methods as each surgeon has his own favourite way of doing this, varying from multiple layer closure to mass closure. It is important to use non-absorbable sutures for each layer in patients at risk, e.g. the elderly, malignant conditions, abdominal distension due to bowel obstruction, potentially contaminated or frankly infected wounds and in the presence of malnutrition. Some surgeons still use deep tension sutures. These are made of non-absorbable material and are usually tied with the aid of a polythene cover to avoid the risk of being tied too tightly. It is important where sutures have been used that the peritoneal stitch, if inserted, should also lift up the tension suture to avoid the risk of loops of bowel being caught, and so cut as with an old-fashioned cheese wire (Figure 10.16). Advocates of mass closure point out that closure of the peritoneum is not required and it is clear this layer does not contribute to wound strength. Certainly the mass closure method has made the use of deep tension stitches virtually obsolete and is associated with a low incidence both of wound dehiscence (<1%) and incisional hernia (5–10%).

Where peritoneal lavage with an antibiotic solution has been used, adequate lavage of the wound edges will have been achieved, but some surgeons do like to apply either povidone-iodine spray, or antibiotic powder or solutions to the wound at that stage. The fascia is closed using large bites of a non-absorbable suture such as Prolene, and the skin is then approximated using either nylon, Prolene, PDS or Michel clips. There is now little evidence to support the practice of leaving the superficial part of the wound open and performing delayed primary suture.

A wound dressing is applied and drainage bag connected to any drains present. Any drains used should be closed, and under certain circumstances, e.g. after mastectomy, a vacuum may be applied to the drain itself.

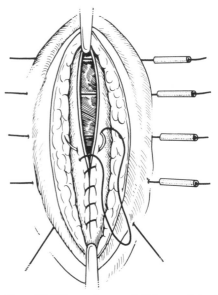

Figure 10.16 Layer closure of all deeper abdominal wall layers with continuous Prolene stitches, strengthened by interrupted tension stitches (now rarely used)

Operation notes

It is important that the operation notes and specific postoperative instructions should be written by the surgeon himself. The patient can then be removed to the recovery room and thence to the ward.

At the end of the procedure it is essential to label any pathological or bacteriological specimens and to fill in the form with as full detail as possible to aid reporting from the laboratory. An operating note should be dictated as soon as possible and when secretarial facilities allow, it is reasonable to write a letter to the patient's family doctor.

In most units where the surgical team is truly a team, all the procedures described above can be carried out with the minimum of effort and maximum amount of success in terms of the satisfactory treatment of the individual patient. The overall responsibility must rest with the surgeon, but it is only if he trains his team sympathetically and carefully that the best possible results will be obtained.

11

Respiratory obstruction and respiratory insufficiency

J. M. Imray and D. C. White

Next to cardiac arrest (Chapter 2), respiratory obstruction and respiratory insufficiency are the two most serious and most common acute disorders encountered. Although respiratory *obstruction* is not usually difficult to recognize, *insufficiency* may steal upon the clinician unawares so that it is only when some disaster, such as cardiac arrest, overtakes the patient that it is recognized that for some time gross hypoxia has existed.

Effects of operation

Abdominal and abdominothoracic operations interfere significantly with the mechanism of respiration chiefly by the pain that the incisions produce. Vital capacity is reduced and in abdominal surgery the diaphragm is usually relatively raised by a combination of intestinal distension and the inhibition to its downward movement produced by pain. As long as vital capacity exceeds needed tidal air, frank respiratory insufficiency will not ensue. However, the raised diaphragm results in breathing taking place in a way that favours the closure of some basal small air passages towards the end of expiration. Thus right-to-left shunting of blood occurs across the lungs and Po_2 will fall. This accounts for most of the hypoxia commonly seen in the immediate postoperative phase and is an indication for the almost routine use of oxygen in the first 24 h after laparotomy, particularly if the surgery has been major. Hypoxia of this type may also contribute to respiratory insufficiency of other primary cause.

Recognition of respiratory obstruction

The circumstances are of extreme importance. The ill-positioned, unconscious patient, the presence of a space-occupying lesion in the neck or mediastinum, damage either accidental or iatrogenic to the neck or the larynx, the possibility of a foreign body, inflammatory disease of the bronchus – all these must be borne in mind for they set the stage for acute respiratory obstruction even if they do not themselves produce it. Often the last straw is some acute incident which precipitates oedema in, or provokes obturation of, an already narrowed airway. Particularly in the accident and emergency department it must be remembered that nothing injudicious should be done which, should it prove unsuccessful, will make worse the patient already teetering on the brink of acute respiratory obstruction. Thus, frantic attempts at intubation which produce damage to an already partially obstructed larynx may precipitate complete fatal, oedematous obstruction; or blood entering the trachea from a hasty tracheostomy may make hypoxia worse.

Clinical features

Activity of the accessory respiratory muscles and stridor are the two cardinal features of incomplete respiratory obstruction. The first merely signifies respiratory effort and is thus not specific; the latter is the consequence of air rushing through a greatly narrowed passage and is not only specific but is usually a harbinger of early doom unless something is done. Indrawing of the intercostal spaces may or may not be present. Incomplete respiratory obstruction does not necessarily imply respiratory insufficiency, although the one is likely to follow hard upon the other. There is not much difficulty in diagnosing complete obstruction – convulsive respiratory effort, cyanosis, unconsciousness, convulsions and circulatory arrest are the sequelae over a period of less than 2 min.

Recognition of respiratory insufficiency

The definition of respiratory insufficiency is bio-chemical and biophysical – an abnormal state of arterial blood gases. It follows that it has no clear-cut symptoms or physical signs – indeed it represents a final common state that results from a wide variety of causes. In surgical patients the usual but not invariable situations are:

1. Inadequate mechanical ventilation from either poor or ineffective movement of the chest wall.
2. Blocked respiratory passage by retained sputum or aspirated vomit with subsequent distal absorptive collapse. To this may be added either the ineffective movement of pre-existing lung disease or the consequent effects of oedema in an infected lung in circumstances where massive inappropriate respiratory efforts are being made.

Given the common underlying causes, the surgeon's job is to recognize the presence of respiratory insufficiency in individual circumstances. When dyspnoea or cyanosis is present there is little difficulty, but before these have supervened respiratory insufficiency is usually well marked. Thus Po_2 may fall from the normal 100 mmHg to 60 mmHg (13 to 8 kPa) before saturation is significantly reduced (and cyanosis consequently apparent); a further small fall may precipitate severe desaturation (see Figure 11.1). This 'slippery slope' of the oxygen dissociation curve should be constantly in the mind of all those dealing with respiratory insufficiency.

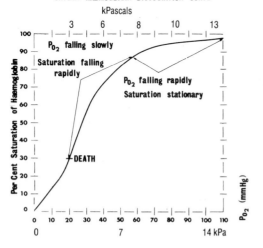

Figure 11.1 The oxygen dissociation curve. Initially Po_2 falls rapidly without change in saturation but at a Po_2 of approximately 60 mmHg, large changes in saturation take place for small changes in Po_2. This is the 'slippery slope'

In the absence of gross signs, what other guides are present for the clinician? Restlessness and disorientation are two of the most valuable. Although both may have many causes, among the commonest in surgical wards is hypoxia. Sudden changes in mental states should at once raise the question: Is hypoxia present or has hypercarbia developed?

Increasingly the so-called adult respiratory distress syndrome or 'post-traumatic pulmonary insufficiency'. This is a complex problem in which pulmonary capillary microaggregates and interstitial oedema combine to reduce compliance, interfere with gas exchange and raise pulmonary artery pressure. The usual cause is sepsis ± trauma.

Respiratory insufficiency may also occur in the surgical patient as a consequence of fatigue. The sequence of events is seen in the malnourished patient with reduced energy stores who is having difficulty in breathing because of some of the factors already listed. Gradually respiratory effort becomes less effective; the ability to generate an explosive cough is also reduced; finally anaerobic metabolism of the respiratory muscles and at other sites may develop. There is a period in such patients when arterial gas tensions are normal.

Warning

It is vital to avoid sedating a restless patient until a diagnosis has been made, for the incautious administration of sedatives to a hypoxic patient is clearly disastrous.

Although *hypercarbia* is mentioned as one manifestation of respiratory insufficiency, it is not commonly encountered as a well-marked syndrome in surgical patients. Consequently, the sweating, vasodilatation and drowsiness that go with a very high Pco_2 (80–90 mmHg; 11–12 kPa) are rarely seen. The explanation is that the surgical patient is not often underventilating in the sense that he has an inadequate stimulus to his respiratory centre or an inadequate mechanical response. Usually he is trying hard to breathe in the face of a situation which involves hypoxia and, because of the free diffusibility of carbon dioxide, he may even produce respiratory alkalosis in association with a low Pao_2 and clinical deterioration.

Aids to the diagnosis of respiratory insufficiency

A chest X-ray is mandatory. It may show: the basal collapse consolidation characteristic of the patient with postoperative sputum retention and raised diaphragm; a fluid collection; or the patchy consolidation increasing to 'total whiteout' of adult respiratory distress syndrome.

The final diagnosis is confirmed by arterial blood gas analysis performed on a sample taken anaerobically and transported rapidly to the laboratory. This will reveal a reduced Pao_2 associated with a $Paco_2$ which may initially also be reduced but inevitably rising above normal as the patient becomes increasingly ill.

Techniques of arterial puncture

Femoral, brachial or radial arteries may be used, but the last is to be preferred in that harm is not likely to follow. A short-bevelled 21 G needle is attached to a 10 ml syringe wetted with heparin 1000 u/ml so that the needle is filled with this solution. The skin is stretched with the thumb and forefinger of the free hand (Figure 11.2), and the artery fixed so that its

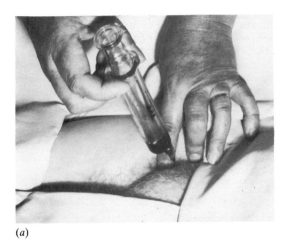

(a)

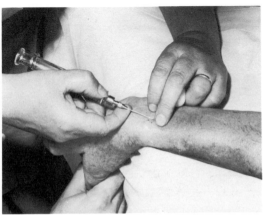

(b)

Figure 11.2 Methods of fixing (a) the femoral and (b) radial arteries for arterial puncture

pulsation can be felt and if possible seen just proximal to the digit of the operator which is pressed against the skin. A quick skin puncture is made at a moderate angle. The needle is then advanced steadily and obliquely into the artery which offers firm resistance. Entry into the lumen of the vessel is signified by a rise of the plunger of the syringe which then fills under arterial pressure alone; failure to detect the added resistance of the arterial wall implies that the needle is lying either to one or other side of the vessel and a fresh puncture should be made. The needle is sharply withdrawn, the syringe capped to avoid aeration of the sample, and firm pressure applied to the puncture site for 3 min by the clock. The results should be available within 5 min.

In complicated circumstances, for repeated sampling, an indwelling cannula, e.g. 20 G Medicut, may be inserted into a peripheral artery, usually the radial. Thrombosis is avoided by using a device e.g. 'Intraflo' which continuously flushes the line with a dilute heparin solution (5000 units in 500 ml of isotonic saline).

Acidosis

Acidosis, a raised blood hydrogen ion concentration in respiratory insufficiency, is the consequence of:

1. Underventilation with a rise in Pco_2, which in turn displaces the equation

$$CO_2 + H_2O = H_2CO_3 = H^+ + HCO_3^-$$

to the right, and
2. The metabolic hydrogen ion production which is the result of anaerobic metabolism in the hypoxic patient with the production of lactic acid.

Both are of particular importance in that they render the patient more susceptible to acute cardiovascular disturbance such as fibrillation, arrest and peripheral circulatory failure. The exact dissection of the relative contributions to acidosis of respiratory and metabolic components rests on the correct application of one of the acid–base nomograms commonly used in hospital practice. Because these vary according to the apparatus used (and also the taste of the resident expert) they will not be considered here. However, circumstances will help: the presence of metabolic acidosis suggests inadequate perfusion, e.g. a low cardiac output; respiratory acidosis is due to inadequate ventilation and is always accompanied by an elevated $Paco_2$.

Oxygen saturation measurement

When facilities for full blood-gas analysis are not available, saturation measurements by pulse oximetry are extremely helpful and obtained with ease continuously and non-invasively. It must be remembered, however, that, as already stated, arterial desaturation is a situation of advanced respiratory failure and requires most urgent and effective management. Absence of desaturation must not lull anyone into a false sense of security.

Prevention and treatment of respiratory obstruction

Predisposing factors should be avoided. The unconscious patient is usually at risk and must be nursed on his side or semiprone. Where this is impossible (e.g. when other injuries such as fractured femur coexist), prophylactic intubation or tracheostomy should be undertaken (see below).

When acute obstruction is diagnosed, an airway must be re-established forthwith. Often this is simple – pulling forward the tongue digitally or with a towel clip (which pierces the tongue without damaging it) and then maintaining forward displacement of the jaw (Figure 11.3). In the deeply unconscious patient an airway may be inserted, but it is far better to insist that someone is delegated to maintain the jaw forward than to insert an airway casually and hope for the best.

Where simple methods do not suffice and total obstruction is present or impending, it is dramatic but unreliable to undertake emergency tracheostomy. In fact, in a dying patient with respiratory obstruction this may prove the *coup de grace,* as often an inexperienced surgeon struggles in the acutely congested neck to expose a windpipe that is gyrating in the storm of respiratory efforts. It is better to carry out one of the following options:

1. Intubate the patient, overcoming trismus with a mouth gag. It should be the pride of every junior doctor to be able to intubate dexterously under direct vision, and the frequency with which endotracheal anaesthesia is used provides ample opportunity for him to acquire the technique. Woe betide the ineffective performer who may well worsen a laryngeal oedema and so lessen the chances of survival. If there is any doubt in the mind as to effective intubation it is preferable to adopt the second option.
2. Plunge a 15 G needle through the thyroid membrane. This apparently fine pathway will maintain oxygenation until more effective measures can be set in hand.

Inhalation of vomitus

The ill-managed surgical patient or the victim of some acute disaster, such as accidental injury or drowning with loss of consciousness, may vomit and inhale. Evidence that this has occurred may be provided by the presence of vomitus on the bedclothes or in the hypopharynx, but the absence of such telltales are of themselves no indication that the event has not taken place: (1) because of the tidy habits of nursing staff or (2) because the amount of regurgitated material is small. There may, on the one hand, be no overt signs of respiratory problems and, on the other, there may be acute pulmonary oedema. The former is particularly true of situations of upper gastrointestinal obstruction where spillover from a full stomach or oesophagus gradually produces bronchopneumonia, often of severe degree. Whenever vomiting has occurred under

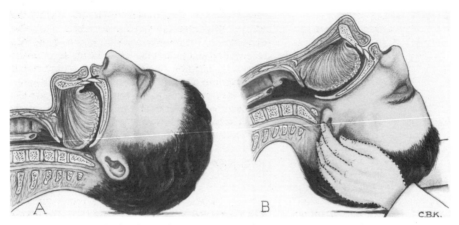

Figure 11.3 Holding the jaw forward to maintain an airway. The same position of head and neck is adopted for bronchoscopy. A shows how the unextended jaw permits obstruction of the airway by the tongue. B illustrates (1) the forward displacement of the jaw by pressure at the angle and (2) the extension of the atlanto-occipital joint which permits direct access to the larynx for toilet or bronchoscopy

questionable circumstances, the hypopharynx and larynx should be viewed directly for signs of vomit and the former cleared by suction. If there is obvious respiratory difficulty, urgent bronchoscopy must be done or the trachea intubated so that suction can be applied through the endotracheal tube. While awaiting intubation or bronchoscopy, the patient is laid on his side or face, oxygen administered and, if necessary, artificial respiration applied.

Re-establishment of an airway in acute respiratory obstruction from any cause is no guarantee that ventilation will ensue. Not infrequently, either some other respiratory condition is present which interferes with normal gas exchange, or hypoxia has been present for so long that partial or complete respiratory paralysis is already present. It is of the utmost importance to satisfy oneself that breathing is adequate once the airway has been restored.

Therapeutic bronchoscopy

Therapeutic bronchoscopy is less used than 10 years ago and now is more often the province of the anaesthetist than the surgeon. However, the ability expeditiously to pass a rigid bronchoscope should, as with an endotracheal tube, be acquired by all surgeons in training as on occasion it will save lives and, more frequently if less dramatically, expand a large collapsed area of lung which threatens to delay convalescence.

Indications

1. Acute severe pulmonary collapse in the postoperative period which is diagnosed by fever, tachycardia, tracheal deviation, bronchial breathing and typical radiological appearances.
2. Retained tracheobronchial secretions in a patient too weak to cough, where time may be gained to permit elective tracheostomy.
3. Aspiration of vomit, including blood.

Technique

An adolescent bronchoscope well lubricated with lignocaine (2%) jelly should be used combined with a large-bore sucker. A venturi high-pressure oxygen source is attached so as to permit inflation of the lungs. The head is extended to a similar position for that of maintenance of the airway (see Figure 11.3) and the instrument gently inserted beside the tongue down to the cords. As the patient inspires and the cords open, it is slipped through the cords and down to the carina. Although uncomfortable, this method is preferable to sousing the cords with local anaesthetic which may then permit inhalation of

oesophageal secretions or vomit before the cough reflex is recovered.

Once the instrument has reached the carina, the patient's head is inclined to either side, so permitting the tip to be slid into each main bronchus. Bronchial toilet is carried out with an oesophageal sucker of large bore and the instrument withdrawn.

This method is not for the tiro. It requires considerable dexterity and sense of timing, but the results are well worthwhile. A chest film is obtained at the end of the procedure.

Fibreoptic bronchoscopy is increasingly being used as an alternative to rigid bronchoscopy but its use demands greater expertise.

Emergency tracheostomy (Figure 11.4)

Very occasionally emergency tracheostomy may be required. The technique used should be the simplest. The head is fully extended on a pillow placed under the shoulders. If necessary 1% lignocaine is infiltrated in the line of the incision from cricoid to manubrium, but the quantity should be kept at the absolute minimum for tissues much distended by liquid are not easy to dissect. A 6 cm vertical incision is made exactly in the midline downwards from just above the cricoid. It appears to lie fairly high in the neck which is extended (Figure 11.4) but this is not so when a normal position is renewed. A horizontal incision is not recommended for urgent tracheostomy. The dissection is carried down to and through the investing fascia. Thereafter blunt dissection spreads the fascia in relation to the thyroid isthmus which can usually be displaced downwards and, by a combination of this and finger palpation, the upper ring of the trachea is palpated. The tube is held ready and a horizontal incision made at the level of the second ring. The lower lip of this incision is grasped and the cut converted into a semi-lune on either side. The tracheostomy tube is then slid over the resulting flap into the trachea while an attendant nurse inserts a sterile, soft, plastic catheter to suck out the blood and mucus that inevitably accumulate during the procedure. 'Burrowing' tracheostomy of this type is infinitely to be preferred to formal dissection, particularly in emergency situations. The thyroid isthmus need never be divided.

Choice of tracheostomy tubes

Most institutions have their own favourite tubes. The old-fashioned silver tube lingers on. Its advantages are minimal irritation and a smooth flowing curve which permits it to lie snugly. Its disadvantages are that it does not usually carry a cuff nor is it suited to adaptation to anaesthetic equipment. The best general-purpose tubes are

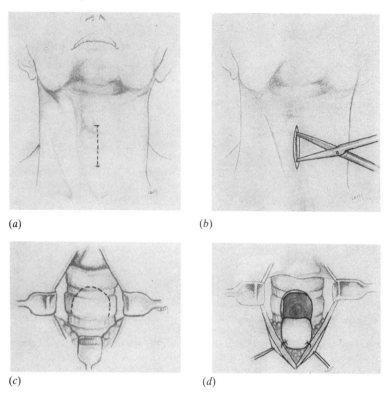

(*a*)   (*b*)

(*c*)   (*d*)

Figure 11.4 The steps in 'burrowing' tracheostomy: (*a*) The incision; (*b*) Midline separation of pretracheal fascia; (*c*) Downward displacement of the thyroid isthmus; (*d*) Formation of distal flap of trachea

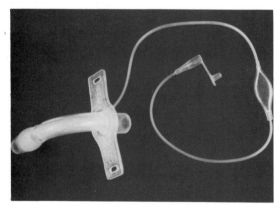

Figure 11.5 A standard cuffed plastic tube for tracheostomy. Anaesthetic connections can be attached directly

plastic, fitted with a cuff, and designed to match standard fittings (Figure 11.5).

Management

The patient is not rendered safe by the relief of respiratory obstruction. Rather he is exposed to new dangers in that the humidifying and filtering mechanism of the nose is bypassed.

The surgeon must ensure that the oxygen-enriched air breathed from pipeline or cylinder is properly humidified. One disposable device, the 'Inspiron' does this with a facility to control accurately the inspired oxygen concentration.

Careful repeated bacteriological control should be kept on the tracheobronchial secretions and therapy promptly instituted as indicated.

Aspiration of secretions

Aggressive high-vacuum suction will damage or even strip the mucosa from trachea and bronchi. The technique shown in Figure 11.6 should be used. The soft, plastic catheter is inserted with the Y-piece open to the atmosphere. With the catheter *in situ* intermittent suction is applied by placing the thumb over the Y. Negative pressure should not exceed 20 cmH$_2$O.

Artificial respiration

Complex methods of external artificial respiration have all been superseded by mouth-to-mouth

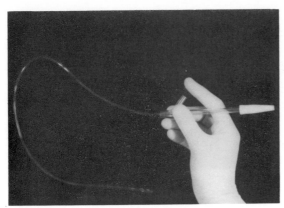

Figure 11.6 A Y-catheter for tracheal suction. Negative pressure can be applied at will by a finger over the end of the Y

breathing – Elisha's technique or as it is sometimes dramatically termed 'the kiss of life'. Mouth-to-mouth breathing (including mouth-to-mask, mouth-to-nose and mouth-to-tracheostomy opening) remains the most effective method of performing artificial respiration yet devised; there is evidence that in terms of maximum passive respiratory exchange mouth-to-mouth artificial respiration is superior to all other methods. Furthermore, the method is simple to learn and to carry out; it requires no apparatus; because it is not nearly so tiring as manual methods of artificial respiration, mouth-to-mouth breathing can be continued for more than an hour by most operators. An inadequate jaw-lift can be detected immediately by inability or difficulty in inflating the lungs – in no other method can the operator be sure that he is effecting respiratory exchange. Mouth-to-nose ventilation is aesthetically more acceptable to some people, and is becoming increasingly popular.

Technique

Rapidly check that the victim's tongue has not fallen back. Wipe away any vomitus from around the mouth. With one hand lift the lower jaw forwards; with the fingers of the other pinch the nostrils together (Figure 11.7). After taking a deep breath, place the mouth over the victim's mouth and blow out strongly. Out of the corner of the eye it should be possible to see the patient's chest wall rise as his lungs are inflated. This forced inflation is continued at a rate of 16–20 breaths/min.

General management of respiratory insufficiency

The surgeon must understand the general principles of respiratory insufficiency which are best addressed by looking at a series of questions.

1. Is the cause of the problem likely to get worse, e.g. the first 2–3 days after an upper abdominal laparotomy or the progression over 10 days to 2 weeks of adult respiratory distress syndrome? If so, consideration should be given to the introduction of respiratory support early (see p. 445).
2. Is the degree of fall in Pao_2 such that the patient is already on the slippery slope (p. 126)? If so, respiratory support is mandatory unless there is an easily reversible cause.
3. Is fatigue a major component? If so, support should be seriously considered.
4. Is there another system disturbance, e.g. cardiac, abdominal (ileus, residual abscess) or renal? If so, consider support earlier because the disturbances often interact.
5. Can it be predicted that something (e.g. a thoracotomy) will bring the patient to the verge of respiratory insufficiency, e.g. because vital

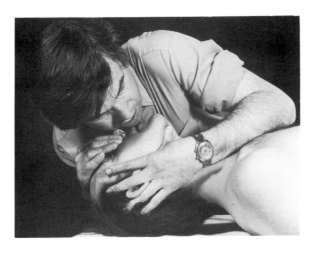

Figure 11.7 Mouth-to-mouth artificial respiration in an adult. Note the position of the left hand of the resuscitator supporting the jaw. His eyes are watching the patient's chest; his right hand should be pinching the nostrils

capacity is less than three times tidal air or because there is obstructive airways disease? If so, respiratory support should be introduced prophylactically before the event.

When the decision is made to provide respiratory support the patient is transferred to the intensive care unit for intermittent positive pressure ventilation via either the endotracheal, nasotracheal or transtracheal route.

While in the unit, the major role of the surgeon is to ensure that the underlying cause of the problem is dealt with – a distended abdomen, a focus of sepsis. Only complete resolution of the cause of the respiratory failure should be accepted as an indication to begin the process of weaning from the ventilator.

A further role for the surgeon can be in ensuring adequate nutrition and normal water and electrolyte balance – matters often inadequately attended to (pp. 25–33).

12

Fractures and dislocations

T. Duckworth

Definitions

A fracture represents a break in the continuity of a bone. Normal bone is more than capable of resisting the stresses to which it is likely to be subjected in everyday use, but if these are exceeded, or if the bone is weakened or *pathological* for any reason, its structure may fail.

Joints vary in their inherent stability but, again, considerable violence is necessary to rupture the ligaments and to overcome the protective function of the muscles. The expression *dislocation* is used to indicate a complete disruption of the joint so that the surfaces are no longer in contact, and *subluxation* to mean that although the surfaces are no longer correctly in apposition, some contact is still maintained. Neither can occur without some damage to the capsule or ligaments, but it is possible for the latter structures to be partially torn (*sprained* or *strained*) or even completely ruptured without significant subluxation occurring. In the case of a complete *rupture* there will, however, be some degree of *instability* which may be detectable clinically, or may only be revealed under anaesthesia when the joint is stressed. Radiographs taken with the joint stressed and unstressed may be valuable in assessing the amount of instability.

Types of fractures

It is helpful in management to try to decide by what mechanism the injury has occurred. A *transverse fracture* is normally caused by a direct blow or impact at the site of fracture. It essentially represents a three-point force system (Figure 12.1). There may be a 'butterfly' fragment which can add to the difficulties of management. A *spiral fracture* is caused by a rotational stress, often due to the weight of the body rotating about a fixed point such as the foot in contact with the ground. In all fractures there is an element of soft tissue damage – either contusion or tearing, and in some cases the soft tissue damage may be more important than the bone or joint injury (see Complications, p. 144). The soft tissue damage tends to be greater with transverse fractures because of the direct nature of the trauma, whereas with spiral fractures the forces have been applied at some distance from the fracture site.

Crush fractures occur in cancellous bone and are caused by direct compression, so that the cancellous substance is impacted into itself. They occur

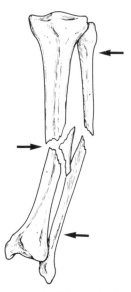

Figure 12.1 Three-point force system producing a midshaft fracture of tibia and fibula

commonly and characteristically in vertebral bodies. Occasionally the compressive forces are so great that the bone almost appears to explode, with fragments being driven outwards – a so-called *burst fracture,* again characteristically seen in certain vertebral fractures.

An *avulsion fracture* is caused by traction – a ligament or tendon tearing off a fragment of bone (Figure 12.2). When the fragment is avulsed by a ligament, the injury is analogous to a complete ligamentous rupture and it is correspondingly likely that there will be some joint instability.

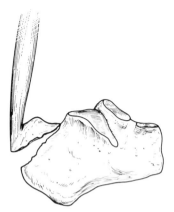

Figure 12.2 Avulsion 'beak' fracture of calcaneum

The soft and pliable bones of children often fracture incompletely, resulting in the characteristic *'greenstick' fracture* which tends to remain in continuity on the concave side.

A greenstick fracture is a good example of a *stable fracture* – in other words, unless further violence is applied, the components of the fracture are unlikely to shift. Fractures which are impacted or those with strong surviving soft-tissue attachments are also usually stable.

The expression *reduction* is used for the process of correctly aligning the fragments of the fracture. A fracture may, in its displaced position, have reached a position of stability but, in general, displaced fractures which have been reduced tend to be unstable, in the sense that they may redisplace to their pre-manipulated position. It is because of this tendency that the complicated question of how to hold the alignment has to be considered. Occasionally after reduction, the fragments may lock together and it is sometimes possible to make use of the soft tissues to help secure stability.

As already mentioned, all fractures involve some soft tissue damage. If there is a surface wound which communicates with the fracture, the expression *compound* or *open fracture* is used. A closed fracture is one in which there is no such connection

with a surface wound. It should be realized that the surface wound may be internal – opening onto a mucosal surface or, for example, into the lung. All such wounds provide a portal for the entry of organisms to the fracture site, with the risk of the fracture becoming infected and of osteomyelitis developing.

The expression *complicated fracture* is normally reserved for the situation in which the damage to the soft tissues involves an important structure such as a major blood vessel, nerve or internal organ. Although not usually included in this definition, the bone ends may occasionally be held apart by soft tissues, particularly muscle and occasionally skin. If

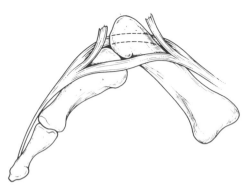

Figure 12.3 'Button-holing' of metacarpal head through extensor expansion

the end of the bone is driven through tight soft tissue or between tendons, it may be impossible to reduce by external manipulation – a phenomenon known as 'button-holing' (Figure 12.3).

The bone may be fractured into two fragments or there may be more than two – in which case the fracture is *comminuted.* This may not be obvious clinically or even on a single radiograph, and it often causes problems in securing and holding reduction.

A fracture may involve a joint, in which case it may be combined with displacement of the joint surfaces resulting in a *fracture-dislocation* or *fracture-subluxation.*

Children are susceptible to a particular type of fracture known as an *epiphyseal displacement* where the fracture runs through the calcifying layer of the epiphyseal line and the epiphysis is displaced on the metaphysis. Fortunately in most cases the germinal layer of the epiphysis remains intact and, after repositioning, growth continues normally. If, however, the fracture line runs obliquely *across* the epiphyseal line, union may occur between epiphysis and diaphysis and growth may be disturbed, with resulting deformity. For the same reason it is important to avoid placing internal fixation devices across the epiphyseal line except in certain very temporary situations.

Fracture union

The process by which fractures unite has received considerable study over the last decade, but there are still gaps in our knowledge, particularly as to why two fractures which appear to be almost identical may, in one individual, unite within a few weeks and, in the other, remain freely mobile after 6 months or more, despite both having been treated in essentially the same way.

The sequence of fracture healing may be compared with that of healing of the connective tissues in general, with the difference that the specialized function of bone requires the laying down, at some stage, of calcium in the regenerating tissues. The process occurs continuously but certain stages can be recognized:

1. Initially, the damaged area bleeds and fills with clot.
2. The inflammatory process is initiated and there is dilatation of capillaries, exudation of fluid and white cells and the process of capillary budding begins.
3. Dead tissue and clot are removed by phagocytes and there is migration of capillaries and osteoblasts from the periosteum and endosteum into the damaged area. The new tissue is essentially similar to granulation tissue and is very vascular.
4. The cellular reaction diminishes and the osteoblasts start to lay down collagen fibres in a feltwork, which at this stage is known as *osteoid*.
5. Vascularity diminishes, the amount of collagen increases and calcification is initiated, the fracture site gradually becoming increasingly rigid.
6. Calcification proceeds to the stage where the fracture ends are essentially held immobile. This stage may be reached within 1 or 2 weeks in a young baby, but may take as long as 3 months or more in a major long bone of an adult. In general the process proceeds more rapidly the younger the individual and the more cancellous and vascular the fracture site.

It has become obvious that the ultimate end-point of fracture healing is that of cortex-to-cortex union. It appears that for this to occur, the fracture must be held sufficiently firmly, so that the repair processes are not destroyed by excessive movement. The body achieves this degree of immobility by forming a temporary cuff of calcified woven bone known as *callus*. In general the more mobile the fracture, the more callus is formed. This is particularly noticeable where movement is not inhibited by muscle spasm as in certain neurological conditions with impaired sensation. The more rigidly a fracture is immobilized, the less need there is for callus and the less callus is actually formed. This is seen at its most extreme when very rigid and mechanically efficient plates are used as internal fixation devices. The plate effectively takes the place of the callus and virtually no callus may be seen on radiographs. This can lead to difficulty in deciding when the fracture is sufficiently united to allow weight-bearing.

The ability of the fracture to bear loads gradually increases as its instability decreases and the decision as to when to allow use of the limb and the degree to which this will be safe is essentially a clinical one. It depends on the disappearance of the original physical signs associated with the fracture, and particularly on the degree of rigidity of the bone when stressed by hand. Obviously, these signs can be masked by a fixation device.

There is evidence that some movement at the fracture site is beneficial in stimulating union and that absolutely rigid fixation may lead to delay in consolidation. Efficient internal fixation devices also absorb some of the stresses which would normally be taken by the bone, reducing the stimulus for the bone to regain its normal strength and leading to a risk of failure of the device. In practice this may mean that the implant would be better removed when the fracture appears to be united, but the problem then arises of having to protect the bone for a further period until it can be assumed to have regained adequate strength. To overcome some of these difficulties there is interest at the moment in making plates and nails of materials which are strong but slightly flexible. Carbon fibre and synthetic polymers offer the prospect of a solution to this problem in the near future.

When cortex-to-cortex union has occurred, the process of remodelling the shape and internal structure of the bone to meet functional needs then proceeds over many months or even years, being particularly effective and rapid in children, but occurring to some extent at all ages. It is important to realize that radiological union, i.e. radiographic evidence of bony continuity across the fracture site, is a late feature and load-bearing can normally be started many weeks before this stage is reached. Even before full load-bearing can be allowed, considerable functional use of the limb is possible by virtue of the temporary fixation provided by the callus or by the alternative fixation provided artificially. This is important in the patient's rehabilitation. It is helpful in avoiding joint stiffness, muscle wasting and the other complications of immobilization.

Diagnosis

The diagnosis of fractures and dislocations should be considered to be essentially clinical, supplemented usually by radiographs and occasionally by special investigations.

History

Certain elements of the history are essential in arriving at a diagnosis and in deciding on the priorities of management. Steps should always be taken to obtain the relevant information even though the patient may not be able to communicate, perhaps being unconscious. Relatives, workmates or observers of the accident may be able to fill in details. The nature of the accident is clearly important and it should always be possible to decide if the alleged accident is compatible with the observed injury – an important medicolegal point. If the injury appears greater than would normally be caused by the circumstances described, suspicions should be directed to the possibility of non-accidental injury, particularly important in children – or to possible underlying pathology resulting in weakening of the bone. The time of the injury should be ascertained as accurately as possible – particularly when the fracture is compound or there are signs of ischaemia or nerve damage. The police or ambulance crew may be able to supply information.

Pain

Pain is the commonest symptom, but varies with the site and mobility of the fracture. In the severely injured patient pain may not be a prominent feature or it may be concentrated at one site, masking an injury elsewhere.

Loss of function

This is almost always present to some degree in the injured area. If the limb is not already splinted, the patient is usually reluctant to move it and may support it with the hand or with clothing. The patient with a fracture of the spine, pelvis or lower limb may stand or even walk, but usually does so with obvious difficulty.

Loss of motor power or sensation

These are particularly important symptoms and enquiry should always be made as to whether the limb is, or has been, numb or felt dead or whether the patient has been unable to move the joints. Pain may, of course, inhibit movement, but most patients can distinguish between the effects of pain and those of neurological weakness.

Physical signs

The classic physical signs of a fracture or dislocation may or may not always be present.

External appearance

The limb may be swollen or bruised and there may be characteristic abrasions suggesting the way in which the injury occurred. There may be deformity, i.e. the limb or the bone may be misshapen. The limb may be bent or shortened, or there may be a step in alignment – particularly in the long bones and the spine. Occasionally the type of deformity will suggest the diagnosis, e.g. the characteristic 'dinner-fork' deformity of a Colles' fracture or the typical internally rotated and flexed position of a posterior dislocation of the hip. Diagnosis should always proceed with caution however, since other injuries may produce very similar deformities.

Tenderness

This is the most valuable and constant physical sign. The tenderness is usually localized over the fracture or the dislocated joint, but with deep structures the localization may be difficult.

Swelling

When the fracture is first seen, swelling may be minimal but it may gradually increase over the first 12–24 h. It is partly due to haematoma, partly due to inflammatory exudate. A large, rapidly appearing swelling should arouse suspicion of a vascular rupture. Early swelling of a joint, for example within the first hour after injury, is almost always due to bleeding into the joint cavity, i.e. *haemarthrosis*.

Marked swelling may be associated with blistering of the skin, particularly around the lower leg and foot and this may increase the risk of sepsis if surgery is contemplated.

An external wound will usually be obvious and some estimate should be made of the likelihood of communication with the fracture and how much bleeding may have occurred.

Local temperature increase

This is part of the inflammatory response and persists for some time after the injury.

Abnormal mobility or crepitation of the fracture ends

These signs may be noticed when moving the limb, but vigorous efforts to elicit them should not be attempted.

Loss of function

This has already been mentioned as a symptom and is almost always detectable to greater or lesser degree.

Note.

In addition to eliciting the classic fracture signs it should always be *essential routine* to examine the limb for evidence of ischaemia and nerve or other important soft tissue damage. Injuries elsewhere should also be suspected and sought.

Records

It cannot be too strongly emphasized that accurate and detailed records should be made as soon as possible after dealing with the patient. In particular the state of the circulation and neurological function *must* be recorded before any intervention takes place.

Radiological examination

This should only be contemplated, as with any non-clinical investigation, if it is likely to give useful information additional to that already obtained. In practice this is usually the case and radiographs are almost invariably needed, whenever possible being taken in two planes. If necessary, anaesthesia may be used to allow important radiographs to be obtained. The radiographs should always include the whole bone which is thought to be fractured, including the joint above and below. The films must be of good quality – if necessary repeat the radiograph.

Radiology provides the following additional information:

1. It localizes the fracture or dislocation accurately and helps to determine the number of fragments.
2. It indicates the degree and direction of displacement.
3. It provides evidence of pre-existing pathology in the bone.
4. It may show an opaque foreign body.
5. It may reveal an unsuspected injury.
6. It may show air in the tissue suggesting a penetrating injury.

Occasionally the radiograph may not reveal a fracture until time has elapsed to allow some resorption of the fracture site and in these cases the fracture may have to be treated on clinical suspicion, and a repeat radiograph taken after an interval of 1 or 2 weeks. Computed tomographic (CT) scanning is now widely available and can be valuable in analysing certain injuries, particularly spinal and pelvic fractures.

Finally, specialized techniques such as cystography, arteriography, arthrography, etc. may be necessary to reveal soft tissue injuries.

Management of fractures and joint injuries

First aid

At the site of the accident the rule should be to do only that which is necessary to keep the patient alive and to minimize the likelihood of further damage occurring. The *maintenance of an adequate airway* and the *control of bleeding* take precedence over other activities. In general, external bleeding can always be controlled by the application of external pressure. This is usually done by fashioning a pad from a handkerchief or item of clothing and bandaging it firmly over the bleeding site. If necessary this can be reinforced by direct manual pressure whilst the patient is moved.

The use of a tourniquet is usually discouraged as it may succeed only in impairing venous return, thus increasing the bleeding. It may not be remembered and thus be left on too long. *N.B.* If a tourniquet is used, the fact should be recorded in a prominent place.

The limb should be splinted by whatever method is available. A simple sling is sufficient for injuries of the arm, and the legs can be bandaged together, if necessary with a splint fashioned from an umbrella or piece of wood. Plastic and wire splints are valuable if available and inflatable splints are often carried by emergency services. In general, if the leg is badly deformed, it may be gently placed in a reasonably anatomical position, but force must never be used and if there are any doubts it is better to splint the limb 'as it lies' rather than to risk causing further damage.

If a spinal injury is suspected the patient must be moved without rotating and flexing the spine – a task which may need several helpers.

Definitive management

Assuming the injury to be adequately diagnosed, with appropriate radiographs and additional investigations if necessary, the management can best be considered as a series of decisions, which follow one another in a logical sequence.

Is there any immediate complication?

Wound closure

Two considerations will govern the degree of urgency of the individual case: (i) the possibility of infection, and (ii) limb ischaemia.

If the fracture is compound the *risks of infection* of the wound increase with every moment which passes. Assuming the wound to be clean, a reasonable estimate of the period during which it can be safely closed is 6 h. There is good clinical and experimental evidence that beyond this time contamination with organisms steadily increases, with the corresponding risk of deep infection. This period should only be used as a guide. A clean incised wound may well be safe to close for several hours longer if protected, and a badly contaminated wound with much necrotic tissue may be better left unclosed, no matter how soon it can be treated. Some authorities argue that the safest course is to avoid closing any wound associated with a fracture. In military situations this is probably best made a general rule, but in civilian practice where the patient can be closely observed, this policy seems unnecessarily cautious.

In either case the decision must be made early and may have to be made in conjunction with a decision as to whether open reduction of the fracture and internal fixation will be required.

Prior to closure, all necrotic tissue, no matter how extensive, and all foreign material, must be excised fully. If the wound edges are badly contaminated or traumatized, they should be trimmed lightly, but, in general, the principle should be to conserve as much viable skin as possible. If the deep fascia is tense, it should be divided longitudinally as it may conceal additional necrotic tissue. In general, bony fragments should be conserved unless small and completely detached. Doubtfully viable tissue, especially if superficial, may be kept but may need excision later. When the wound is closed, the deep fascia should, in general, be left unsutured.

The decision to close the wound or not will depend on the availability of adequate viable skin. Closure by apposition of the skin edges using sutures, or with adhesive tape or clips, is the ideal and should be attempted whenever possible, provided the wound is not going to be under excessive tension. If skin has been lost or is obviously non-viable, closure by means of a primary skin graft should be considered. For almost all purposes, partial thickness or split skin sutured over the defect provides the safest technique and the 'take' is usually well over 90%. For some sites, full thickness skin may be more suitable but this requires plastic surgical techniques in the fashioning of flaps and pedicles and needs considerable expertise. It is often better held in reserve as a secondary procedure. Occasionally bone may be sacrificed to allow primary wound closure, e.g. over the finger tip.

Every endeavour should be made to cover exposed tendons and articular cartilage with full thickness vascularized skin, even if this involves rotating or displacing flaps, leaving a defect elsewhere to be covered by split skin.

If primary closure is considered inadvisable, the wound is left open, packed with petroleum jelly gauze or preferably saline-soaked packs, and closed at a later stage when infection has been avoided or overcome. Secondary suture may be possible but

skin grafting is more likely to be necessary. If a limb swells to such an extent that the skin, although intact, will not close, it may be possible to close it by delayed primary closure at 24–48 h.

Limb ischaemia

The second feature which makes treatment urgent is evidence of ischaemia in the limb. Here every minute counts in restoring the circulation either by manipulation of the fracture or, if this fails, by operative intervention. As a rough guide, if the circulation can be restored within 8 h, the chances of the limb surviving are good.

Will reduction be necessary?

Not all fractures need reduction even if displaced. Reduction will be necessary if the displaced position would result in:

1. Union with impairment of function.
2. Cosmetic impairment even if function might be satisfactory.
3. Difficulties with union. Some fractures impair the blood supply to one or more fragments so that union may be delayed or uncertain. In these cases union may be helped by accurate reduction, which may give the few remaining vessels a chance to function. A subcapital fracture of the femur is a good example.
4. Trapping of soft tissue between the fracture surfaces.

If none of these factors are likely to be important, the fracture may be left displaced.

The accuracy required for reduction may depend on the fracture site and the extent to which function and appearance will be impaired. Some types of displacement are more important than others. A little overlap of a fracture of the shaft of a long bone may not matter, provided it will not show, but when good alignment is necessary for movement, much greater accuracy will usually be necessary. Fractures of the shafts of the radius and ulna will need to be accurately aligned if rotation of the forearm is to be adequate and most injuries involving joint surfaces and joint alignment require anatomical reduction for satisfactory short and long-term function.

How will reduction be achieved?

If it is decided that reduction is necessary this may be achieved either by a closed technique or by open operation.

Closed reduction

1. *Manipulation.* This is usually carried out with anaesthesia, either local, regional or general.

The manipulation usually requires relaxation and, in principle, involves reversing the mechanism by which the fracture occurred, as analysed clinically and from the radiographs. It often relies on hinging the fractures on the intact soft tissue and must be carried out carefully to avoid causing further soft tissue damage.

2. *Traction.* It is occasionally appropriate to avoid an immediate anaesthetic and to reduce a fracture slowly by traction applied to the limb. This may be particularly appropriate if the position is eventually going to be held by continuous traction. Subluxation of the cervical spine and, occasionally, femoral neck fractures may, for example, be reduced by this technique.

Operative or open reduction

Operating on fractures carries the considerable risks of increasing the soft tissue damage, stripping the bones of periosteum and possibly introducing infection, so the indications should be considered carefully. They are:

1. When the desired position cannot be achieved by a closed technique.
2. When internal fixation is likely to be necessary. It should be noted, however, that the use of internal fixation does not always involve opening the fracture site itself, e.g. pin and plate fixation of a femoral neck fracture. Nor does open reduction necessarily imply that internal fixation must be used.

How will the position be maintained?

As mentioned above, some fractures are inherently stable either before or after reduction. In these cases, immobilization is used, not to hold the position but for comfort and to reduce pain.

If the position is unstable, again two techniques are available, external and internal fixation.

External fixation

Splintage

Many types of splint are available for different purposes, ranging from simple polythene, plastazote or cardboard splints, bandaged or taped in position, up to elaborate external braces requiring considerable expertise in manufacture and fitting.

The most widely used material for fashioning splints is, of course, plaster of Paris, which is used to make open or closed casts, jointed casts, jackets etc. It has the considerable advantages of being cheap, easily available, fairly strong and very versatile and readily applied. It is reasonably comfortable and absorbs secretions to some extent. It has disadvantages, however, being rather heavy, warm and unyielding, so that it may cause pressure problems. It is not waterproof and may conceal trouble such as sepsis or ischaemia. Nevertheless its advantages outweigh these disadvantages for most purposes. Newer types of casting material based on plastics, remove some of these disadvantages, but introduce other problems, notably cost and difficulty of application. They are, however, in relatively affluent societies, gradually gaining favour.

Traction

In addition to being used occasionally to secure reduction, traction can be very useful in maintaining a position. It may be applied to the patient either through the skin or directly to bone.

Skin traction is applied by means of adhesive strapping and applies a tangential force to the skin. It is adequate for small traction forces but damage to the skin, sometimes with sensitivity problems and infection, make it unsuitable for high traction loads and traction over long periods. In these circumstances *skeletal traction* is more satisfactory, and is applied by means of metal pins driven through the bone with weights attached to the pins by caliper devices. The insertion of these pins is described later. It carries the disadvantage of allowing infection along the pin tracks, particularly if the pins move within the bone and threaded pins which are screwed into the bone are better in this respect. The pins may be incorporated into plaster casts to give greater stability.

Fixed traction is applied to the limb by one of the techniques described above, and the counteracting force is applied against the patient's body. This is best illustrated by the Thomas splint, a useful splint for the lower limb frequently used during warfare. It consists of a ring fitting round the upper thigh and bearing against the ischial tuberosity, with a U-piece extending down the sides and beyond the leg to the end of which the traction cords are attached and tightened (see Figure 14.7, p. 163).

A simple sling for the arm is also a device acting on the same principle of fixed traction. The advantage of these systems is that the patient is relatively mobile and can be transported with the traction still applied.

Sliding or balanced traction is applied by means of a weight attached by a cord or 'extension' to the limb and the counter force in this system is the weight of the patient and the friction of his body against the bed. The disadvantage is that the patient is confined to bed, but movements of the joints of the limb may be possible if the traction is carefully devised. Several commonly used methods of applying traction are described elsewhere.

Internal fixation

There has been, in the past 20 years, an enormous increase in interest in internal fixation techniques, brought about by considerable improvements in the mechanical efficiency of internal fixation devices and their instrumentation.

The *advantages* of internal fixation are considerable:

1. It should allow accurate reduction and maintenance of position.
2. It should allow the patient and possibly the involved joints to be mobilized, encouraging rehabilitation.
3 It may be a factor in encouraging union.
4. It may diminish hospital time.

There are, however, considerable *disadvantages,* not to say *dangers* of internal fixation:

1. Infection is always a possibility and severe infection may prejudice union and lead to longstanding morbidity, with sinuses and recurrent flares of infection.
2. Operative complications are common and fixation may be inadequate. It is often said that the 'bad results of internal fixation are the results of bad internal fixation'. In other words, the operation must be possible and must be within the technical capability of the surgeon.
3. The device may have to be removed and the limb subsequently protected for a while.
4. If fixation is inadequate, mobilization may not be possible and the patient may then be saddled with the disadvantages of both internal and external fixation and few of the advantages of either.

The *indications* may be summarized as follows:

1. When the position required cannot be held by an external technique.
2. When it is particularly desirable to avoid a long period of immobilization in bed.
3. When it is particularly desirable to move the affected joints early in the recovery period.
4. Multiple injuries and certain pathological fractures may be internally fixed to allow other important treatment to be carried out. There is some evidence to suggest that early internal fixation of fractures in the patient with multiple injuries improves the chances of survival and reduces the overall morbidity.

Accurate reduction is often required for fractures involving joints and it is here that internal fixation tends to be widely used. The question of internal fixation of compound fractures is controversial. The old attitude, that it is dangerous to introduce foreign material into a wound, has to some extent been superseded. Experience has shown that the benefits of firm fixation of the fracture can outweigh the theoretical disadvantages. Assuming the wound to be reasonably uncontaminated and well within the 6 h period, and with antibiotic cover, good results can be achieved. Nevertheless, it remains a hazardous procedure and should be embarked upon *only in circumstances where the patient will be kept under close postoperative supervision.*

Intero-external fixation

This technique has become popular over the last few years because it combines some of the advantages of rigid internal fixation, in allowing mobility of the patient and the joints, whilst avoiding the introduction of foreign material directly into the fracture site. It relies upon the introduction of fixation pins through the sound bone above and below the fracture and these are connected together by rods to form a rigid frame. It has the considerable advantage of securing fixation of the fracture, whilst allowing access to the fracture site for wound dressing or for skin grafting (Figure 12.4).

Unfortunately some of the frame devices are expensive. A rough but adequate frame can be fashioned from Steinmann's pins connected together by rods embedded in orthopaedic acrylic cement at

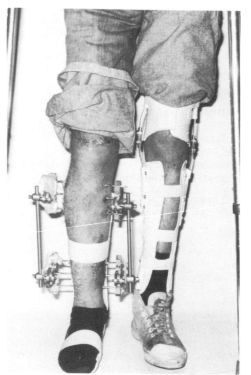

Figure 12.4 Intero-external fixation frame on the right leg and cast brace on the left leg

the junction points. This is not recommended for general purposes as it lacks the adjustability which is a feature of the better systems. The severe and badly contaminated compound fracture is the most likely indication for this technique.

There is a growing belief that strong, rigid fixation frames may actually inhibit union of the fracture and modern designs allow a small amount of movement at the fracture site. This is usually allowed to occur after 2 or 3 weeks of rigid fixation. The process is sometimes graced by the ugly term 'dynamization'.

Internal fixation devices

As mentioned above, the mechanics of fracture fixation have been much studied and modern internal fixation techniques have been refined considerably. It is important that the fixation device should be as simple in design and in use as is consistent with the security of fixation required. The newer techniques, although efficient, are quite demanding in terms of operative skill and frequently fail because this skill is lacking. The Swiss-based AO/ASIF group has been responsible for popularizing its own technique which is based on sound mechanical principles – particularly emphasizing the stability given by compression and the neutralization of tension forces. It is beyond the scope of this work to describe these fixation techniques in detail but some of the concepts are illustrated in Figures 12.5, 12.6 and 12.7. Less expensive and, given careful use, perfectly adequate fixation devices are still widely used.

Screw fixation

Screws are widely used to attach small fragments, e.g. the malleoli and epicondyles. The screw may have a large self-tapping thread which is wider than the shank to give a good grip on cancellous bone, or it may be designed with a standard thread, in which case it is usually necessary to penetrate the opposite cortex. This type of screw may be self-tapping but the AO/ASIF design requires the hole to be tapped – giving better mechanical strength and making removal easier. A single screw placed across a fracture can be used to compress the fragments if the thread is arranged to bite into the opposite cortex only. This is only sufficient to hold the alignment, and will require additional internal or external fixation.

Plate fixation

Many shapes and sizes of plates, sometimes coupled with nails and held with screws and bolts, are available. The principle of compression has been widely adapted by AO/ASIF.

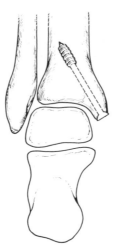

Figure 12.5 Cancellous screw fixation of medial malleolus (AO/ASIF)

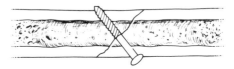

Figure 12.6 Single screw compression of oblique fracture (AO/ASIF)

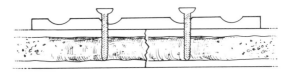

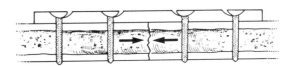

Figure 12.7 Compression plating – the compression is obtained by the shape of the screws and the countersunk hole in the plate (AO/ASIF)

Intramedullary nailing

The Küntscher nail has stood the test of time. A hollow rod which is trefoil-shaped in cross section and slotted along its length to allow it to be compressed a little, is passed down the medullary cavity and across the fracture site. Since most bones have a slight curve, it acts on the principle of three-point fixation. It is usually inserted by opening the fracture site and passing the nail back along one fragment to emerge through a separate incision, then opposing the fracture and driving the nail across it. Given suitable X-ray equipment, a more recent technique known as 'blind nailing' involves inserting the nail into one end of the bone and manipulating the fracture into line, then driving the nail across, without at any stage opening the fracture.

One of the difficulties about conventional intramedullary nailing is that, particularly with fractures in the lower half of the femur, the device may not control rotation adequately and very comminuted fractures tend to 'telescope' along the nail, with the nail tending to back out. These problems can be overcome by using one of the newer types of so-called 'interlocking' nails, which have provision for one or more cross screws passing through the nail (Figure 12.8). The cross screws may be used at one or both ends. Where control of length is likely to be the main problem it is usual to use the screws at both ends of the bone and this also gives very good control of rotation. If it is considered desirable to allow a little movement at the fracture site, the upper screws may be removed when the fracture becomes 'sticky', for example at 3 weeks, and this allows the fragments to compact to some extent when the patient bears weight. These nails require careful technique of insertion and image intensification is usually needed for accurate location of the screws.

Infection following intramedullary nailing is usually more difficult to treat than with other methods of fixation. If infection occurs the nail is usually left *in situ* until the fracture has united, then removed. Unfortunately, removal of the nail does not always lead to complete resolution of the infection. Intramedullary nailing is used mainly for femoral fractures, less commonly in the humerus and tibia.

Wires

Small fragments may be held temporarily or permanently in position by wires passed across the fracture line or encircling the fracture. Stiff Kirschner wires are often used for this. The tension-banding technique of the AO/ASIF system is a refinement of this (Figure 12.8).

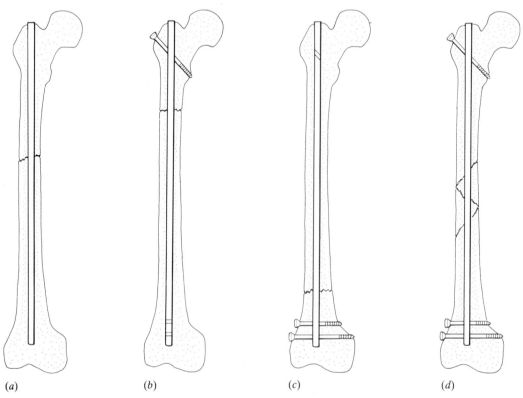

(a)   (b)   (c)   (d)

Figure 12.8 Interlocking nail for femoral fractures: (a) conventional nail; (b) proximal locking; (c) distal locking; (d) locking both ends for comminuted fracture

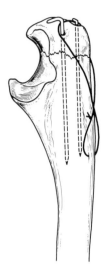

Figure 12.9 Tension-band wiring of olecranon fracture (AO/ASIF)

It should be repeated that, attractive though many internal fixation techniques are, they require considerable expertise and judgement if they are to be used safely, and many fractures can be quite adequately treated by external methods. The essence of good therapy is that it should be directed towards assisting the natural process of healing.

How long should the fracture be held?

As mentioned previously, assessment of fracture union is essentially clinical, depending on whether the original physical signs have disappeared. The presence or absence of pain and tenderness, a feeling of movement on stressing the fracture, and the ability of the patient to use the limb are the essential features involved in making the decision. The appearance of callus on the radiograph may be helpful in deciding if union is occurring but is not in itself a particularly helpful sign. Some impairment of function will usually still be present following the period of immobilization and again cannot be considered a particularly reliable indication. When an external fixation method is used, it is usually necessary to remove this to check the state of the fracture, supplementing the clinical testing, as necessary, with radiographs. As a rough guide to when union may be expected, a fracture of the shaft of a major long bone in an adult will take approximately 12 weeks to become sound, and fractures of the cancellous ends and of the short bones will take 6–8 weeks, depending on the loads they will have to bear. The range of variation is considerable from individual to individual and from

bone to bone – the clavicle for example usually being united in as short a time as 3 weeks in an adult. In children up to the age of 12 years, healing times can be halved, and below the age of 2 years, they can be halved again. In a neonate a fractured femur will unite in 1–2 weeks.

If the fracture has been fixed internally, these tests are not readily applicable and the joints will often have been mobilized early in the course of treatment. Radiographs again are not of great help. Here it is only possible to allow a gradual programme of increased load-bearing on a 'trial and error' basis, bearing in mind the union times mentioned above.

Some fractures require a further period of protection from full load-bearing, even when apparently united, and here hinged and moulded casts and braces can be invaluable in allowing movement whilst relieving some of the applied load.

Rehabilitation

There is always a conflict of interests between the need to immobilize a fracture and the desirability of keeping the patient fully mobile and active. Whenever possible the treatment should encourage as much active participation on the part of the patient as possible. Encouragement and instruction from the beginning of treatment helps to avoid fear of pain and of attempting activities which the patient fears may be harmful. This, in turn, avoids the development of joint stiffness and contractures, and helps to prevent an attitude of excessive dependency on help from others. Wherever possible, the splinted limb should be used, not simply exercised, and an early return home and to work is undoubtedly beneficial in achieving a positive attitude. Many patients benefit from a course of physiotherapy and, where appropriate, occupational therapy, the elements of personal supervision and encouragement often being more important than the actual physical treatment. Inevitably, some injuries will be so severe as to leave permanent disabilities which may make a return to the patient's original work impossible. This should be anticipated early wherever possible so that preparations can be made for re-training and re-settlement with the minimum of delay.

Unfortunately the possibility of financial compensation does play a part in delaying recovery in a small proportion of cases and the legal disputes, which can be protracted, can lead to considerable bitterness and a feeling of reluctance to adapt to changed circumstances. There is no doubt that the psychological make-up of the patient and his attitude and capabilities can play at least as large a part as the purely organic components of the injury in deciding the ultimate end result.

Complications of fractures

These can be conveniently considered as *immediate,* i.e. occurring at the time of injury, *early* or occurring during the initial period of treatment and *late,* occurring after the initial treatment period. These latter may be delayed many years.

Immediate complications

Haemorrhage

The extent of external haemorrhage can be difficult to estimate, particularly if there are several wounds. Lacerations of the face and scalp are particularly deceptive in terms of the blood which may be lost over a period of time. The amount of internal haemorrhage into the limb at the site of a fracture is frequently over-estimated. A simple fracture of the femoral shaft in a fit adult is unlikely to lead to sufficient internal bleeding to induce a state of shock – rarely exceeding, or even approaching, 1 unit (500 ml). If the patient is, in fact, in a state of circulatory shock, another site of bleeding must be sought, usually either intra-abdominal or intra-thoracic. Very serious bleeding can occur with pelvic fractures and since the blood tends to collect in the pelvis and retroperitoneal areas it may not be appreciated. Here the pulse, blood pressure and central venous pressure may be the only reliable indicators. Extreme distension of a limb, particularly the thigh, usually indicates rupture of a major vessel and arteriography may be indicated. The idea of estimating the total blood loss by adding up published figures for average blood loss at each site of injury should be approached with caution, since on occasions it can lead to an estimate which is greater than the total blood volume, an absurdity which will be avoided if the state of the circulation is used as a more realistic guide.

Injury to important internal organs

The soft tissue damage which accompanies certain fractures may be of greater importance than the fracture itself and the possibility of severe internal injury should always be considered following major trauma. If the diagnosis is not initially obvious, a period of observation may clarify the situation. A knowledge of the likely associations between certain fractures and corresponding soft tissue injuries, for example those between injuries to the bladder and urethra with fracture of the pelvis, and lacerations of lungs, spleen and liver with rib fractures, should lead to an early diagnosis. The management of the soft tissue injury will frequently take precedence over that of the fracture, although both must be considered together.

Injury to local nerves or vessels

It is damage to important structures in association with the fracture itself which usually merits the term 'complicated' fracture. Again anatomical awareness will often lead to recognition of the nerve or vascular injury, but the value of a thorough clinical examination of the circulation and neurology as *an essential routine* must be stressed.

The effects of vascular injuries can develop insidiously and may be exacerbated by swelling of the limb. In general, elevation of the limb, the avoidance of constricting dressings or tight plaster casts, with occasional recourse to fasciotomy, will avoid ischaemic consequences, but where there is suspicion that a major vessel is divided, early investigation and exploration may save the limb.

Many nerve injuries associated with fractures are due to stretching or contusion of the nerve and there is often potential for recovery. If the patient has noticed some function in the relevant nerve territory after the accident, complete division is unlikely and exploration is rarely indicated. Indeed, immediate exploration of damaged nerves, except in the case of compound injuries, is rarely justified. Severe injuries of the brachial plexus may be an exception to this, since some workers are claiming improved results following early surgery.

The majority of nerve injuries may be left for later exploration if recovery does not occur or if there is reason to suspect complete rupture. Nerve repairs when combined with a difficult fracture have a poor prognosis.

If nerve or vascular damage is detected or suspected every effort must be made by careful management to avoid causing further damage. Nowhere is this more important than in the case of spinal injuries with cord or cauda equina damage, where careless handling may have devastating effects.

Skin loss or damage

The importance of securing early wound closure has been explained above and skin loss can make this a difficult problem. In general terms dead skin should be excised, but doubtfully viable skin may be left and observed carefully. This is particularly important where the skin is specialized, e.g. over the palm of the hands and sole of the feet. Tension on the skin should be avoided and, occasionally, relieving incisions may allow the skin to be closed over an important site such as exposed tendons which tend to slough if not covered.

Early complications

Immediate complications are not usually avoidable, except by the patient taking preventive precautions during dangerous activities. Many of the complications arising in the early treatment period are avoidable with good management. They may conveniently be classified as *local* and *general* complications.

Local complications

Skin and soft-tissue necrosis

Skin which appeared viable or borderline immediately after the injury may declare itself as non-viable within the first few days. A definite boundary line will usually become obvious and at this stage the dead skin is better excised and the area grafted or, if infection has occurred, grafting may follow a period during which the wound is allowed to granulate.

A granulating surface forms almost as good a bed for a skin graft as freshly exposed bleeding tissue. Skin will 'take' on almost any surface (even bone) with the exception of cartilage and bare tendon.

Ischaemia from vascular damage or external pressure

The former of these may be unavoidable. Local gangrene due to vascular injury may not be preventable by vascular surgery. Again, as with skin, it is soon obvious where the line of demarcation lies and when this is obvious amputation should not be delayed as spreading sepsis and necrosis due to small vessel thrombosis may lead to unnecessary further tissue loss.

Gangrene from external pressure should not occur and can be avoided if constricting dressings and complete encircling plaster casts are not used in circumstances where swelling may develop or where the circulation is already prejudiced. All patients at risk should be kept under observation, if at all possible in hospital. A useful test is to check the return of blood flow to the digits after compression of the skin. Any complaint of pain, numbness, change of colour, etc. of the extremities should be investigated immediately. If a plaster cast has been used this should be split, with the underlying dressings, *down to the skin* throughout its whole length and, if necessary, removed. Moderate oedema of the extremities is common and provided the circulation remains intact is of little significance except in so far as it may discourage movements and lead to stiffness. It is best treated by elevation of the limb and vigorous active exercises of the fingers or toes. Blistering of the skin is also common, particularly of the ankle. It should be anticipated if surgery is contemplated and the operation carried out before the blistering develops. The blisters are best treated by pricking with a sterile needle and then by dry dressings.

Compartmental syndrome is caused by a rise in pressure within one or more of the fascial compartments. It may occur as a direct consequence of the swelling associated with trauma, usually from a fracture, but occasionally from soft tissue injury. If the swelling develops within a closed compartment, the pressure rise may be sufficient to occlude the circulation in the venous system and capillaries. This may lead to tissue ischaemia, particularly of the muscles, which in turn may cause more fluid loss and a further rise in pressure. If the pressure is not relieved, extensive tissue necrosis may occur within a very short time. The most vulnerable tissues are the muscles themselves and the nerves which pass through the affected compartment. The problem tends to arise within the first 12–24 h after the accident and may be masked by plaster of Paris or other dressings. There is usually a complaint of pain in the affected compartment, although this may become less as the tissues become effectively denervated. The extremity may be oedematous, although this is not always the case, and the pulses may persist beyond the block for some time before eventually diminishing in volume. The segment of the limb will usually feel tense and tender. Of particular significance is evidence of impairment of function in the nerves running through the compartment. When the signs suggest increased pressure, the safest course is to decompress the compartment by splitting the fascia from end to end. When this is done, the ischaemic muscle will bulge through the split and the vascularity should quickly return to normal. If facilities are available and there is doubt about the diagnosis, the intra-compartmental pressure can be measured, but if this is likely to cause delay then surgery should be preferred.

Volkmann's ischaemic contracture is a rather rare complication of certain vascular injuries, the best known of which is to the brachial artery at the elbow as a result of a supracondylar fracture of the humerus in a child. This can result in ischaemia of the flexor muscles of the forearm with eventual scarring within the muscle, which in turn becomes contracted and draws down the fingers into a flexed position. A similar but less dramatic condition probably occurs much more frequently following tibial shaft fractures, affecting the deep calf muscles and producing flexion contractures of the toes.

The classic forearm Volkmann's ischaemia is to some extent preventable. It is such a notorious complication of a supracondylar fracture of the elbow, that any child who has had such a displaced fracture manipulated should be admitted overnight for observation, the limb elevated and the pulse and circulation in the fingers checked hourly. The radial pulse may disappear following the fracture and it may fail to reappear after the manipulation. This in itself is not necessarily significant provided the fingers are well vascularized and the circulatory return is satisfactory following compression of the finger tips.

The *warning signs* are pain in the forearm, particularly if this is made worse by passively extending the fingers, pallor of the fingers and possibly disturbance of sensibility in the fingers, which may be due to ischaemia or to associated nerve damage.

If the condition is suspected, all encircling bandages and splints should be removed and the degree of flexion of the elbow reduced. If there is no improvement following these measures, most authorities favour an immediate surgical exploration of the brachial artery. The artery may appear to be in spasm and there may indeed be spasm extending to the smaller branches. There is usually an intimal tear, even if the outside wall of the vessel seems intact and it may be necessary to resect the damaged segment and replace it with a vein graft. This is a task for an experienced vascular surgeon and the time available before irreparable damage is caused to the muscles is short, probably being no more than 8 h.

Pressure sores and nerve palsies from splintage or traction

One of the disadvantages of plaster-of-Paris and similar occluding materials is that ridges and projections may produce sufficient pressure on the skin to cause ischaemic necrosis. This is particularly liable to occur over bony prominences and where there is an element of sensory disturbance. Developing sores are not necessarily painful as the ischaemia renders the part insensitive. They can be avoided by good technique, with care being taken to protect the vulnerable areas. Most patients experience at least some discomfort, but may fail to mention this, being unaware of its significance.

Warning signs are: discoloration of the plaster, an area of local warmth, and a persistent smell. Unexpected oedema of the extremity may also be significant. Whenever there is discomfort or any other suspicious signs, either the plaster or splint should be removed or a 'window' cut to enable inspection of the area.

Patients occasionally push foreign objects down the inside of the plaster in order to scratch, and coins, knitting needles, etc. may be lost and cause pressure problems.

Nerve palsies are also avoidable, but still commonly occur, often from splintage or traction, the most common and most important being a paralysis of the common peroneal nerve at the head of the fibula from pressure by the side bar of a Thomas splint. All such traction devices, many of which require long periods of recumbency in bed, carry the risk of skin damage and pressure sores, the heels and sacral areas being particularly at risk. Careful nursing and protection of the skin, together with the avoidance of continuous pressure, will prevent the majority of these. In the debilitated patient a period of continuous pressure of 2 h may produce a sore which could take weeks to heal.

Infection and wound breakdown

Infection of a closed fracture or dislocation is extremely uncommon, but all open fractures and fractures which have been treated operatively, particularly when an internal fixation device has been used, are at risk of contamination and infection. Inadequate wound cleaning and debridement contribute significantly to this risk. It is usual to cover all patients at risk with suitable broad-spectrum antibiotics, the nature of which will vary with local circumstances.

Infection may be difficult to detect if the fracture is encased in plaster. The warning signs are pain, increasing rather than decreasing oedema of the extremity, malaise and fever. If the area can be inspected, redness and increasing tension at the suture line may be evident.

The wound may break down and discharge. If the infection appears superficial and early, antibiotic treatment may be effective, but if antibiotics are to be used some attempt should be made to obtain a culture of the organisms either by swabbing the wound or by aspiration, or if there appears to be a collection of pus, by removing some or all of the sutures and laying open the abscess. A specimen of the pus is sent for microbiological examination. Any dead or necrotic tissue must be removed but a metal implant may have to be left *in situ* until the fracture is united. Serious deep infection undoubtedly delays union and may actively prevent it. Nevertheless in many cases, the wound, if left open, will eventually heal and the implant may be removed when the fracture appears united. A sinus may persist until the foreign material is removed and may indeed fail to heal even then if there are areas of unseparated necrotic bone.

Gas gangrene and tetanus are serious complications and are considered on pp. 53–54.

Loss of position of the fracture

It is not uncommon, when the early swelling has subsided, for the splintage to become inadequate and for the position of the fracture to move. This should be anticipated and the position checked on radiograph at weekly intervals for the first 2–3 weeks. Most fractures will be difficult to remanipulate after the end of the second week, and in children the opportunity may be lost well before this.

General complications

Many of these are the complications of long periods of bed rest and are particularly common in the elderly and the debilitated.

1. Deep venous thrombosis and pulmonary embolism.
2. Pulmonary collapse and hypostatic pneumonia.
3. Renal calculus, acute retention and other urinary tract problems.

Two conditions which occasionally follow trauma require separate consideration since their consequences can be serious or fatal.

Fat embolism

This complication, which may occur more commonly than used to be thought, tends to occur 3–10 days after fractures, usually of the long bones and particularly after major trauma. Its cause is unknown. It was originally thought to be due to fat released into the circulation from the bone marrow of the fracture site but it was always difficult to explain how such emboli could reach the brain, having to pass through the lung filter first. It is now thought to be, at least in part, a metabolic phenomenon associated with hypovolaemia and the shock syndrome.

The principal manifestations are confusion and respiratory difficulty and a petechial rash which tends to occur on the face, neck and upper trunk but varies in severity. Fat may be detectable by filtering the urine and the emboli may be visible in the retinal vessels. At post-mortem, multiple deposits of fat with small infarcts are found in the brain, lungs and other organs.

Diagnosis may be difficult and blood gas analysis may be necessary. In the fully established case, death is not uncommon and treatment requires the resources of an intensive care unit to maintain the circulation and respiration.

'Crush syndrome'

This is an uncommon complication usually associated with extensive soft tissue damage, or ischaemia of a large volume of tissue, for example following occlusion of the femoral artery. Various factors enter into its causation – fluid loss, release of toxic materials from the site of damage, possibly disseminated intravascular coagulation, all contributing to an effect on the kidneys, resulting in acute tubular necrosis with renal failure. It may be prevented by removal of the damaged tissue before severe renal changes have occurred or by amputation of the limb. If the renal damage occurs, renal dialysis may be necessary, in anticipation of recovery of renal function after several days.

Late complications

Malunion

Despite attempts to hold the position of a reduced fracture, union may occur in an unsatisfactory position, resulting in functional or cosmetic impairment. This is likely to be particularly important in fractures involving joints. The joint surfaces may be disturbed, with potential stiffness and the likelihood of later development of osteoarthritic changes. Fractures which do not actually involve the joint surfaces may also carry this risk if the alignment of the joint relative to the rest of the limb is disturbed.

Moderate degrees of malunion with angulation or shortening may be compensated and in children there is remarkable potential for re-modelling during growth, even quite major degrees of malalignment gradually being corrected.

In children, however, epiphyseal damage may occasionally lead to growth disturbance and increasing deformity or length discrepancy. There is, in these circumstances, the risk of secondary complications due to stretching of nerves, a phenomenon well seen in the development of the so-called 'delayed ulnar palsy' caused by a valgus deformity developing at the elbow after a fracture of the lateral condyle of the humerus, the nerve being stretched round the medial side of the elbow.

Malunion may occasionally be severe enough to require corrective osteotomy or leg length correction.

Delayed and non-union

The expression 'non-union' is usually reserved for the situation where there are definite radiographic appearances suggesting that union is unlikely to occur. Rounding of the bone ends and closure of the end of the medullary cavity with sclerosis suggests that a fibrous union has occurred. These are late signs, however, and although union may be delayed beyond the expected normal time, in the absence of such signs there is still a chance that union will occur if the fracture is suitably immobilized. It is not possible, however, to wait indefinitely and, in general, if there are no signs of union occurring after 5 months for a shaft fracture in an adult, it is usual to take steps to stimulate healing. The factors which contribute towards delay are not fully understood, but they include (i) infection, (ii) relative avascularity of one or more of the fragments, (iii) inadequate immobilization, (iv) underlying bone pathology, and (v) distraction of the bone ends. It has been increasingly realized that the amount of energy involved in producing the fracture (which influences the amount of soft and bony tissue necrosis and the degree of comminution), does to some extent determine the likelihood of union, severe violence often being associated with delay.

The management of delayed union depends to some extent on whether the fracture site is infected or not. The wound associated with an infected non-union usually fails to heal on antibiotic treatment alone because of the presence of dead tissue, either as a separate sequestrum or still attached to the living tissue. Excision of the dead tissue may allow the wound to heal, but this is more likely to occur when assisted by firm internal or external fixation.

If on the radiograph there is much callus around the bone ends, but still an obvious gap, this is often called a *hypertrophic* non-union. If callus is almost absent it may be called an atrophic non-union. To some extent the two types behave differently.

If non-infected, the first type will often unite if the fracture is rigidly immobilized, usually by internal fixation with a plate or intramedullary nail. A compression plate gives particularly firm fixation, although external protection may also be necessary. The atrophic type also usually requires firm fixation, but union tends to proceed more quickly if a bone grafting procedure is carried out.

Cancellous bone strips or chips of the type described by Phemister, taken usually from the iliac crest, may be packed around the fracture site, without breaking down the fibrous union. Internal or external fixation may be used, although it may be impossible to secure adequate internal fixation without re-aligning the fracture. Corticocancellous grafts are sometimes useful, often fashioned into plates and held with screws, to provide both stabilization and an osteogenic stimulus.

The infected fracture does not usually lend itself to the implantation of foreign material and in these circumstances large cortical grafts tend to be rejected. Firm fixation of the fracture with excision of dead tissue will often eliminate or reduce the infection, enabling a bone graft to be inserted later with more safety and likelihood of success. If the defect which remains is large, a considerable quantity of tissue may be needed to bridge the gap and for this purpose cancellous bone chips are normally used. In these circumstances an intero-external fixation device of the type described on p. 140 can be extremely valuable.

In the last few years attempts have been made, with some success, to stimulate healing in long-standing non-unions using electrical fields produced either directly, via electrodes implanted into the bones, or by externally applied coils which induce an electromagnetic field at the fracture site. These techniques are currently being evaluated and may offer promise for the future.

Failure of internal fixation

If a fracture does not unite and the bone is continually stressed, metal implants can cut out or may break as a result of metal fatigue. In these instances the implant may migrate or cause pressure problems and may need to be removed.

Joint stiffness and contracture

It is difficult to avoid some stiffness in the joints close to a fracture site and failure to use the limb may result in stiffness in joints at some distance away. It is not uncommon for stiffness to develop in the shoulder following injuries to the wrist and hand, particularly after prolonged use of a sling. Older patients are more prone to stiffness and the importance of instruction and supervision in exercising the joints has already been stressed. Fractures and dislocations involving joints are particularly prone to stiffness and internal fixation often has the great advantage that early mobilization is possible.

Sudeck's atrophy

Occasionally, following almost any fracture in adults but particularly following fractures around the wrist, the limb becomes more, rather than less, painful and, when taken out of splintage, the hand is swollen, mottled and shiny, the radiographs showing a diffuse, patchy, 'moth-eaten' type of osteoporosis. Its cause is unknown, but it is thought to be due to a sympathetic malfunction. The pain leads to a vicious circle of decreased use, with further porosis and the only treatment appears to be to encourage vigorous movement despite the pain, in which case improvement usually occurs over the course of many months. There is some evidence that thyrocalcitonin injections may shorten the time course of this troublesome condition.

Compensation neurosis

This has been mentioned previously as a factor in delaying satisfactory rehabilitation. Unfortunately the solution of the medicolegal problems does not necessarily result in a resolution of the psychological manifestations which have been partly caused by them.

13

Injuries of the spine and pelvis

T. Duckworth

Fractures of the spine

The essential similarity between all the intervertebral articulations is that each consists of a secondary
cartilaginous joint represented by the intervertebral
disc and two posterolateral synovial articulations,
with the whole bound together by a strong group of
ligaments. However each region of the spine has its
own anatomical characteristics which make it
susceptible to a particular pattern of injury. The
posterior ligament complex, consisting of the
intertransverse, interspinous and supraspinous ligaments, is at least as important as the disc in
maintaining the stability of one vertebra on the next.
In the cervical region the synovial facet joints lie in a
horizontal plane, in the lumbar region they are
vertical and almost in a parasagittal plane, and in the
thoracic spine they are intermediate in alignment,
giving this region more stability. The ribs also
contribute to the stability of the thoracic spine,
whose mobility is extremely limited.

Essentially, stability is lost when both the
intervertebral disc and the posterior bone and
ligament complex are disrupted. The significance of
most injuries to the spine depends on two factors –
displacement and stability. The degree of displacement determines the extent to which the spinal cord
and cauda equina are subjected to pressure and
again the different regions vary in their vulnerability
in this respect. In the cervical region, the canal is
relatively large and surprising degrees of displacement can occur without cord damage. In the lumbar
region, below the lower border of L1, the theca is
occupied by the roots of the cauda equina, which are
relatively less susceptible than the cord itself. The
canal is narrowest in the thoracic region and the
cord almost fills it, making this the most vulnerable

region in terms of serious cord damage. The *stability*
of the spinal segment after injury will determine the
likelihood of further displacement, causing cord
damage where none had previously occurred, or
perhaps rendering complete a previously partial
lesion. Radiological displacement is not necessarily
a good index of how much displacement is possible
or has occurred. In some cases the displacement
may have been considerable but the spinal elements
may have returned to their original position, giving a
misleading impression of stability. Clinical judgement of stability can be difficult. In the thoracic and
thoracolumbar spines, there may be a palpable gap
or step between the spinous processes, a valuable
sign that the posterior ligament complex is ruptured.
A careful examination of good radiographs, perhaps
taken in the flexed and extended positions (with
care) may be necessary to assess stability. *N.B.* The
radiographs must be of high quality and an expert
radiologist's opinion should be obtained.

In many centres computed tomographic (CT)
scanning is now available for the investigation of
acute spinal injuries. It can be useful for working out
the precise configuration of the fractures and
dislocations and it has been particularly useful in
demonstrating the extent to which the spinal canal
can be encroached upon by fragments of bone,
usually from the vertebral body. It is now clear that
surprising degrees of penetration of fragments into
the canal can occur without much neurological
damage. It is not yet clear whether, or in what
circumstances, removal of such fragments is justified. Nuclear magnetic resonance (NMR) scanning
offers the promise of better visualization of the soft
tissues and should help further in understanding the
nature of the neurological damage.

Emergency management of suspected spinal injuries

Any patient who is suspected of having a spinal injury should be handled and transported with extreme caution to avoid causing unnecessary cord damage. The unconscious patient is particularly at risk and any patient with a severe injury must be regarded as having a possible injury of the cervical spine. It will be particularly important for the person responsible for the ultimate management of the patient to know if movements of the limbs were possible immediately after the accident and whether the patient was able to feel the limb normally. This information should be recorded before any attempt is made to move the patient. Wherever possible, moving and transporting the patient should be delayed until expert help arrives, the only movements allowed being those which may be necessary to ensure that respiration is adequate. The principle in moving the patient is that he should be lifted and supported 'in one piece' without either flexing, extending, laterally flexing or rotating the spine. This usually requires many helpers and a suitable firm stretcher or improvised platform. If the cervical spine is thought to be injured, the head should be carefully supported during lifting and further protected by sandbags on either side to prevent rolling on the stretcher. On reaching hospital it is usually best to avoid further lifting until the necessary radiographs have been obtained.

Cervical spine

Injuries of the cervical spine are commonly the result of road accidents, or sustained during sporting activities. The usual cause is a fall on the head with forcible flexion of the neck. Hyperextension injuries are also common, in particular the so-called 'whiplash' injury, characteristically sustained by the driver or front seat passenger of a car, who is sitting in a stationary vehicle when a second vehicle runs into the rear. In this type of injury the neck is first hyperextended, then tends to whip forward. The main damage is to the anterior longitudinal ligament of the spine. Radiographs may look normal, although occasionally there is a small telltale fragment of bone avulsed from the upper or lower margin of the anterior surface of the vertebral body. This type of injury, despite sometimes having involved considerable displacement, is not grossly unstable and there is little risk of cord damage.

The most serious injuries are usually caused by flexion and rotation and these result in subluxation or dislocation of one or both posterolateral facet joints, with disruption of the intervertebral disc – an unstable injury (Figure 13.1).

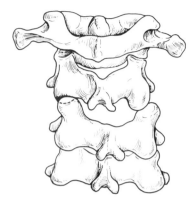

Figure 13.1 Subluxation of second cervical vertebra on the third. The left facet joint is dislocated

Clinical features and diagnosis

The patient is often unconscious following a head injury, so the injury to the cervical spine may not be immediately apparent. This possibility should be considered in all patients who are unconscious following an injury and if there is any suspicion of cervical damage, radiographs of the neck should be obtained.

In the conscious patient, a cervical injury is usually suggested by pain and muscle spasm, sometimes with torticollis and localized tenderness. If the tenderness is maximal in the suboccipital region, with obvious limitation of movements, a fracture of the axis or atlas should be considered. In these upper fractures, a haematoma may develop under the mucosa of the nasopharynx. Neurological loss may be gross, minimal or absent, but a full neurological examination of the limbs must be carried out in all cases.

Radiology

Radiographs should be taken in any suspected case, the risks of missing an important injury being greater than those involved in actually obtaining the films. Even in the unconscious patient, the procedure is safe if reasonable precautions are taken when moving the neck.

The radiographs required are: (i) a lateral film of the whole cervical spine, (ii) including one taken with firm traction on the head, with an assistant applying traction to the arms to draw down the shoulders, allowing an adequate view of the C7–T1 region; (iii) an anteroposterior view, (iv) including one through the open mouth; and (v) 30° oblique views to show the facet joints in detail.

If one body is displaced forwards on the one below by less than half a diameter on the lateral film, this usually means a subluxation of one facet joint. More displacement than this means a subluxation or dislocation of both joints.

If the film appears normal, a hyperextension injury or a flexion injury which has reduced fully may be suspected. In these circumstances, lateral views with the neck held in flexion and extension may be advisable but these must be carried out with great care.

N.B. Fractures of the axis and odontoid are uncommon and easily missed. The fracture of the odontoid is usually at its base and the peg may be considerably displaced along with the first cervical vertebra, while still allowing survival of the patient.

Treatment of cervical injuries

Management depends essentially on whether the fracture is considered to be stable or unstable. In order to render the segment unstable, there will normally have had to be disruption of the disc (or odontoid), together with significant damage to the capsules of the facet joints and the posterior intervertebral ligament complex.

Extension injuries are rarely unstable in this sense, and many flexion injuries, together with fractures apparently produced by longitudinal compression and often having a burst appearance, are also stable.

Treatment of these injuries normally consists of immobilization of the neck in a surgical collar for up to 6 weeks, followed if necessary by physiotherapy to regain motion. The whiplash injuries, in particular, often remain intermittently painful for months and sometimes years.

Treatment of all cervical fractures will, of course, be very much influenced by the presence or absence of neurological damage.

The unstable injury, particularly if there is no significant neurological loss is, of course, potentially the most dangerous. It is usually accepted that any dislocation or subluxation should be reduced whether there is neurological loss or not. This may be achieved by manipulation under anaesthesia with radiographic control. General anaesthesia is necessary, with particular care being taken during induction and intubation. The manipulation is carried out with the patient supine, the operator supporting the head over the end of the table. The head is held between the two hands and traction applied whilst the spine is inclined to the side away from the locked facet. The head is then brought back to the neutral position first by rotating and secondly by correcting the lateral flexion. Check radiographs are obtained immediately.

Alternatively, reduction may be achieved by applying continuous and gradually increasing traction, using calipers of the Crutchfield or more modern types applied to the skull. Again, radiographs are used to check the reduction.

Whichever method is used, following reduction, traction is usually maintained with the skull calipers until signs of bony fusion start to appear on the radiograph, normally at about 3–4 weeks. If this does not occur, it is usually safer to carry out a fusion operation on the involved segment to ensure long-term stability. Atlantoaxial and odontoid fractures often unite and become stable with conservative treatment, or traction followed by a protective collar for up to 3 months. If non-union of the odontoid occurs, then a surgical fusion may be carried out through the mouth or by a posterior approach.

Thoracic and thoracolumbar injuries

Flexion injuries are common in the thoracic spine. They may occur as a result of a definite injury, but also commonly occur more or less spontaneously in pathological conditions affecting the vertebrae. They are particularly common in postmenopausal osteoporosis when they may be multiple, but myeloma or secondary carcinoma should always be considered as possible underlying disease. Characteristically these fractures take the form of a wedging of the normal rectangular vertebral body when seen on a lateral radiograph. They are usually stable, often not associated with neurological damage and they heal well, if non-pathological, or if the pathology is non-neoplastic.

Symptomatic treatment, with a short period of bed rest and analgesics followed by mobilization as the pain settles, is usually adequate. Occasionally with more severe displacement, paraplegia may occur and is usually complete.

Fracture-dislocations of the thoracolumbar spine are much less common, but also much more serious. They are almost always caused by flexion and rotation of the spine, either by a fall on to one shoulder or by a heavy object, such as a rock, falling onto the flexed back. The injury occurs most commonly at the junction of the fixed thoracic spine and the mobile lumbar spine. In the typical case, the intervertebral disc is disrupted and the posterior ligament complex is also completely ruptured, sometimes with a fracture of one articular process (Figure 13.2). Such an injury is unstable and frequently associated with complete or partial paraplegia.

Clinical features and diagnosis

The characteristic history is often obtained and further evidence of the mechanism of injury may come from the fact that there may be abrasions over

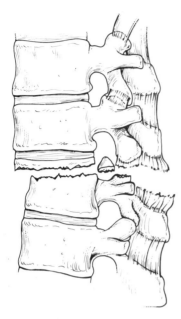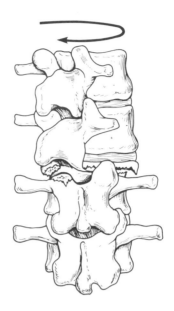

Figure 13.2 Fracture-dislocation of thoracolumbar junction. One articular process is fractured

the back of one shoulder or of the chest. If a gap is felt on palpating along the line of the spinous processes, the fracture is unstable and great care should be taken in moving the patient as described above. A full neurological examination is, of course, mandatory and this may need to be repeated at intervals over the next 24–48 hours.

Management of the unstable injury

The treatment depends on the presence or absence of paraplegia. If there is only minimal or no significant neurological loss the patient can be nursed on a plaster bed in the expectation of union of the fracture occurring – usually by fusion of the two vertebrae involved. This normally takes up to 12 weeks. Internal fixation, either with plates or using the techniques of scoliosis surgery, has its advocates. If carried out successfully, it has the advantage of allowing early mobilization and less reliance on nursing care.

If the patient is paraplegic, the problem is complicated by the risks of developing pressure sores, urinary tract and chest complications. In these circumstances some authorities recommend internal fixation of the spinal fracture, which has the advantage of minimizing the risks of deformity of the spine, which can lead to pressure problems later in life. Internal fixation makes the regular 2-hourly turning, which is necessary in the early weeks, easier and less painful. Others rely simply on careful nursing to avoid the complications, thereby avoiding the risks of spinal surgery.

Lumbar and sacral injuries

Transverse processes are frequently fractured as a result of violent crushing or lateral flexion injuries. The fractures are often multiple and they essentially represent the radiological signs of a severe underlying soft tissue injury, with considerable tearing of muscles and ligaments and, not uncommonly, injury to the kidney. If haematuria follows such an injury, an intravenous pyelogram is usually advisable to ascertain the extent of renal damage.

The patient with fractures of this type is normally treated symptomatically with rest in bed and analgesics, but symptoms often persist for a long period after mobilization.

Flexion injuries, with typical wedging, and vertical compression injuries, which may have a 'burst' or exploded appearance, also occur in the lumbar spine. Paraplegia is relatively less common than in the thoracolumbar region and at the lower levels the neurological damage is to the roots of the cauda equina, making recovery a more likely possibility. In the absence of paraplegia most of these injuries, which are essentially stable, can be treated symptomatically by bed rest until the patient is able to be mobilized, wearing a polythene or plaster lumbosacral support until union occurs.

Fractures of the sacrum and coccyx

These usually arise as a result of direct impact and can produce neurological problems, with the risk of the bladder being affected if the upper and middle sacral segments are involved. Treatment is purely symptomatic but these injuries, particularly the coccygeal fractures, can produce long-term pain.

Coccygeal pain or coccydynia can be a troublesome long-term problem following a fracture of the coccyx, but it can also occur spontaneously and occasionally after childbirth. It causes pain when sitting and is difficult to treat. Injections of local anaesthetic and hydrocortisone into the tender area can be helpful and manipulation of the coccyx via the rectum and with general anaesthesia can also give relief. Rarely, excision of the coccyx may be necessary.

Traumatic paraplegia

Cervical injuries

The patient with cord transection above the level of C4 is unlikely to survive because of paralysis of all the respiratory muscles including the diaphragm. Artificial ventilation may prolong life but there will be no motor function below the level of the lesion. With lesions below this level varying degrees of quadri- and paraplegia occur – often complete, with a sharply defined neurological level, but occasionally incomplete, with sensory or motor sparing below the level of section. The cervical nerve roots emerge horizontally at the disc above their correspondingly numbered vertebrae, except for the eighth roots, which emerge above the first thoracic vertebrae. The roots tend to emerge horizontally from the spinal cord so that a complete transection of the cord usually produces a clear cut, neurological level.

Incomplete lesions in the cervical cord may lead to diagnostic difficulties, e.g. the Brown-Séquard syndrome, where partial loss of function may occur in one arm with neurological disturbance in the opposite leg; and the so-called 'central-cord' syndrome, in which flaccid weakness of the arms is associated with spastic weakness of the legs. This type of injury, thought to be caused by hyperextension, usually occurs in late middle age and in patients who already have degenerative changes in the spine.

Transection of the cord in the lower cervical spine may leave a good deal of useful function in the arms.

Thoracic and thoracolumbar injuries

As mentioned above, transections at these levels tend to be complete with a well-defined neurological level, but at the thoracolumbar level the picture is complicated because the cord terminates at the lower border of L1 vertebra and the lumbar and sacral roots in the upper part of their course pass downwards alongside the cord to their foramina. Transection at this level may produce various combinations of cord and root section, giving a mixture of upper motor neurone and lower motor neurone phenomena in the legs.

Diagnosis of neurological conditions

The prognosis depends entirely on whether the cord lesion is complete or incomplete, and whether the transection involves the cord itself or the cauda equina roots. In general, recovery does not occur from complete cord transection, but incomplete lesions frequently recover to a degree and root lesions are also capable of some recovery.

Accurate neurological testing must be carried out as soon as possible after the accident and usually several times during the first 24–48 hours, recording the findings carefully. Sensory testing is best carried out with a pin, starting from the area of likely normal sensation and working down to the abnormal area. Other modalities may be tested in the complicated case. Motor power is tested and graded according to the MRC scale. If some residual sensation or voluntary movement is detectable below the likely level of cord damage, then recovery is possible because the lesion must be incomplete.

The spinal reflexes are valuable in reaching a diagnosis and prognosis, the usual stretch reflexes being supplemented by two additional reflex responses:

1. The anal reflex is manifested by a contraction of the anal sphincter when the skin around the anus is stimulated with a pin.
2. The bulbospongiosus reflex is elicited by squeezing the glans penis, causing a contraction of the cremasteric muscle. These reflexes are often the first to return and if they do so in the early hours after injury, particularly if the spinal reflexes also return *without* return of voluntary motor power or sensation, the prognosis is likely to be bad.

Management

Wherever possible, paraplegic patients are best nursed and rehabilitated in special Spinal Injury Units. Until transfer can be arranged, the patient should be nursed carefully to avoid pressure sores. The mainstay of treatment is to turn the patient from side to side, every 2 h, day and night. This must be started immediately the patient is received. This can be most conveniently done by having the patient lie on a firm bed on a draw sheet which can be used to pull the patient from side to side, allowing an inspection of the pressure areas, the new position being maintained by carefully placed pillows behind

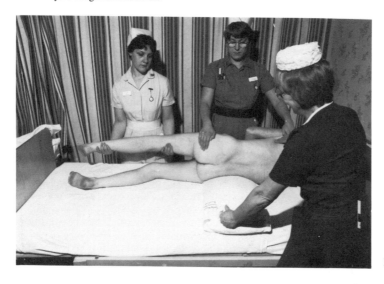

Figure 13.3 Turning a paraplegic patient

the shoulders and between the legs (Figure 13.3). Catheterization is usually necessary and must be carried out with full aseptic care. Current thought favours intermittent catheterization, twice daily, rather than continuous drainage which tends to produce a small contracted bladder.

Transfer to the specialized unit is usually arranged as soon as the acute period is over – long-term rehabilitation being a skilled and prolonged operation, with supervision usually being necessary throughout life.

Fractures of the pelvis

As with the spine, fractures of the pelvis tend to be important because of the commonly associated soft tissue injuries. Serious pelvic injuries have become more common in the industrialized nations, resulting from high-speed motoring accidents and occupational hazards.

Stability of pelvic fractures

The pelvis behaves as a ring structure which, of course, is intrinsically stable. Certain fractures do not break the ring at any point and others only enter the ring at one point. Fractures of the iliac wings and

of the ischiopubic rami are examples of these and all these injuries are stable and usually minimally or undisplaced.

The system becomes unstable if the fracture disrupts the ring in two places, particularly if one is above the hip joint (Figure 13.4). The upper disruption may be through the sacrum, the sacroiliac joint or the ilium and may, of course, be bilateral. Various combinations of these, with a second disruption through the lower part of the pelvis, i.e. ischiopubic and iliopubic rami, pubic bone or pubic symphysis are also possible and these combinations are often grossly unstable. If disruption occurs in two places *below* the level of the hip joints, the pelvis may usually be regarded as stable and long periods of immobilization avoided.

Depending on the position of the fractures, the pelvis may open like an oyster, or one side may be displaced bodily upwards relative to the other – so-called 'hind-quarter dislocation'. Complications are common with both these fractures e.g. urethral damage, rupture of the bladder or diaphragm.

Management of pelvic fractures

The stable fractures, if uncomplicated, are easily managed by allowing the patient to rest in bed until

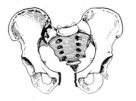 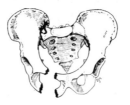 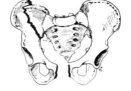

Figure 13.4 Types of unstable pelvic fractures

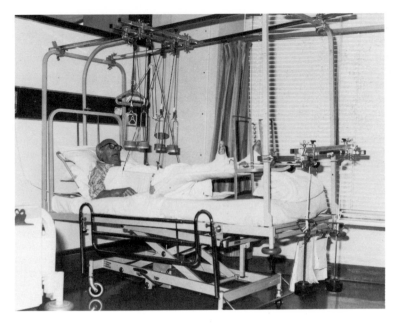

Figure 13.5 Use of slings for unstable pelvic fracture

the symptoms settle sufficiently to allow walking, usually after 2–3 weeks.

The unstable fractures, which are frequently complicated, can themselves usually be managed fairly simply. The 'oyster' type of displacement can be closed by nursing the patient on a system of pelvic slings (Figure 13.5) with the hips flexed and the legs elevated on Braun frames to prevent the hips tending to roll into external rotation. The legs are usually held on longitudinal traction to keep the frames in position. The pelvic slings are so arranged that the weight of the patient with the slings underneath his buttocks and lower spine causes the sides of the sling to compress the pelvis. Sufficient weight is applied just to support the patient off the bed. The hindquarter dislocation may be manipulated under anaesthesia and the patient then nursed in the same way. The patient will usually require up to 12 weeks on traction before union is sound.

There is a move towards open reduction and internal fixation of pelvic and acetabular fractures, using plates and screws. There is no doubt that excellent reconstitution of the pelvis can be achieved, but the surgery can be difficult and considerable expertise is necessary if the obvious dangers are to be avoided. If surgery is to be attempted, it is important that the fracture be fully analysed so that the operation can be planned in detail. In addition to conventional AP and pelvic inlet radiographs, special oblique views taken with the patient rotated through 45° in both directions are usually needed, together with further intermediate oblique views as necessary. CT scanning has now become almost mandatory for this type of surgery. Because of the expertise required, it is likely that in

the future patients will be transferred to special centres when the acute phase is over and the immediate complications have been dealt with. If such expertise is not available, the majority of patients are still likely to be better served by conservative management, rather than being subjected to heroic surgery in the hands of the inexperienced surgeon.

Although reconstructive surgery may not be readily available for many patients, fixation of the unstable pelvic fracture may often be safely achieved by the use of an external fixation frame, with the pins usually inserted into the iliac bone. This technique can be used even with severely compound injuries and has the considerable advantage of allowing the patient to be mobilzied at an early stage (Figure 13.6).

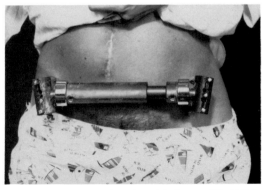

Figure 13.6 Frame fixation of a pelvic fracture (Orthofix)

Complications

Haemorrhage

The commonest complication, particularly of the unstable pelvic fracture, is haemorrhage from the large plexus of pelvic vessels, usually occurring internally, the blood tending to track up the posterior abdominal wall outside the peritoneum. The bleeding can be catastrophic and also difficult to estimate. Internal bleeding can be recognized by the usual signs of impending hypovolaemic shock and a mass may be palpable in the suprapubic region and also on rectal examination. The progress of the haemorrhage can be checked by marking the level on the anterior abdominal wall of the upper border of the palpable mass.

Management

Blood transfusion is the mainstay of treatment, with the situation monitored by measuring the central venous pressure. The bleeding usually lessens if the patient is put on pelvic slings and this can often be done almost as soon as he arrives in the emergency department, before full investigations are carried out. If transfusion does not succeed in controlling the situation, surgical exploration, with attempted ligature of the bleeding vessels, may be necessary. If a major bleeding point is not found, the wound may have to be packed. Surgery is often unsuccessful in controlling the bleeding and the mortality is then high.

Injuries to bladder and urethra

These are common, particularly with injuries around the symphysis. The bladder may be ruptured, either intra- or extraperitoneally. The urethra tends to rupture at the junction of prostatic and membranous parts, the prostate and bladder often being displaced upwards to a considerable degree.

Management

Most patients with severe pelvic fractures also have multiple injuries and may be in a state of shock or great pain. For these reasons alone, they may not readily pass urine. After the immediate emergencies have been dealt with, the patient may be asked to attempt to pass urine, but advised not to persist if the attempt fails. Bleeding from the urethral meatus may signify a urethral rupture and bruising along the course of the urethra may be obvious. Rectal examination is helpful in deciding if the prostate is in its normal position or displaced upwards.

There are essentially two schools of thought as to subsequent procedure:

1. An attempt is made to pass a soft rubber catheter gently along the urethra. If this passes easily into the bladder and an adequate quantity of clear or slightly bloodstained urine is recovered, the chances are that there is no serious damage and the catheter may be left *in situ*. If the catheter passes into the bladder, but only a small quantity of urine or blood is obtained, this may mean that the bladder itself is ruptured and a cystogram is advisable. If the catheter fails to pass, the urethra is probably ruptured. If either type of damage is suspected or confirmed, a surgical repair may be carried out if the patient's general condition will allow this.

2. The second school considers catheterization to be dangerous in that it may increase the existing damage or introduce infection, and therefore recommends suprapubic drainage if the patient fails to pass urine. Surgical repair of bladder or urethra is carried out at a convenient time, as before.

Injuries of the rectum and vagina

These are relatively uncommon, usually presenting as rectal or vaginal bleeding. The rectal injuries can be fully diagnosed by sigmoidoscopy and usually require suture and a temporary defunctioning colostomy. Vaginal injuries can usually be repaired surgically.

Sciatic nerve injuries

Perhaps surprisingly these are uncommon and there is a reasonable chance of recovery. Occasionally, if sciatic pain is persistent, exploration may be necessary to free the nerve or roots which may have become trapped between the fracture surfaces.

Traumatic rupture of the diaphragm

When the pelvis has been run over, the sudden upward force may burst the left leaf of the diaphragm. There may be acute respiratory distress but sometimes the signs of herniation may be long delayed.

Fractures and dislocations of the hip

Pelvic fractures involving the acetabulum and the hip joint are conveniently considered together with fractures of the head of the femur and dislocation of the hip. Like other pelvic fractures they have become relatively common as a result of motoring accidents. The ordinary driving position, with hips and knees flexed, is compounded by the tendency for the driver and passengers (if not wearing seat belts) to continue moving forwards after the vehicle has suddenly decelerated. Striking the knees on a parcel shelf or other projection tends to drive the femoral head against the back wall of the acetabulum. Depending on the degree of hip flexion at the time, the hip may be dislocated posteriorly or the acetabulum fractured to a variable extent. The acetabular fracture may be through the posterior wall, the centre or floor, or less commonly, through the anterior wall.

Dislocation of the hip

Simple dislocation of the hip is usually posterior, anterior dislocation being a rare injury. The position of the leg after dislocation is very characteristic, the patient presenting with the leg flexed, adducted and shortened, the femoral head often being palpable in the buttock. The only common complication is damage to the sciatic nerve which lies directly behind the joint. The lateral division of the sciatic nerve appears to be more vulnerable in this respect than the medial, and the patient may be left with a drop foot, but with other components of the sciatic nerve functioning normally.

Simple dislocation of the hip is rare in children.

Management

As with all dislocations, the sooner reduction can be attempted the easier it tends to be. General anaesthesia is necessary. The patient is laid supine, preferably on a low couch or table (Figure 13.7). The hip and knee are then flexed to a right-angle, and by gentle upward traction and slight internal and external rotation, the head usually slips into

place without force. If the first attempt fails, traction may be applied with the hip first in flexion, then with gradual extension together with abduction and external rotation and finally internal rotation into neutral. If neither of these manoeuvres is successful, it is likely that there is a fragment of bone from the head or margin of the acetabulum blocking reduction. In these circumstances open reduction via a posterior approach will usually be necessary, replacing the displaced fragment and, particularly if (as is usually the case), the fragment represents the posterior margin of the acetabulum, holding the reduction with a screw. Fragments from the head, if completely detached, may have to be discarded. The same procedure will be necessary if a fracture-dislocation has reduced easily by manipulation, but equally easily redislocates when tested in the flexed position. In these circumstances fixation of the marginal fragment is necessary to restore stability. This latter type of injury is particularly likely to be associated with sciatic nerve injury and the nerve may have to be released in the course of the open reduction. It is usually contused, but not completely divided, and considerable recovery may occur.

Following reduction of a hip dislocation, the patient is usually nursed on longitudinal traction for 3 weeks, then allowed to mobilize, non-weight-bearing, for a further 3 weeks. Stiffness of the joint is rarely a problem, but late osteoarthritis may occur.

Fracture-dislocation of the hip

The acetabulum can be regarded as being formed from a strong roof, an anterior or iliopubic column, and a posterior or ilio-ischial column. Judet has

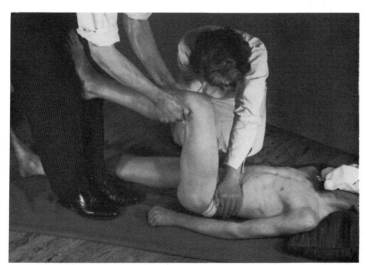

Figure 13.7 Reduction of a traumatic dislocation of the hip

classified fractures of the acetabulum on this basis into four broad groups:

1. Fracture of the posterior rim, as mentioned above.
2. Fracture of the ilio-ischial column (Figure 13.8).
3. Transverse fracture (Figure 13.9).
4. Fracture of the iliopubic column (Figure 13.10).

In each case the head loses its normal relationship with the pelvis considered as a whole, frequently being displaced inwards, the condition then being rather loosely called a 'central dislocation'.

Management of fracture-dislocation

Before attempting any kind of manoeuvre, the situation should be assessed fully by taking antero-posterior, lateral and oblique radiograph views, taken with the patient rotated through 45° towards and away from the film plane. Without these, diagnosis is likely to be incomplete.

Fracture of the posterior rim has been considered above in association with simple dislocation of the hip.

Some fracture-dislocations may be treated quite adequately by manipulation under anaesthesia and the application of traction to the limb. In effect, an attempt is made to pull out the head to its normal position. The head will often reduce suddenly and, provided the capsular attachments remain reasonably intact, the other fragments may also fall back into place. Occasionally the head will reduce to its normal position under the roof of the acetabulum, but the other fragments may remain displaced. In these circumstances, even after a long period of immobilization, the head may redisplace. If reduction is inadequate or incomplete, consideration should be given to open reduction of the fracture. As with other pelvic fractures, the operative techniques involved are by no means easy and should not be attempted by the inexperienced. If the patient cannot be transported to the care of someone with the necessary expertise, the alternative of accepting the position and simply maintaining the patient on traction for the necessary 12 weeks may be safer. Even severe degrees of residual displacement of acetabular fractures, provided the head is stable, can give surprisingly good function. It should be mentioned that, as an adjunct to simple longitudinal traction, the tendency of the head to redislocate centrally can sometimes be overcome by passing a Steinmann pin from front to back through the greater trochanter and attaching lateral traction to this. This can only be expected to succeed, however, if the pelvic fragments have been pulled into alignment along with the head.

All these injuries can be difficult to manage, as they are often accompanied by other severe injuries, when the various requirements of treatment may conflict.

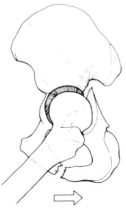

Figure 13.8 Fracture of the ilio-ischial column

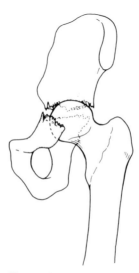

Figure 13.9 Transverse acetabular fracture

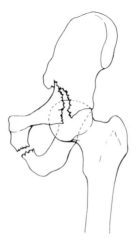

Figure 13.10 Fracture of the iliopubic column

14

Injuries of the limbs

T. Duckworth

Injuries of the lower limb

Fractures of the femoral neck

The majority of femoral neck fractures occur in the elderly and, particularly in the West, a steadily ageing population has made this a major sociological problem, with many hospital beds permanently occupied by patients who have had this type of injury. There is good evidence that in these patients the bone structure is deficient as a result of matrix or mineralization defects, so the fracture is essentially pathological. This being the case, the fracture may occur after a relatively trivial injury, such as a minor fall or even a stumble. There is indeed reason to suppose that in some patients the fracture occurs spontaneously and may precede the fall.

The incidence of the condition is steadily rising in many countries and, at least in the UK, the rise far exceeds the increase in the number of elderly in the population. The reason for this remains obscure but may relate to the fact that many old people now live alone and may be taking powerful drugs for various medical conditions, resulting in a chronic confusional state which makes them prone to fall and reluctant or unable to summon help. As a consequence, it is not uncommon for such patients to present to hospital with a fracture which is several days old, with a correspondingly worse prognosis for the survival of the femoral head. There is currently a good deal of interest in the possibility of preventing femoral neck fractures by management of the underlying osteoporosis. There is as yet, however, no form of treatment which is generally accepted as making a significant difference to the condition. There is no doubt that the osteoporosis can be influenced by factors such as exercise, hormones such as oestrogens and anabolic steroids and drugs such as fluorides, but it has yet to be demonstrated that the incidence of femoral neck fracture can be influenced by these measures.

Management

As the injury is often minor and the patient frequently confused, diagnosis can be difficult. The main complaint is of pain in the groin or hip region and difficulty in standing or walking. Occasionally walking may be possible, but the gait is usually poor and restriction of hip movements almost invariable. Any patient in this age group complaining of hip pain and with appropriate physical signs, must be assumed to have a femoral neck fracture and radiographs should be taken (Figure 14.1). Good quality AP and lateral films are necessary and the undisplaced fracture can even then be difficult to diagnose on a first film. In these circumstances the patient may have to be treated by bed rest and perhaps repeat radiographs taken each week later when slight displacement may have occurred. Tomography and magnified radiographs can be useful.

Intracapsular fractures

Sometimes called subcapital fractures, these occur through the upper femoral neck within the capsule of the hip joint. Typically, the head tends to displace backwards and the hip to fall into external rotation and adduction.

The anatomy of the blood supply of the femoral head – the main supply being derived from vessels which pass along the neck into the head – makes the head vulnerable to ischaemia of varying degree. With the greater degrees of displacement, the head may be rendered completely avascular and, although union may still occur, given adequate fixation, from vessels growing in from the distal

159

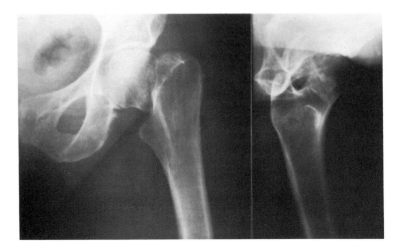

Figure 14.1 Subcapital fracture. AP and lateral radiographs

fragment, ischaemic necrosis is still liable to occur and causes fragmentation and collapse of the head.

Classification of the fracture into different types is relatively unhelpful. Many fractures which appear to be impacted will displace if not managed carefully. An estimate of the degree of displacement is, however, more useful. The minimally displaced fracture with only slight angulation of the trabecular markings across the site of the fracture will usually be reducible to a fairly accurate position. If the head is significantly displaced, rather than angulated on the neck, considerable disruption of vessels must have occurred. In the most severe degrees of displacement, where the head is bodily displaced downwards relative to the neck and the trabeculae come to lie parallel in the proximal and distal fragments, reduction will be difficult and probably incomplete, and the prognosis for the head is poor.

Unfortunately it is not possible with current techniques to assess accurately the extent of residual blood supply to the head, the only reasonable guide being the degree of displacement. Grossly displaced or long-standing, unreduced fractures are presumed to have a poor prognosis.

Management

The patients who usually sustain this type of fracture have a precarious hold on life and the mortality is high – approaching 30% over the 6-month period following the accident. There is general agreement that early mobilization should be the aim if possible, to avoid the complications of long periods in bed. This is usually achieved by either reducing the fracture and holding it by an internal fixation device which is sufficiently strong to allow the patient to bear weight, or, alternatively, by removing the head and replacing it with a prosthesis of the Thompson or Austin Moore type. The choice may be made on the basis of the degree of displacement, the patient's

age, or a combination of the two. At the ends of the spectrum, most surgeons will elect on the one hand to fix the undisplaced or minimally displaced fracture after manipulation, and on the other hand to remove the head if displacement is severe or the injury more than a few days old. Some surgeons tend to elect routinely for replacement in the older patient, arguing that the risk of further surgery is thereby lessened. In the best hands internal fixation, providing reduction is good, can give over 90% union, but a proportion of those that have united will develop ischaemic necrosis and some of them will require a further operation because of this.

Whichever technique is preferred, the mortality of immediate operation is high and it is now usual to spend 2–3 days assessing the patient's general condition and correcting any medical problems. During this time, if the fracture is to be fixed, it can be reduced gradually and simply by applying traction and internal rotation as described by Wainwright. With this technique, a Steinmann pin is passed through the upper tibia. Hamilton–Russell traction is then set up, but with the vertical cord of the traction system attached to the outer end of the tibial pin to produce an internal rotation force. Check radiographs then make it possible to make a decision, prior to taking the patient to theatre, whether to fix the fracture or replace the head.

If internal fixation is to be undertaken, the final degrees of manipulation can be carried out on the orthopaedic table, gentle traction and internal rotation usually securing adequate reduction. Many methods of internal fixation are used. The simple trifin Smith-Petersen pin is not now generally considered adequate. Various types of screws, sliding nails and pins are available. One of the most effective, but requiring good technique and accurate reduction, is the double-screw technique described by Garden (Figure 14.2). This is designed to compress the fracture and to prevent rotation of the

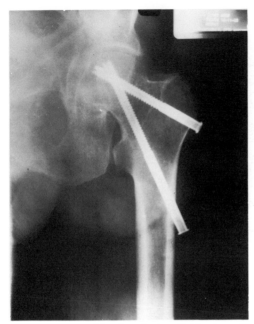

Figure 14.2 Internal fixation of subcapital fracture with Garden screws

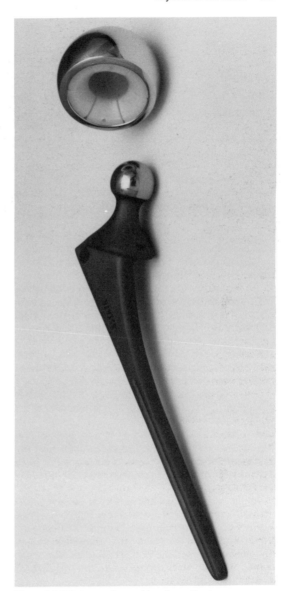

Figure 14.3 Bateman femoral head prosthesis

head. The alternative technique is to remove the head and replace it with a femoral prosthesis. The Thompson type, designed to be used with orthopaedic cement, is most widely used. This type of prosthesis is satisfactory in the older patient with limited mobility and expectation of life, but in the younger and more active patient the prosthesis has a tendency to wear its way into the acetabulum, which may fracture. For this type of patient it may be more appropriate to consider a total hip replacement with a Charnley-type prosthesis. This is, however, a more major operation with an increased complication risk and there is currently interest in the use of so-called 'bi-polar' prostheses. These have a metal-backed polyethylene acetabular component, which is free to move in the patient's own acetabulum, articulating with a Charnley-type metal femoral component. This has several advantages. The insertion is relatively simple and comparable with that of a Thompson prosthesis. The tendency for the head to bore into the pelvis appears to be less and if wear of the polyethylene occurs the loose cup can be replaced relatively easily or can be exchanged for a conventional cemented Charnley cup, without disturbing the femoral component. The Bateman prosthesis (Figure 14.3) is of this type and was designed to be used with the femoral component either cemented or uncemented.

Whichever technique is used, following surgery, the patient is usually allowed to sit out of bed next day and, if satisfactory fixation has been achieved, may begin walking almost immediately.

Extracapsular or basal fractures of the femoral neck

This type of fracture tends to occur in somewhat younger patients than the intracapsular fractures, although many of the difficulties associated with a serious fracture in old age still apply. The fracture line tends to run across the base of the neck between the greater and lesser trochanter and is frequently called intertrochanteric. The blood supply of this

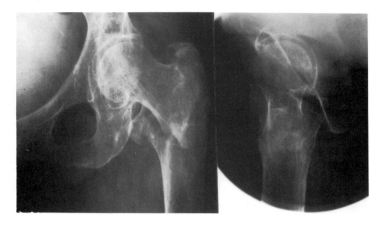

Figure 14.4 Intertrochanteric or basal fracture of femoral neck. AP and lateral radiographs

area is adequate to ensure satisfactory union in most cases. The outcome depends to a large extent on the amount of comminution around the calcar femorale. If the lesser trochanter is split away from the calcar, then, even if the neck and shaft are restored to their normal relationship, the direct line of weight transmission up the neck cannot be properly reconstituted and the fracture becomes difficult to fix securely. It then tends to drop into a varus position on weight-bearing, with the fixation device cutting out or failing.

Management

The history and physical signs are usually very similar to those of the intracapsular fracture. Radiographic diagnosis presents no problems, but a lateral view of the neck should always be obtained (Figure 14.4).

In the younger patient, bed rest on Hamilton–Russell traction is quite satisfactory but now seldom used. The fracture will usually unite securely after 10–11 weeks and the patient may then bear weight. In the older patient the arguments for early mobilization become stronger, and internal fixation is usually preferred.

The operation is carried out as soon as the general condition of the patient permits. Gentle manipulation of the limb into internal rotation and abduction is sometimes necessary, but occasionally internal rotation may result in opening the fracture posteriorly, so radiographs should be taken before proceeding.

The trifin nail and plate (Figure 14.5) has now been largely superseded.

The failure rate with the potentially unstable fracture described above is high and many alternatives have been tried. Currently in favour, although expensive, are devices which utilize a sliding principle to allow some compression of the fracture surfaces. The Richards and AO types are the most widely used (Figure 14.6).

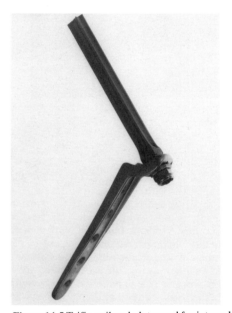

Figure 14.5 Trifin nail and plate used for internal fixation of intertrochanteric fracture

Rehabilitation following femoral neck fractures

Relatively few patients return to full mobility following these injuries. The aim of internal fixation is to allow early mobilization and this should be started as soon as possible after surgery. The patient may normally get out of bed on the day after operation and begin walking with a Zimmer-type frame and with assistance on the next day. Partial or non-weight-bearing is rarely possible and the operative procedure should be designed to allow full weight-bearing wherever possible. Many patients are confused and an early return to home surroundings may help to alleviate this. Full attention should

is often compound and frequently severely contaminated.

Management

The diagnosis is normally self-evident, but radiographs in two planes are, of course, always necessary and the not uncommon association of this injury with a dislocation of the same hip should be remembered.

The aim of treatment is to secure union, in good alignment, with length restored and with early rehabilitation. Many different techniques are employed, depending on the fracture itself and on local circumstances. Manipulative reduction under anaesthesia is usually the initial procedure. Strong traction is required. In general, reduction simply involves securing alignment and length. Perfect anatomical reduction is rarely necessary. Overlap of less than 1 cm is not harmful. Occasionally the fracture ends will obviously not come into contact and, in these circumstances, there is likely to be muscle between the fracture surfaces. If this is the case, open reduction will usually be necessary to extract the muscle and allow apposition.

Having achieved reduction by closed or open manipulation, various possibilities may then be considered for fixation.

1. A widely used technique involves the use of the Thomas splint (Figure 14.7), which employs

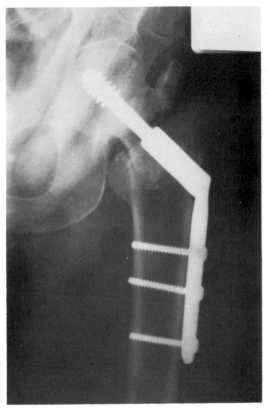

Figure 14.6 Richards dynamic hip screw and plate

be paid to any medical and nutritional problems. Several studies have shown that the eventual outcome depends more on the mental and social state of the patient at the time of injury than on the method of treating the fracture. As mentioned above, the social problems are formidable, particularly where family support is not available, as is increasingly the case in the developed world.

Fracture of the shaft of the femur

This type of fracture is one of the commonest and occurs in all age groups. Considerable violence is necessary to fracture the non-pathological femur and the fracture is frequently associated with other injuries. The fracture occurs at various levels in the shaft, the lowest levels being described as supracondylar. Neurological and vascular complications are, fortunately, relatively uncommon, but gross swelling of the thigh should always arouse suspicion of a femoral artery rupture. Blood loss in the uncomplicated, closed fracture is seldom more than one unit and often much less, so that shock is unlikely in the absence of other injuries. The injury

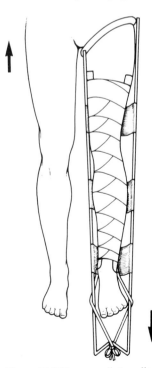

Figure 14.7 Thomas splint applied with skin traction

counter-traction against the ischial tuberosity. In the young patient with powerful thigh muscles, skeletal traction may be needed and, in these circumstances, the Thomas splint is modified with a Pearson knee attachment (p. 185).

2. Sliding traction with the femur supported on a frame or pillows and using a Steinmann pin through the upper tibia (p. 185) offers an alternative, but is somewhat more difficult to manage successfully.

3. The fracture may be immobilized in a plaster hip spica, extending from the toes on the affected side to the upper chest. The fixation achieved is relatively poor and the cast is uncomfortable, but a long stay in hospital may be avoided.

4. A technique known as cast-bracing has achieved some popularity. This involves an accurately fitting full leg plaster cast hinged at the knee. Its fitting requires considerable expertise but it has obvious advantages. It may be made of plaster of Paris or one of the newer casting materials. It can normally be applied after 3–4 weeks on traction.

5. Internal fixation offers considerable advantages in giving good alignment, early mobilization of the patient and the joints, and a very high union rate. The most commonly used device is the Küntscher intramedullary nail which is usually introduced by opening the fracture, reaming the medullary canal and passing the nail upwards and out through a separate incision in the gluteal region, then aligning the fracture and driving the nail down into the distal fragment. The most troublesome complication of this technique is sepsis, which may delay union and lead to persistent wound discharge until the nail is removed, and sometimes indefinitely. A newer technique, which can be used when suitable equipment and X-ray facilities are available, does not require the fracture to be opened, but simply manipulated, the nail then being passed downwards from above. In skilled hands this gives a very high union rate with few complications.

The lowest level fractures are difficult to fix by intramedullary nailing because the medullary canal widens considerably. Even higher fractures may tend to rotate around the nail if this is not a tight fit and a small plate may be necessary to control this tendency.

These problems can now be dealt with better by the use of the so-called 'interlocking nails'. Even the most difficult comminuted fractures of the femoral shaft can be controlled adequately by these devices and early weight-bearing is usually possible.

At supracondylar level, internal fixation may require a transverse nail attached to a plate extending up the side of the femur similar to the system used for intertrochanteric fractures. Traction on a Thomas splint with a pin through the upper tibia may be more appropriate for the comminuted supracondylar fracture.

Whatever method of fixation is chosen, 12 weeks is the average time for a shaft fracture to unite in an adult and if external fixation has been used, a further period of protected weight-bearing, using a weight-relieving caliper or cast brace is usually advisable. An intramedullary nail will normally allow full weight-bearing after about 6 weeks.

Physiotherapy is often necessary to relieve knee stiffness, which is particularly common following external fixation of the fracture.

Fractures and dislocations of the knee and tibia

Dislocation of the patella

This injury tends to occur in children and young adults, usually from a blow on the inner side of the knee, causing the patella to dislocate laterally. The medial expansion of the quadriceps mechanism is torn and the patella and patellar tendon come to lie along the lateral side of the joint, which is held in a flexed position until the dislocation is reduced. In some patients, usually adolescent girls, once the dislocation has occurred it tends to recur easily and sometimes spontaneously. It is likely in these cases that there is an anatomical abnormality of the patellofemoral joint. These patients may describe the incident as 'locking' of the knee, and may be unaware of the true nature of the condition. A helpful diagnostic sign is the so-called 'apprehension' sign, elicited by an attempt to dislocate the patella laterally.

Management

The acute dislocation will usually reduce easily when the knee is extended. An anaesthetic is not always needed. The knee is then immobilized in a plaster cylinder in extension for 3 weeks, followed by a period of physiotherapy to regain movements. The recurrent dislocation may require surgery to stabilize the patella. Various operations are available, but a generally successful procedure in the skeletally mature patient is to transplant the insertion of the patellar tendon, with an attached block of bone, to a more medial and slightly more distal position. It has become obvious, however, that although this and similar procedures will usually correct the tendency to dislocate, they are associated with a high incidence of patellofemoral arthritis in later life.

Rupture of the quadriceps tendon and the patellar tendon

These injuries tend to occur in middle age, rupture of the patellar tendon affecting a slightly younger age group than rupture of the quadriceps tendon. In both cases the injury usually occurs when the knee is flexed suddenly against a contracting quadriceps, sometimes simply as the result of a stumble. Active extension of the knee is lost and the gap in the tendon is usually easily palpable and may be visible as a translucent shadow on a lateral radiograph.

Management

In general, the importance of the quadriceps mechanism is such that surgical repair is justified, followed by a period of 3–6 weeks in a plaster cylinder. Knee flexion may be difficult to regain after removal of the plaster cast.

Fractures of the patella

Two types of patellar fracture are usually recognized, the star-shaped or comminuted fracture and the transverse fracture.

The star-shaped or comminuted fracture is caused by a direct blow, e.g. on a parcel shelf in a car (and not uncommonly associated with a dislocation of the hip). The underlying femoral condyles may also be damaged. The quadriceps mechanism is essentially intact, the fracture occurring within the substance of the patella. A tense haemarthrosis should be aspirated. A minimally displaced stellate fracture may be treated conservatively by 3–4 weeks in a plaster cylinder, but if displacement is severe, patellectomy is usually advisable. Following both methods of treatment a course of physiotherapy will be necessary to restore flexion.

The transverse fracture which is caused by the same type of violence as that which causes a rupture of the quadriceps or patellar tendon produces two large fragments and with a tear of the extensor expansion, extending horizontally to a considerable distance on each side of the patella. Open reduction and internal fixation are usually preferred, either with a circumferential wire suture, a longitudinal screw or a tension-banding procedure as described by the AO/ASIF group. The lateral expansions must be carefully repaired. After 3 weeks in a plaster cylinder, mobilization and flexion of the knee may be started under supervision.

Osteoarthritis of the patellofemoral joint is a well recognized late complication of many patellar fractures.

Injuries of the ligaments and menisci of the knee

The principal ligaments of the knee – the collaterals and the two cruciates – are frequently injured, particularly in road traffic and sporting accidents. The subject of acute ligamentous injury and the chronic instability which may result has received a great deal of attention in the last 10 years and has become very complicated, suggesting that considerable expertise is needed to reach an accurate diagnosis. Only a few points of guidance will be considered here.

Injuries of the menisci and capsule are frequently combined with damage to the specific ligaments, the combination of a medial meniscus tear and a rupture of the anterior cruciate ligament being particularly common.

Acute strains of the collateral ligaments, particularly the medial, are common, often the results of sporting accidents, notably during football and skiing. The knee has usually been forced into a position of varus or valgus and reproducing this movement passively causes pain in the damaged ligament. With this type of injury the knee usually shows some swelling, although this may take several hours to develop. The radiograph is usually normal, but is helpful in distinguishing a strain from a complete rupture. Occasionally the AP radiograph may show a small flake of bone avulsed from the femoral or tibial condyle.

In order to diagnose a complete rupture with any certainty, a film taken with the knee stressed to open it medially or laterally is needed, and a general anaesthetic will usually be necessary to achieve this. Clinical diagnosis of acute ligament injuries without anaesthesia tends to be difficult and inaccurate.

Rupture of the cruciate ligaments is diagnosed on the basis of the anterior and posterior 'draw' signs, performed with the knee flexed to a right-angle. In principle, a rupture of the anterior cruciate allows a positive anterior draw sign and a rupture of the posterior cruciate (and capsule) makes it possible to push the tibia backwards on the femur.

More refined clinical tests are claimed to improve the diagnostic accuracy. The most widely used are the Lachman and the so-called 'pivot-shift' tests. Lachman's test involves trying to draw the tibia forwards on the femoral condyles with the knee flexed to about 10–15°. It can be useful in the swollen painful knee. The test is positive with an anterior cruciate ligament disruption. There are various 'pivot-shift' tests and tests for rotatory instability. Pivot-shift tests are performed by flexing the knee slowly whilst valgus or varus stresses are applied, with the tibia in internal or external rotation. The test is positive in each case when there is a sudden subluxation at 30–40° of flexion and can be used to diagnose combinations of cruciate, collateral ligament and capsular injuries.

In practice, ligament injuries tend to occur in combination and this can make diagnosis difficult. It is helpful to remember that an *isolated* anterior cruciate ligament rupture causes only very minimal anterior laxity. Wide opening of the joint on either side when stressed implies a complete rupture of the corresponding collateral and also one or both cruciates (usually the posterior). In these circumstances damage to the meniscus can rarely be diagnosed accurately purely on clinical grounds.

With complete medial or posterior cruciate ruptures, swelling of the knee is rarely gross because the blood tends to leak out of the joint through the torn capsule.

The acute sprains and strains may be immobilized in a plaster cylinder for 2–3 weeks with the knee in a few degrees of flexion, if severe, or otherwise treated by early supervised exercise. Complete ruptures require specialist management – often by surgical repair, but the end results usually leave much to be desired.

Injuries of the menisci

Meniscal tears are among the commonest of knee injuries. Many tears probably occur in menisci which are degenerate and this is particularly the case with the knees of miners and other manual workers who spend much time crouching. The nature of the game makes soccer a very common cause of meniscal injuries.

The patient, who is typically a young male (although the degenerate type of tear occurs in a somewhat older age group), twists the knee forcibly whilst bearing weight on the leg with the knee flexed. He experiences pain in the side of the knee corresponding to the tear and the knee may lock, i.e. refuse to extend fully. Occasionally the knee may 'unlock' spontaneously or be 'unlocked' by a colleague. Swelling may occur within minutes due to a haemarthrosis, often signifying an associated anterior cruciate tear, or it may take several hours, in which case it is due to an effusion. The acute injury of tearing a normal meniscus is a severe one, and walking may be impossible. Typically the swelling and pain subside over the next few days and the knee may then return to normal, only to give rise to intermittent symptoms, such as 'giving way', pain, locking and swelling, over the course of the next few months. This is the classic history, but the diagnosis can be made much more difficult by the history being atypical, particularly if there has been no definite injury.

In the acute stage the knee is usually swollen with an effusion or haemarthrosis, may lack extension, i.e. be 'locked' and there is usually localized tenderness over the damaged meniscus. In the chronic stage signs may be minimal – perhaps a little tenderness over the meniscus and a degree of wasting of the quadriceps muscle. McMurray's sign (a test for a posterior tear) may be positive. This test is performed by flexing the knee fully, gripping the joint with middle finger over the medial joint line and thumb over the lateral joint line, and rotating the tibia on the femur whilst slowly extending the knee and feeling for a 'catch' as the torn meniscus displaces.

Management of meniscal injuries

In the acute phase, diagnosis is not always easy and the history and signs of a ligament tear can be very similar to those of a meniscus tear, even the phenomenon of 'locking' being mimicked by muscular spasm. At this stage the knee is best supported in a Robert Jones compression bandage, i.e. alternating layers of cotton wool and crêpe bandage wrapped around the knee and extending to just above and below the limits of the joint cavity. Care should be taken to avoid pressure of the lower part of the bandage on the calf. After a few days the swelling usually subsides and spasm relaxes. If the knee is still locked, examination under anaesthesia is usually advisable and if it remains locked, either an exploration or, preferably, arthroscopy is carried out.

The knee with chronic symptoms may be investigated either by arthrography, if facilities are available, or by arthroscopy, which usually clarifies the diagnosis. Sometimes the knee may have to be explored purely on the history and physical signs, and this will obviously be necessary if arthroscopy is not available.

The torn meniscus is usually excised in part or as a whole if the tear is extensive. Techniques have been developed for performing meniscectomy using the arthroscope, but considerable expertise is required for this procedure. The advantage is that recovery is usually much more rapid than with the conventional open technique.

Complete dislocation of the knee

This is a rare injury, sometimes associated with a rupture of the femoral artery, and always involving considerable ligamentous damage.

Reduction under anaesthesia is usually possible if the femur has not 'button-holed' through the capsule. The knee may then be left in a Thomas splint or in a plaster cylinder or back splint for 4–6 weeks, then mobilized. Function can be surprisingly good following this relatively simple line of treatment.

Fractures of the upper tibia

The cruciate ligaments may be avulsed from their attachment to the intercondylar eminence of the tibia. The fragment of bone which is torn off may be visible on radiograph in the intercondylar notch and a lateral film will identify which ligament is involved. If there is significant displacement, the knee is usually best explored and the fragment sutured or pinned into position.

It is common for the weight-bearing knee to be struck on either side, forcing the joint into varus or valgus. The car bumper or fender injury is an example of this. In these circumstances, one or other femoral condyle may be compressed against the corresponding tibial condyle producing a depressed and usually comminuted fracture of the latter. The knee usually fills with blood and if an attempt is made to stress it sideways there is usually a degree of instability.

Minor degrees of depression of one tibial condyle, i.e. less than 0.5 cm may be left unreduced and the knee mobilized on a sliding traction system. More severe depression, particularly in the young active individual, should be treated by operative elevation of the joint surface to its normal level, the underlying defect being filled with cancellous bone. A transverse screw may be used to maintain reduction.

The joint surface is usually badly damaged and the meniscus may be torn. Mobilization as soon as possible should be encouraged as stiffness is a likely complication.

Osteoarthritis may be a late sequel of this type of fracture.

Fractures of the shafts of tibia and fibula

The two bones essentially function as one unit and frequently both are fractured. If the tibial shaft is fractured and the fibula remains intact, it can be difficult to reduce the tibial fracture and the risks of non-union are increased. It is occasionally necessary to divide the fibula to secure an adequate reduction of the tibia.

Fractures of the two lower leg bones are common at all ages, and often occur as a result of road traffic or sporting accidents. Because of the subcutaneous position of the tibia, the fracture is frequently compound and often comminuted.

Management of tibial and fibular shaft fractures

Diagnosis is usually easy. The state of the circulation and peripheral nerves should be noted carefully. Fractures with severe vascular injury may require primary amputation.

Oblique and spiral fractures (Figure 14.8) tend to be unstable in that they easily shorten or angulate after reduction. Any wound is examined carefully and closed where the likelihood is that this can be accomplished safely and the patient can be kept under observation. Except for undisplaced fractures, reduction under anaesthesia is usually necessary to restore length and alignment. Even minor degrees of angulation can be cosmetically unacceptable. Tibial shaft fractures, particularly the severely comminuted and compound ones (Figure 14.9),

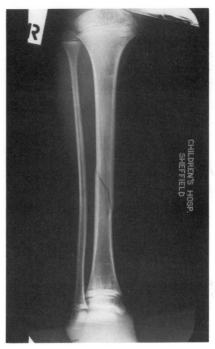

Figure 14.8 Undisplaced spiral fracture of tibial shaft

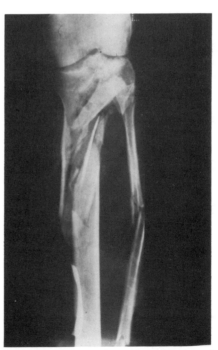

Figure 14.9 Compound comminuted fracture of upper tibia and fibula

have a high rate of non-union, and this is made more likely if the fracture is (a) inadequately immobilized, (b) over-distracted, or (c) becomes infected. A clean transverse shaft fracture will usually be stable when reduced and can normally be held adequately in a full leg plaster cast, extending from the groin to the base of the toes, with the knee flexed to 20–30°, to prevent rotation at the fracture site. The fracture may be conveniently manipulated by allowing the leg to hang over the end of the operating table. Angulation and rotation are corrected and a below-knee cast applied whilst the fracture is held and the plaster is moulded so that it appears slightly angulated medially. Check radiographs are taken and, if satisfactory, the plaster is completed to full leg length and a final set of check radiographs is then obtained. If the fracture is slightly angulated after applying the plaster, this can be corrected by wedging the plaster after it has dried.

A full leg plaster alone is rarely sufficient to prevent shortening of an oblique or spiral fracture, and additional steps must be taken in these cases. Various methods can be used:

1. Traction may be applied, with the leg supported on a frame, through a pin inserted through the calcaneum or lower tibia. After 3 weeks a degree of stability will have been achieved, and a full leg plaster cast may then be applied.
2. Two Steinmann pins may be passed, one through the upper tibia and one through the lower tibia or calcaneum and both of these embedded in a full leg plaster cast.
3. A close fitting cast brace as described by Sarmiento may be used to allow knee movement. The technique of fitting the cast brace is not easy, but good results can be achieved.
4. Internal fixation has become popular as it allows accurate reduction, early mobilization and the union rate is good. Compression plating is frequently used, although intramedullary nailing tends to be safer for open fractures. Considerable expertise is necessary to obtain good results and many fractures can be extremely difficult to fix adequately. If adequate expertise or equipment is not available, closed techniques may offer a safer, if in some respects, slightly less satisfactory alternative.
5. A useful technique, because of the ready accessibility of the bone, is to use an external fixation frame. This is particularly valuable for the severely compound fracture with skin damage or loss. It gives good fixation and allows easy access to the wound. Generally speaking, the pins should be removed after about 8 weeks and the limb immobilized in a plaster cast until final union occurs.

Whichever technique is chosen, the fibular fracture is usually ignored. Time to union ranges from 3–4 weeks in a baby up to 12 weeks and sometimes much longer in an adult.

There are differences of opinion as to when weight-bearing may be allowed. The internal or intero-external fixation techniques, together with cast bracing, allow early knee movement. If the fracture is stable, weight-bearing in a plaster cast can be started almost immediately, otherwise it is usually delayed for at least 6 weeks. The cast is provided with a rubber or plastic heel, or in elderly and unsteady patients, a pad of sorbo rubber may be used to form a sole. The patient's ability to bear weight is usually an indication of the state of union of the fracture.

In addition to non-union, as mentioned above, stiffness of knee, ankle and foot may delay rehabilitation. Ischaemia of the calf and anterior tibial muscles is common and may result in ischaemic contractures of the toes which can produce long-term problems.

Injuries of the ankle and foot

Ligament strains

The lateral ligament of the ankle is a complex structure, consisting of an anterior talofibular component running almost horizontally, a talocalcaneal or deep component, and a calcaneofibular component. It is commonly damaged, usually in the anterior talofibular region, by the patient going over on the foot and sustaining an inversion strain, usually with a rotational component. A more severe degree of the same type of violence may cause a complete rupture of the lateral ligament.

Clinical features and management

The history is usually characteristic. In the lesser strains the ankle is swollen only over the outer side. In the more severe injuries with complete rupture of the ligament, the swelling is often severe and may involve the whole ankle including the medial side.

Fractures of the ankle may produce identical physical signs and fractures of the lateral malleolus can be impossible to differentiate clinically from lateral ligament strains. In general, with the ligament strains the tenderness tends to be below and anterior to the lateral malleolus and stressing the joint into inversion is painful. Plain AP and lateral radiographs of the ankle are useful in excluding a fracture, but will not normally reveal a complete lateral ligament rupture. It is a useful rule that if swelling is severe and the ankle 'ought' to be fractured but the radiograph looks normal, then stress films should be taken either under general anaesthesia or using local anaesthetic injected into the lateral ligament. If the lateral ligament is torn, the ankle will open widely on the outer side, a minor

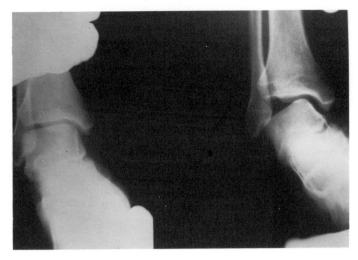

Figure 14.10 AP radiograph with the ankle stressed into adduction – rupture of lateral ligament

degree of tilt being normal (Figure 14.10). This degree of instability is sometimes detectable clinically, but not usually when swelling is severe. The ankle may also be stressed by pulling the foot forwards and backwards to detect anterior and posterior instability – the former caused by a rupture of the anterior talofibular ligament.

Simple strains may be protected by elastic adhesive strapping. The strapping should be applied firmly from the base of the toes to the head of the fibula, wound in such a way that it tends to evert the foot. Severe swelling may require a period of elevation in bed on a frame for a few days and in these cases a below-knee walking plaster may then make the patient more mobile. Three weeks of protection is usually sufficient.

Complete ruptures of the lateral ligament need careful treatment if chronic instability of the ankle is to be avoided, hence the need for accurate diagnosis. Treatment may consist either of surgical repair, followed by plaster immobilization, or plaster alone without surgery. Differences in results from the two methods of treatment are relatively minor. Six weeks' immobilization is usually adequate, followed by physiotherapy to restore ankle and subtalar movements.

Long-term instability tends to give rise to persistent 'giving way' of the ankle, often with recurrent strains. Various operations are available to correct this, but most limit subtalar movements to some extent.

Medial ligament injuries are uncommon and can usually be treated conservatively, either by strapping or in a below-knee walking cast.

Fractures and dislocations of the ankle

There have been many attempts to classify fractures and fracture-dislocations of the ankle. These are usually based on an analysis of radiographs taken after injury and usually without any stress applied to the joint. It is currently fashionable to try to work out the mechanisms by which the fracture occurred. The common mechanisms are considered to be forced inversion, forced eversion, inversion and external rotation, eversion and external rotation, and vertical compression. There are problems, however, in that the exact mechanism of injury is rarely known, and has to be presumed from the radiographic appearances, and many fractures stubbornly refuse to conform to such classification systems. Most ankle injuries are, understandably, caused by the foot becoming fixed and the weight of the patient applying a force to the ankle, usually with a rotational component.

The primary reason for attempting to classify these injuries is to make it possible to treat them in a logical and consistent manner. For most purposes the subject can be simplified by regarding the ankle joint as a hinge joint whose stability depends on the shape of its bony components and on the ligamentous complex on each side, the anterior and posterior capsular ligaments being relatively weak. It can be reasonably assumed that successful treatment will need to ensure that the joint surfaces are as congruent as possible and that the system has been restored to normal stability. Many fractures and ligamentous injuries are associated with a degree of subluxation or dislocation of the joint. This is not, however, always obvious because the components may have returned to their original alignment after the injury, but are nevertheless capable of redisplacing if stability is not restored.

Essentially, the ankle can be injured on one or both sides, and in the most severe rotational injuries the posterior, or more rarely the anterior, lip of the tibial joint surface may be fractured and displaced as the talus rotates out of the mortice. The posterior lip

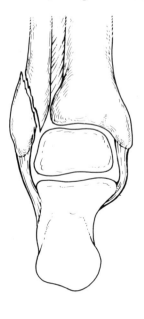

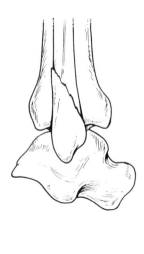

Figure 14.11 Spiral fracture of lateral malleolus – unimalleolar injury

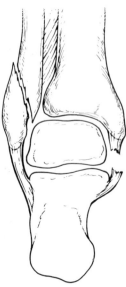

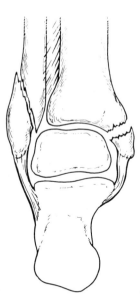

Figure 14.12 Two types of bimalleolar injury

is often called the 'third malleolus'. Fractures of the medial or lateral malleolus tend to have the same effect on the stability of the joint as a rupture of the corresponding ligament. The latter may not be obvious from the radiograph unless stress is applied.

The least degree of instability occurs when one side only is disrupted. This occurs most commonly on the lateral side, either the lateral ligament being ruptured as described above, or the fibula being fractured (Figure 14.11). The tip of the lateral malleolus may be avulsed when the adduction component of the force predominates or the fracture

may be spiral in type, implying a rotational stress. Major degrees of subluxation are not seen with unilateral or unimalleolar injuries.

Bimalleolar injuries involve disruption on both sides, either of which may be a fracture or ligament rupture (Figure 14.12). It is common for a patient to 'go over' on the ankle, producing violent inversion, but it can be demonstrated that when this happens there is a 'torque-convertor' effect which causes the talus to rotate outwards within the ankle mortice. It is suggested that this is why rotational fractures of the lower fibula, as described above, are so

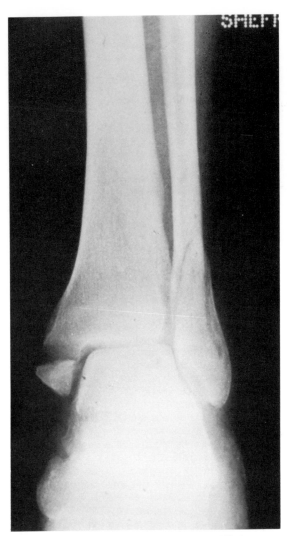

Figure 14.13 Bimalleolar fracture, the tibia and fibula remaining bound together

common. As the violence continues, the medial ligament or the tip of the medial malleolus may be avulsed, producing the commonest type of bimalleolar injury. The level at which the fibular fracture occurs may depend on whether the foot is inverted or everted at the time of the external talar rotation.

It is believed that when the foot is inverted and the 'torque-convertor' mechanism operates, the fibula tends to fracture in a spiral fashion below or through the interosseous tibiofibular ligament, leaving the ligament at least partially intact so that tibia and fibula remain bound together (Figure 14.13).

If the foot is everted when the external rotation occurs, it is suggested that the fibula is more likely to fracture at a higher level, even near the upper end of the bone and, in these circumstances, the interosseous tibiofibular ligament may be completely ruptured, together with part of the interosseous membrane, allowing the tibia and fibula to separate, widening the ankle mortice – a condition called 'diastasis'. This needs to be recognized as it is an important factor in allowing talar subluxation.

If the violence to the ankle involves *adduction*, the lateral ligament may be ruptured or the tip of the lateral malleolus avulsed, and the medial malleolus tends to fracture along a line running upwards from the corner of the ankle joint, producing a larger malleolar fragment than is seen with the avulsion fracture.

The most unstable injuries of all tend to be *rotational* and involve disruption on both sides, together with a fracture of the posterior or 'third' malleolus (Figure 14.14). These are the so-called trimalleolar fractures and oblique radiographs of the ankle joint may be necessary to diagnose them accurately.

Finally, and certainly to be classified separately, are the relatively uncommon *vertical compression* fractures, usually caused by a fall vertically onto the

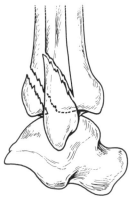
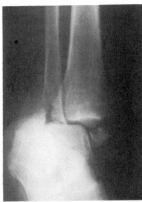
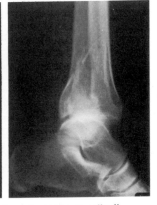

Figure 14.14 Trimalleolar fractures showing the fractures of the lateral and 'third' malleoli

foot, sometimes with the ankle being forced into dorsiflexion, the talus being driven upwards into the lower end of the tibia causing a fracture with severe comminution and extensive damage to the joint surface. These fractures carry a bad long-term prognosis.

In summary then, before deciding on treatment, the radiographs should be studied carefully and the information they give supplemented by examining the joint under anaesthesia, taking additional oblique or stress views as necessary.

Management of ankle injuries

In general, unimalleolar injuries (either bony or ligamentous), produce a degree of instability which can be controlled by external fixation, following manipulation if necessary. Manipulation under anaesthesia is usually simple if the mechanism of injury has been worked out – either involving a gentle rotational movement or simply squeezing the joint from side to side. It is best carried out with the foot hanging over the end of the table (Figure 14.15). A closely fitting below-knee cast is then applied with minimal padding, the fracture re-moulded as the plaster sets and a check radiograph taken.

If rotation has not been a feature, a below-knee walking plaster cast is usually adequate, this being retained for at least 6 weeks. If the fracture is spiral, rotational displacement may recur so that a full leg plaster cast with the knee partly flexed is required. Again, 6 weeks is usually sufficient.

Bimalleolar fractures are usually associated with more subluxation and require precise analysis. This type of fracture has received much attention recently, and there is a school of thought which believes that internal fixation, with plates and screws, should always be recommended, arguing

that anatomical reduction is essential and can only be achieved by operative techniques. Others believe that minor degrees of incongruity may not prejudice good function, and treat these fractures by manipulation and plaster immobilization.

There is no doubt, however, that this can be difficult, since the foot is usually swollen and the fractures themselves often very unstable. If the medial malleolus is intact or there is a sufficient lip of it left intact, then manipulation is often successful, and the plaster cast can be moulded to hold the talus up against the intact medial malleolus. If this is not the case, internal fixation is usually more successful. Current thought is that accurate reduction of the fibular fracture, and its fixation with compression screws and a plate, is the 'key' to a satisfactory overall reduction. A medial malleolar fragment, if large enough, may also be successfully fixed with a screw or by tension wiring. The medial ligament is rarely repaired.

The trimalleolar fractures are extremely unstable, and if the posterior malleolar fracture bears one-third or more of the tibial articular surface, it is usually best reduced at operation and secured with a screw, in addition to whatever other fixation is required for the lateral and medial side.

Following internal fixation, if the joint has been rendered completely stable by the fixation technique, it can be useful to allow the patient to mobilize the ankle with help from a physiotherapist for up to 2 weeks. It is usually wise then to protect the ankle in a below-knee cast for at least 6 weeks. It may be 12 weeks before full unprotected weight-bearing is considered safe.

It should be emphasized that the operative management of ankle fractures requires considerable judgement and skill. Decisions about treatment should be made as soon as possible. Many of these badly swollen ankles will develop severe skin

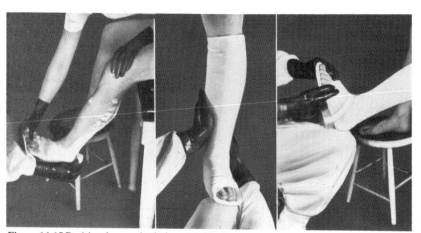

Figure 14.15 Position for manipulating an ankle fracture, and applying a below-knee plaster cast

blistering within a matter of hours, making operation more risky. Whatever the eventual treatment, for the severely swollen and obviously for the postoperative ankles, a period of elevation of the leg either at home or under observation in hospital is recommended.

Fractures and dislocations of the talus

Talar fractures are uncommon. Those affecting the body are often undisplaced, although fragments may be chipped from the edge of the ankle articular surface. Fractures of the neck are of greater importance and, since these may also be combined with subluxation or dislocation of the subtalar joint, avascular necrosis of the body may follow due to interruption of vessels passing through the neck and through the sinus tarsi. This is a serious complication leading to stiffness and pain in the ankle with the early onset of osteoarthritis. Undisplaced neck fractures are of less importance, carrying a greatly reduced risk of avascular necrosis.

Management

Fracture of the talar neck is usually caused by forced dorsiflexion of the ankle, for example, by impact against a car pedal. Characteristically, if displacement occurs, it is best corrected by putting the foot into steep plantar-flexion, which aligns the two halves of the bone and corrects the subtalar subluxation. The foot is held in this position in a plaster cast for 6 weeks, after which the position of the ankle can be corrected to neutral and the cast retained with a walking heel for at least a further 6 weeks. Even if union occurs avascular necrosis may not be avoided.

Following severe violence, the neck may be fractured and the body of the talus rotated completely out of the ankle mortice and the subtalar joint. The body then usually comes to lie on the medial side of the foot and may damage the posterior tibial artery, particularly if the injury is compound. Closed injuries carry the risk of skin breakdown. Open reduction is usually necessary and the fracture may need to be stabilized with pins or screws. A plaster cast is needed for 12 weeks. Not surprisingly, this injury carries the highest risk of avascular necrosis of the body, a figure of 85% being usually quoted.

An equally severe injury is combined dislocation of the subtalar and midtarsal joints. This often impairs the circulation to the foot and must be reduced as soon as possible. Manipulation is usually successful and stability may be improved by using Kirschner wires passed across the joint surfaces. The wires are removed at 6–8 weeks. The end result is usually a stiff and somewhat painful foot, which can occasionally be helped by manipulation under anaesthesia after physiotherapy has achieved its maximum benefit.

Fractures of the calcaneum

The majority of fractures of the calcaneum arise as a result of falls from a height onto the heels, and are frequently bilateral. Multiple injuries are common in falls from a height and crush fractures of the spine are frequently associated with os calcis fractures. The severity of the calcaneal injury depends on whether the fracture enters the subtalar joint. Since the wedge-shaped lower surface of the talus tends to be driven downwards into the calcaneum, this is frequently the case, and in particular the 'thalamus' or area between the subtalar articular surfaces may be driven into the substance of the bone.

Management of calcaneal fractures

The heel is usually grossly swollen and tender, and there is bruising, particularly on the medial side and extending to the attachment of the plantar fascia. The heel may be flattened, wide and somewhat valgus. The usual lateral and AP radiographs should be supplemented by an axial view of the calcaneum taken with the film at 45° to the vertical.

Those fractures not entering the subtalar joint may be managed conservatively and indeed many of those which do enter the subtalar joint may also be managed in the same way. The patient is usually admitted to hospital and the limb enclosed in a compression bandage of cotton wool and crêpe, and elevated on a frame. When the swelling goes down, usually after 1–2 weeks, a lighter bandage or a plaster cast with a sorbo sole may be applied. The patient may attempt walking as soon as the pain permits. Rehabilitation may take many months and complete freedom from pain may never be achieved.

One particular type of fracture which does not enter the subtalar joint, but merits special attention, is the so-called 'beak' fracture which produces a large posterosuperior fragment pulled upwards by the attachment of the tendo Achillis. This may need reduction and immobilization in equinus or, alternatively, internal fixation with a single screw.

If the subtalar joint is severely displaced as evidenced by flattening of Bohler's angle (Figure 14.16), and particularly if there is a central depressed fragment, some surgeons recommend open reduction and elevation of the fragment, using a cancellous bone graft to fill the space below. Better results are claimed than for conservative treatment.

If the foot remains painful and stiff 18 months to 2 years after the accident, triple arthrodesis may be necessary for pain relief. Heavy manual work is rarely possible for patients who have suffered a severe calcaneal fracture.

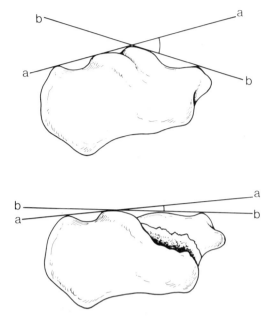

Figure 14.16 Fracture of calcaneum – flattening of 'Bohler's angle'

Dislocation of the tarso-metatarsal joint

Known as a Lisfranc dislocation, this injury is rare and may produce ischaemia of the medial ray of the forefoot. The second metatarsal bone is usually fractured and the forefoot tends to be displaced laterally. The displacement should be reduced, if necessary by operation, as soon as possible. It is usually stable after reduction and may be treated in a plaster cast for 6 weeks. Unstable reduction may require pin fixation.

Crush injuries of the foot

The foot is vulnerable to crushing, particularly in heavy industry. Protective shoes may prevent the worst damage, but the edge of a steel toe-cap may itself cause considerable damage. The injuries are frequently compound and the underlying fractures are often of much less importance than the soft tissue damage. Ischaemia of the toes is common.

Management

The foot is usually grossly swollen and the toes may be obviously ischaemic. More often the circulation is impaired rather than completely absent. The radiographs should be analysed carefully and any dislocations and displaced fractures should be gently manipulated under anaesthesia. No attempt is made to secure accurate alignment of all fractures, but if the alignment of the metatarsal heads in the sole is abnormal, this should be corrected if possible. Kirschner wires may be useful in maintaining reduction. The patient is admitted, and the foot elevated on a frame. If the circulation is suspect, the foot is kept cool to reduce the metabolic demands, but the patient himself is kept warm. It is occasionally necessary to carry out relieving incisions either in the sole and through the plantar fascia, or less commonly on the dorsum of the foot. The wound caused by this procedure may be closed after a few days. Toes which become obviously gangrenous should be amputated as soon as the demarcation line has become evident. When the swelling and ischaemic problems have been overcome, the foot may be immobilized in a below-knee plaster cast which will be required for at least 6 weeks.

Fractures of metatarsals

These usually occur as a result of crushing of the foot as described above.

Isolated fractures may be treated in a below-knee walking cast, as may the common fracture of the base of the fifth metatarsal which is an avulsion fracture caused by forced inversion of the foot; 3–6 weeks in plaster is sufficient.

March fractures usually affect the metatarsal necks, particularly the second, and are caused by the stress of long periods of walking. They are often showing signs of healing when first diagnosed and 3–6 weeks in a below-knee cast is usually curative.

Fractures of toes

These are common injuries. The big toe is particularly vulnerable and the injuries are often compound and with considerable comminution of the phalanges. Occasionally circulation may be impaired, necessitating amputation, but usually a simple, protective dressing and a metatarsal pad is sufficient for comfort and the patient is advised to wear a shoe as soon as possible, as this protects the fracture to some extent.

Dislocations of the toes are usually very easily reduced, and tend to be stable when reduced, but can be fixed with a Kirschner wire if this is not the case.

Injuries of the upper limb
Fractures of the clavicle

This injury is common, occurring at all ages, but particularly in the young and active. It may result either from a fall on the shoulder or on the outstretched hand. The bone may fracture anywhere along its length and, because its action as a strut is lost, the shoulder tends to drop, carrying the outer fragment downwards and forwards.

Management

Diagnosis is usually readily made; the patient comes in supporting the weight of his arm with his other hand or an improvised sling. The fracture is often palpable. Complications are rare, but occasionally brachial plexus or axillary artery damage occurs. The clavicle usually unites extremely rapidly, and only minimal treatment is necessary. For most patients, a simple broad sling for comfort, with analgesics for the first 2–3 days, is perfectly adequate. If displacement is severe, a traditional figure-of-eight bandage, bracing back the shoulders may be used, but its value is uncertain.

Fractures and dislocations of the shoulder and humerus
Fractures of the acromion and scapula

These are usually caused by a fall on the shoulder or by a direct blow. They heal quickly. A simple sling is sufficient, with active movement of the shoulder as soon as the pain permits.

Dislocation of the acromioclavicular joint

This injury tends to occur from a fall in which the tip of the shoulder is struck forcibly, forcing the shoulder downwards. If the outer end of the clavicle is significantly displaced and lying well above the acromion, the important coracoclavicular ligament is likely to have been ruptured. The displacement is revealed best in an AP radiograph taken in the standing position, with the limb unsupported.

Management

The results of conservative management of this injury are good, although reposition of the acromioclavicular joint may not be achieved.

The arm is supported in a broad sling supplemented, if the displacement is severe, by strips of elastic strapping applied from front to back over a felt pad overlying the outer end of the clavicle. After

3 weeks, mobilization may begin. Full function is usually achieved, although the appearance of the shoulder may leave something to be desired.

Dislocation of the shoulder

Falls on the arm and shoulder not infrequently result in a dislocation of the head of the humerus from the glenoid. The commonest dislocation results from the head displacing forwards, coming to rest in front of the glenoid and below the coracoid process – a so-called subcoracoid dislocation (Figure 14.17). Posterior dislocation is much less common and downward displacement rarest of all, this latter producing a curious and characteristic position with the arm held elevated above the head.

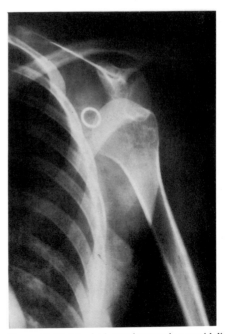

Figure 14.17 A typical anterior or subcoracoid dislocation

Management

Diagnosis of the typical anterior dislocation is usually obvious because of the flattening of the deltoid muscle, the contour of the shoulder dropping in a straight line from the tip of the acromion. The arm is usually held against the chest and supported by the other arm. A full neurological examination is, as always, essential since damage to the axillary nerve is not uncommon and produces paralysis of the deltoid muscle. The muscle itself may be difficult to test, but if the nerve is damaged this produces a patch of sensory blunting over the deltoid insertion. Recovery is usual, although this may take several weeks. Rarely, a brachial plexus or axillary artery injury may occur.

As with any dislocation, reduction is easier the sooner it is carried out. There are many techniques, of which the following are most consistently effective and safe:

1. The patient is given a full dose of an analgesic such as pethidine and is positioned face down with the arm hanging over the end of a couch. As the muscles relax, the weight of the arm tends to relocate the shoulder joint, and it is usually easy with a gentle rotational movement to slip the head into the joint.
2. If the above fails, or the patient is not suitable for the treatment, the Hippocratic method is usually successful. Under general anaesthesia, the patient lies supine on the couch or operating table. The operator removes his right shoe when reducing the right shoulder and, whilst exerting traction on the arm, uses the toes of his right foot to manoeuvre the head into the joint. The procedure is usually easy and, once achieved, reduction is almost always stable. If reduction does not occur with either of these techniques, a fracture of the glenoid or head should be suspected.

A posterior dislocation can usually be reduced by a similar technique.

After reduction, the arm is supported in a broad sling and may be strapped to the chest with elastoplast. The clothes are worn over the sling which is left in place for 3 weeks, then physiotherapy is prescribed to regain shoulder movements. The temptation to remove the sling early should be resisted except in the elderly where stiffness is likely to be a greater problem than recurrent dislocation.

Recurrent dislocation of the shoulder

This may follow one or more traumatic dislocations, but some patients seem to have a developmental predisposition. After a time, the dislocation occurs with minimal trauma or simply as a result of externally rotating the shoulder. The episodes are painful, but the patient may sometimes be able to reduce the dislocation himself.

It is important that the shoulder should actually be seen dislocated before treatment is decided upon, as dislocation may be anterior or posterior, and the operative procedure required for one may actually worsen the other. After a number of dislocations, a defect may be visible in the head or on the margin of the glenoid on suitable lateral radiographic views. CT or NMR scanning may be helpful in diagnosing the uncertain case.

Management

After a number of dislocations, conservative treatment cannot be expected to be successful, and operation will be necessary. The most widely used procedures are the Putti–Platt and Bankart operations which involve tightening and reinforcing the anterior capsular structures. They inevitably produce some restriction of external rotation of the shoulder, but are usually successful in controlling the instability.

Fractures of the neck of the humerus

These can be some of the most difficult injuries to manage. They occur at all ages from late childhood on, but are particularly common in the elderly, where a stiff shoulder is the usual outcome. They are often complicated by severe bruising, gravitating down the back of the arm to the elbow.

Management

Displacement may be severe, particularly in younger patients, and in these circumstances reduction may be achieved by manipulation under anaesthesia, traction being applied to the arm, usually with some adduction, and with pressure on the inner aspect of the humerus. If this is unsuccessful, open reduction may be necessary, particularly if the head is rotated within the glenoid. These are, however, difficult fractures to stabilize, even when reduction has been achieved. Traction, with the patient lying supine in bed and the arm suspended at 90° to the body, is often convenient and effective. After 3 weeks of traction of this type, the fracture will usually be sufficiently stable to allow the arm to be brought down and supported in a broad sling and gentle mobilization exercises begun.

In the elderly, even when displacement is severe, manipulation and particularly open reduction are rarely justified. Fortunately many of these fractures are impacted so that, following a short period of rest in a broad sling until the immediate pain has settled, physiotherapy can be started, the patient beginning to move the limb by swinging it like a pendulum and later attempting to abduct the shoulder and to rotate it by reaching behind the neck and behind the back. Rehabilitation may take many months and permanent stiffness, with inability to reach above the head, is a common end result. Where the shoulder remains painful a shoulder prosthesis, e.g. of the Neer type, may have to be considered but these rarely restore abduction to more than 90°.

Fracture-dislocation of the shoulder

This is fortunately uncommon, being a particularly difficult injury to treat. The fracture often makes reduction of the shoulder impossible, and operative reduction may be necessary.

Fracture of the shaft of the humerus

This is a common injury and may be caused by a direct blow or fall on the arm. Except with direct violence, there is usually a rotational element and the fracture is spiral. The radial nerve is vulnerable because of its position relative to the fracture. The other major nerves and brachial artery are occasionally damaged.

Management

Manipulation is rarely necessary. The arm is supported in a collar-and-cuff sling to allow the weight of the arm to align the fracture. This is not sufficient by itself to give adequate comfort, particularly when the patient is lying down, and alignment is further maintained by enclosing the upper arm in three metal or plastic 'gutter' splints cut to the correct length, a short one down the inner aspect of the arm and two longer ones applied in anterolateral and posterolateral positions – the three held in place with strapping and forming a triangle. These need to be re-applied weekly at first, as the swelling of the arm diminishes. An alternative method is to use a long plaster slab extending as a U from the axilla, under the elbow and up the outer side of the arm and over the shoulder. This is held in place with a circumferential bandage round the humerus. Perfect alignment is rarely necessary and, even if there is some residual shortening, function is usually good.

Union may take 12 weeks, but non-union is uncommon. Patients with other injuries who have to lie in bed are not suitable for this technique, and balanced skin traction may be more appropriate or even internal fixation with a metal plate.

Supracondylar fractures of the humerus

Fractures occurring just above the elbow, transversely above the epicondyles, happen at all ages but are particularly common and important in children when they are usually the result of a fall from a height (Figure 14.18). In adults, the situation may be complicated by an additional vertical fracture extending downwards between capitulum and trochlea – the so-called T-shaped fracture.

Management

Considerable swelling is common with all these fractures, but the bony landmarks of the elbow usually retain their normal relationships. In the adult with a simple or T-shaped fracture, displacement may be minimal and support in a collar-and-cuff sling may be satisfactory. The more displaced or unstable fractures may require open reduction and internal fixation, but this can be difficult. A Y-shaped plate is available and is applied to the posterior surface of the humerus. It may be sufficient to fix together the two lower fractures and treat the transverse fracture conservatively. Mobilization of the elbow should be started as early as possible, but 6 weeks is usually necessary to secure adequate stability in the fracture.

The supracondylar fracture in a child deserves separate consideration. The condylar fragment is usually rotated and displaced backwards, and the sharp edge of the humeral fragment may impinge on and damage the brachial artery, leading to ischaemia of the forearm (Figure 14.19). The muscles are particularly vulnerable and if this complication is allowed to occur, Volkmann's contracture may result. Fortunately, the complica-

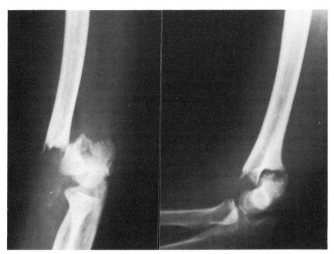

Figure 14.18 Supracondylar fracture of the humerus in a child

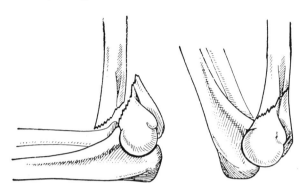

Figure 14.19 Typical displacement of a supracondylar fracture and its therapeutic reposition

tion is rare, because a fully established Volkmann's contracture produces considerable disability.

When the child first presents with the fracture, the radial pulse may be absent, but this is not necessarily a danger sign provided the circulation is obviously adequate. The usual neurological examination should be carried out, the median nerve and ulnar nerves being particularly at risk.

The fracture is usually manipulated under anaesthesia and this should be done as soon as possible, before the swelling becomes very severe. The elbow is kept flexed to about 60°, and the two epicondyles are held between the operator's fingers and thumb, whilst the distal fragment is pulled downwards and forwards. The line joining the epicondyles should be kept at right-angles to the humerus, otherwise the fracture may unite with a tilt. Reduction is usually relatively easy and is checked immediately with AP and lateral radiographs. The arm is then held in a collar-and-cuff sling against the chest, to which it may be held by strapping as this position usually gives satisfactory correction of rotation of the fragments. Flexion above 90° is not necessary and should be avoided if swelling is severe. Check the radial pulse.

The patient is admitted for overnight observation and the circulation is checked carefully at hourly intervals. The radial pulse may not return, but again this may be of little significance provided the circulation remains adequate as judged by return of blood flow to the skin of the fingers after compression, and there is normal sensibility and absence of forearm and hand pain. If there is pain in the forearm flexor region and particularly if this is intensified by passively extending the fingers, the elbow should be allowed to extend somewhat and if this does not relieve the symptoms the brachial artery should be explored.

The method of treatment summarized above is satisfactory for most supracondylar fractures in children, but occasionally the fracture is unstable when flexed and may need to be held in extension or may even need to be held on balanced traction or, occasionally, internally fixed.

Fractures and dislocations of the elbow

It is a feature of injuries around the elbow that, irrespective of the severity of the injury, stiffness may be the end result and a long course of physiotherapy with graded active and passive exercises may be necessary to regain movement.

Extension is the movement which is most likely to remain restricted. Fortunately for most purposes, the last 20° of extension are not essential.

Dislocation of the elbow

This is an uncommon injury, usually occurring from a fall on the hand when the elbow is flexed, the radius and ulna dislocating backwards on the lower end of the humerus.

Management

Immediately after the injury the elbow lies in a flexed position; the three bony landmarks of the elbow, the two epicondyles and the tip of the olecranon, which normally form an equilateral triangle in the flexed position, are obviously displaced. There is usually considerable swelling. Complications are unusual, but the median nerve and brachial artery may be damaged. Neurological recovery tends to occur in most cases.

Reduction is accomplished by manipulation. The elbow is kept flexed and the operator grips the elbow from behind with both hands and pushes forward on the olecranon with his thumbs. Reduction can sometimes be achieved without an anaesthetic. A collar-and-cuff sling is worn for 3 weeks and the elbow can then be mobilized. Physiotherapy is not always required as stiffness is relatively uncommon with this injury.

Fracture-dislocation of the elbow

This is usually a severe injury, often compound and with considerable comminution. An example of this is the 'side-swipe' injury caused by a violent blow to the elbow hanging out of a car window.

Management

Much will depend on the precise nature of the injury. Manipulative reduction may restore alignment but open reduction and internal fixation may be required. Paradoxically, sometimes the most severely damaged elbows give relatively good function, although stiffness is the usual outcome.

Fractures of the epicondyles

These injuries occur in childhood and may be missed on radiographs because the epicondyles at this age are largely cartilaginous with only a small ossification centre.

Lateral epicondylar fractures usually separate off a large fragment bearing the capitulum, the actual fragment being much larger than appears on the radiograph. Internal fixation with a wire or screw may be advisable since the fragment tends to displace upwards, and may lead to a growth defect leading to late development of a valgus deformity. This in turn predisposes to traction damage to the ulnar nerve as it is stretched around the medial side of the elbow (late or 'tardy' ulnar palsy).

The importance of fractures of the medial epicondyle lies in the fact that the fragment may be pulled into the elbow joint by the common flexor origin which is attached to it, this being essentially an avulsion fracture.

If the fragment appears to lie between the olecranon and the trochlea on a lateral radiograph, it will be found to be within the joint and, although manipulation may be possible by putting the elbow into valgus and extending the wrist and fingers to draw out the fragment, open reduction is more likely to be needed. After reduction the fragment may need only to be sutured into position as redisplacement is unlikely.

After 3 weeks in a collar-and-cuff sling the elbow may be mobilized, but even in children long-term stiffness is not uncommon.

Fracture of the olecranon

Fractures extending transversely across the olecranon into the trochlear notch (see Figure 12.9) tend to occur in adults, usually in middle age. Depending on the amount of surrounding soft tissue damage, the proximal fragment tends to be pulled upwards to a variable extent by the triceps muscle. The injury sometimes occurs as part of a dislocation of the elbow.

Management

If displacement is minimal, the elbow may be supported in a collar-and-cuff sling until pain and swelling subside, then gradually mobilized. With more severe degrees of displacement, open reduction and fixation with a single screw or by tension-band wiring gives good results and may make it possible to move the elbow almost immediately. In the elderly, even with displaced fractures, it is sometimes more expedient to rely on immediate movement without operation. Function can be surprisingly good, although full power of extension is rarely regained.

Injuries of the radius and ulna
Fractures of the radial head

The radial head is usually damaged by being forced against the capitulum as a result of a valgus stress on the elbow. Not surprisingly, it may be combined with a strain or rupture of the *medial* ligament.

Management

Swelling is variable, but if the medial side is swollen the medial ligament is likely to be damaged, and the elbow may be quite unstable. There is usually well localized tenderness over the radial head itself and pronation and supination may be limited or impossible. The degree to which the patient can pronate or supinate the arm is a useful guide to prognosis and may also be used as a guide to the selection of the method of treatment for the more severe fractures.

Simple cracks and undisplaced fractures of the head may be treated conservatively, the arm being supported in a collar-and-cuff sling until movement becomes possible. The comminuted and displaced fractures usually restrict rotation more severely, and if this is the case, excision of the head is usually the most satisfactory procedure. If, at the time of presentation, rotation is good, then a conservative policy may be prescribed with a reasonable expectation of a satisfactory end result. In the severe, comminuted fractures, displacement of the head fragments can be surprising, sometimes isolated pieces being found in the forearm.

Following excision of the head, a collar-and-cuff sling is used to support the arm and physiotherapy started as soon as pain will allow. Ossification in the capsule and ligaments occasionally adds to the tendency to stiffness. Late removal of a damaged radial head is rarely successful in restoring rotation to a stiff elbow.

In children, the displaced head should be retained as it represents the upper radial epiphysis. It can usually be manipulated either by applying pressure through the skin or by open reduction and is then usually stable.

'Pulled elbow'

This is a common injury in young children who have been pulled forcibly by the arm. The radial head slips out of the annular ligament. The child presents with a painful elbow which he is reluctant to use. Rotation of the elbow often produces a click as the head reduces and function then normally returns rapidly.

Fractures of the shafts of the radius and ulna

These injuries are usually caused by direct violence but may result from a fall on the outstretched hand. They are frequently compound and, in severe cases, may be complicated by nerve, tendon and vascular injury. It should be remembered that if one bone only is fractured and the fracture is significantly angulated, then either the superior or inferior radioulnar joint must be disrupted. With ulnar shaft fractures it is characteristically the superior joint which is dislocated (Monteggia fracture), and with radial shaft fractures it is usually the lower joint (Galeazzi fracture). More commonly, both bones are fractured.

Management

Diagnosis is mostly obvious, angulation being usual. It is important to secure accurate alignment of these bones as this is essential if forearm rotation is to be restored. Although below the age of 10–12 years remodelling will usually correct any minor deficiencies, above this age it is difficult to hold the fracture sufficiently accurately. This being the case, it has become almost universal practice to open these fractures and fix them with plates, six-hole plates usually being necessary for adequate fixation. Even compound fractures can be internally fixed if treated early, provided the wound is not too severely contaminated and the skin is viable. If the fracture is not suitable for immediate internal fixation, the wound is allowed to heal and internal fixation then performed as a secondary procedure. When the shaft fractures are reduced, a dislocation of either radio-ulnar joint usually reduces spontaneously. After internal fixation, it is usually safer to allow 4–6 weeks in a long-arm plaster, followed by exercises to regain rotation, but avoiding heavy weight-bearing for at least 12 weeks.

Greenstick fractures in children heal readily and should be manipulated carefully to avoid completing them. They are then held in plaster extending from knuckle to axilla with the elbow flexed to 90° and the

forearm in the position of rotation which best controls the fracture. If the distal fragment is angulated backwards, full pronation is usually necessary, and if the distal fragment is angulated forwards, full supination is more appropriate. Six weeks are usually sufficient and subsequent mobilization is usually rapid.

Fractures of the lower end of the radius

Colles' fracture

This term has come to be applied to a specific type of fracture of the lower end of the radius, occurring within 2.5 cm of the articular surface and with characteristic backward tilt, backward displacement and radial deviation of the distal fragment. The fracture is one which occurs in adult life and is most common in women of postmenopausal age, where there is evidence to suggest that it is a pathological fracture, occurring in bone which is osteoporotic.

Management

This fracture is well known for its tendency to produce the characteristic 'dinner-fork' deformity of the forearm and wrist. Nevertheless, many undisplaced and some displaced Colles' fractures do not produce a significant deformity. In addition to the dinner-fork appearance, there is frequently obvious displacement of the wrist towards the radial side, causing the lower end of the ulna to be prominent. It is common for the ulnar styloid to be avulsed by the interarticular disc, which remains attached to the displaced lower end of the radius – this represents a disruption of the lower radio-ulnar joint and is frequently a cause of long-term morbidity.

The need for reduction of the fracture should be assessed from the appearance of both the AP and lateral radiographs. On the lateral film a line drawn between the anterior and posterior lips of the radial articular surface is a useful guide (Figure 14.20). If this line is tilted slightly forwards relative to the line of the radial shaft, or is at right-angles to the line, reduction is probably unnecessary. Similarly on the AP film, if there is no significant radial displacement of the radial fragment and the ulnar styloid, then again the fracture is probably satisfactory. If the line is tilted backwards, or if the fragment is significantly displaced backwards or to the radial side, reduction should be considered (Figure 14.21). Other factors may be relevant, such as time after injury, age and general fitness of the patient, although many of these fractures can be manipulated under local anaesthesia, thus avoiding the risks and complications of general anaesthesia. Nevertheless, the temptation should be resisted to try to manipulate these fractures without anaesthesia or simply with analgesics. Adequate relaxation is necessary, other-

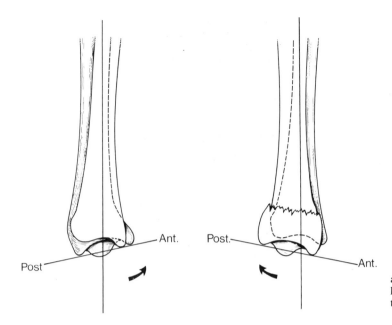

Figure 14.20 A line drawn through the anterior and posterior margin of the lower end of the radius demonstrates the backward tilt of a Colles' fracture

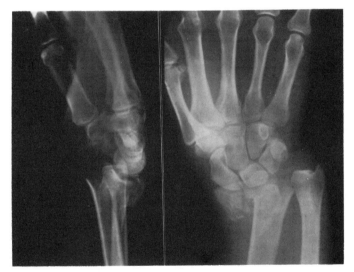

Figure 14.21 Typical Colles' fracture

wise reduction is likely to be incomplete. Local infiltration, regional block or Bier block anaesthesia can all be satisfactory in experienced hands. This is an exceedingly common fracture and in almost all cases there should be no excuse for unsatisfactory reduction.

Whilst the patient is being anaesthetized a dorsal plaster slab is prepared from a 15 or 20 cm plaster bandage. It should be long enough to cover the back of the hand, wrist and forearm from a point just proximal to the metacarpophalangeal joints, to just below the point of the elbow, and wide enough to stretch slightly over half way round the circumference of the arm. The slab should be somewhat wider at the proximal end than the distal.

The upper arm is held by an assistant or by a traction loop attached to a wall and traction is applied to the distal fragment to disimpact it from the proximal. This fragment is then flexed, pushed forwards and towards the ulnar side. This can conveniently be done using the thenar eminence of the same-sided hand of the operator (Figure 14.22). Having moulded the fracture into correct alignment, the hand can then be slid over the back of the hand

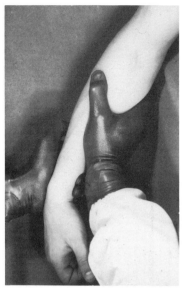

Figure 14.22 Reduction of Colles' fracture. Correction of backward displacement after traction

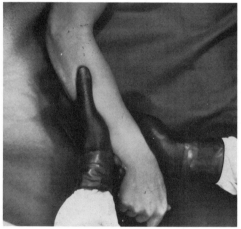

Figure 14.23 Reduction of Colles' fracture. Correction of radial displacement

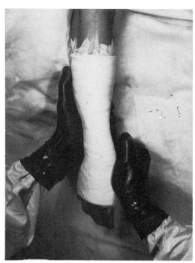

Figure 14.24 Reduction of Colles' fracture – final moulding of plaster cast

stockinette tubing. The slab is bound into place before it begins to set with a wet gauze bandage (a dry bandage may shrink and cause constriction).

As the plaster begins to set, the operator transfers his grip to mould the fracture into its final position (Figure 14.24). When the plaster has set hard, check AP and lateral radiographs are taken, and if manipulation is unsatisfactory, it must be repeated. After manipulation, the arm is supported in a broad sling and the patient is allowed home, with instructions (preferably printed) to report back to the hospital at once if the fingers are discoloured, very swollen, painful, or feel numb. The patient is also instructed to begin exercising the fingers and to practise movements of the shoulder.

The following day, a plaster check is carried out and the instructions reinforced. The fingers tend to swell and stiffen if vigorous active exercises are not started immediately. After 24 hours, the sling can be discarded and use of the limb encouraged.

One week later, the patient is seen again and a further set of check radiographs obtained. If the fracture has slipped, a further manipulation may be necessary. Otherwise the plaster may be completed to a circumferential cast, although this is not always necessary. Physiotherapy may be advisable even at this early stage if mobilization is poor.

After 5–6 weeks, the plaster is removed. If tenderness is not extreme, the arm may be left free and further exercises allowed, concentrating on finger and wrist movements, pronation and supination, and shoulder movements. Recovery may take several months in severe cases.

Median nerve symptoms are common, but usually recover spontaneously. Sometimes Sudeck's atrophy may occur as a late complication. An inadequ-

of the patient (Figure 14.23), still exerting traction, and over the thumb, which can then be grasped and used to maintain the alignment. Pulling the thumb in line with the forearm gives the necessary amount of ulnar deviation. A minimal degree of palmar flexion of the wrist is usually sufficient. Extreme palmar flexion is now regarded as unnecessary, and tends to inhibit use of the fingers. With the fracture still held in this position, an assistant moulds the preprepared slab over the back of the wrist and the hand, with no underlying padding other than a single layer of

ately reduced fracture, particularly if comminuted, may result in long-term pain, often from the subluxated lower radio-ulnar joint. If symptoms in this joint do not settle, excision of the lower end of the ulna may be considered.

Displacement of the lower radial epiphysis

This is almost the same injury as a Colles' fracture, but occurring in a child, the epiphysis displacing backwards. Only severe degrees of displacement need be reduced; in either case 3 weeks in a plaster back slab is sufficient.

Smith's fracture

This is a fracture of the lower end of the radius, similar to a Colles' fracture, but with forward displacement. It is caused by a fall on the back of the wrist, which causes a pronation force. Occasionally, only the anterior lip of the lower end of the radius is fractured allowing forward subluxation of the carpal bones – Barton's fracture.

Management

Manipulation under anaesthesia usually reduces the fracture easily. The forearm should be held in supination and this position is maintained by using a full arm plaster cast, with the elbow at right-angles. Occasionally, the fracture is very unstable and tends to slip forwards, in which case internal fixation with a small specially designed plate (Ellis) may be necessary to maintain reduction. Immobilization may be necessary for 2–3 weeks longer than is usually necessary for a Colles' fracture, and the precautions regarding exercise of fingers and shoulder still apply.

Injuries of the wrist and hand

Fractures of the scaphoid

Injuries of the wrist are common and are frequently dismissed as sprains or strains, and not radiographed or treated. They often settle and a later radiograph, perhaps taken for some other purpose, reveals that there has been a scaphoid fracture which has failed to unite. The *diagnosis of a sprain of the wrist is a dangerous one and is rarely accurate.*

Fractures of the tubercle of the scaphoid are of little importance, but fractures through the waist of the scaphoid may, depending on the exact vascular anatomy, deprive the proximal fragment of its blood supply, because of damage to vessels entering through the distal half. This may make union uncertain and is particularly likely to occur when the fracture surfaces are displaced. In these circumstances, non-union may occur and the proximal fragment may collapse and become distorted due to avascular necrosis. Osteoarthritis of the wrist with troublesome pain may then be a late sequel.

Diagnosis is not always easy, a fall on the hand or severe blow in the palm as used to occur following a strike-back from a car starting-handle, being the usual history. Characteristically, the wrist is swollen, particularly on the lateral side, causing the scaphoid fossa to be partly filled in, and with tenderness at this site. Wrist movements are diminished and longitudinal pressure on the thumb causes pain. If the fracture is suspected, then in addition to the standard AP and lateral views of the wrist, extra oblique scaphoid views are taken, as the fracture may appear as little more than a hairline across the waist of the bone (Figure 14.25). Radiological diagnosis is not always certain, and in these circumstances, it is usual to treat the injury as a scaphoid fracture on clinical suspicion.

Management

The wrist is immobilized in a scaphoid plaster, with the wrist in a neutral position, the plaster extending from the point of the elbow to the knuckles, *including the thumb to the base of the nail.*

If the original diagnosis was not certain, the plaster is removed after 1 or 2 weeks and the radiographs repeated. The fracture may then be obvious, but if not, and the signs have disappeared,

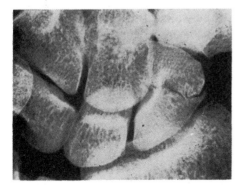
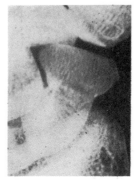

Figure 14.25 Recent fracture of the carpal scaphoid bone

the wrist may be left free. The established case is left in plaster until the clinical signs have disappeared and there is some radiological evidence of union. This may take from 6 weeks to several months. If non-union occurs (Figure 14.26) this may be treated either with a screw placed across the fracture line (a technique which should also be considered as initial treatment for the badly displaced scaphoid fracture) or by means of a bone graft. Mobility is usually quickly recovered after union.

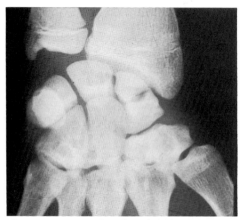

Figure 14.26 Non-union of scaphoid fracture

If the wrist remains painful due to long established non-union and osteoarthritis, excision of the necrotic fragment or of the radial styloid, or more commonly arthrodesis of the wrist, may be necessary. Nevertheless, many non-unions remain undiscovered with the patient symptom-free or minimally handicapped.

Fractures of the carpus

Various types of carpal dislocation and subluxation, often combined with fractures of the scaphoid or other wrist bones, are encountered, but all are rare. Unfortunately, because they are uncommon and not easily spotted on radiographs, they are commonly missed and can lead to considerable disability.

The possibilities of these injuries should always be considered with wrist injuries, and radiographs of the wrist carefully compared with the normal side.

The whole carpus may be dislocated forwards or backwards on the lower end of the radius and one or other of the carpal bones may be left behind *in situ*, usually the lunate or the proximal pole of the scaphoid if the latter has also fractured (trans-scaphoperilunate dislocation). Single carpal bones or fragments may be dislocated out of the carpus – the lunate being the commonest – and this latter is very prone to compress the median nerve in the carpal tunnel (Figure 14.27).

Management

Simple dislocation of the carpus can usually be reduced by closed manipulation under anaesthesia. If a carpal bone is dislocated or there is a trans-scaphoperilunate dislocation, manipulation often fails and open reduction is necessary. In the latter condition many surgeons believe that the incidence of scaphoid non-union is so high as to merit internal fixation of the scaphoid fracture as a primary procedure.

Following reduction, 6 weeks in plaster is usually sufficient. Median nerve symptoms usually recover after reduction.

Bennett's fracture

This is a particular type of fracture-dislocation of the base of the thumb in which the metacarpal fragment displaces away from the trapezium, leaving a small fragment still in position (Figure 14.28).

Management

The thumb is swollen at the base, and the metacarpal itself is usually prominent at its proximal end. Gripping with the thumb is impossible. The fracture-dislocation can be treated by applying a

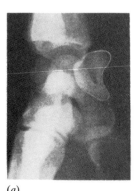

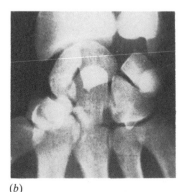

(*a*)   (*b*)

Figure 14.27 Dislocation of the carpal lunate bone. (*a*) On a lateral view the cup of the lunate is tilted forwards and the capitate lies behind it. (*b*) The AP view shows the normal quadrilateral-shaped shadow of the lunate is now triangular

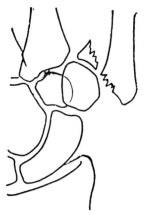

Figure 14.28 Bennett's fracture-dislocation of the thumb metacarpal

plaster cast, with the thumb extended and applying pressure over the base of the metacarpal whilst the plaster sets.

Four to six weeks in plaster is usually sufficient for union. Open reduction is occasionally necessary, the fragment then being pinned in position.

Fractures of metacarpals

The hands are often struck or crushed so that metacarpal fractures are common, frequently compound and complicated by injuries to tendons and nerves.

Isolated metacarpal fractures are rarely severely displaced and with multiple displaced fractures, the soft tissue component of the injury tends to be more important than the fractures themselves. The fifth metacarpal neck is often fractured and angulated forwards as a result of a blow with the fist.

Management

In general, isolated fractures, unless severely displaced, are simply protected by a dorsal plaster slab for 2–4 weeks. The fifth metacarpal neck fracture, if severely displaced, may be manipulated under anaesthesia and the dorsal plaster slab is extended to include the little finger with the metacarpophalangeal joint in extension. Severely displaced metacarpal fractures with extensive soft tissue damage may need internal fixation, usually with Kirschner wires, to give stability to enable hand and finger movements to be carried out. It is essential, whenever possible, to leave the fingers free and to encourage immediate active movements.

Fractures of phalanges

Although the phalanges are small bones, they are important for finger function and these must be regarded as serious injuries. Not surprisingly they are frequently compound and comminuted, with tendon, nerve or vascular damage.

Management

Fractures of intermediate phalanges, if displaced, can often be aligned by flexing the finger over a malleable metal splint, padded with orthopaedic felt. If undisplaced, strapping the finger to the adjacent one allows movement to occur but controls the tendency for the fracture to rotate, because if this is allowed to happen, the finger may flex in a plane which is out of alignment with the others.

Fractures of the shafts which are difficult to control may be treated by internal fixation with small metal plates, and pins may be used to fix small basal fractures which are important for joint function.

Fractures of terminal phalanges are often compound and skin loss is common. The nail may be lifted off its bed by haematoma, a painful injury which may be made more comfortable by boring a hole through the nail with a red hot paper-clip to let out the haematoma, or by removing the nail, which is often shed later anyway and usually regrows.

Partial amputation of the tip in children may be treated simply by dressing the wound and making no attempt to close the defect. In adults, primary split skin grafting may be suitable, or occasionally flap grafting using the thenar eminence as a donor site may be worthwhile. It is often more satisfactory to remove part of the terminal phalanx and close the end with full thickness anterior and posterior skin flaps.

Dislocation of finger joints

These are usually easily reduced without anaesthesia and may be mobilized immediately. Rarely, a phalanx may 'button-hole' through the joint capsule or tendon, in which case open reduction will be necessary.

Mallet finger

This injury is caused by stubbing the finger tip, resulting in avulsion of the extensor tendon insertion from the base of the terminal phalanx. The deformity is characteristic.

Management

If a fragment of bone is avulsed from the terminal phalanx, prospects for union are good and the finger should be splinted with the terminal interphalangeal joint in extension, and the proximal interphalangeal joint in flexion, to relax the lateral slips of the tendon. Special splints are made for this purpose and are simply slipped over the end of the finger and taped in position. Alternatively, a splint may be fashioned from a wooden spatula with a layer of orthopaedic felt to fit under the finger pulp, the splint being taped to lie along the palmar surface of the finger. This needs to be replaced weekly, and is less satisfactory because the whole finger is splinted in extension. Six weeks' splinting is necessary and it is important that splintage is started from the day of injury and is uninterrupted.

If the tendon itself has ruptured, the failure rate is much higher. The same method of treatment may be used, but at the end of the period of splintage many patients will still have a deformity. They can be told that this will usually improve or 'take up' somewhat over the first year. The finger which can be extended passively but not actively tends to 'catch', but most patients learn to compensate for this and arthrodesis of the terminal interphalangeal joint is rarely necessary.

Rupture of the middle slip of the extensor tendon

This is an uncommon injury and sometimes occurs spontaneously in rheumatoid arthritis. The middle slip of the extensor tendon, which is normally inserted into the base of the middle phalanx, is avulsed, leaving the lateral slips intact, causing the finger to flex at the proximal interphalangeal joint, and hyperextend at the terminal interphalangeal joint – boutonnière deformity.

Management

The prognosis for this injury is poor. Surgical repair of the tendon is a specialized procedure, but gives the best chance of success.

Principles of management of hand injuries
(see also Chapter 26)

Stiffness of the hand and fingers is a common outcome following injuries to the hand and fingers, and can often be avoided if immediate movement is encouraged, usually with a physiotherapist's supervision. Swelling is often the forerunner of stiffness and any significant hand injury should be treated by admitting the patient to hospital if possible, elevating the hand in a sling supported from an overhead stand, and even at this early stage, encouraging movements.

Wherever possible, uninjured fingers should be left free. Severely damaged fingers are often better amputated if the likely outcome is a long period of treatment which prejudices the rest of the hand, and may still at the end leave a stiff and painful or anaesthetic finger. As much of the thumb as possible should always be preserved.

A digit lacking sensation, particularly on the palmar aspect, is useless and very liable to further damage.

The index and little fingers contribute most to the power grip. If the intermediate fingers are amputated at the metacarpophalangeal joints, small objects tend to fall out of the hand.

Severe crush injuries of the hand require specialist treatment, and are best treated in Hand Units, where decisions on surgery, fixation, rehabilitation and reconstruction, can be based on wide experience.

15

Orthopaedic techniques

T. Duckworth

Application of the Thomas splint

Although originally designed as a knee splint, the Thomas splint now tends to be used mainly to treat fractures of the femoral shaft. It still, however, has a place in splinting a knee which needs to be kept under close observation as, for example, with a septic arthritis.

The application of the splint is straightforward, but attention to detail is necessary if complications are to be avoided. If the splint is being applied to a recently sustained femoral fracture, general anaesthesia is usually necessary. Manipulation of the fracture simply consists of aligning the fragments and applying traction to maintain the alignment and length. If the fracture ends are not obviously in contact, there may be muscle separating the ends and, in these circumstances, it is usually advisable to open the fracture to extract the muscle. The splintage may then be used as before.

1. The splint is selected by measuring the circumference of the thigh at the level of the groin. This gives the size of ring. The length is that of the good leg from crotch to the underside of heel plus 15–25 cm.
2. The splint is prepared by covering it with three slings made from non-stretch bandage, held in place with safety pins, or with commercially available slings fitted with Velcro tape. One is placed under the thigh, one under the knee and one just above the tendo calcaneus.
3. The limb is shaved, the fracture manipulated, and skin 'extensions' are applied on each side (see Figure 14.7). Elastoplast strapping 7.5 or 10 cm wide, specially made for this purpose, is

now widely used. Skin sensitivity occasionally occurs, and this may be avoided by the use of Holland strapping which is warmed to make it stick. This material is not, however, widely available now, although it has many advantages. The extensions are applied directly to the skin and arranged so that the outer strip is placed slightly towards the back of the limb and the inner strip slightly to the front. This has the effect of counteracting the tendency for the leg to lie in external rotation at the fracture site. The extensions are held in place with circumferential crêpe bandages which end just above the malleoli. The ends of the extensions are held away from the malleoli by pads of orthopaedic felt.
4. The tapes are secured by passing the outer one over the lateral bar and the inner one under the medial bar, again to counteract the tendency to rotate.
5. The tapes are tied over the end of the splint and, if necessary, a wooden bar may be used as a 'windlass' to increase the traction. Pads and small aluminium 'gutter' splints may be used under the thigh to secure the correct position of the fracture.
6. If the splint is to be on for a long time it may be suspended by overhead slings and a weight may be attached to the end to relieve pressure on the groin. It should be remembered, however, that in using it as it was originally designed, the pressure on the ischial tuberosity provides the counter traction force.

The exact position of the groin ring and the state of the slings and tapes must be checked carefully every day, adjustments being made when necessary.

The Thomas Splint with Pearson knee attachment

If the patient is a young fit man, the pull of the thigh muscles is difficult to overcome with skin traction alone and, in these circumstances, it is usual to employ skeletal traction with a Steinmann pin through the upper tibia (see below). This is more conveniently applied with the knee flexed and to achieve this, a second, smaller Thomas-type splint is attached to the full length splint to support the lower leg (Figure 15.1). It is applied with slings as with the straight splint, but the skin extensions are, of course, not required. The angle of the knee can be altered by adjusting the two splint components. A balanced traction system can then be used attaching the extension cord to a loop which fits over the ends of the Steinmann pin (Figure 15.2). It is rarely necessary to apply more than 10 lb weight to the system since over-distraction is harmful. After 2–3 weeks, the traction can often be reduced to 5 lb with the bed horizontal.

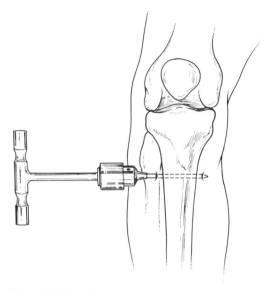

Figure 15.2 Insertion of Steinmann pin from the lateral side, upper tibia

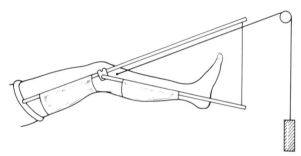

Figure 15.1 Thomas splint with Pearson knee attachment and skeletal traction

Insertion of Steinmann pin

This procedure should be carried out with full aseptic precautions, preferably in a theatre, but at least in an acceptably clean environment. The surgeon should wear full operating clothing and gloves. General or local anaesthetic may be employed and the procedure is, of course frequently carried out at the same time as the fracture is being manipulated. The usual sites for insertion are (a) through the upper tibia, just below the level of the tubercle and 2 cm behind the sharp anterior border; (b) through the lower tibia, 4–5 cm above the tip of the medial malleolus and 2 cm behind the anterior border; (c) through the calcaneum, 3 cm in front of and 3 cm above the point of the heel. All these measurements are, of course, average and relate to an adult.

The skin is cleaned and a small skin incision, just larger than the thickness of the pin, is made on the lateral side. The pin is then inserted through the skin incision and the tip is used to push back the muscle from the lateral surface of the tibia so that an area is cleared to allow the pin to penetrate the bone. The pin is then driven through the bone, care being taken to align it at right-angles to the line of the limb and in the coronal plane when the limb is held in neutral. The pin may be bored through using a specially made handle (see Figure 15.2) or, in hard bone, may be drilled through. It should be allowed to penetrate the soft tissues on the far side carefully, and when it begins to emerge through the skin, a second incision is made. The wounds may be covered with small pads soaked in benzoin tincture. It is important that the stirrup through which the traction is applied should move freely on the pin, otherwise the pin rotates in the bone and sepsis and loosening are inevitable. Threaded pins (Denham) are now available and avoid this type of loosening. These are widely used with intero-external fixation frames. Particularly firm fixation, suitable for long periods of fixation, can be achieved by the use of tapering threaded pins.

Application of skull callipers (Figure 15.3)

Several types of callipers are available. The Crutchfield type, although somewhat outdated, is widely used and its application will be described as an example of the technique. Blackburn's callipers are attached to the side of the skull about 6–7 cm above the external auditory meatus.

General anaesthesia or local infiltration anaesthesia may be used. The head is shaved either completely or in a wide strip across the centre of the skull. The operation is carried out in a theatre with full aseptic precautions. The patient lies on the operating table with the head at the top end resting on a ring or small pillow. The skin is marked with an indian-ink marker (Figure 15.3). The sagittal

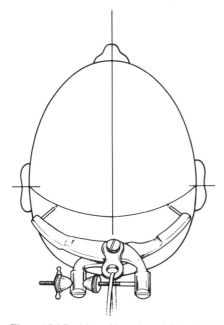

Figure 15.3 Position of insertion of Crutchfield callipers

midline is drawn first. A second line is drawn in a coronal plane over the skull from one external auditory meatus to the other. The callipers are opened out fully and centring the appliance on the midline, the points where the tips contact the skin are marked. At these points, incisions approximately 1.5 cm long are made, along the coronal line. The incision is deepened without widening to the skull, whilst an assistant applies pressure to the edges of

the incision with fingers and a swab. The periosteum is slightly elevated, sufficiently to allow the insertion of the special drill. The position of the drill hole in the bone should be checked by re-applying the calliper before drilling. The drill is designed to penetrate the outer table of the skull only. It is driven in a direction towards the centre of the skull. When both holes are drilled, the calliper is inserted and tightened. Two or three skin sutures may then be used on each side and benzoin tincture dressings applied on small pads. Bleeding usually stops with pressure, but an infiltration of adrenaline, 1 in 250 000, may be used with the local anaesthesia if required. The weights necessary for traction are attached. The callipers should be checked and, if necessary, tightened gently daily for the first few days.

More modern types of calliper are available, each with its own fixation technique. They have the advantage of being less likely to be dislodged and may be be left in place for long periods.

Traction systems

Commonly used systems are illustrated in Figures 15.4–15.7. Each may be applied either with skin or skeletal traction as required. Hamilton–Russell

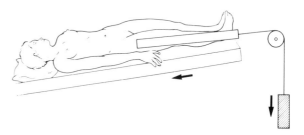

Figure 15.4 Longitudinal skin traction. The bed is tilted towards the head

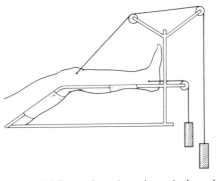

Figure 15.5 Femoral traction using a pin through the upper tibia and a second pin through the calcaneum. The leg rests on a Braun–Böhler frame

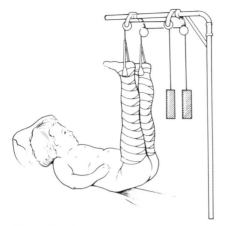

Figure 15.6 'Gallows traction' used for treating a femoral shaft fracture in children up to the age of 2 years. The traction is arranged so that the buttocks are lifted off the bed

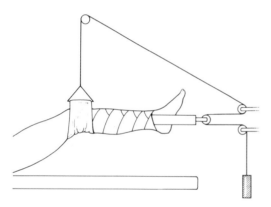

Figure 15.7 Hamilton–Russell traction using skin extensions. The traction may be applied via a pin through the upper tibia

traction is designed to give a resultant pull in line with the femur, whatever the position of the limb. It is normally used for fractures of the upper femur and hip conditions.

Aspiration of a joint

The knee is the joint most likely to need aspiration, but from time to time other joints may have to be aspirated and the needle should be introduced after due study of the anatomy. The hip, being a deeply placed joint, presents some difficulty. It may be approached by inserting the needle either two finger-breadths lateral to the pulsation of the femoral artery just below the inguinal ligament and

directing the needle slightly medially or, alternatively, by inserting a larger needle above the greater trochanter and running it along the upper border of the femoral neck.

Aspiration of the knee will be used to describe the technique:

1. The procedure should be carried out in the operating theatre with full aseptic precautions, the limb draped and the surgeon gowned and masked.
2. General anaesthesia may be used or, alternatively, local infiltration anaesthesia. If the latter is used, care should be taken to anaesthetize the skin and deep tissue, and particularly the synovium, which is acutely sensitive when inflamed. Adequate time should be given for the anaesthetic to take effect before proceeding.
3. A wide bore needle will be necessary, particularly if the joint contains blood. A 00 gauge needle or larger, attached to a 20 or 50 ml syringe is usually satisfactory.
4. The joint will usually be distended and the needle is introduced just medial to the border of the patella near the upper margin. The point is directed laterally and slightly backwards to pass behind the patella, with care to avoid the articular cartilage. It is usually obvious when the synovium has been penetrated and aspiration may then proceed.
5. After aspiration, the knee is wrapped in a Robert Jones bandage of alternate layers of wool and crepe. The aspirated specimen may be sent for culture or histology, as required.

Casting techniques

Many substitutes have been suggested for plaster-of-Paris, but it remains the most widely used splintage material because of its obvious advantages. It is reasonably cheap, versatile, widely available and easy to use, requiring very little in the way of apparatus. If carefully applied, it is comfortable and, being somewhat porous, absorbs perspiration and secretions. Its strength is adequate for most purposes and it is radiotranslucent. Nevertheless, it does also have disadvantages and many new materials are currently being developed as possible substitutes. Even when carefully built up to give maximum strength for weight, plaster tends to be heavy and warm and its unyielding nature makes it liable to produce pressure problems. A complete plaster cast makes inspection of the limb difficult, so it may conceal trouble and its rigidity can lead to uncertain immobilization, particularly when it is applied to a swollen limb. Finally, it is not waterproof and, for this reason, quickly disintegrates if allowed to get wet.

Plaster-of-Paris is made from gypsum and it used to be the practice for hospitals to make their own plaster bandages by impregnating wide-mesh gauze bandages with dry plaster base. These were then carefully rolled by hand and used before they deteriorated. Almost all plaster casts are now made from commercially produced bandages which are supplied in varying widths and are uniform in their spreading and setting characteristics.

The material can be used in several different ways:

1. As a simple splint. The splint is fashioned by laying strips of wet plaster along the limb to form a 'gutter', enclosing the limb to a variable degree. A better fit will be obtained if a completely circumferential plaster is made and allowed to dry and is then cut into two halves longitudinally. Both halves can be used individually or together. Slabs of plaster for the purpose of making splints can either be made by folding a plaster bandage along its length to form several layers (Figures 15.8 and 15.9), or are available ready-made from

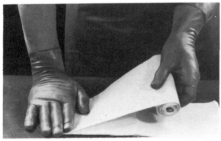

Figure 15.8 Method of making a plaster slab. Preferably the bandage should be dry

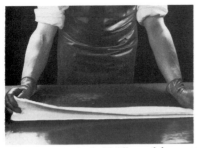

Figure 15.9 Method of folding a slab on end

special dispensers. The folding can be done dry or wet, the advantage of the dry technique being that the resulting slab can be tested for size and can be ready prepared before the manipulative procedure is carried out. The slabs can be increased in width by slightly overlapping each layer on the one below.

2. As a complete plaster cast, the type and extent of the cast depending on the immobilization required, e.g. half-leg, full-leg, etc. As a general rule, for adequate immobilization, the joint above and the joint below a fracture need to be incorporated in the plaster, although occasionally, if the fracture is very close to one end of a long bone, this rule may be broken. A plaster cast which is designed to immobilize the hip or shoulder is often known as a 'spica'.

3. As a functional cast. This type of application is becoming very popular and has the advantage that it allows greater use of the joints and greater mobility of the patient, avoiding stiffness and many of the other complications of disuse. Function is provided for by the incorporation of hinges or springs. The so-called 'cast brace' is a sophisticated, hinged and closely fitting plaster cast which requires considerable expertise and careful technique if it is to be successful.

4. As a plaster bed, in which the patient can lie for long periods without developing pressure sores, a technique which again requires careful workmanship.

Application of plaster-of-Paris

Everything required should be assembled before starting to apply the plaster, and the limb should be suitably supported to make the application as easy as possible. Assistants are usually required, but with careful planning and the use of slings and supports, much can be done to avoid the need for the limb to be held, often in an uncomfortable position, for long periods of time.

Generally speaking, the more closely the plaster fits and conforms to the limb, the more accurate the immobilization. If swelling of the limb is not expected, the plaster cast may be applied without padding and will be skin-tight. In order to prevent it sticking to the hairs of the skin, and to make removal easier, a single layer of stretch stockinet is usually applied to the skin before applying the plaster. Where swelling is expected or already present, some padding is necessary, usually a single layer of plaster wool wrapped evenly around the limb, with care being taken to ensure that pressure points and prominences are well covered. If the swelling is likely to be extreme, it is usually advisable to avoid a completely encircling plaster and to use instead a plaster slab held in place by a wet gauze bandage which will have reached its maximum shrinkage by virtue of being wet before application.

The plaster is activated by soaking in water, the temperature of which to some extent governs the setting speed. Approximately 35°C will prove to be suitable for most purposes, i.e. a comfortable lukewarm temperature. A good sized bowl or bucket should be used as the water soon becomes thick with shed plaster. A standard roll of plaster bandage is approximately 3 m long and available in widths from 5 cm to 20 cm. The end of the bandage is slightly unrolled and held with one hand whilst the bandage is held in the water (Figure 15.10) until bubbles cease to emerge from the ends of the roll. Surplus water is then squeezed out by gently rotating the ends (Figure 15.11) and the bandage is rolled onto the limb, without applying any tension and carefully avoiding any folds and wrinkles. The turns should be kept even and, if a change of direction is necessary, a small tuck should be made so that the plaster still lies flat. The plaster is rubbed to distribute the material evenly between the layers and is finally smoothed off. The assistant may need to hold the plaster whilst it is setting but must be careful to avoid pressure with the finger tips on the cast until it is set. The plaster wool or stockinet may be folded over the ends of the cast to give a neat and comfortable finish.

If a slab is being used, it should be held at the two ends and drawn slowly through the water. It can then be held vertically by one end and the water

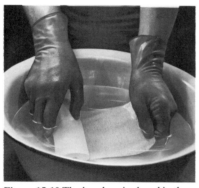

Figure 15.10 The bandage is placed in the water. The end is free

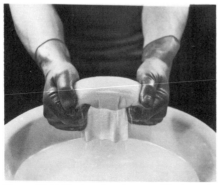

Figure 15.11 The bandage is grasped by its end and excess water is expelled

allowed to drain off. Finally, the slab is allowed to collapse into the palm of the hand and is gently compressed to remove surplus water. It is then spread out on a flat surface and air bubbles are squeezed out with the palm of the hand. It is an important point in plaster technique that the layers should be well bonded together without air bubbles and dry areas otherwise the strength of the plaster will be adversely affected. If required, the plaster slab can be strengthened by drawing the wet plaster up into longitudinal ridges, taking care to avoid irregularities on the inner surface.

A cast made using lukewarm water will normally set in about 4–6 min, but will not be fully hard until 24 h later. Trimming of the cast can be carried out immediately after setting, whilst the plaster is still wet. A sharp plaster knife with a curved blade is useful for this purpose and care must be taken at all times to cut away from the skin. When the plaster is fully hardened, it may be cut for the purpose of wedging or a heel or iron may be incorporated to allow weight-bearing.

Warning. The patient should be given printed instructions to watch for changes in the circulation and sensation in the limb and to report immediately to hospital if these occur. Specifically, the instructions should state that if the fingers or toes become painful, blue or swollen and this does not improve rapidly with elevation of the limb, then medical help should be sought. It is sometimes suggested that, rather than delay, the plaster should be removed with a knife or saw. If this instruction is felt necessary, perhaps in remote areas, it should be emphasized that this should be done with great care, cutting the plaster a little at a time to avoid damage to the skin, particularly when sensation is impaired. The author has seen a limb almost completely amputated by the patient's own efforts, using a carpenter's saw, the limb having been rendered completely anaesthetic by the overtight cast.

Following treatment of an acute fracture or in any circumstances where there is likely to be swelling the patient should be seen on the following day to allow any modifications to be made to the cast. Where there is a serious risk of circulatory occlusion the patient should be admitted overnight for observation.

Cutting the plaster cast

If there is any suggestion that the plaster is too tight, it should be split with a plaster saw and the opening spread. The split should be made *down to the skin throughout the whole length of the plaster cast* and the limb elevated.

A fracture which has been manipulated but is in slight malalignment may often be improved by wedging the plaster. This can be done by making a cut around half the circumference of the plaster and holding the cut open with a wooden block. The position for the cut can be judged by putting a line of drawing pins along the edge of the cast and taking a radiograph to relate the level of the fracture to the pins on the surface. Occasionally, it is more satisfactory to take out a wedge of plaster on the convex side of the deformity and to close this, rather than to make an opening wedge on the concave side, the latter sometimes tending to result in complete displacement of a very unstable structure. After wedging, if the check radiograph is satisfactory, the cast is completed again with a roll of plaster.

Removal of plaster casts

The instruments normally used for removing a cast are shown in Figure 15.12. The electric Desoutter saw has an oscillating blade and provided it is not dragged forcibly along the skin it does not cut the limb (Figure 15.13). It has the disadvantage when dealing with children of being very noisy and frightening. A plaster which is not too thick can often be cut with heavy scissors of the type shown, which have one blade longer than the other and curved upwards. Stille's shears, which have a lever action, will cut through thicker plaster and with care

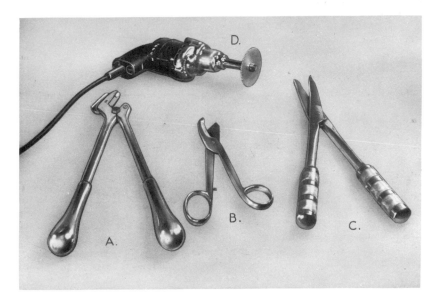

Figure 15.12 Instruments for removing a plaster. A, Stille's shears; B, Böhler's scissors; C, Lloyd's plaster opener; D, Desoutter's plaster cutter

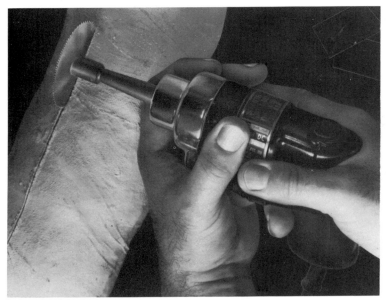

Figure 15.13 The Desoutter electric plaster cast cutter in use

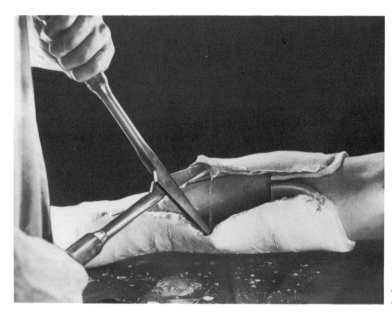

Figure 15.14 When a plaster has been cut through, Lloyd's plaster opener, by spreading apart the cut edges, facilitates removal of the cast

are very safe to use. Having split the plaster along its length, it is prised open using a spreader of the type shown (Figure 15.14), and the plaster wool is either cut with scissors or torn apart a little at a time. The plaster should normally be cut at diametrically opposite points on the circumference and consideration should be given to using the two halves of the cast as a splint which can be bandaged back in position, a procedure sometimes called 'bi-valving'. Occasionally, it is known in advance that the cast will need to be split as soon as it sets, in which case it is convenient to lay a copper strip along the skin and to apply the wool and plaster over this. When the plaster is set but still wet, a knife can be used to cut down onto the metal strip, which is then removed.

Application of common types of plaster casts
The dorsal slab for the wrist and hand

This type of cast is often used where critical immobilization is not required, or where swelling is anticipated. It is very useful where pain relief is the main reason for immobilization. Perhaps its most common use is in the treatment of a Colles' fracture. It may, if required, be extended to include one or more fingers.

Counter-traction is often necessary when manipulating a fracture, and even when this is not the case it can be convenient to use a simple sling as illustrated

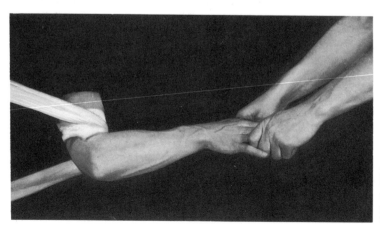

Figure 15.15 A counter traction band is applied to the upper arm over a pad of wool. Manual traction is maintained on the fingers and thumb

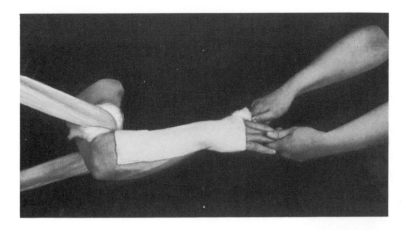

Figure 15.16 The slab extends from elbow to knuckles, and is moulded to the contour of the wrist

in Figure 15.15. A traction band is passed around the upper arm over a pad of wool and is fixed to a wall hook or other immovable object. The fingers are than grasped by an assistant and the arm and hand are left completely free to allow application of the plaster. If a Colles' fracture has been manipulated, the correct position for the wrist can readily be achieved by applying traction to the thumb with the latter in line with the forearm. This gives the necessary degree of ulnar deviation of the wrist to ensure correct radial and ulnar alignment. A plaster slab is prepared from a 15 cm wide plaster bandage. The arm is measured from the tip of the olecranon to the knuckles and the slab is arranged to be 5 cm longer than this measurement. If required, the slab can be made slightly wider at the elbow end by allowing it to fan out somewhat when folding. Depending on the circumstances, the slab is applied over a layer of well-fitting stockinet or over a single layer of plaster wool applied as a bandage. The slab is laid along the dorsum of the forearm, wrist and hand, and is moulded carefully to the limb (Figure 15.16), taking particular care to ensure that the radial border of the wrist and hand are well covered and that the cast does not extend beyond the knuckles themselves. The slab is bandaged on with a wet gauze bandage, care being taken not to pull this tightly (Figure 15.17). Finally, the ends of the slab are folded back obliquely to leave a neat finish and to avoid restricting elbow and finger movements. The plaster should never be so wide that the two edges touch and the palm of the hand should be free from plaster, a few turns of the gauze bandage being taken across the palm. Whenever possible, the thumb and first metacarpal should be completely free. If it is later decided to complete the cast, this can be done without disturbing the gauze bandage, simply by wrapping around one or two turns of plaster bandage. If the slab is extended to immobilize a metacarpophalangeal joint, the extension should only reach a point just proximal to the first interphalangeal joint.

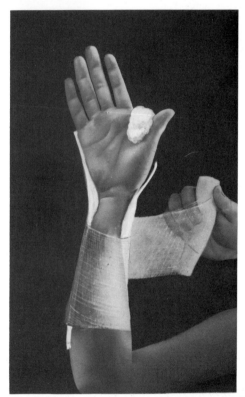

Figure 15.17 Application of a dorsal slab. *Note*: (1) Pad of wool separating index finger and thumb; this helps to keep the thumb abducted and therefore permits full flexion of fingers; (2) The slab does not include anterior one-third of wrist; (3) Wet gauze bandage used to fix the slab

The complete below-elbow and scaphoid plaster

When swelling is not expected, the dorsal slab can be replaced by a complete plaster cast and for adequate immobilization of a fracture of the scaphoid it is usual to include the thumb as far as the level of the first interphalangeal joint. The plaster will usually be applied over a single layer of stockinet, but plaster wool may be used if preferred. If stockinet is used a hole is cut for the thumb and the thumb itself is covered with a single layer of plaster wool. The cast is formed by applying a 10 cm wide plaster bandage in a circular fashion around the hand and wrist and taking several turns round the thumb. If required, a dorsal slab may be applied first and the circular layers applied over this. This has the advantage that fewer circular turns are required and the plaster can easily be cut along the anterior midline for removal.

The full-arm plaster cast

This type of plaster cast is often used for fractures of the forearm bones, particularly in children, and also for Smith's fractures and comminuted and unstable Colles' fractures. The position of rotation of the forearm will depend on the particular type of fracture being treated, a Smith's fracture normally requiring full supination, a Colles' fracture full pronation and forearm fractures requiring various positions depending on the angulation of rotation of the fracture. The elbow will usually be at a right-angle to control rotation of the forearm.

It is usually convenient to have the patient lying supine and to apply traction to the arm with a loop of crêpe bandage as shown in Figure 15.18. The spreader is useful to provide sufficient room for a slab to be applied along the back of the upper arm, behind the elbow and along the back of the forearm and wrist. This is measured from the knuckles to the level of the lower fold of the axilla. This type of plaster is usually applied over a single layer of plaster wool, but if swelling is likely, the complete cast is better replaced by a dorsal slab fixed with a wet gauze bandage and later changed or completed. The slab is made from a 10 cm wide, 3 m long plaster bandage or the equivalent ready-made unit, and is applied as described. If the plaster is to be complete, no gauze bandage is required and the cast is formed using 10 cm plaster bandages in a circular fashion, the turns passing through the traction loop and including it in the completed plaster. When the cast has set, the loop is cut off flush with the cast and a final turn is made to produce a neat finish.

The U-slab for fractures of the humerus

This type of plaster is usually used for the treatment of fractures of the shaft of the humerus, the fracture being held out to length by gravity, with the arm supported at the wrist by a collar and cuff sling. The collar and cuff sling is applied first and the patient is treated sitting in a chair, leaning slightly forwards. A pad of adhesive felt is placed over the acromion and the outer end of the clavicle. The length of the slab is estimated by measuring from the axilla down the inner side of the arm, around the elbow, up the outer side of the arm and over the shoulder to just beyond the acromioclavicular joint. The slab is made by folding two 15 cm wide plaster bandages and making it 5 cm longer than the measured length. It is applied over a single layer of wool which is applied in circular fashion around the arm and carried as far as possible over the shoulder. The slab is applied and carefully moulded to the contours of the arm and bandaged in place either with a wet gauze bandage or, often more conveniently, with a dry crêpe bandage. This type of cast tends to loosen and usually needs adjustment at weekly intervals. The upper end of the cast tends to come away from the shoulder and after carefully turning back the upper end to produce a neat and smooth finish, this end may be taped down with a strip of adhesive

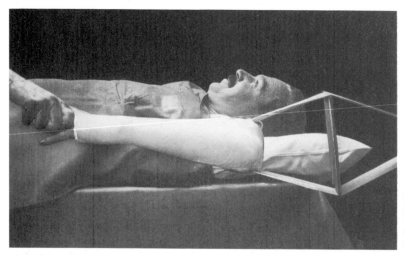

Figure 15.18 Application of full-arm plaster cast. *Note*: (1) Manual traction; (2) Fixed counter traction; (3) Spreader separating loop of traction band

plaster applied from front to back. The cast must also be carefully finished in the axilla to prevent discomfort, and the patient should be advised to sleep in a reasonably upright position whenever possible.

The shoulder spica

There are relatively few indications for this type of plaster. For many purposes, abduction splints are more convenient and more comfortable. Occasional fractures around the shoulder and operative procedures such as tendon transplantation require the reliability of immobilization which only a spica can give. The requirements are usually that the shoulder be immobilized in a position of abduction as shown in Figure 15.19.

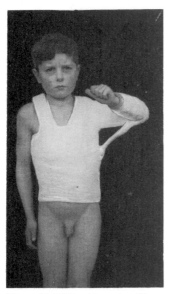

Figure 15.19 Shoulder spica. The cast should extend lower over the iliac crests. The bar over the free shoulder can often be omitted

The plaster is usually applied with the patient sitting on a stool or standing. Applying this type of plaster with the patient anaesthetized can be particularly difficult and usually needs a number of assistants. The elbow is normally flexed to a right-angle and with the arm placed about 30° in front of the coronal plane. Pads of orthopaedic felt, about 5 cm wide, are placed over the length of the iliac crests and a length of wide stockinet is cut sufficiently long to reach from the neck to the pubis. Holes are cut to allow the arms to pass through. A second length of narrow stockinet is cut to cover the arm from the shoulder to the knuckles and pads of wool or thin sorbo rubber are placed over the whole

length of the spine and over each shoulder outside the stockinet. These can be taped in place with adhesive strapping.

In an adult, the body part of the spica is made mainly from 20 cm wide plaster bandages; in a child 15 cm wide bandages usually suffice. Using the wide plaster bandages, the lower part of the spica is formed by using circular turns ensuring that the iliac crests are covered but that the plaster does not reach the groins. The turns are then taken gradually up the body, applying them firmly and moulding the cast around the waist. When the shoulder is reached, the turns are taken in spiral fashion around the shoulder and under the axilla. Careful moulding in this area is necessary if the spica is to be comfortable. A plaster slab made from two 15 cm wide bandages, measured for length before wetting, is taken from the opposite anterior superior iliac spine across the front of the chest, over and around the back of the shoulder, finishing around the inner aspect of the arm. A second slab is taken in the opposite direction from the back of the opposite iliac crest, diagonally across the back, under the axilla and over the front and top of the shoulder. Finally a slab of the same width is taken in the midaxillary line from the iliac crest up the side of the trunk and is moulded under the axilla to reach the inner aspect of the arm. A full-arm plaster is applied as described previously and continued over the shoulder in spiral fashion and on to the chest. A further one or two turns of wide bandage are used around the chest and abdomen to produce a smooth final surface. If required, a stay can be formed from a short aluminium rod covered with plaster and bandaged in position at each end, or simply by using a rolled plaster bandage pulled out to form a rod and using the loose ends to attach it to the spica, as shown in Figure 15.19.

If the patient is not too heavy, and the cast is carefully formed, this strut can be dispensed with and this makes it easier for the patient to wear normal clothes. The plaster strap extending across the opposite shoulder shown in the figure can also usually be dispensed with and the opposite shoulder left completely free. Care must be taken in moulding the cast around the iliac crests and the lower edge must be trimmed to allow the hips to flex fully without the thigh contacting the lower margin. Similarly, the upper borders must be carefully finished off by folding the stockinet over the edge to avoid pressure on the neck and axillary folds. It should be noted that this type of cast is supported essentially by the iliac crests and not by the shoulder or arm.

The below-knee plaster cast

This is one of the most commonly used plaster casts, being suitable for many injuries of the ankle and foot and frequently used for supporting the foot after operative procedures. It may, if required, be reinforced for weight-bearing by incorporating a heel or iron.

The plaster is most conveniently applied if the patient sits on a high chair or lies on a table with the lower leg hanging vertically so that the operator can support the foot on his knee. It is helpful to place a small pad or sandbag under the thigh. A piece of orthopaedic felt is placed around the leg immediately below the flexed knee joint (Figure 15.20A). The plaster is applied over a layer of stockinet or over a single layer of plaster wool. A long slab is prepared from two 15 cm wide bandages and is applied from the medial condyle of the tibia along the medial

Application of a weight-bearing heel or sole

A satisfactory sole can be prepared from a pad of sorbo rubber cut to a pattern of the outline of the sole of the cast (Figure 15.21). As a foundation for the rubber sole a wet plaster bandage is unwound back and forth over the plaster sole, and is rendered rugged (Figure 15.22) deliberately, in order that its craggy exterior will bind better with the sorbo sole laid upon it. The sorbo sole is lashed to the foundation with a moist plaster bandage (Figure 15.23). When the cast is moderately dry, that portion covering the foot is covered with elastic adhesive strapping (Figure 15.24), which protects the thin shell binding the sponge to the sole, and it

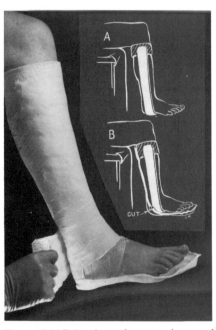

Figure 15.20 Below-knee plaster nearing completion. Showing also, inset **A**, position of the rim of felt and the first slab; Inset **B**, the same with second slab superimposed

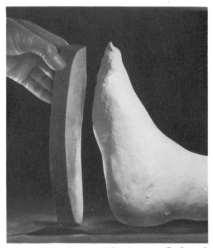

Figure 15.21 Sorbo rubber is cut to fit the sole of the cast

aspect of the leg, beneath the heel, and along the lateral aspect of the leg to the lateral condyle of the tibia (Figure 15.20A). Another slab is made long enough to extend from the back of the knee joint passing behind the heel to the base of the toes. After this has been applied (Figure 15.20B), a transverse cut is made on either side of the heel and the cut edges are imbricated upon one another evenly. These slabs are fixed in position by rolling on moist plaster bandages from above downwards. The cast is usually extended to form a platform underneath the toes, but is trimmed so that the dorsal surfaces of the toes are free.

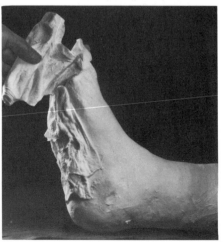

Figure 15.22 The sole of the cast is reinforced with a deliberately rough foundation

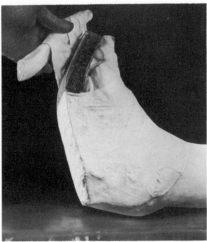

Figure 15.23 The rubber sole is incorporated in the cast by the superimposition of a further plaster bandage

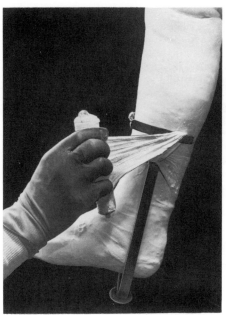

Figure 15.25 Application of an iron heel. The long axis of the heel must be in the line of the leg

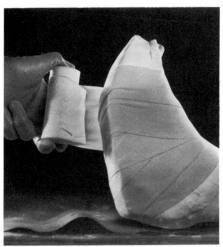

Figure 15.24 When the cast is dry, the application of elastic adhesive strapping helps to prevent wear and is 'non-skid'

also renders the surface upon which the patient will walk less slippery.

A heel or rocker gives better protection for the plaster and tends to last longer, but gives the patient slightly less support and is tricky for the older patient who finds balancing difficult. Ready-made heels are available in various materials and are easily attached to the finished cast. They should be fixed directly under the line of the tibia.

Application of an iron heel

The iron heel consists of a stirrup on which the patient walks; it extends about 3–4 cm below the plaster cast. It must be attached to the cast exactly in

the line of the leg, and not tilted backwards or forwards. To fix the iron heel in place, a turn of moist plaster bandage is taken around the leg. The iron is then placed in position, and the next turn of bandage passed once around the leg over the side bars, and then the bandage is hitched over the free end of one of the cross-bars, as shown in Figure 15.25, the direction of the encircling bandage being then reversed. One and a half more turns will bring the bandage to the cross-bar on the opposite side, over which the bandage is hitched and reversed. This process is repeated until the iron frame is stabilized. At this stage, the soft cross-bars are moulded firmly against the cast. Two turns of bandage are taken over the cross-bars and the bandage is continued over the side bars down the leg to the ankle. The remaining length of bandage is taken through the loop and finally bound round the extended legs of the iron.

The full-leg plaster cast

This cast is frequently used for fractures of the tibia and fibula and for those fractures of the ankle which require the knee to be held flexed to control rotation of the lower leg. This can be a difficult cast to apply successfully. It is usually applied over a layer of stretch stockinet or over a single layer of plaster wool. It is commonly made by extending a below-knee cast applied as described above. The layer of felt around the upper tibia and fibula is omitted and, of course, the wool or stockinet is applied as a continuous length from toes to groin. Having completed the below-knee component, an assistant holds the still wet but solid plaster in a horizontal position to control the angle of the knee, which is usually 20–30°, and the plaster is completed by taking turns of 15 cm wide bandage up to the level of the groin. Care should be taken to ensure that a good bond is formed at the knee and the upper end of the cast should be finished in the usual way by folding over the stockinet or wool in an outwards direction and incorporating this in the final turn of plaster.

The plaster cylinder

This type of cast is often used for injuries around the knee, where rotation does not need to be controlled and the foot can be left free. It is applied over the usual layer of stockinet or plaster wool. A pad of orthopaedic felt is applied over each malleolus and the wool is extended to cover this. The cast may be built upon two slabs of 15 cm wide bandage applied on each side of the limb from malleolus to groin and completed in the usual way by circular turns. It must be carefully moulded above the malleoli otherwise it will tend to slip down. Except in certain special cases, the knee is not immobilized in full extension, a few degrees of flexion being more comfortable.

The hip spica

To immobilize the hip using a plaster cast, the shell needs to extend from just below the nipples to a point either just above the knee or, in certain circumstances, to include the lower leg and foot. This type of cast is no longer in common use for adults, but is still frequently used for the later treatment of femoral shaft fractures and certain hip conditions in children.

If a spica is to be applied to an adult, it is usually best, if possible, to suspend the patient on an orthopaedic table so that the position can be completely controlled. A small child can be managed on a removable rest (Figure 15.26), on which the spine is supported, and which can be covered by the stockinet or wool and plaster and is removed at the end of the procedure.

If an orthopaedic table is used the feet are bandaged to the sole-plates. The knee is suspended by a bandage from the cross-bar to avoid extension of the hip and hyperextension of the knee. The table is then 'let-down', so that the patient is suspended by the shoulders, pelvis and feet (Figure 15.27).

The trunk is covered with a length of wide stockinet extending from the groin to the nipples. A second length is applied over the leg to overlap the first at the groin. Small pads of wool may be placed

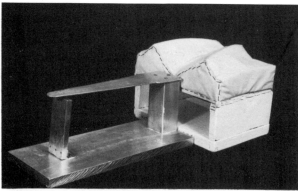

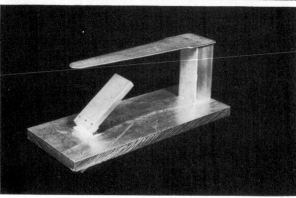

Figure 15.26 Stand and headrest for application of hip spica to a small child. The horizontal metal bar would be covered with a layer of plaster wool and the spica would enclose the stand, which would then be removed at the end of the procedure

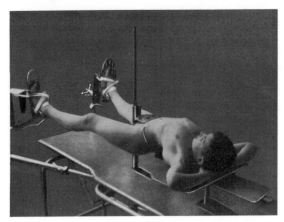

Figure 15.27 Patient on an orthopaedic table for application of hip spica. The knees have not yet been suspended

over the iliac crests and the sacrum, and held in place with adhesive tape.

Plaster bandages 15 cm wide will usually be most suitable for a small child and 20 cm wide for an adult. The bandages are applied in circular fashion around the upper chest and trunk, working from above downwards and putting rather more tension on the bandage than is usually required. The turns should be continued in spiral fashion around the hip and thigh. After two or three layers have been applied, preprepared slabs, made from one or two bandages, are used to reinforce the cast, the first one being taken from the opposite axilla, diagonally across the chest and trunk, around the front and side of the hip, behind the buttock and finishing on the inner side of the thigh. The second slab extends from the back of the thigh, around the inner aspect and front of the thigh, around the iliac crest and diagonally across the back to the opposite axilla. A third slab is placed across the buttocks, around the iliac crest on the side which is to be left free, and on the side to be included is carried as a spiral round the hip and thigh. The leg part of the plaster is most conveniently formed by simply continuing the turns of plaster down the thigh and, if required, down the lower leg to the foot, an assistant holding the knee and foot in the required position if an orthopaedic table is not used. If the opposite hip is to be left completely free, an additional slab is applied on the enclosed side, along the side of the trunk from axilla to knee. All the slabs are bound in place with one or two turns of plaster bandage, folding the stockinet over at top and bottom and incorporating the turned ends in the plaster. In the adult, slabs may be used on the legs to reduce the number of circular turns.

It is often helpful, particularly in small children,

to incorporate the opposite hip and thigh, at least to knee level, a so-called 'double hip spica', and the cast can then be reinforced with a bar extending between the thighs, as described for the shoulder spica. With all hip spicas care should be taken to ensure that there is sufficient thickness of plaster behind the buttocks as this area is often left rather weak and may crack. If the spica has been applied rather tightly, it will be found that when the patient is taken off the stand and the spinal or sacral support is removed from within the plaster, there will then be sufficient room for comfort and the spica will be reasonably close-fitting. After taking all the supports out, the cast is trimmed around the genitalia and between the legs and buttocks. If both hips are included in a spica, it is essential that they should be abducted to at least 25 or 30°. A plaster hip spica is very liable to cause some discomfort for 2 or 3 days after application, particularly in adults. Nausea and abdominal pain are common and, occasionally, paralytic ileus may develop. If this occurs, it may be necessary to split the upper part of the cast down the sides as far as the lower ribs, spreading the cuts in the usual way. This is generally sufficient to relieve the symptoms. If a full scale paralytic ileus develops, the usual conservative regimen of gastric aspiration and intravenous fluids will normally result in a return of bowel function within 24–48 h, and it is rarely necessary to remove the cast completely. The plaster can be reconstituted when the symptoms have settled.

The plaster jacket

The newer types of lightweight casting materials are tending to replace plaster-of-Paris as a support for the spine. The plaster jacket is rarely used now for spinal fractures, but still has a place in the conservative and operative treatment of a number of spinal conditions and in scoliosis surgery, where the requirements may be very specialized. For most purposes, the plaster jacket will consist of a shell enclosing the trunk and extending from iliac crests to the level of the nipples. Occasionally, to provide immobilization for the thoracic spine, it may be appropriate to extend the cast over the shoulders.

The ordinary body jacket is applied with the patient sitting or standing. The procedure is essentially as described for the shoulder spica, the cast being designed to rest on the iliac crests. It is applied over a single layer of stockinet used as a vest and felt pads are placed over the iliac crests. Heavy slabs need not be used, as the cast does not have to take heavy loads, but one slab applied in the axillary line on each side makes it possible to use fewer turns of bandage. The cast must be carefully moulded round the waist and iliac crests and must not extend so low that it catches the thighs when sitting.

The plaster bed

This is no longer popular but once was widely used in the treatment of infective conditions of the spine. For conservative management of spinal fractures which are not complicated by paraplegia, the plaster bed is a most effective way of immobilizing the spine, but requires very careful attention to detail if it is to be comfortable for the long periods for which it is likely to be used.

The posterior shell is made by applying preprepared or ready-made slabs to cover the patient, who is placed in the required position, face down on pillows or other suitable supports. Care should be taken to avoid a position of hyperextension of the lumbar spine, and supports should be provided under the shoulders to brace them back a little. The hips should normally be flexed 10 or 15° and the knees flexed to about 20°, and it is important to abduct the hips sufficiently to allow toilet functions to be carried out. The plaster is applied over a single layer of stockinet which covers the head, the whole of the trunk, the buttocks and the thighs and legs. A single or double layer of plaster bandage is first applied over the whole area which is to be covered by the shell, avoiding folds and ridges, and carefully smoothing this down to form a base for the slabs which are applied edge to edge, extending as far as the midaxillary line on the trunk and halfway around the legs. A single wide slab extending from the occiput to the lower thoracic spine is moulded around the head and neck and separate slabs are used on each side of this for the shoulders and chest. A single large slab, if available, is placed across the lumbar spine extending to the loin on each side. Further slabs are used for the buttocks and the thigh and lower legs. About 5–6 layers of plaster will normally be sufficient for the slabs, and all must be carefully smoothed down. Additional strength can be provided by applying ridges of plaster lengthwise down the outer surface of the cast. When this has hardened it is carefully removed from the patient and set aside for at least 24 h. When completely dry, the inner surface is inspected for irregularities and, if any are found, these are smoothed off with wet and dry emery paper. The patient may be allowed to lie in the shell if it is supported on pillows to check that it is a comfortable fit. If it appears satisfactory, the inner surface is finally rubbed smooth with talc and is lined with wool or thin foam which is taped in place using waterproof adhesive tape around the edges of the cast. The shell is finally mounted on a wooden frame with cross-bars provided at the points of maximum load-bearing. It is often convenient to make a second front shell, which need not be mounted on a frame, and which can be used for short periods to allow the patient to lie face downwards to provide a change of position and to enable the back-shell to be properly maintained.

Alternative plaster materials

Over the past few years a number of new products have appeared on the market, with claims that they overcome some of the disadvantages of, and are more efficient than, plaster-of-Paris. They tend to be based on a plastic material which is activated in various ways according to the product. Most use water as the activator, the trend being towards using cold water, although some require high temperatures and consequently need some kind of water bath and special lining materials to protect the limb. The advantages claimed usually include greater strength per unit weight than plaster-of-Paris and a resistance to water to an extent that makes it possible to actually immerse them in water. They vary in their ease of application and in the degree to which they can be made to conform to the limb, and it would be fair to say that in both these respects they have, so far, left much to be desired. They also suffer from the very important disadvantage that they are much more expensive than plaster-of-Paris, and this has limited their use to situations where their particular characteristics justify the extra cost. It is undoubtedly sometimes an advantage to use a waterproof material, and strength coupled with lightness can make it possible to mobilize a patient who might otherwise be confined to bed. They have proved particularly useful for splint and brace making, but they have found little favour for the management of acute fractures, difficulty in moulding them and, once again, cost, tending to rule them out. Nevertheless, they are constantly being improved and there is little doubt that they will become more versatile and probably cheaper and they may prove to be serious competitors for traditional methods.

It is beyond the scope of this publication to describe in detail the technique of using these materials. The manufacturers' literature will describe their applications, but it is suggested that any potential user should compare the different characteristics of the various materials and the ease of using them and overall cost before embarking on their large-scale use.

16

Head injuries

H. A. Crockard

The toll of deaths and suffering caused by trauma continues to rise. Trauma is the commonest cause of death of young people in modern society, and a major cause of morbidity and of loss of productivity. Road accidents are the commonest source of trauma and well over half have a head injury; statistics show that almost three-quarters of fatal road accidents have a significant head injury. About one-third of these die at the scene of the accident, and another one-third within 24 h of hospital admission. While many of these injuries are incompatible with survival, there are a great number who are adversely affected by secondary pathophysiological changes which develop shortly after injury. Thus, optimum treatment of head injuries is not solely the domain of the neurosurgeons, but the responsibility of all involved from the scene of the accident to the hospital administering primary care. Management of any head injury is always a serious responsibility, requiring sound judgement, a correct sense of priorities, detailed and frequently repeated assessments and awareness of the possibility of injury to other systems. There are a large number of patients with relatively trivial injuries who require reassurance more than treatment when seen in the emergency department but the few serious injuries tax the ability and resources of all concerned. Constant vigilance is essential.

Pathophysiology

A head injury may be localized or generalized (Figure 16.1). The localized injury is usually caused by a small object moving at moderate velocity. It expends most of its force upon a small area of scalp and skull, and may even penetrate skull, dura and cortex without causing loss of consciousness or change in vital signs. The generalized injury

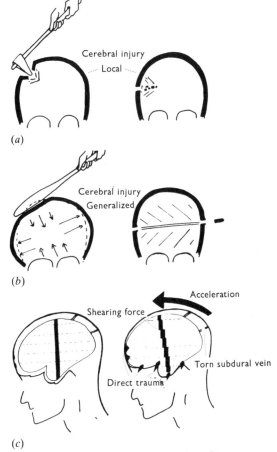

(a)

(b)

(c)

Figure 16.1 Types of injury: (a) local injury. Damage limited to a small area of cortex; (b) generalized crushing and explosive injuries. Damage widespread; (c) generalized accelerating or decelerating injury. Damage widespread

203

damages the whole brain by compression or, more commonly, by acceleration/deceleration forces which set up shearing strains within the brain, contuse the surfaces against the skull's bony ridges and avulse bridging veins. The 'whiplash' mechanism also distorts the midbrain and brain stem, usually resulting in a loss of consciousness and often alterations in vital signs. The bullet will produce a local injury but, in addition, will damage all the intracranial contents. Many injuries have a variable degree of brain swelling, but about 1% will develop a significant intracranial clot, extradural or intracerebral, the early removal of which will reduce morbidity and may prevent mortality.

Following injury, the primary damage will produce secondary brain swelling, either focal or generalized, and as there is a limit to the intracranial capacity, the increase in brain or blood volume will soon cause an increase in intracranial pressure (ICP), causing cellular hypoxia, increasing oedema and intracranial volume. Inadequate or irregular respirations, due to brainstem damage or associated thoracic injury, will compound the error; coughing and straining will raise the ICP in the 'tight' brain situation. Once established, brain swelling is life-threatening and resistant to treatment. If these basic concepts are foremost, then the vital roles of the care of the airway and, if possible, reduction of ICP will not be forgotten.

Definitions

Closed head injury is one in which the scalp is intact and there is no communication between the intradural contents and the outside.

Open head injury implies communication between the intradural contents and the atmosphere.

A minor head injury is one in which there is no loss of consciousness, or only a brief loss of consciousness, with return to normal function and no clinical or radiological evidence of fractures or dural tears.

The severe head injury is one in which there is prolonged or profound loss of consciousness. In retrospect, the patient who has been unconscious for 24 h or who cannot remember anything for a week after the injury is also considered to have had a severe head injury.

Coma is a state of complete loss of consciousness from which the patient cannot be roused even by the most powerful stimuli. Using the Glasgow Coma Scale it may be defined as 'no eye opening, no comprehensible verbal response and not obeying commands'.

The Glasgow Coma Scale quantifies the severity of injury by the best response to stimuli in terms of eye opening, motor response and verbal response. Its great advantage is that it is universally accepted

Table 16.1 Assessment of level of consciousness using the Glasgow Coma Scale

Eye opening		
Spontaneous	4	
To speech	3	E
To pain	2	
Nil	1	
Best motor response		
Obeys	6	
Localizes	5	
Normal flexion	4	M
Abnormal flexion	3	
Extensor response	2	
Nil	1	
Verbal response		
Orientated	5	
Confused conversation	4	
Inappropriate words	3	V
Incomprehensible sounds	2	
Nil	1	

and observation charts based on this system allow a graphical representation of the change in neurological condition, the significance of which can be appreciated by all who are caring for the patient (Table 16.1).

The unconscious patient
Initial management

Immediately and sequentially the patient needs:

1. A good airway.
2. Control of bleeding and restoration of circulating blood volume if necessary.
3. Examination of the whole body to assess or exclude other injuries.
4. Detailed assessment of head and facial injury.

When his condition is stable, he should have

5. X-rays of the involved areas, and then
6. A decision as to the priority for treatment of each injury.

Finally, if it has been decided to

7. Transfer him to a specialist unit, this must only be done when the vital signs are stable and he is
8. Accompanied by trained personnel or, if severely injured, or requiring ventilatory assistance, a medical practitioner.

Before handing over to another medical practitioner, there should be

9. Full documentation of the history, vital signs, gross neurological findings and all drugs and intravenous fluids administered.

Some of these steps are self-explanatory, others will be amplified in the following paragraphs.

On admission to the Accident and Emergency department, staff teamwork will greatly improve efficiency and the quality of care. At the very beginning a note should be made of:

1. Level of consciousness.
2. Reaction and size of pupils.
3. Blood pressure.
4. Pulse.
5. Respiratory rate.

The injured patient who is unconscious should be completely stripped so that his whole body, back and front, can be carefully examined, in a good light. When moved from stretcher to trolley or bed, or turned on his side for examination of his back, he should be *handled as if his neck or spine were broken;* thus, head, shoulders and pelvis must be supported and turned at the same time. With multiple injuries it is important to reduce to an absolute minimum the number of transfers from trolley to trolley as movements of fractured bone ends increase shock and internal haemorrhage may recommence. It is essential to obtain a history from relatives, accompanying bystanders, police or ambulancemen; without this it is difficult to determine whether the unconsciousness is as a result of the impact, or due to a pre-existing medical condition which led to the accident. The roles of alcohol and drugs in the patient's presentation must also be evaluated and, again, a history may be the only clue.

Adequate airway

This is of the utmost importance. The tongue of the comatose patient in a supine position must be regarded as a foreign body in the oropharynx. Extension of the head and elevation of the mandible by its angles will raise the tongue out of the posterior oropharynx. Stove-in fractures of the middle third of the face and double fractures of the mandible constitute special hazards requiring continuous clearing of the airway of blood, and early assistance from a maxillofacial specialist. Beware of loose teeth and food in the pharynx. Secretions are removed by nasopharyngeal and oral suction; to prevent vomiting and aspiration it is wise to pass a nasogastric tube and empty the stomach. All unconscious patients should have an oropharyngeal airway inserted to maintain a good airway even if the patient clenches his teeth. If there is any depression of the cough reflex or level of consciousness, a cuffed, non-kinkable endo- or nasotracheal tube should be inserted. Patients who have aspirated pharyngeal secretions or gastric contents should have an endotracheal tube passed for very careful pulmonary toilet. This applies to the drowsy patient also and so this procedure is best performed by a competent anaesthetist who may have to use a short-acting anaesthetic. Large doses of steroids (1 g hydrocortisone i.v.) and antibiotics should be given if the respiratory system has been soiled. Emergency tracheostomy is only rarely required in cases of crushed larynx or massive posterior pharyngeal bleeding; an endotracheal tube can usually be passed. The care of the airway cannot be over-emphasized; too often apparently moribund patients with dilated pupils are seen to improve dramatically with this simple manoeuvre.

Bleeding and shock

Brain injury does not cause oligaemic shock. If shock is present other sources must be found. Scalp haemorrhage has usually stopped by the time of hospital admission, but sufficient blood may have been lost to cause shock, especially in the elderly. Fractures of major long bones may be associated with shock and may cause reflex lowering of the blood pressure, and it is common experience to find an improvement in the condition with correct splintage. Bleeding into the body cavities is always a diagnostic problem, a potent cause of shock and rarely obvious in the unconscious patient. Replacement of circulating volume is of paramount importance (see pp. 25, 34), for oligaemic shock, when severe, will cause coma due to insufficient blood supply to the brain. Throughout the period of resuscitation it is important to have repeated (every 5 min at least) observations of blood pressure and pulse.

A low blood pressure is sometimes present without loss of blood. A neck fracture with cord compression and interruption of sympathetic fibres carrying vasomotor tone may cause pooling of blood in dependent parts of the body. Controlling continuing haemorrhage from the scalp may be accomplished by local pressure held for 5 min by the clock. A spurting artery, if visible, may be caught in a sterile haemostat.

Examination of head

A systematic examination of the external surface of the head may reveal lacerations and haematoma of the scalp. Haematomas are circular or oval and have an elevated edge, with a fluctuant centre. This must not be confused with a depressed fracture. A soft swelling in the temporal region should alert the clinician to the possibility of a temporal fracture and extradural haematoma.

Subconjunctival haemorrhages extending back behind the eye suggest an anterior fossa fracture. Two black eyes may indicate anterior fossa fractures. Continued bleeding or loss of cerebrospinal fluid from the nose or external auditory meatus represents fracture of the base. Skin discoloration behind the ear, which may or may not be obvious at an early stage, is a sign of a fractured temporal bone. Undisplaced fractures of the mandible or cervical spine are not uncommon but are frequently overlooked. Zygomatic and malar fractures will be overlooked unless the orbital rims and mandibular movements are tested. Failure to recognize and treat them early may result later in diplopia and facial asymmetry. Apart from a gross, compound depressed fracture, diagnosis should only be made by radiography. Palpation may damage more underlying brain and start bleeding from cortical vessels. No wound should be blindly probed with a haemostat.

Neurological examination

The nuances of good neurological examination are lost in the presence of unconsciousness. Examination consists of observing spontaneous movements and movements elicited by painful stimuli, and also tendon reflexes and size and reaction of the pupils to light. Respiratory rate, rhythm, pulse rate and blood pressure are also vital pieces of information.

From the start it is important to determine whether or not the patient is conscious, and if the level of consciousness is altering. There are many words used like stupor or semicoma, and while these may convey an exact description of the patient's state to one group, they may not mean the same to others, particularly if the patient is transferred to another unit. It is much better to describe in words the patients mental state and response to various stimuli. Is he alert, fully orientated in place and time? Does he respond briskly and accurately to questions? Will he only swear or use monosyllables when painfully stimulated and not respond to simple commands? Or will the patient not respond in any way to pain? While it may be time-consuming to document all of this, it is more helpful to others involved in the patient's care and, in addition, it reminds the examiner to evaluate specifically the level of consciousness. Of course, it is important that the clinician be aware of the spectrum of conscious level and the vegetative changes associated with changes. Drowsiness is the earliest change from full consciousness, the patient loses interest in questions and yawns frequently, yet with some stimulation, for instance a pin prick, will waken up and give full and accurate responses. This state then merges into confusion, with disorientation for place and time, and then as unconsciousness deepens it becomes more difficult to rouse the patient to say anything.

Many patients with head injuries display cerebral irritation, in which they are restless, attempt to get off the examination trolley, shouting, swearing and even attacking bystanders; and yet a few minutes later they may be quite docile, cooperative and lie quietly. Children often vomit in this state, so beware of airway problems; they may have an epileptic convulsion and again there must be effective airway care and also an awareness that the resulting unconsciousness may be post-ictal rather than a sign of a developing intracranial haematoma.

When in coma the patient responds now only to painful stimuli with appropriate movements in the first instance. As coma deepens there is no response even to the most severe pain. In coma, vegetative signs of the brain damage are also apparent, there may be changes in respiratory rate and rhythm, a tachypnoea, rather than hyperventilation *per se* is common in head trauma, and this gives way to irregular gasping breathing, Cheyne–Stokes or phasic respiration, and, finally, periods of apnoea. It must be emphasized here that careful monitoring or observation of the respiratory pattern will display changes which may precede any gross alterations in conscious level or neurological deficit. The clinician should ask himself 'What is the respiratory pattern, rate and rhythm and has it altered during the period of observation?' The blood pressure may be raised and pulse slow and, with deterioration, further slowing of the pulse with rising blood pressure. The pupils may become more sluggish in their response to light and finally become fixed and dilated; at this stage the blood pressure may suddenly fall and the pulse accelerate. These are terminal changes.

There are motor changes as the level of unconsciousness deepens. Initially the patient will display numerous spontaneous purposeful movements, scratching his face, covering himself with blankets, etc. but with deterioration these movements disappear and may only be provoked by painful stimuli. Later still, the response to pain may cease to be purposeful and becomes extensor and finally there is no response to pain. Focal neurological signs may be produced by the injury. Basal skull fractures may often injure one or more cranial nerves: I, II, III, IV, VI and VII are especially vulnerable. Damage to the motor cortex will produce a contralateral weakness (hemiparesis) with loss of tone, usually most pronounced in the face and arm. The eyes in the early stages may be conjugately deviated towards the side of the lesion. Midbrain and brainstem damage will also produce a hemiparesis or hemiplegia; often the leg is involved and tone is usually increased. It is important to document carefully all neurological findings for any neurological deterioration must raise the possibility of an intracranial haematoma. Some patients may seem to be worse than they actually are; no movements in a limb or one side of the body may be due to a fractured long bone, or extensive bruises. An unresponsive pupil may be due to direct damage to the eye or optical nerve. The patient may not speak, not because he is unconscious but due to facial injury, damage to lower cranial nerves or the cortical motor area.

Ingestion of drugs or alcohol will make the assessment of conscious level very difficult, and it is important to ask oneself repeatedly 'Would I expect this degree of unconsciousness, etc. or neurological signs from an injury of this severity?' Unless all the signs and symptoms match, the clinician should determine if there is any chance of ingestion of tablets or drinks, etc. This clinical problem is particularly common in children. Pre-existing disease is another problem, and diabetic coma, cerebrovascular accidents and myocardial infarctions are infrequent causes of head injuries.

Management in the first few hours

At this stage, the patient's circulatory responses should have stabilized due to resuscitation and adequate airway, and the extent of his injuries will be assessed. Investigations can now be undertaken and decisions made as to the priority in treatment of the various injuries. The general care of the unconscious patient is still the most important aspect regardless of his injuries. The steps to be taken during this period are given below.

Maintenance of airway

In the uncomplicated injury this is accomplished by turning the patient into the three-quarter prone position. The patient is turned on to the other side at least every 2 h as shown in Figure 16.2. An oropharyngeal airway should also be used so long as the patient tolerates it. If an endotracheal tube was inserted during resuscitation and the patient tolerates it, the tube should be kept in place. The inflated cuff should be released 5 min in every hour for as long as the tube is *in situ*. The same applies to cuffed tracheostomy tubes.

If there is a chest injury or extensive pulmonary soiling then this patient requires controlled ventilation. Some of the indications for controlled ventilation in head injury management are given in Table 16.2.

Table 16.2 Indications for controlled ventilation in head injury management

Missile injuries
Associated chest trauma
Respiratory and pulmonary pathology, e.g. aspiration; fat
 embolism
Generalized brain swelling
Status epilepticus
Acute reduction in intracranial pressure
For CT scanning in unconcious patient
For all surgery

Catheter

During the first few hours it is usually wise to insert an indwelling Silastic catheter into the bladder. A fluid balance chart is started and a rough estimation of renal function can be made by noting the volume of urine produced hourly.

Restlessness

Restlessness is managed by padding the sides of the bed and by covering the hands with a soft bandage in

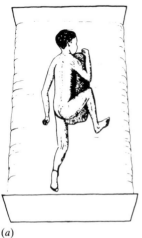 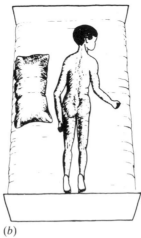 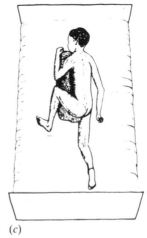

(a)   (b)   (c)

Figure 16.2 The three-quarter prone positon (a) The right arm and leg are supported by a large pillow or pillows. The head automatically assumes the three-quarter position. (b) To turn the patient, pull out the pillow. This allows the body to fall completely prone. (c) Next turn the head to the left side, raise the left arm and leg upon the pillow, and the head will again assume the three-quarter position. One person can turn a heavy patient in this manner without help

a manner to prevent the patient grasping his catheter, intravenous lines, etc. No sedative drugs should be used.

Medication

Antibiotics

Patients with basal skull fractures and cerebrospinal fluid leaks should have a broad-spectrum antibiotic (ampicillin, 500 mg, 6-hourly). Any suspicion of aspiration pneumonitis should be vigorously treated with pulmonary lavage and ampicillin, 500 mg i.v. 6-hourly or a cephalosporin 750 mg i.v.

Anticonvulsants

Status epilepticus is best managed by controlled ventilation. Prophylactic anticonvulsants are not so popular now, except in patients with a high probability of fits, e.g. extensive compound injuries. Phenytoin, 100 mg orally or i.v., will provide adequate blood levels in 48 h; immediate control is by 1 g i.v. administered slowly, with ECG monitoring.

Hyperpyrexia

This is often seen in children and in those with extensive brainstem injuries. The body temperature can be controlled by using a cooling mattress.

Serial neurological examination

The frequency depends on the skill of the doctors and nurses present. Full observations must be documented at least every 15 min. The attending nurse should call the house-doctor if:

1. The degree of restlessness changes.
2. The level of consciousness deepens.
3. The respiratory rate or rhythm alters.
4. The pulse rate either quickens or slows.
5. The blood pressure changes.
6. Pupillary size and response to light alters.

7. The temperature exceeds 39°C.
8. A convulsion occurs.

Subtle changes can be demonstrated graphically using the Glasgow Coma Chart (see Table 16.1).

Radiographs

It must be emphasized that all radiology and computerized tomography (CT) should be considered only when the basic care of the patient has been completed. All unconscious patients should have radiographs of the skull; well-penetrated true lateral and true anteroposterior views will demonstrate most fractures. A complete cervical spine radiograph *must* be obtained to identify any cervical fracture and a chest radiograph is desirable on all unconscious patients.

CT scans

The availability of CT has revolutionized the diagnosis of intracranial pathology, and if the system is available, it allows the clinician at an early stage to identify an intracranial mass with precision and allows exact surgery to be performed when required (Figure 16.3). By the same token, the absence of any intracranial clot will allow the clinician to proceed with controlled ventilation, if it is indicated, with some confidence. Like all investigations, unless it is performed correctly and interpreted by experts, the results may be dangerous. Also, there may be a risk to the patient in that he is required to lie still during the procedure, and the temptation to give sedation to obtain perfect pictures may result in cerebral anoxia. The restless patient may require an anaesthetic for the investigation and thus it should not be requested before careful assessment of the patient. Some indications for CT in the first few hours following head injury are given in Table 16.3.

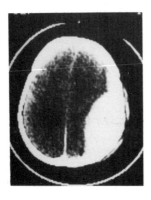 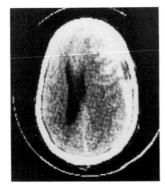

Figure 16.3 CT scans will demonstrate accurately intracranial pathology: (*a*) the biconcave shape of an extradural haematoma; (*b*) an acute subdural haematoma with underlying brain contusion

Table 16.3 Indications for CT scan in head injuries

History and/or physical signs of injury to the head together with one or more of the following:

1. Sustained reduction in Glasgow coma score (<6) after resuscitation. (Mistakes are made when a reduced level of consciousness is entirely attributed to alcoholic intoxication)
2. Focal or lateralizing neurological deficits
3. Deteriorating level of consciousness
4. Post-traumatic epilepsy
5. Depressed skull fracture
6. Penetrating wounds – bullets, sharp objects, etc.
7. Persisting cerebrospinal fluid leak
8. Local scanning of facial bone and orbit fractures
9. Suspected development of complications, such as chronic subdural haematoma, infection or hydrocephalus
10. When a patient with multiple trauma, including a significant head injury, is to be ventilated for reasons of inadequate gas exchange or to control pain

Blood-gas analysis

This is invaluable in assessing the patient's respiratory state; the tachypnoea usually leads to a low Pco_2 with normal Po_2 levels. High Pco_2 and low Po_2 indicate a respiratory problem which should be treated.

Anaesthetics

Unless there is a real indication for surgery during this period, when the intracranial dynamics are so labile, then operation should be delayed for 24 h. If however, a general anaesthetic is required during this time, this is no task for the inexperienced anaesthetist for anoxia, coughing and laryngeal stridor will all augment the brain damage. Controlled ventilation with moderate hypocapnia ($Paco_2$ 25–30 mmHg), using muscle relaxants (pancuronium bromide, 8 mg i.v.), is the method of choice. It is wise to avoid all volatile anaesthetic gases (halothane) and depend on local (lignocaine) or intravenous agents (phenoperidine, etc.) for anaesthesia.

Management during the first week

If the patient is not conscious within 24 h, he may remain unconscious for several days or even weeks. The main problems are the care of the unconscious patient and management of cerebral swelling. Deterioration from late extradural and from subacute haematoma must be watched for; details of treatment are given in a subsequent paragraph.

Airway

It is difficult to maintain a good airway over a prolonged period; continued nasopharyngeal and oral suction traumatize the oral pharynx with swelling and haemorrhage and thus increase obstruction. Thus, if there are no signs of an early awakening a tracheostomy is advisable. An endotracheal tube should also be replaced by a tracheostomy after 5–7 days. Chest physiotherapy is of the utmost importance in prolonged unconsciousness. Without it mucous plugs will obstruct lobular bronchi, produce atelectasis and infection will supervene.

Blood-gas analysis daily and chest radiographs every 48–72 h are important monitors of pulmonary function.

Position

Throughout the period of unconsciousness it is important to change the patient's position 2-hourly. All pressure areas must be massaged routinely to prevent ulcer formation.

Fluids and feeding

In the first few days care must be taken not to overhydrate the patient. Parenteral feeding should commence early for the injury will promote catabolism. Initially the nasogastric tube is inserted to empty the stomach and prevent aspiration. After 2 or 3 days, motility is normal in the alimentary tract and so it is possible to provide all the fluid and caloric requirements via a nasogastric tube. The large tubes are irritating; therefore when gastric function is restored a narrow gauge tube (Clinifeed) should be used to provide the daily fluid (150 ml) and calorie (2500 cal) requirements.

Many head injuries have acute gastric erosions (stress ulcers) and occasionally may have extensive blood loss from them. To prevent these it is advisable to give all unconscious patients cimetidine, 200 mg, t.d.s. and 400 mg at night. This provides much more effective protection than oral alkalis.

The indications for controlled ventilation to reduce ICP are given in Table 16.2.

Enema

To prevent massive faecal impaction it is well to use olive oil retention enemas.

Treatment of cerebral oedema

Cerebral oedema following trauma occurs for a number of reasons. Firstly, the impact will cause local tissue damage and release of local vasoactive substances; secondly there is almost always an associated hypoxia/ischaemia event which will cause the oedema consequent on altered cerebral metabolism; and thirdly, there is a component of increased vascular permeability secondary to the injury. As well as cerebral oedema, there may be an element of *cerebral swelling*; by this is meant vascular engorgement due to an increase in intracranial blood volume secondary to venous obstruction and lost autoregulation. For the latter, controlled ventilation is indicated in severe cases. For the treatment of cerebral oedema, an intravenous bolus of mannitol 0.5–2 g/kg body weight may reduce intracranial pressure. Steroids have no effect on traumatic cerebral oedema. Hypothermia and massive cerebral decompression operations will not improve the outcome.

Acute intracranial haematoma

With extradural haematomas as many as 25% are not found in the classic temporal position, but may occur subfrontally or in the posterior fossa. In the latter cases the signs may occur much later and a diagnosis made only by CT or, if this is unavailable, angiography. Early removal of the clot will give a good chance of recovery. Acute subdural haematomas are usually associated with extensive brain damage and the prognosis is very poor even if the clot is removed. They may occur on the convexity, subfrontally or subtemporally. Traumatic intracerebral haematomas are also associated with severe brain damage. For all haematomas, evacuation of the clot and occasionally removal of a temporal or frontal lobe will reduce the intracranial volume and hence the pressure. Medical management of the swelling must be instituted as well, but the outlook for all but the acute extradural is poor.

Fat embolism

The second to fourth days are the likely times to see evidence of fat embolism. A high temperature, tachypnoea, restlessness, decreasing oxygen levels and later a macular rash best seen in the axillae are the hallmarks of this complication in a patient with multiple injuries. Symptomatic treatment is the standard therapy.

Serial neurological examination

As the patient's state becomes more stable, observations are needed less often, but if there is any change or deterioration then they must be increased to every 15 min. If the patient's condition cannot be easily explained, for instance a progressive hemiparesis or deterioration in level of consciousness, then angiography should be performed.

Medication

Antibiotics and anticonvulsants are continued as required.

Management during subsequent weeks

Airway problems have now stabilized and if the patient is still unconscious all the treatment, turning and chest physiotherapy must be continued. Nutrition must be carefully maintained and caloric requirements may change quite suddenly, so that a patient who was losing weight in the first few weeks may quite quickly become obese. During this time it is important to provide adequate physiotherapy, especially to paretic limbs; failure to do so will allow contractures to develop which will greatly inhibit future rehabilitation. All fractured bones must be treated as if the patient were fully conscious for the same reasons.

The alert patient who has been previously unconscious

Even a short period of unconsciousness indicates that a significant brain injury was sustained and the possibility of developing an acute extradural or subdural haematoma exists. The patient should have a radiograph of his skull and if there is a fracture line it is essential that he remains in hospital for 24 h and then be reviewed by an experienced clinician. Intracranial haematoma is 100 times more likely in the presence of a skull fracture. Observation consists of determining if the patient is becoming drowsy and must be made at least every 30 min. This means that the patient gets little sleep for 24 h in most instances. The patient who has been unconscious, but now is fully recovered, with no fracture on good quality skull radiographs, may be discharged into the care of informed relatives on the understanding that he comes back if drowsiness or headache increases. Not all patients who deteriorate after this interval of consciousness have a haematoma. Many, as already noted, have a swelling or have a pulped lobe. CT scan or, if unavailable, arteriography, will be required.

The patient who has never been unconscious

The vast majority require simple reassurance. There is no need for radiographs unless there is a scalp laceration and a depressed fracture is suspected. A depressed fracture can be present in an infant (and very rarely in an adult) without a scalp laceration.

The history of the trauma is important. Small sharp objects such as a pencil or nail can penetrate deeply into the skull of a child, especially in the temporal region, leaving a minimal stab in the skin. A penetrating fracture of this type may not always be evident upon radiographs. Patients without fracture are allowed to go home. They are told that a small amount of headache and some lack of energy are not unusual after a mild bump upon the head and that these symptoms may last a few days or a few weeks. If the headache is severe and not relieved by simple analgesics they should return for examination. Patients with unusually severe post-concussion headaches must be suspected of developing signs and symptoms of a *chronic subdural haematoma* at a later date. Most do not and they lose their headache in a few weeks. A few, motivated by factors of industrial compensation and fears of mental function, develop functional headaches. The cause of many post-concussional headaches, dizziness and loss of memory is not understood. Recent work suggests they may be related to changes in cerebral circulation.

The clear indications for immediate admission to hospital are set out in Table 16.4.

Table 16.4 Indications for admission to a general hospital

1. Confusion or any other depression of the level of consciousness at the time of examination
2. Skull fracture
3. Neurological symptoms or signs
4. Difficulty in assessing the patient, e.g. alcohol, epilepsy, or other medical condition
5. Lack of a responsible adult to supervise the patient; other social problems

Note: Brief amnesia after trauma with full recovery is not sufficient indication for admission. Relatives or friends of patients sent home should receive written advice about changes that would require the patient to be returned urgently to hospital

Depressed fractures

The patient with a depressed fracture often has not lost consciousness and the diagnosis is made by radiograph only if the injury is a closed one with intact skin. The decision to operate is best left to a neurosurgeon but, in general terms, if the depression is less than the thickness of the skull bone then it may not need correction. It is important to remember that the closed depressed fracture is uninfected and care should be taken to keep it so. There may be little or no brain damage. The compound depressed fracture by contrast is already infected and the brain has already been damaged. No attempt should be made to remove obvious bone fragments or stop bleeding by blindly inserting haemostats, for both manoeuvres will provoke cortical vessel bleeding and further damage the brain.

A bacteriological swab should be taken of the damaged area and this must be sent for culture and a light gauze dressing applied. Broad-spectrum antibiotics should be given immediately (ampicillin 500 mg or flucloxacillin 500 mg 6-hourly), and then the patient should be transferred to a neurosurgical unit for debridement, dural repair and skin closure. The bacteriological results should quickly follow the patient to ensure that the appropriate antibiotic is being used. Any evidence of bacterial resistance will require a change in the antibiotic. Following injury, oedema will develop around the area of contusion or laceration, and if the injury is in the parietal cortex it may make the neurological deficit worse. Steroids (dexamethasone, 4 mg i.m. 6-hourly) may be effective in this type of focal oedema. If the brain injury is extensive there is a 50% chance of an epileptic fit and so this should be prevented by giving diphenyl-hydantoin 100 mg 8-hourly, following a loading dose of 1 g i.v.

Bullet injuries

Like the previous injury described, the bullet will produce extensive focal brain damage, but because of the high energy imparted by the missile, it literally causes an explosion within tissue. The whole brain is to some extent affected, and is extremely vulnerable to any insult, the slightest cough or struggle will cause bleeding, extrusion of brain and irrevocable rises in ICP. For this reason our experience has shown that the best method of treatment is to anaesthetize any patient who is not fully conscious, pass an endotracheal tube and institute controlled ventilation (see Table 16.2). This is begun in the resuscitation period and continued until after surgery. If the patient is treated in a peripheral hospital, he should be similarly treated and then transferred, still anaesthetized and accompanied by a medical practitioner, to a specialist unit.

Unlike head injuries due to road traffic accidents, many patients with missile injuries require a lot of intravenous fluid, due to bleeding and a central neurogenic type of hypotension. Whatever the cause, the blood pressure must be raised to maintain perfusion. Surgery for such injuries is aimed at haemostasis and removal of all necrotic tissue and bone fragments; the metallic fragments are less important. The dura must be closed with fascial patches if necessary. Good skin cover is also essential. Antibiotics, anticonvulsants and antacids as well as anaesthetic drugs will all be mandatory.

Cerebrospinal fluid leaks

Most cerebrospinal fluid leaks are obvious early after injury and many stop spontaneously within a few days of injury. Some will appear some time after injury, often heralded by a damp patch on the pillow. The most common sites of leak are from the nose (rhinorrhoea) or ear (otorrhoea) and these areas should be specifically examined and note made of the findings. Unclotted blood in the ear or a clear serous discharge from the nose or ear which gives a positive reaction to Dextrostix is good evidence of a leak. A bacteriological culture should be made of the discharge from the orifice in question and then broad-spectrum antibiotics given, ampicillin or flucloxacillin for rhinorrhoea and the addition of chloramphenicol in otorrhoea, due to the high incidence of Gram-negative organisms in the ear.

If there is a displaced maxillary or nasal fracture, the leak may stop following reduction and fixation. For the rest, they should be treated expectantly. The patient should be forbidden to blow his nose and should lie propped up. If, after a few days, the leak persists then neurosurgical advice should be obtained regarding possible surgery to repair the dural tear. Fully conscious patients with no neurological signs must be kept in hospital and observed carefully for signs of meningitis. If, after discharge from hospital, the leak returns, the patient should be re-admitted for consideration of surgical treatment.

Intracranial infections

Following injury the intracranial contents may be infected early, usually by direct spread from a compound wound or later by blood-borne infection to a damaged area or activation of bacteria on a long forgotten bone fragment or piece of shrapnel. Infection causes a meningitis, a cerebritis or a brain abscess.

Meningitis is usually the result of an undetected or untreated cerebrospinal fluid leak affording entrance to nasal or aural pathogenic bacteria. Classically, 2–4 days after injury, the patient's level of consciousness deteriorates, his temperature rises and his neck becomes stiff. The main differential diagnosis is a subarachnoid haemorrhage and to make a diagnosis and obtain cerebrospinal fluid for bacteriological examination a lumbar puncture must be performed. In both conditions the fluid may be xanthochromic but the finding of numerous polymorphonuclear corpuscles and Gram-staining bacteria is diagnostic of meningitis. Rigorous therapy is essential; large doses of intravenous antibiotics (whichever are appropriate) and daily intrathecal doses are used. Particular care must be taken with intrathecal antibiotics; the dose and contraindications must be carefully studied.

Cerebritis is an infection of damaged and necrotic brain following its injury. With adequate debridement this should not be seen nowadays. It is often accompanied by a meningitis. A brain abscess may be very difficult to diagnose because the original head injury may be long since forgotten. It may present weeks or months after the injury with vague ill-defined mental signs. If poorly treated, it still carries a very high mortality and so if there is any suspicion a CT scan and neurosurgical advice are essential.

Technical procedures
Scalp laceration

The hair should be widely shaved (at least 7.5 cm) from the margins of the incision. The adjoining hair should be matted with soap or petroleum jelly so that it will not float loosely into the clean area. Using full aseptic techniques, the wound is loosely packed with gauze and the surrounding area cleansed by gentle washing with soap and water for a period of about 10 min. Using a new set of gloves, gowns and instruments, an ellipse of skin surrounding the wound is anaesthetized by intracutaneous injection of 1% procaine or 1% lignocaine which is injected into the skin and not subcutaneously. An intradermal injection blanches the skin, whereas a subcutaneous injection merely elevates it. The patient need feel only one pinprick during this process. Each subsequent needle puncture is made into the periphery of the blanched analgesic area and the fluid spreads from that point into the adjoining skin without pain. The wound is draped with self-adhesive plastic or with skin towels sewn into the anaesthetized margins. The operator dons new sterile gloves and gown (Figure 16.4). The

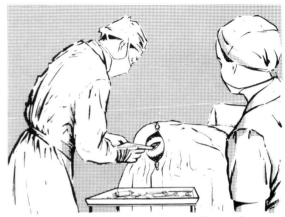

Figure 16.4 Exploration of a head wound. The area is isolated with sterile towels. Surgeon and instrument nurse masked and wearing sterile gloves

wound is now painless and is cleansed by sterile saline and sponge. Devitalized tags of skin are trimmed away (Figure 16.5). If the wound is more than 12 h old or if it is grossly contaminated with dirt that cannot be washed away, then the skin edges should be excised. This will start fresh bleeding for the control of which artery forceps on the galea or cautery to the bleeding points is required. Underlying periosteum should not be disturbed unless there is some ingrained dirt. If periosteum is removed, bleeding from the bone is best stopped by packing and waiting for at least 5 min. If it still persists, bone wax and cautery may be used, but neither of these is desirable. One remains as a foreign body, the other produces necrotic tissue in a potentially infected wound. Underlying temporal muscle may have to be trimmed of devitalized fragments. Penetrating injuries should be traced through the muscle to the bone. Scalp injuries are

usually closed in one row of inverted mattress sutures so that no foreign body will be left in a potentially infected wound. Haemorrhage from the scalp is sometimes better controlled by a stitch which grips the galea (Figure 16.6). A braided nylon is most useful. If the wound is extensive, vacuum drainage may be used but ordinarily this is not necessary; corrugated drains are not used on the head. Haemostasis must be adequate. Patients with severe contusion of underlying muscle or with neglected wounds involving muscle should have a tetanus booster if previously inoculated (p. 52). If some skin is missing, the wound cannot be closed easily. It is possible to approximate the edges by various plastic procedures, but it should be remembered that the scalp is extremely vascular and it is better for the inexperienced operator to pack the wound and await expert help rather than get involved in extensive vascular mobilization of skin.

Subcutaneous haematomas

If soft, fluctuant and painful their contents may be aspirated but usually it is best to leave them alone.

Compound depressed fractures

The primary care of such an injury has been outlined (pp. 211); it has been stressed that removal of bone fragments or unskilled elevation may further damage the brain and cause profuse haemorrhage. Ideally, then, the procedure is best left to a neurosurgeon, but it is recognized that there will be situations in some areas where this is a counsel of perfection. In such a case the medical practitioner should consult an operative neurosurgical textbook.

Emergency burr holes

Occasionally a situation arises where a patient suddenly deteriorates and the signs suggest an

Figure 16.5 A method of excising a wound of the scalp

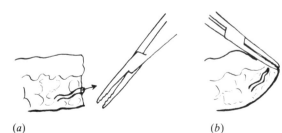 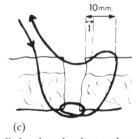

(a)   *(b)*   *(c)*

Figure 16.6 Control of scalp haemorrhage. (*a*) The haemostat is applied to the galea deep to the spurting artery. (*b*) It is then turned back over the skin. The artery is compressed between the haemostat and the galea. (*c*) Single-layer closure with tight galea approximation. The needle follows the direction of the arrow. This is particularly useful if scalp haemorrhage persists. Otherwise a simple mattress stitch is sufficient

intracranial haematoma. The most important thera-peutic manoeuvres are to intubate, paralyse and ventilate the patient, administer mannitol intra-venously and obtain a CT scan and neurological help. The occurrence of a pure extradural haema-toma is very rare; more commonly the deterioration is due to an acute subdural, a 'burst' lobe or a combined extradural and subdural haematoma. For these a burr hole is useless and time organizing this procedure in unfamiliar surroundings by untrained surgeons will cause more damage than the transfer to neurosurgery for a craniotomy. Very occasional-ly, if there is a classic extradural haematoma or if specialist help is unobtainable, then the procedure described below might be life-saving.

If an extradural haematoma is suspected, a straight 10 cm incision is made, 2.5 cm in front of the external auditory meatus, extending down to the zygoma. Skin bleeding is controlled by artery forceps on the galea. The muscle is incised in the line and skin and muscle separated by a mastoid retractor. The temporal bone is penetrated by a perforator and then by a burr. The end-point of penetration of each of these instruments is deter-mined by a tactile feeling of increased resistance which is learned by experience. The inexperienced should remember that these instruments may plunge excessively and should concentrate upon the rota-tory rather than the perforating aspect of the instrument. Further bone is removed by a rongeur and the clot removed by suction. The bleeding point should be located and controlled by cautery or clip, or wax if from bone. If the bleeding cannot be located or controlled, the wound may be packed lightly until competent help arrives. If very little or no clot is found temporally then the other sites of

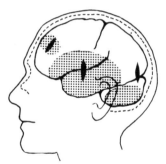

Figure 16.7 Sites of predilection of extradural haemorrhage

extradural haemorrhage must be explored (Figure 16.7). If a temporal burr hole is made and there is no extradural clot but the dura is tense and bluish, a subdural and/or cerebral contusion is likely. To evacuate a subdural haematoma other burr holes will be required in the parietal area 3.5 cm from the midline and, if possible, the clot removed. The subacute subdural will usually be solid and so in a desperate situation a wide craniectomy will be needed to evacuate the clot. The dura is incised in a cruciate fashion. Beware of the sagittal sinus and bridging veins during this procedure.

With a chronic subdural haematoma, the clot is liquefied and all that will be required for decom-pression is a parietal burr hole and gentle suction to remove the liquid.

For all subdural clots it is important to make bilateral burr holes as there is a very high incidence of haematoma on both sides.

17

Management of cardiothoracic cases

G. H. Smith

In the early days of thoracic surgery, operations were mainly concerned with diseases of the lungs. Later, cardiac and oesophageal disease began to involve surgeons and there are now two broad areas of interest in the specialty. Pulmonary and oesophageal surgeons share with the cardiac surgeons a common interest, however, since both disease and surgery of any intrathoracic organ have effects on all other organs in the chest. Also, the whole body is affected by chest disease and surgery, thus adding to the complexity of the clinical problems.

The role of the house surgeon on a cardiothoracic unit is, therefore, the management of the whole individual whilst giving special attention to the specific disease involved. Modern cardiothoracic surgery is supported by a large number of individuals in different medical specialties, by highly skilled nursing staff and by specialized paramedical and technical staff. To manage his patients successfully, the house surgeon will need to communicate well with all these groups and help to coordinate their efforts.

Informed consent

Very few chest operations are minor and nearly all are potentially lethal. Sometimes the patient may feel virtually normal and yet will accept surgery on trust. That trust has to be bought by constant and frank discussions with the patient and his or her family. The risks and benefits of surgery have to be carefully and fully described. This process cannot be hurried and must be completed before the patient makes the decision whether an operation should be performed or not. Often, this consultation may distress the patient and his or her family because no evasions can be allowed to insulate them from the full truth. A careful and sympathetic manner usually

helps, but often the facts are difficult to bear. Afterwards, however, the confidence of the patient in his doctors increases and should the surgery lead to death or disability, then no acrimony follows. Time spent with the patient before operation usually leads to a saving of time and distress later. Obviously, by his constant presence in the hospital, the house surgeon is the key figure in this matter.

History-taking

Nearly all patients are referred after seeing several doctors and by the time of referral are practised historians. The temptation to rely on previous histories should be resisted and whilst a final history is taken, particular attention must be made to the drugs taken by the patient and to his smoking habits.

Nearly all cardiac drugs and anticoagulants are highly effective and, therefore, dangerous. For each drug there will be a firm hospital policy on whether it should be stopped before operation and if so when. Certain drugs such as beta-blockers and diuretics may have to be continued up to the moment of anaesthesia.

Many surgeons will not willingly operate on the patient who is still smoking regularly at the time of admission to hospital. Not only is cigarette smoking a major cause of cardiothoracic disease, but it also adversely affects the postoperative condition. A period of several weeks without cigarettes is beneficial.

Examination

Cardiothoracic disease frequently affects the nutrition of the patient and during clinical examination both under- and overnutrition and the state of hydration of the patient should be noted. There are no esoteric tricks in the examination, however, which uses the conventional clinical techniques. Sepsis of the skin should be sought for. A full examination of the central nervous system is important so that a baseline of normality can be determined.

Investigation of patients for cardiothoracic surgery

During their illnesses, patients with cardiothoracic disease will have seen many doctors and have had many investigations performed. An important duty of the house surgeon is to impose some order on this chaos and to select the investigations which are germane to individual patients. Experience and knowledge are valuable in this process, but the following investigations are important and need to be summarized in a readily accessible form.

For *all* cases having cardiothoracic surgery:

1. Full blood count and haemoglobin level.
2. Blood group.
3. Full blood chemistry, including screening tests of liver and kidney function.
4. Chest radiograph (both postero-anterior and lateral).
5. Electrocardiogram.
6. Bacteriological examination of the sputum.
7. Routine analysis of the urine.

For those patients having *lung* or *oesophageal* surgery:

1. Contrast radiographic studies (e.g. barium swallow or bronchogram).

2. Endoscopy (bronchoscopy, oesophagoscopy, mediastinoscopy or pleuroscopy).
3. Tissue diagnosis based on histological report.
4. Sputum cytology.
5. Respiratory function tests. (These may be of a greater or lesser degree of complexity. Few tests, however, surpass the ability of the patient to walk quickly over a moderate distance accompanied by a fit young doctor.)
6. In some hospitals further tests may be available, such as radioactive scans of lung, brain or bone, CT scans or magnetic resonance imaging.

For those patients having cardiac surgery:

1. Clotting studies.
2. Cardiac catheterization and cardio-angiography.
3. Echocardiography.
4. In some hospitals only, radioactive scanning investigations, e.g. thallium or technetium.
5. The patient's height and weight to allow calculation of surface area. This will give an indication of the ideal cardiac output for that patient and will determine the dosages of certain drugs.

All patients having a surgical operation are anxious beforehand. This anxiety may be blunted by the premedication given by the anaesthetist. However, in patients undergoing cardiothoracic surgery, such anxiety and sympathetic over-activity can be damaging and most units try to abolish these by heavy sedation the night before an operation, in advance of the premedication.

Many patients will not tolerate being taken to the operating theatre lying completely flat. The house surgeon on the ward has to state specifically which patients must be taken to theatre in a sitting position.

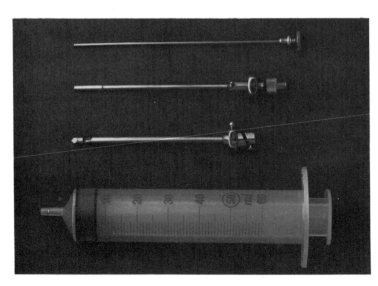

Figure 17.1 The Abrams needle – used for pleural aspiration and biopsy

Chest aspiration

Fluid collections in the pleural cavity are always abnormal. The clinical detection of such collections is only possible when at least 250–300 ml of fluid are present. A chest radiograph is much more sensitive and will show collections of over 50 ml in volume.

Chest aspiration is a diagnostic and a therapeutic procedure. Examination of the fluid will show whether it is an exudate or a transudate. Cytological examination may show abnormal or malignant cells and bacteriological tests will detect any organisms.

The diagnostic efficiency of chest aspiration can be increased by taking a pleural biopsy at the same time. Aspiration should, therefore, be performed using a large bore needle which has the capacity to take a bite of parietal pleura (Figure 17.1).

As a therapeutic procedure, chest aspiration has a limited value. Fluid can be removed easily only if it is of fairly low viscosity. Reaccumulation or an increase in viscosity are best treated by intercostal tube drainage (see below).

The prudent house surgeon performs chest aspiration with a chest radiograph taken both before and *afterwards*.

Technique

1. Location. The majority of chest aspirations are performed in the *triangle of safety*. As Figure

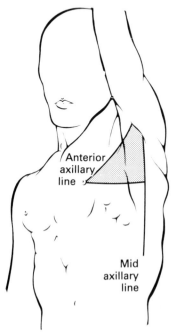

Figure 17.2 Diagram showing the triangle of safety used during insertion of chest drains and chest aspiration

17.2 shows, this is a triangle situated in the anterior half of the axilla above the level of the fifth intercostal space. The boundaries of the triangle are: (a) anteriorly: the anterior axillary line; (b) posteriorly: the mid-axillary line; (c) inferiorly: a horizontal line drawn posteriorly from the level of the nipple in a man or fourth interspace in a woman.

Certain localized and loculated effusions may need different sites of aspiration, but preliminary radiographs with markers to show the exact location are then necessary.

The triangle of safety contains no important or dangerous structures in the chest wall. Furthermore, the chances of inadvertently perforating the diaphragm, even if it is raised, are very low indeed.

2. Position of the patient. The most comfortable position is for the patient to be in bed. A bed table with a pillow on it allows him to lean forward with his arms across the table and his head resting on the pillow looking away from the operator (Figure 17.3).

3. Local anaesthetic should be infiltrated after cleansing of the skin and before the operator 'scrubs up'. About 15–20 ml of 1% lignocaine are injected down to and including the parietal pleura. Ideally, the track should pass just above a rib, thus avoiding the intercostal neurovascular bundle. This injection takes at least 3 min to work: the impatient surgeon should, therefore, spend this time scrubbing his hands and putting on sterile gloves.

4. The procedure is now conducted by an aseptic technique. The aspiration apparatus is connected. An Abrams biopsy needle is attached to a disposable three-way tap and a 60 ml disposable syringe (Figure 17.4). A sterile tube leads off the side arm of the three-way tap.

5. The skin is cleaned with a suitable chemical (0.5% chlorhexidine in spirit) and surrounded by sterile towels.

6. The needle is passed into the pleural cavity by a combination of pressure and a twisting motion (Figure 17.5). In male adults, a small incision in the skin will make passage through this tissue easier. The inexperienced operator rightly worries about the needle suddenly penetrating too deeply. This danger can be avoided by attaching artery forceps to the needle about 5 cm from its tip, thus limiting penetration to that distance. As the needle passes through the parietal pleura, a distinct lessening of resistance can be felt.

7. By aspiration on the syringe, fluid is withdrawn.

8. The three-way tap is turned and the fluid forced out of the syringe's side arm into a suitable sterile container (Figure 17.6).

9. This sequence is repeated until all fluid has been

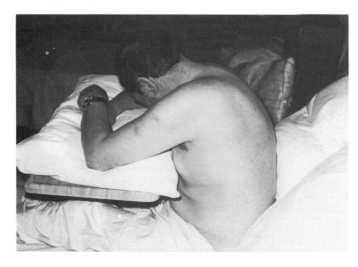

Figure 17.3 The ideal position of the patient during chest aspiration or insertion of a chest drain

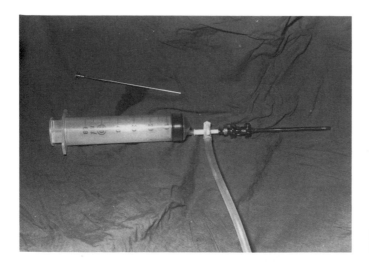

Figure 17.4 The Abrams needle, three-way tap and aspirating syringe

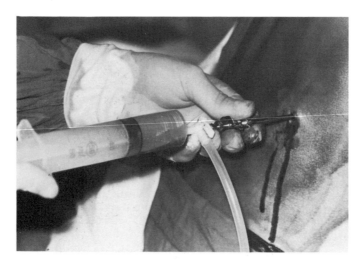

Figure 17.5 Aspirating needle entering the chest wall

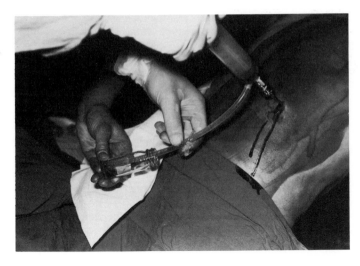

Figure 17.6 Aspiration in progress

aspirated. At this point, the patient may feel some discomfort as the visceral pleura on the expanding lung comes into contact with the sensitive parietal pleura.

10. Before the needle is withdrawn the side channel on it is brought to the level of the parietal pleura and the cutting edge closed. The needle is then totally taken out and pressure applied to the puncture wound. Meanwhile, the small fragment of parietal pleura is placed in preservative and sent to the laboratory, along with the pleural fluid.

11. A further chest radiograph is then taken to rule out a pneumothorax and to show how much fluid remains.

Chest drainage

The pleural cavity is normally a potential space only since the parietal and visceral pleura are in contact throughout the whole of their area. Accumulations of fluid (Figure 17.7) or air (Figure 17.8) create a real space, compressing the underlying lung at first and later, because of positive pressure, causing a shift of the mediastinum away from the affected side. This, in turn, causes compression of the opposite lung. Depending on the size of the abnormal collection and the speed with which it gathers, varying degrees of disturbance of the function of the lungs occur, leading to hypoxia and cardiac depression in the most severe cases.

The causes of fluid or air accumulation are dealt with fully in standard texts and will not be reproduced here. Instead, the principles and practice of the treatment will be described in an attempt to relate the issue of chest drainage to simple physical principles.

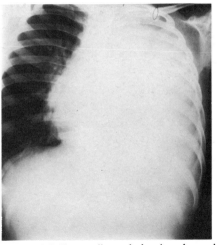

Figure 17.7 Chest radiograph showing a large pleural effusion

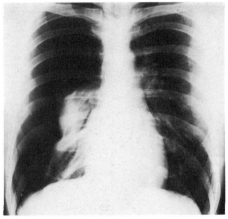

Figure 17.8 Chest radiograph showing a pneumothorax

The aim of chest drainage is to remove the abnormal pleural collection as completely as possible in order to allow apposition of the visceral and parietal pleura. This, in turn, leads to normal expansion of the underlying lung and return of the mediastinum to its normal position, thus permitting normal lung function.

The clinical diagnosis of abnormal collections in the pleural cavity is very difficult and sometimes misleading.

Except in cases of very severe chest injury where the patient may be only seconds away from dying (see later), chest radiographs, both postero-anterior and lateral, are essential before the final diagnosis is made and treatment begun. The practice of separate inspiratory and expiratory films in an attempt to increase the reliability of diagnosing pneumothorax has been largely abandoned by thoracic surgeons.

Chest radiographs will always show some deviation of the mediastinum to the opposite side and

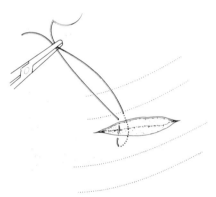

Figure 17.9 Diagram of the incision made in the chest wall for insertion of a chest drain

will, therefore, by themselves not be able to distinguish the patient with a 'tension' pneumothorax, hydrothorax or haemothorax. Tension is a clinical term and is applied when the patient is distressed and showing signs of respiratory or circulatory embarrassment. Clearly, the size and speed of accumulation necessary to produce this clinical picture will vary from patient to patient. However, the diagnosis of tension implies the need for very early action to relieve the abnormal pressure.

Technique of inserting a chest drain

1. Preliminary erect anteroposterior and lateral chest radiographs are obtained.
2. The patient is positioned as described in the section on chest aspiration and local anaesthetic infiltrated down to the parietal pleura. At the same time the diagnosis is usually confirmed by aspirating on the same syringe after the needle is pushed into the pleural cavity. The site of infiltration and insertion is in the triangle of safety previously described. Thoracic surgeons deplore the use of the second interspace anteriorly, mainly because they are frequently asked to deal with complications arising from its use. The anterior site is deeply situated over the bulk of the pectoralis major muscle. It leaves a scar just above the breast in a woman. Occasionally, this site may lie over an abnormally lateral internal mammary artery which can lead to a severe haemorrhage if lacerated. In contrast, the lateral chest wall above the nipple is very safe and there is no risk of perforating the diaphragm, the liver or the spleen.

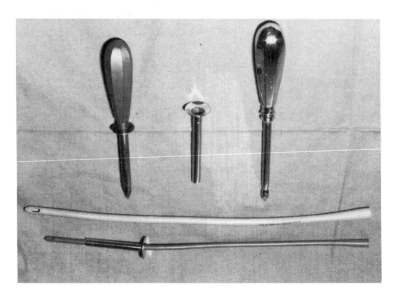

Figure 17.10 Trocars and catheters for chest drainage

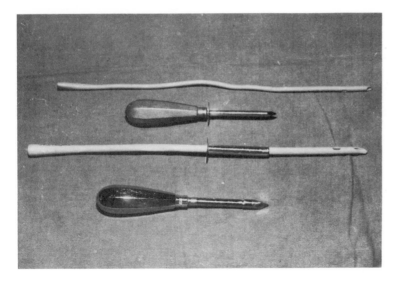

Figure 17.11 Chest drain being passed through the cannula

3. The operator now washes and puts on sterile gown and gloves. The infiltrated areas are cleaned and draped. Using a scalpel, an incision about 3 cm long is made in the line of the skin crease and deepened to subcutaneous fat (Figure 17.9). Using a thick, non-absorbable suture (e.g. No. 2 nylon) on a cutting needle, a vertical mattress suture is placed about half of the way along the incision. This is left long and will eventually be tied when the drain is removed.

4. Using the trocar and cannula shown in Figure 17.10, a track is formed down to the parietal pleura and through this into the abnormal collection of air or fluid. The trocar is withdrawn and an appropriate-sized plastic or rubber tube passed through the cannula into the pleural cavity (Figure 17.11). Holding the drain securely, the cannula is pulled out of the chest wall and over the drain. The drain is then clamped by a pair of large artery forceps.

5. A further thick suture is then placed through the larger portion of the incision and tied around the chest drain so as to hold it in position (Figure 17.12).

6. The chest drain is then attached to an underwater seal and unclamped.

7. A further chest radiograph is then performed to assess the position of the drain and to confirm that no damage has been done.

A common query is 'What is the best size of chest drain?' Since the major hazard of this procedure lies in the introduction of a sharp pointed instrument through the intercostal space and not in the size of the drain, the answer is obviously as large a tube as will pass comfortably through the intercostal space. To undergo the hazards of the procedure and have an inadequately small drain inserted is illogical.

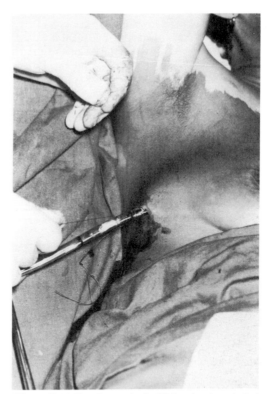

Figure 17.12 Showing method of fixing the chest drain in position

Dangers

There is always some hazard in passing the trocar and cannula through the chest wall even when all the precautions outlined above are followed. The unknown factor is the presence of pleural adhesions which may cause the lung to be adherent to the chest wall in the site chosen for insertion of the drain. If there is any doubt about this, the trocar and cannula should not be used. Instead, more local anaesthetic is used and the track for the tube formed by blunt dissection with the gloved finger and large artery forceps. In this way, the precise location of the pleural cavity may be found and adhesions located. Many units now use this as the method of choice.

Recently, a commercially available system has been available which consists of a metallic trocar within a plastic chest drain. The insertion of this device is just as dangerous as using a trocar and cannula separately and all the precautions above should be observed.

Removal

Chest drains are removed when they have achieved their objective and ceased to function. In the case of fluid, apart from pus, this is when the fluid both clinically and radiologically has disappeared and there is not more than 20–30 ml per day discharge.

In those patients with pus in the pleural cavity (empyema thoracis), abrupt removal of the drain will lead to a poorly drained track which will then become another abscess. In these cases, the tube is removed gradually when repeated sinograms show that there is no cavity remaining at the end of the tube.

The removal of chest drains in patients with pneumothorax leads to much confusion of thought and deed. Such confusion may be avoided if the following points are agreed:

1. Apposition of the two layers of the pleura is essential. Whilst this apposition may be insecure at first, within a few days it will be made permanent by fibrosis between the two layers. In the meantime all air accumulation must be vigorously removed by suction.
2. Only when air leaks stop spontaneously and trial clamping of the tube causes no recurrence of pneumothorax on chest radiograph after 8 or 24 h should the tube be removed abruptly.
3. If air leaks persist and for some reason the patient does not have surgery to stop them, the tube may be removed slowly (as in empyema) when pleural fusion has occurred.

To clamp the drainage tube in order to stop an air leak is as illogical as plugging the rectum to stop diarrhoea. All air leaks will eventually cease if the lung can be kept in a fully expanded state. However, this may take up to 6 weeks and most thoracic surgeons will advise thoracotomy to stop such leaks at source before that time. However, the principle is clear – expand the lung and keep it there until pleural fusion occurs either spontaneously or by surgical intervention.

Chest drainage bottles

The lungs contain elastic tissue and unless the pressure within the pleural cavity is below that of the atmosphere they will contract to an airless state. Chest drainage tubes, therefore, cannot be left open to the air and must be attached to a device which will allow fluid or air to escape from the pleural cavity and yet prevent the entry of air in a reverse direction.

There are two methods of achieving this.

Underwater seal (Figure 17.13)

The chest drain is connected to a tube passing below a column of water. The bottle containing this water is sealed at its top and apart from the tube passing under the water has a much shorter tube passing through the cork seal. This lies well above the level

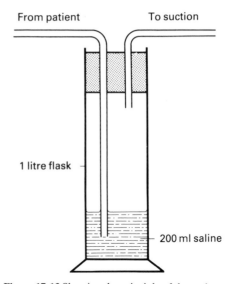

Figure 17.13 Showing the principle of the underwater seal

of fluid. This arrangement permits air and fluid to leave the chest and yet prevents air returning in the opposite direction. The natural tendency of the lung to collapse is balanced by the hydrostatic pressure of the column of fluid in the longer tube.

Flutter valves

These are commercially available in some countries and although expensive do permit the patient to be mobile. The one-way system is created by a soft, plastic diaphragm within the device which permits air to escape from the chest and yet maintains full expansion of the lung. They are used for pneumothorax only.

Problems of chest drainage

Suction

Drainage of air or fluid from the pleural cavity is clearly made easier by the application of suction to the shorter tube of the drainage bottle. Some surgeons believe that all chest drains are best attached to suction. Usually −25 mmHg pressure is applied for air leaks and −5 mmHg for fluid leaks. Other surgeons believe that suction is painful and actually prolongs drainage. First principles, however, mean that the primary objective must be to re-expand the lung and clearly this is best achieved by suction. In the experience of many, pain is not a problem after the first few minutes of full re-expansion.

Failure of the lung to re-expand fully

This problem is rarely due to blockage of the drainage tube and re-positioning of the tubes is usually ineffective. The most common causes are:

1. Bronchial blockage leading to collapse. The blockage is usually due to sputum. Less commonly an underlying bronchial neoplasm is found and, sometimes, a foreign body, especially in children. Bronchoscopy will provide the diagnosis and usually the treatment.
2. The presence of a fibrinous 'peel' over the lung. A 'peel' usually develops in patients with empyema and is due to delay in drainage. Surgical removal is necessary.

Removal of the chest tube

Again, radiographs before and immediately after removal are necessary. Removal is a four-handed procedure. Whilst one operator cuts the retaining suture and removes the drain, the second operator ties the first stitch which has been left untied during insertion. A soft dressing is applied afterwards. Most patients will need some analgesic for this procedure.

Speed of removal of pleural fluid

The rapid evacuation of a large collection of fluid within the pleural cavity may sometimes cause pulmonary oedema to occur. The causes of this complication are unknown. Large effusions should not be drained abruptly but over several hours, say 4–6 h.

Pulmonary surgery

There are a limited number of surgical procedures which can be carried out on the lungs and most of these involve resection of lung tissue. This may vary from a simple removal of localized disease with a small surrounding area of lung (wedge resection), through removal of a segment and a lobe to the removal of the whole lung. If the disease causing the need for surgery is non-malignant, then a smaller volume of lung is removed than in the radical operations performed for malignant disease. All lung surgery is major and associated with long periods of bed-rest. During recumbency, subcutaneous calcium heparin, 5000 units 8-hourly, begun before operation will help to reduce the incidence of pulmonary embolism.

Inflammatory lung disease

The commonest causes of surgery for inflammatory lung disease are:

1. Acute inflammation, e.g. lung abscess.
2. Chronic inflammation, e.g. bronchiectasis, tuberculosis.

In Great Britain and Western Europe, bronchiectasis is more common than the other causes. In other parts of the world, tuberculosis remains a problem and lung abscesses are often uncontrolled by medical means in communities and individuals where a low level of nutrition and resistance to infection exists.

Lung abscess

In Western Europe, lung abscess occurs very rarely except as a result of bronchial obstruction or in the immunosuppressed patient. In other parts of the world, lung abscess is more common and often due to parasites.

Usually, adequate chemotherapy over a prolonged period will allow resolution of the abscess by limiting its systemic effects and allowing its eventual drainage via the bronchial tree. This process may take several weeks and frequent observation is required. During this time bronchial obstruction must be excluded by bronchoscopy.

Very rarely, however, surgery may be indicated for the abscess. Two reasons make intervention necessary:

1. Overwhelming systemic disturbance uncontrolled by antibiotics. Usually resection of the abscess at thoracotomy is indicated, but only simple tube drainage may be allowed in the very ill patient.
2. Empyema necessitatis. This condition arises when the abscess points and threatens to discharge from the chest wall. Early insertion of a drain will relieve discomfort.

The general medical care of a patient with lung abscess can be extremely demanding and close cooperation with the physicians and bacteriologists is important. In particular, nutrition and fluid balance have to be closely observed (see p. 25).

Bronchiectasis

This disease is the result of a severe parenchymal lung infection in the past. The resulting fibrosis of the lung and bronchi leads to their dilatation. This causes an impairment of the normal resistance to infection and impaired ability to clear infected secretions. Over the years, repeated infections increase the damage and recurrent ill health, pneumonia and haemoptysis cause considerable disability to the patient. Ultimately haemorrhage, respiratory failure or amyloidosis may kill.

Bronchography

The definitive diagnosis is made by bronchography which involves the introduction of a viscid radio-opaque liquid into the bronchial tree, following which radiographs are taken. This liquid causes some chemical irritation of the bronchial tree and often leads to an exacerbation of the symptoms.

Certain precautions should be taken before bronchography to reduce these effects:

1. Iodine sensitivity must be excluded.
2. Physiotherapy (see below) will help to clear the secretions which accumulate before and after the procedure.
3. If possible, the investigation is performed under local anaesthetic so that vigorous coughing is possible immediately.
4. In children, where a general anaesthetic is usually necessary, only one lung should be studied at one time.

The final diagnosis is made using the broncho-gram. Usually this will show localized severe disease in one part of the lung, usually the left lower lobe and lingula (Figure 17.14). However, less severe, but more diffuse disease is usually present else-where. Although the operation will remove the most diseased area, the beneficial effects may well be reduced by the residual disease. The wise doctor will emphasize to each patient before operation that this is the case and that the operation may produce a disappointing result.

Physiotherapy

Before surgery, the lungs must be as 'dry' as possible of bronchial secretions. Physiotherapy including postural drainage and percussion is the most effective way of achieving this and a severely

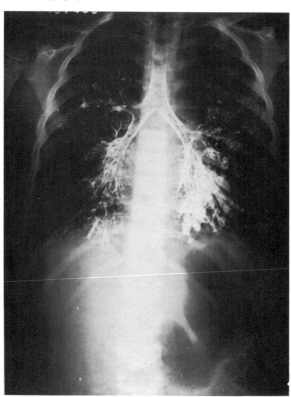

Figure 17.14 Bronchogram showing bronchiectasis of the left lower lobe

affected patient may need 2 weeks' preparation. Failure of adequate preparation will lead inevitably to morbidity and mortality after surgery.

Sputum

Bacteriological examination of the sputum usually reveals a variety of organisms. Their respective sensitivities should be determined. Since the underlying problem is one of dilatation and inadequate drainage, it has been our practice not to give antibiotics until the time of surgery. Earlier administration will only alter the nature of the flora in the respiratory tree and make subsequent problems more difficult to treat.

The respiratory function should be measured before operation. However, the segments of lung removed during operation for bronchiectasis are usually functionless and their removal unimportant.

Postoperative care

The patient returns to the ward and particular emphasis is placed on the following:

1. Usually two drainage tubes are attached to individual underwater seals. The convention is that the drain at the *Back* drains *Blood* and is situated at the *Base* of the pleural cavity. Conversely, the drain *Anteriorly* drains *Air* and is situated with its tip at the *Apex* of the pleural cavity. The management of each drain is along the principles laid down previously.
2. Pain must be controlled (see below) so that early effective coughing and full cooperation with the physiotherapist is possible.
3. Severe bleeding may occur. If this is more than 500 ml an hour for more than three consecutive hours, the patient should be returned to the operating room and explored. Usually the cause is a bleeding bronchial artery.

As soon as the drainage tubes are removed rapid mobilization is encouraged and many patients will benefit by a daily visit to the physiotherapy department for general body exercises.

Pulmonary tuberculosis

In Great Britain, surgery plays a steadily diminishing role in the treatment of tuberculosis. Reasons for this include the variety and effectiveness of chemotherapy, early diagnosis and a high state of resistance in the community which is mostly well fed and housed. However, tuberculosis of the lungs remains a very common condition elsewhere in the world and surgery still has an important role in the total treatment of patients living in areas where it is rife.

The operations for tuberculosis are indicated: (1) when the organism responsible becomes resistant to the antibiotics and other drugs; (2) when a cavity either inside or around the lung threatens to cause persistence of infection in spite of adequate medical treatment; and (3) when secondary haemorrhage threatens the life of the patient.

The aim of surgery is to remove the affected areas of lung. This may be accompanied by simultaneous resection of a chronic tuberculous empyema. The operations of thoracoplasty and pleural plombage have been largely abandoned.

Lung resection in the tuberculous patient is extremely demanding. The surgeon faces a fibrosed lung and dissection is extremely difficult and often bloody. At least 8 units of blood should be available for transfusion. Bronchopleural fistula may be the result of poor bronchial healing and will have to be managed on its merits (see below).

The patient has a demanding experience also. Surgery is usually advised after a prolonged period of ill health and a background of chronic lung disease is usually present. A long period can usefully be spent in preparing the patient for surgery. Intensive physiotherapy is essential and should produce improvement in respiratory function. The nutrition of the patient should be improved by a high protein diet. Careful monitoring on a frequent and regular basis of the organisms in the sputum should be performed and their sensitivities to antibodies constantly measured. After surgery adrenal function may be insufficient to cope with the extra demands and an Addisonian crisis will occur.

The extra efforts of coughing up sputum after surgery may be too much for the patient and, before exhaustion sets in, a therapeutic bronchoscopy and suction of secretions will greatly aid the speed of recovery.

Neoplasms of the lung and bronchi

Neoplasms of the lungs and bronchi are the most frequent indications for lung surgery in Great Britain. No attempt will be made in this book to describe the pathologies and clinical presentations of the various neoplasms. Instead, the principles of surgery and the practical management of patients will be described.

The first problem in the management of patients who may be suffering from a neoplasm of the lungs or bronchi is to establish a diagnosis and the ease of doing this may vary. The demonstration of a 'shadow' on the chest radiograph or perhaps an abnormality of a radioactive scan should be treated as inferior evidence. The constant need is to establish the diagnosis by the histological examination of abnormal tissue. This tissue may be obtained by one of the following methods:

1. Bronchoscopy with a rigid bronchoscope.
2. Bronchoscopy with a flexible bronchoscope.
3. Needle biopsy from outside the chest well.
4. Cytological examination of the sputum.

The need to establish a cytological diagnosis is cardinal to the assessment of candidates for operation. However, to pursue a diagnosis relentlessly in a patient who is unsuitable for surgery is not good medicine.

Bronchoscopy with a rigid instrument is simple, cheap and effective. In addition to providing a diagnosis on most occasions, a judgement as to the mobility of the major bronchi and to the ideal operation can be made. A large piece of tissue is removed and this is examined histologically.

Flexible bronchoscopes are expensive to buy and use and although more of the bronchial tree can be examined the tissue removed is small in bulk and subject to histological error. Great caution is needed, therefore, when introducing the flexible bronchoscope to an institution. The same caution applies to needle biopsy and to the cytological examination of the sputum. In all three methods, the histological skills needed for an accurate diagnosis will take time to be learned.

Every patient with a proven lung neoplasm should be considered for surgery. Between this consideration and the operation, however, a number of increasingly fine filters are placed.

The clinical filter

The patient may be too old (in the experience of many surgeons, the patient of 70 years or more responds badly to lung resection). There may be poor respiratory function or clinical evidence of spread of the neoplasm – superior vena caval obstruction, laryngeal palsy or an obvious cerebral lesion are examples. There may be major disease of another organ in the body.

The radiological filter

The plain chest radiograph may show phrenic paralysis (which may only be shown on sniffing during screening). There may be bony metastases or lesions in the opposite lung. The mediastinum may be grossly widened and distorted. A barium swallow in a patient with dysphagia will often show distortion caused by enlarged mediastinal lymph nodes.

The investigation filter

Bronchoscopy will show if the lesion is removable. Examination of the lymph nodes in the mediastinum is possible by mediastinoscopy. (This is mostly a digital examination performed through a small suprasternal incision. Right-sided lymph nodes are easily felt down to the level of the right main bronchus; those on the left are mostly inaccessible).

Various radioactive scans may show visceral involvement, thereby ruling out surgery.

Computerized tomographic (CT) scans are now widely available and should be used to detect the presence of intrathoracic and distant metastases.

The surgical filter

When the patient eventually comes to surgery, a further filter remains: it may be impossible to remove the growth. Between 5 and 30% of patients who have a thoracotomy do not have a resection. The hospital mortality of a failed resection is quite high and the objective of every surgeon is to keep his non-resection rate very low. Therefore, any information which will enable the patient to avoid a fruitless operation should be used.

The aim of surgery in neoplasms of the lung is the same as that for neoplasms in any other organ. Benign neoplasms are removed with a small surrounding area of normal tissue. Malignant neoplasms are removed intact with a wide margin of healthy tissue and the associated lymph drainage in one specimen (radical resection). In the lungs a radical resection may be performed either by removal of a lobe or by removal of the whole lung, depending on the site and size of the cancer. Lobectomy and pneumonectomy carry the same long-term cure rates.

The operations are performed through identical incisions. The patient is placed with the affected side of the chest uppermost. Strapping and pillows are used to avoid movement and to cushion vulnerable areas of the body (heels, lateral popliteal nerve, buttocks and arms) (Figure 17.15).

The incision is situated in the skin crease below and behind the scapula. The muscles of the chest wall are divided (Figure 17.16) and the chest cavity entered by incision above a rib or its complete removal. Removal of the lung tissue is performed by dissection.

Usually the chest is closed with drains (see above). However, many surgeons do not use drains if a pneumonectomy has been performed. Antibiotics are given throughout the operative period. Liberal analgesia is essential. The care of those patients having lobectomy is much the same as the care given to patients who have had resection for bronchiectasis. Important differences are found in the care given to patients after pneumonectomy, however.

Patient care after pneumonectomy

Removal of one lung leaves behind an empty hemithorax and the patient survives on one lung. Besides all the other aspects of patient care,

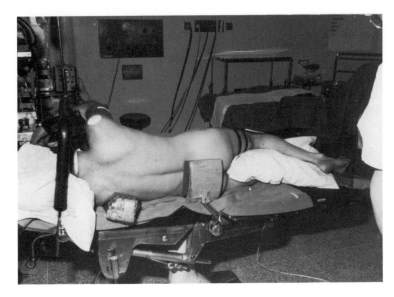

Figure 17.15 Showing the position of the patient prior to thoracotomy

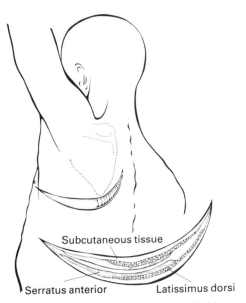

Subcutaneous tissue

Serratus anterior   Latissimus dorsi

Figure 17.16 Diagram of the thoracotomy incision, showing the muscle layers

therefore, these two factors determine the specific needs of the patient after pneumonectomy. The care of each will influence the other, and this applies whether or not the empty hemithorax has a temporary drain in it or not.

The empty hemithorax is a hazard until such time when it becomes occupied by living fibrous tissue. To achieve this, the space must first fill with blood. This clots and then becomes organized, through the stages of granulation tissue and immature scar tissue, into mature fibrous tissue. Until the space is occupied by living tissue it may become infected since an empty space or blood clot will permit any bacterial contamination to become active infection. Therefore, the space must be encouraged to obliterate as quickly as possible. This is the rationale of not using a drain at all. If a drain is used, it is removed after 24 h. In that period, it is usually released every hour to allow blood to drain.

The opposite lung must clearly remain fully expanded to work properly. The expansion of this lung will be affected by changes in pressure in the empty hemithorax causing mediastinal shift. In particular, the pressure may rise because of accumulation of blood – an objective desirable from the point of view of filling the space, but undesirable because of compression of the opposite lung. In practice, the maintenance of a slightly negative pressure in the empty hemithorax will encourage the obliteration of the cavity without impairing the function of the remaining lung.

Clinically and radiologically the ideal state is to have the mediastinum slightly towards the empty cavity. Clinically the position of the trachea is a useful sign. The distance of the mediastinum from the chest wall on the preoperative chest radiograph may be measured and compared with the distance seen on postoperative films (Figure 17.17).

Should the pressure rise when there is no drain in the empty pleural cavity, it is necessary to remove either air or blood or both from the cavity depending on the radiographic appearances. Accurate adjustment of the pressure may be obtained by the use of the Maxwell box – originally intended as a device for inserting air into the pleural cavity. However, this instrument is not essential, providing accurate clinical and radiological observations are frequently made.

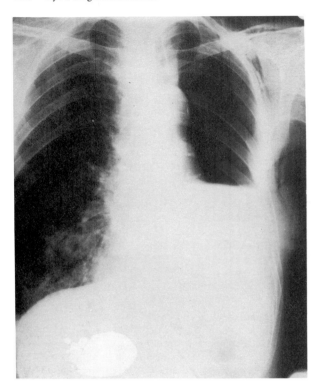

Figure 17.17 Chest radiograph after an uncomplicated pneumonectomy

Probably the most common error in the care of patients after pneumonectomy is to attribute the cause of shortness of breath to causes other than mediastinal shift compressing the remaining lung. Similarly, sudden onset of atrial fibrillation or 'bronchitis' in the remaining lung or mental confusion due to hypoxia may all be due to this relatively simple cause, the treatment of which is dramatically effective. Earlier assumptions that the mediastinum becomes 'fixed' and immovable within 24 h of surgery are demonstrably incorrect.

Bronchopleural fistula after lung resection

A communication between the bronchial tree and the pleural cavity will usually lead to a pneumothorax. Provided the cavity is obliterated by expansion of the lung by means of tube drainage, the fistula becomes unimportant and heals. This is true after a partial lung resection. Maintenance of full expansion in the remaining lung obliterates any cavity and very quickly fusion of the parietal and visceral pleura occurs. Even if the tubes are still draining air at that time, slow removal will lead to healing of the fistula.

Bronchopleural fistula becomes dangerous when a space in the pleural cavity persists. This, of course, is bound to happen after a pneumonectomy.

After lung resection the bronchus, which has a poor blood supply, may fail to heal. There are a number of surgical techniques which minimize this possibility but, in spite of these, fistula formation may occur. The bacteriological contamination which is physiologically present in the bronchial tree then infects the pneumonectomy space causing a severe systemic reaction. In addition, the onset of the fistula may lead to the liquid contents of the pneumonectomy space emptying into the remaining lung, leading to acute severe impairment of respiratory function and death. Smaller leaks may merely cause 'bronchitis' at the base of the remaining lung.

The difficulty in making the diagnosis of postpneumonectomy bronchopleural fistula may vary. A patient who suddenly coughs up a litre of brown fluid a few days after pneumonectomy is easily diagnosed. Smaller leaks, however, may cause considerable problems of diagnosis and a high degree of suspicion is necessary.

The cardinal sign of a small bronchopleural fistula is the occurrence of a positive air space in the operated side. This is semicircular in shape, instead of the triangular shape of the normally negative space. Because of varying rates of fluid accumulation and loss, the level of fluid in the thorax may not vary as much as one might expect. The presence of positive pressure in the air space may or may not

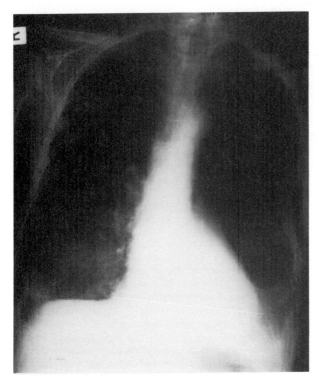

Figure 17.18 Chest radiograph after pneumonectomy complicated by a bronchopleural fistula

be accompanied by shift of the trachea, detected clinically (Figure 17.18).

Thus, the diagnosis of a small bronchopleural fistula may be indicated by this rather subtle radiological sign. Attempts at introducing dye into the hemithorax may fail to confirm a fistula because of loculation and bronchoscopy will detect only the larger lesions.

Therefore, any patient with an impaired course after pneumonectomy should be regarded with the suspicion of having a bronchopleural fistula. If the only sign of this is the presence of a positive pressure air space, sufficient is present for diagnosis.

The treatment of bronchopleural fistula is surgical and although more difficult can be accomplished successfully even years after pneumonectomy.

Chest injuries

Injuries to the chest may be 'blunt' or 'penetrating'. The former condition is present when there is no external wound penetrating the chest and most commonly is the result of a motor vehicle accident. Penetrating injuries are accompanied by an external wound which causes a variety of intrathoracic lesions depending on the extent of penetration. Knife and gunshot wounds are the most common causes.

Blunt chest injuries

These injuries usually occur in the multiply injured patient. Unless the other injuries are the cause of severe haemorrhage, the management of the chest injury is given the first priority because of the effects on the lungs and circulation.

Blunt chest injuries are caused by direct trauma to the chest or by deceleration causing damage to the thoracic viscera. Attention must be given to the possibility that any intrathoracic organ may be damaged.

Low cardiac output syndrome will accompany many of the more severe injuries and the usual diagnostic criteria should be applied. Similarly, the insertion of a central venous pressure line (p. 242) is cardinal to the management of the more severe injuries. Finally, care must be taken in the assessment of the adequacy of the patient's oxygenation. Cyanosis itself is unreliable and sweating, confusion and agitation more common. If facilities for measurement of the blood-gas levels are available, they should always be used.

Most chest injuries (with certain exceptions) need urgent chest radiographs. The supine portable film is often misleading, particularly in the presence of a haemothorax, and it is essential to tilt the patient's head up as much as possible when the film is taken. The severely injured patient can be moved very little, but even a 5° head-up tilt will improve the diagnostic quality of the chest radiograph.

Broken ribs

Isolated fractures of the ribs follow direct injury to the chest wall. They always heal without difficulty but cause severe pain. This pain impedes full respiratory movement and hence usually impairs the ventilation and removal of secretions in the underlying lung. Retention of secretions causes segmental collapse and these areas may become infected. In the young, healthy adult no consequence will arise. In the older patient, often with chronic lung disease, the pathological process may cause severe illness.

Pain relief will avoid all these effects. In minor injuries in the young simple oral analgesics may be sufficient. More severe pain is controlled by the direct injection of local anaesthetic into the fracture site(s). Usually 5 ml of 1% lignocaine injected into the site of maximum tenderness will give instant relief. The injection usually has to be repeated at 24 h and then at 48 h. Nerve blocks are less satisfactory; the quality of analgesia is less predictable and the insertion of the local anaesthetic demands higher skills.

Strapping of the chest wall in the affected area is virtually useless. It neither relieves pain effectively, nor does it avoid the pulmonary complications.

Flail chest

When several ribs are each broken in more than one place, the chest wall in that area becomes unstable. Respiration causes the segment to be forced inwards and expiration pushes it out. Thus, depending on the size of the segment, there is a varying degree of respiratory inefficiency because the underlying lung fails to be adequately ventilated.

A flail segment about 10 cm in diameter can be easily tolerated by a fit adult. Increasing age, however, and especially accompanying chronic lung disease will reduce this size and then respiratory insufficiency will occur and be a threat to life.

The diagnosis of flail chest is clinical. Detection of the abnormally moving segment may be difficult in the immediate period after the injury owing to tissue oedema: repeated examinations will help to avoid mistakes.

If the flail segment is tolerated by the patient, it should be treated as for isolated rib fractures. Respiratory embarrassment will, however, need urgent treatment.

As a first aid measure, the flail segment should be immobilized by a pressure dressing. This does no good whatsoever to the underlying lung, but at least ensures that the rest of the lungs will continue to be ventilated.

In hospital, stabilization of the flail segment is necessary. Attempts at operative stabilization are usually useless because of the associated soft tissue damage. The only method of proven success is internal fixation of the segment by artificial positive-pressure ventilation. This is continued until the chest wall has healed sufficiently to permit stability. This may take up to 3 weeks. Attempts at correcting any bony deformity are unnecessary.

Pulmonary damage

The lungs may be damaged by penetration by fragments of broken rib, direct contusion or by deceleration forces.

Penetration of the lung will result in a haemo-pneumothorax and this should be diagnosed and treated as described in the section on chest drainage. Clinical evidence of surgical emphysema around a rib fracture should always raise the suspicion of underlying lung damage. Surgical drainage of the pleura in traumatic haemopneumothorax should never be delayed as tension complications may rapidly follow. As emphasized in the section on chest drainage, the insertion of a drain should normally follow a chest radiograph. In a small number of patients, however, the speed of accumulation of blood and air in the pleural space is so great that the patient may be only a few seconds away from death when first seen by the surgeon. Urgent drainage is clearly needed but delay for a chest radiograph is fatal. The dilemma is solved by judging the position of the mediastinum. Clinically, there is a large collection of blood or air in one pleural cavity, then the trachea will be grossly deviated away from that side. In these desperate circumstances only, a chest drain should be inserted into that side of the chest – opposite to the side to which tracheal deviation has occurred. This is an exceptional circumstance and in no way negates the general rule of insisting on a chest radiograph before insertion of a chest drainage tube.

Pulmonary damage, from whatever cause, will produce respiratory insufficiency. The diagnosis of this is often very difficult and repeated and frequent assessments are necessary. Ideally, measurement of the arterial blood gases is performed frequently and provides the only sure method. Clinical signs are subtle and varied. Tachypnoea, tachycardia, sweating, confusion and anxiety are useful signs especially if they worsen on repeated examination. Ultimately, mechanical ventilation may have to be used in order to see if improvement will occur. Unnecessary ventilation is preferable to death from respiratory failure untreated because of scientific scepticism.

When is thoracotomy performed in blunt chest injuries?

The following complications are treated by thoracotomy:

1. Ruptured bronchus or trachea. Suspected by a pneumothorax which is uncontrollable by chest drainage and confirmed by bronchoscopy.
2. Uncontrollable haemorrhage. A litre of blood drainage per hour for 3 h should lead to exploration.
3. Ruptured aorta. This is suspected by the finding of a wide mediastinum on the chest radiograph and confirmed by aortography. *Any* patient with a wide mediastinum should have urgent aortography.Centres with the appropriate equipment may perform echocardiography, CT or MRI scanning. The important feature to recognize is that *no* one test is 100% sensitive in detecting a traumatic rupture of the aorta and even aortography which is probably still the best test may occasionally fail to detect the lesion. A few negative investigations are preferable to missing a single rupture since delay in treatment is lethal.

Low cardiac output syndrome ('shock') is commonly found in severe 'blunt' chest injuries. The syndrome is characterized by cold skin, poor urinary output and acidosis. The blood pressure may or may not be low. Measurement of the central venous pressure is essential since oligaemia is only one of the causes of the syndrome. Cardiogenic low output may occur separately or with oligaemia, and appears as a result of a variety of insults to the heart. Sometimes the heart may be compressed by a haemorrhage into the pericardium. There may be a direct cardiac contusion. Finally, a number of metabolic causes such as hypoxia and acidosis may depress cardiac function (Figure 17.19). In cases of oligaemia, the central venous pressure is low and in those cases suffering from cardiogenic low output, the venous pressure is normal or high.

Measurement of the central venous pressure is essential also during the transfusion of blood. If the level is brought to and maintained at about 10 cmH$_2$O, pulmonary oedema is unlikely to occur.

Cold skin
Poor urinary output (0.5 ml/kg/h)
Usually a low BP
Acidosis

Low CVP	High or normal CVP
Haemorrhage	Cardiac contusion
(may be concealed)	Myocardial depression
	Cardiac tamponade

N.B. More than one cause may be present

Figure 17.19 Low output syndrome (shock) in chest tissue

Penetrating wounds of the chest

In certain parts of the world where guns and knives are used to settle arguments, these injuries form the bulk of chest trauma.

A high level of suspicion is necessary if all the damage done by a penetrating wound is to be identified. Vascular injuries should always be assumed and the palpation of the peripheral pulses is essential. Similarly, any wound may end in the heart or pericardium. The anatomy of the diaphragm means that an abdominal injury may complicate even a high stab wound. Finally, both the major air passages and the oesophagus in the mediastinum may be damaged.

As in blunt chest injuries, a chest radiograph is important and can only be omitted in the most desperate circumstances in the manner already outlined.

After resuscitation of the patient by infusion of blood and the insertion of appropriate chest drains, the wound should be explored and the chest opened in the appropriate area. This advice is given because even the most experienced surgeon can be misled as to the extent of the injuries internally and often catastrophic haemorrhage is being prevented only temporarily by blood clot. The interests of the patient and the protection of the surgeon, therefore, demand that the exact extent of the penetrating wound is determined and this can only be done by thoracotomy.

This practice, however, is not universally accepted. In countries where many penetrating injuries of the chest are frequently seen, a 100% operation policy is logistically impossible. Moreover, the continuing experience of these centres makes it possible for many penetrating injuries without excessive bleeding (500+ ml every hour) to be treated by intercostal drainage and careful clinical and radiological control

Tamponade

Cardiac injuries of this type are frequently accompanied by tamponade caused by the accumulation of blood in the pericardium. Owing to the speed of collection, only a small volume is necessary to cause fatal tamponade. Tamponade should be suggested by a penetrating wound over the middle of the anterior aspect of the chest, by low output syndrome and by a pulse which decreases in volume on inspiration (pulsus paradoxus) together with a high and moving central venous pressure.

The definitive treatment is to evacuate the blood by a left anterior thoracotomy. This operation should be performed in the operating theatre, but is often performed in the Accident and Emergency department if the heart is in asystole when the patient arrives in hospital or if time does not allow removal of the patient. Whilst preparations are being made to do this, a large-bore needle attached to a syringe may be passed into the pericardium and constantly aspirated. The needle is inserted to the left of the xiphisternum and passed at 45° upwards and backwards into the pericardium. This manoeuvre will often fail, however; emergency thoracotomy is then the only way of relieving the cardiac compression.

The general principles of management of penetrating wounds are observed. Dead or unviable tissue is removed, together with fragments of bone or foreign material. Antibiotic prophylaxis should be given and antitetanus measures taken (p. 52). Most penetrating wounds of the heart can be controlled by simple sutures. Cardiopulmonary bypass is rarely required.

Oesophageal surgery

Only certain principles of management of oesophageal cases can be outlined here. The oesophagus is the most inaccessible organ clinically and specific signs of diseases are few. Nearly all diseases of the oesophagus cause difficulty in swallowing and this may be accompanied by pain. The failure of enough food to get into the stomach leads to a progressive loss of weight and nutritional deficiencies of all types. The food which fails to pass naturally is usually vomited, but inevitably, especially in the later stages, regurgitation into the respiratory tract occurs and leads to episodes of pneumonia and ultimately, if the disease permits, to lung fibrosis.

Therefore the doctor has three problems – the disease, the inanition and the lung complications resulting from regurgitation.

Inanition results in a physical appearance which suggests terminal carcinomatosis. Until nutrition is improved the distinction between starvation and carcinomatosis is impossible.

The nutrition of the patient may be improved in several ways. An entirely liquid, high-protein, high-calorie diet may well pass an obstruction while solid food impacts in the limited orifice available. Failing this, it is possible to pass a very fine polythene tube across the oesophageal lesion and to give liquid nutrients slowly but continually down this. Intravenous feeding regimens are the final way in which nutrition may be improved before surgery (p. 30).

Aspiration lung disease often improves once the above measures are taken. However, a prolonged programme of physiotherapy will help matters further and should include postural drainage exercises.

Oesophageal lesions are mainly investigated by contrast radiographic studies, by endoscopy and by specialized investigations performed in an oesophageal laboratory. Two observations of a practical nature may help the house surgeon:

1. If gastro-oesophageal reflux is suspected always inform the radiologist who will then undertake special provocative measures to show this.
2. Oesophagoscopy carries a risk of perforation. The possibility should be considered in every patient who has had the investigation. Perforation of the thoracic oesophagus usually causes pain. Immediate chest radiographs should be taken and, if necessary, a contrast study performed. The preferred medium of radiologists is thin barium as this substance causes the least irritation in the mediastinum should it pass through a perforation. Finally, the prudent house surgeon will order a check radiograph of the chest on any patient who has had a 'difficult' oesophageal examination for whatever reason.

Oesophageal perforations of the spontaneous or iatrogenic type can be repaired by direct suture with a low risk, provided the repair occurs within a few hours of surgery. Delay in diagnosis will lead to dangerously late surgery with very much higher morbidity and mortality. Efforts put into the early diagnosis of oesophageal perforation will, therefore, reduce the mortality of this condition.

Thus the management of a patient before surgery is in two equally important parts. First, the diagnosis must be made. Barium swallow radiographic studies and oesophagoscopy usually provide the diagnosis but some motor disorders of the oesophagus may need pressure and pH measurements made in a specialized laboratory.

Secondly, the patient must be made as fit as possible for surgery. Malnutrition has to be corrected and the lungs improved by physiotherapy. This part may take days or weeks to achieve and clearly the time available may be shortened by the need to treat the underlying disease. The major causes of death after resection of the oesophagus are related to leaks from oesophageal anastomoses and malnutrition contributes to this hazard. Regardless of the underlying condition, malnutrition is 'malignant' in this respect and its correction is of major importance to the success of surgery.

Cardiac surgery

Surgical operations on the heart are a consequence of the concept that the heart is a sophisticated pump and that diseases cause damage to the pumping action. Most diseases cause mechanical or hydraulic disturbances and are, therefore, ideally treated by mechanical solutions: hence surgery.

Cardiac operations are in two groups – 'closed' and 'open'. Closed operations are performed upon the heart whilst it is supporting the circulation and these were the first cardiac operations to be performed. Open operations, conversely, are done on the heart whilst it is not supporting a circulation. Thus, more complex and multiple procedures can be undertaken under direct vision. The techniques of open heart surgery are outlined later in this chapter.

The patient presenting in the cardiac surgery clinic usually comes with a diagnosis which has been formulated by the cardiologist, surgeon and radiologist in consultation. In arriving at the diagnosis, evidence is gathered from many sources. Clinical features of the history and examination remain important, but often complete information may be obtainable only by cardiac catheterization, cardioangiography, echocardiography and recently by nuclear studies. There will be no further description of these, but clearly, the prudent admitting surgeon will bring together all the pertinent facts about a particular patient and have them available for a final review by the operating surgeon.

When admitting a patient for cardiac surgery, particular emphasis is placed on the following:

1. The level of maximum physical activity. Many patients with chronic heart disease minimize their disability and only careful questioning about specific disabilities will reveal the true level. This is important to establish as a baseline against which the operation may be judged afterwards. In children, for the same reasons, a measurement of height and weight is made.
2. Nearly all patients are taking cardiac drugs on admission. Some of these may cause problems during surgery and yet to stop other drugs might create equal troubles. Full documentation is, therefore, essential. At the same time, drug allergies, particularly to antibiotics, are noted.
3. Many patients smoke cigarettes and, depending on the policy of the particular unit, surgery may be delayed or cancelled. The smoking habits of every patient are, therefore, of interest.
4. Examination of the patient should not be confined to the heart and circulatory system. The general appearances and nutrition should be noted and the teeth carefully examined. Caries carries the slight risk of causing a bacteraemia during or immediately after surgery. If the surgical operation involves the implantation of a foreign body, e.g. an artificial valve, then this bacteraemia may cause endocarditis which carries a high mortality.

Most patients will have had the opportunity to discuss their problems with the surgeon before admission and the patient's informed consent has been obtained at that time. Informed consent implies that the patient, amongst other things, be aware that any open heart procedure carries the risk of brain damage occurring as a result of the artificial circulation and that in 2% of all operated cases, such damage will have residual effects. In the United Kingdom, legal advice has determined that this hazard should be specifically mentioned to each patient who is about to have surgery. Further explanation and the opportunity to pose further questions are welcomed by the patient on his surgical admission, especially since there is growing apprehension on his part. Time spent at this stage is always richly rewarded later and because of all the medical time which has already been spent on a patient, it is probably the most important function of the admitting surgeon. Similarly, the patient's next of kin are seen, either at the same time or later, and equal importance must be given to this interview. Often, parents of children about to have operations may need to be seen more than once.

Techniques of open heart surgery

Whilst the details of techniques are inappropriate in this chapter, the principles of open heart surgery are important because they create special problems and situations after the operation. Proper management will depend on an accurate appreciation of the techniques.

In open heart surgery, either the circulation can be maintained artificially or the metabolic needs of the body tissues so reduced that the circulation may be stopped for a short time.

Artificial maintenance of the circulation is the most common technique and this is performed mechanically by the heart–lung machine. The procedure is termed cardiopulmonary bypass. Earlier techniques of bypassing only the heart and allowing the lungs to function have mostly been abandoned because of technical complexity.

Cardiopulmonary bypass

The heart and great vessels are exposed, usually through a vertical sternal splitting incision. Heparin is then given to the patient to prevent blood clotting in the apparatus. After bypass, this will be reversed by protamine sulphate. Either the great veins or the right atrium are then cannulated and blood allowed to drain by siphonage with the heart–lung apparatus.

In the machine, four major events occur:

1. The blood is oxygenated and carbon dioxide removed. This is usually done in a disposable plastic device which allows oxygen to froth with the blood. The same device has settling chambers in which the froth can again become blood. The device is a 'bubble' oxygenator (Figure 17.20) and many different types are commercially available. Alternatively, the blood may be oxygenated by exposing it to oxygen on the other

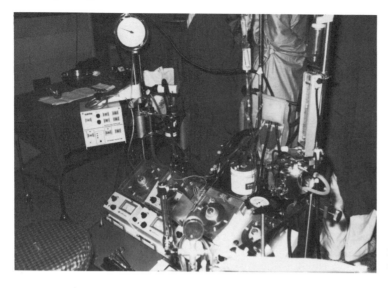

Figure 17.20 The heart–lung machine during use

side of a very thin membrane. This is called a 'membrane' oxygenator and clearly has no foaming problems.

2. The newly oxygenated blood now passes through a pump on its way back to the patient. The standard type is the roller pump shown in Figure 17.21. The output of this is variable according to the speed of the electric motor.

3. After oxygenation and pumping, the blood has usually cooled considerably below 37°C. There-

fore it is passed through what is essentially a large water bath called a heat exchanger.

4. Finally, the blood is filtered through a very fine mesh, with a pore size of 20–30 μm in order to remove debris (Figure 17.22).

The warmed, oxygenated, pressurized blood is now directed back into the patient's arterial system. The point of entry is usually the ascending aorta, but sometimes a femoral artery may be cannulated. The

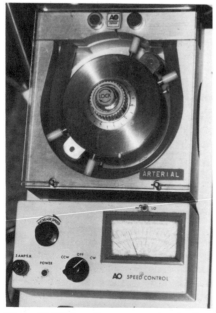

Figure 17.21 The roller pump used to circulate blood in the heart–lung machine

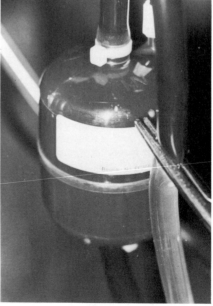

Figure 17.22 A microfilter – in this case in the arterial line of the cardiac bypass circuit

blood flows backwards in the aorta and stops at the closed aortic valve, perfusing the coronary arteries and all other arteries of the body.

Clinical problems following cardiopulmonary bypass

The above summary of cardiopulmonary bypass shows that the process is unphysiological and will create certain problems which can make the care of patients after surgery difficult.

Haemorrhage

The clotting cascade of blood may be disrupted at several points. Heparin is given and then neutralized by protamine and the dosages may be difficult to match, leading to impaired clotting of the blood. Exposure of the labile protein elements of clotting function to oxygen bubbles will degrade the protein and thus further impair clotting. Platelet function and numbers are both diminished by bypass and lead to more troubles. The net effect is for a haemorrhagic tendency after surgery which can usually be made safe by sound surgical techniques. However, bleeding after surgery is commonly a problem. Usually 500 ml loss in any one hour after operation or 300 ml for 3 consecutive hours should lead to exploratory re-operation and surgical haemostasis. However, in those cases where no obvious bleeding vessel is found, clotting studies may show a remediable defect. Appropriate specific therapy is then given in consultation with the haematologist. Usually transfused platelets are effective. However, often a specific problem cannot be identified or bleeding persists in spite of appropriate treatment. Most surgeons believe that fresh blood (less than 8 h old) is the answer to this problem and the weight of experience convinces even the most ardent advocate of specific blood component therapy.

Organ dysfunction

Impaired function of almost every organ can be demonstrated after cardiopulmonary bypass. Many studies have shown that there is imperfect perfusion of the tissues in spite of what would appear to be a satisfactory output from the pump. This impairment appears to lie at the level of the precapillary arterioles and functions as a partial obstruction to blood flow into the capillaries.

The nature of flow in cardiopulmonary bypass is non-pulsatile and this triggers the renin-angiotensin system leading to arteriolar vasoconstriction. Further, small emboli of about 20–40 μm in diameter may be created by the bypass. These can be of air, fatty debris or aggregated blood cells.

The combined effect is to limit capillary blood flow, leading to mild tissue hypoxia. In the brain, this may lead to anything from unconsciousness to nightmares after surgery. Kidney and liver function are temporarily or, very rarely, permanently diminished. Tests of virtually every body function show derangement – often so mild as to be detectable only in the laboratory. The lungs show impairment of oxygen uptake, the heart shows diminished function. Even an intestinal ileus is common for a day or two after surgery.

Most of these problems can be avoided by removal of the particles by filters – hence the inclusion of a filter somewhere in the bypass circuit. Priming the pump with a non-blood fluid such as a balanced electrolyte solution is a further help.

However, even with all possible precautions, some organ damage will occur and will increase with time. Damage which is mild at 2 h of bypass may be lethal at 4 h. The aim of the surgeon therefore is to perform accurate corrective surgery as quickly as possible. In practice, there are few procedures needing more than 2 h bypass.

Surgical cerebral air embolism

If the heart is opened, air replaces the blood in it. The surgeon spends a lot of time at the end of the cardiac operation removing this air. If any remains, however, and this is common, air will be pumped into the arterial circulation when the heart resumes its function. Air emboli are particularly damaging to the brain. According to the number of emboli, their size and the type of cerebral artery in which they impact, cerebral damage of a varying degree will occur. At one extreme, the patient may die of irreversible and widespread cerebral damage. At the other, the patient may just take a long time to wake up after the anaesthetic.

Surgical cerebral air embolism is the major hazard of cardiac surgery in spite of the most strenuous efforts made to reduce its incidence. Once it has occurred, there is little that can be done apart from waiting and nursing the patient. Steroids may reduce some of the cerebral oedema, but the initial neuronal insult will not change. Ultimately, the patient may be able to compensate for the nerve loss and in all cases of air embolism to the brain, good general medical and nursing care will promote this.

Myocardial damage

The heart is no exception to the generalized organ dysfunction. In addition, it is handled and cut and is already diseased. Consequently, it may fail to function properly. Again, the degree of this may vary from a fixed ischaemic contracture ('stone heart') found immediately after bypass through mild cardiac failure in the early hours after operation to a mild chronic damage which impairs the patient's function and detracts from the ultimate benefits of surgery.

During cardiopulmonary bypass, the surgeon is at all times aware of the need to avoid damaging the contraction of the heart muscle. The many techniques involved are grouped together as 'myocardial protection'. They form two main groups. First, the function of the myocardium may be preserved by supplying the heart with all its metabolic needs. This means that the coronary circulation has to be continually perfused with oxygenated blood at the correct pressure. Secondly, the metabolic needs of the myocardium may be reduced virtually to zero with the prospect of full function when those needs are restored to normal. This is accomplished by the infusion into the coronary circulation of cold (4°C) hypokalaemic (30 mmol/l) asanguineous solutions. Because of the ease of operating on a cold stationary heart, this technique is widely practised.

Other methods of open heart surgery

A patient may be cooled down to 30°C and then the circulation arrested for about 8 min without harm. In this time many simple cardiac defects can be repaired. This technique was the first successfully used in humans but the limitations on time and difficulty in cooling adults by external means led to it becoming obsolete. The technique has been reintroduced in the past few years for open heart operations on infants. The small body size of these babies makes cooling to 15–20°C easy and quick and allows 60 min of circulatory arrest. Conventional cardiopulmonary bypass in these children is very difficult because of their small size.

Congenital heart disease

Most congenital heart defects are repaired in childhood and there is a tendency for these repairs to be performed earlier rather than later. The major surgical task lies in the operating theatre, where the aims are to correct the defect fully and to avoid myocardial damage. If these objectives are attained, then the heart usually improves immediately and the postoperative course of the patient is smooth and rapid.

However, not all operations are corrective and many do unavoidably damage the myocardium. Therefore, there may be signs of low cardiac output after surgery. The management of the syndrome of low cardiac output is discussed later. Children have specific problems in that alterations in cardiac output may happen very rapidly and indirect measurements have less validity than in an adult. Thus, the management of these children is very

demanding and the close cooperation of the paediatrician and the anaesthetist is essential.

Certain groups of paediatric patients are identifiable as being at high risk before surgery:

1. Cyanosed patients usually have more complex disease. The cyanosis arises from unoxygenated blood (which should stay in the right side of the heart until it has passed through the lungs) being shunted into the systemic oxygenated circulation. Clinical cyanosis may be difficult to detect in artificial light. It causes clubbing of the toe and finger nails. In addition, complex haematological abnormalities arise and often blood clotting is impaired after surgery. Fresh blood for transfusion is desirable for any child under 8 years having cardiac surgery and more should be ordered (say 8 rather than 4 units) if cyanosis is present.
2. The management and surgery of the neonate and infant has virtually become a subspecialty because of the unique and difficult problems involved. In Great Britain there are several centres where these small children have surgery and there is broad agreement that any such centre is most safe when performing 100 operations or more per year.
3. Pulmonary vascular disease may occur when the cardiac disorder leads to the flow of blood through the lungs being much greater than normal. The disorders are usually those permitting high-pressure left-sided blood to pass into the pulmonary artery (viz. ventricular septal defect). The excessive flow will lead to reactive and later organic changes in the pulmonary arterioles. At first reactive spasm limits the flow of blood through the lungs but later, organic changes in the arteriolar walls create permanent obstructions to flow. The fully developed changes virtually preclude surgery. The objective in performing early surgery is to avoid this complication. However, the surgeon who has to operate on a child with less severe changes knows that troubles of right heart failure and low output will be encountered after surgery.

Valvular heart surgery

Disease of a cardiac valve causes regurgitation, stenosis or a combination of both, regardless of the underlying aetiology. Clearly, valve disorders which suddenly happen, such as aortic regurgitation due to infective endocarditis, are more poorly tolerated than those disorders which progress over a number of years.

There is a clear distinction between the stenotic and regurgitant valves, however, in their clinical presentation, precision of objective diagnosis and results of treatment.

Stenotic valves impose a pressure load on the pumping chambers of the heart. This load is often well tolerated with few symptoms until sudden and severe deterioration occurs leading to death in a short time. At cardiac catheterization, the pressure difference across a valve can easily be measured and the degree of obstruction assessed. Surgical relief of the obstruction, either by valve repair or by replacement, carries a very good result in length of life and function.

Regurgitant lesions of valves are associated with minor symptoms initially. The rate of progression of these is very variable and timing of surgery less easy to determine. Objective measurement of the degree of regurgitation through a valve is inaccurate and very difficult. Finally, the late results of surgery are less predictable and worse than those following surgery for stenotic valves.

Valve disease is rarely 'curable' by surgery; essentially, severe valve disease is replaced by minor disease. This is true whether valve repair or replacement is performed. Thus, at some time in the future all such patients will have further valve problems and require more surgery. Clinical assessment of these patients, therefore, has to be very detailed and repeated frequently after operation. Particular emphasis is placed on *symptoms*.

Shortness of breath on exertion and the precise level of activity when the symptom occurs is noted. Ability to work and in what capacity are important facts. Sleeping habits and the number of pillows used will give some idea of the severity of cardiac failure. Tiredness is a prominent symptom and frequently ignored by doctors because it seems to be so vague. Chest pain is an important feature before operation because it may indicate coronary artery disease and, therefore, affect the nature and risk of the operation.

Examination of this group of patients usually provides accurate diagnosis and details of this are available in most cardiological texts. From the surgeon's point of view, however, certain points need emphasis:

1. In the late stages of valvular heart disease, there may be a reduction of body weight and general poor nutrition. Sophisticated tests of metabolic function merely confirm the clinical impression. Probably correction of this problem helps to improve the risk of the operation to follow.
2. The malar flush associated with mitral valve disease carries prognostic importance. The back pressure on the pulmonary venous circulation resulting from mitral valve disease causes similar changes to those resulting from overflow in congenital heart disease. The presence of ele-

vated pulmonary vascular resistance in mitral valve disease does not usually bar surgery, but certainly increases its risk.
3. Valve disease often affects more than one valve and the alert surgeon will spend some time assessing other valves apart from the obviously diseased one.
4. The liver and the kidneys may be affected by the valvular heart disease. Clinical and biochemical assessment of their function is essential.

The chest radiograph and the electrocardiogram are regarded as part of the clinical assessment of every cardiac patient. The chest radiograph should always be in the postero-anterior and lateral planes and preferably in the ·erect position. In this way comparable films are obtained and precise measurements of the cardiothoracic ratio made. Change in heart size is useful in the repeated assessment of leaking valves before surgery and in all patients after surgery. The electrocardiograph is used as a baseline before surgery and is most useful in detecting ventricular hypertrophy and rhythm changes.

Coronary arteriography in valve surgery

An important cause of operative mortality during valve surgery is undiagnosed or untreated coronary artery disease. All adult patients above 40 years have coronary arteriography as part of their assessment before surgery. Some centres have a lower age limit.

However, there is less agreement about the extent of routine pressure measurements and angiography. Some surgeons will demand detailed catheter information from every cardiac chamber and others in certain circumstances will accept the data from clinical examination and coronary angiography. Others will accept the diagnosis which has been made by echocardiography alone, in certain cases.

Types of valve operation

Valve-preserving operations

These are performed as 'closed' or 'open' operations. The surgical objective is to correct the leak or the obstruction, not to eradicate the disease. The procedures vary from a single split of fused commissures to difficult and complex repairs of cusps and chordae and removal of calcium. These operations are most frequently done on the mitral and tricuspid valves.

Valve-replacement operations

There is no ideal valve substitute – to replace a diseased valve with a prosthesis is to change severe valve disease into minor valve disease.

Types of prostheses

Valve prostheses are of two types, depending on the materials from which they are made. Each type has specific advantages and disadvantages.

Mechanical valves (Figure 17.23) are made of non-organic substances – usually a metallic alloy or specially prepared carbon. A variety of ingenious designs exist, but the most common are the ball and cage type and the tilting disc type.

'Biological' valves (Figure 17.24) are made of animal tissue mounted in a metallic or plastic frame. All valves of this type are either animal aortic valves or built so as to resemble the design of the normal aortic valve.

The surgeon advising valve replacement has to decide (or ask the patient to decide) which sort of valve to use (Table 17.1). Mechanical valves are

Table 17.1 Comparison of the main features of mechanical and biological valves

	Mechanical	Biological
Function	Fair	Good
Thrombus formation	High	Low
Durability	High	Unknown

very durable, but patients need to take anticoagulants for life. This may cause problems in patients wanting to become pregnant or those with peptic ulceration. Certain groups may find proper control of anticoagulants difficult because of inadequate local laboratory facilities.

Patients with biological valves usually need anticoagulants for 3 months after surgery. Degeneration of these valves, however, is probable and very rapid in children or patients with renal disease, because of calcium deposition.

However, *all* valves may fail and the rate of failure in mechanical valves is very fast and surgical help must be rapidly sought. Biological valves tend to fail more slowly and allow the patient time to get to a surgeon. The choice of valve, therefore, depends on many factors and each doctor will have to consider each case on its merits, usually in discussion with the patient.

Ischaemic heart disease

Atheromatous obstructions to the coronary arteries are a common cause of disability and of death in Western countries. Other parts of the world, however, have a much lower incidence for reasons which are unclear. Probably environmental factors, diet and cigarette smoking are important.

The effect of atheroma in the coronary arteries is to limit the amount of blood flowing to the myocardium. This limitation may be small, causing myocardial pain (angina pectoris) during exercise, or may be so severe as to lead to death of muscle (myocardial infarction).

There is no specific treatment which is directed towards removing the obstructing lesions. Instead, the aim of all treatments is to modify the effects of ischaemia on the myocardium. Drug treatment, such as glyceryl trinitrate, or one of the beta-adrenergic blocking drugs, tries to reduce the myocardial oxygen demand. Surgery aims to bypass the obstructions, thus increasing myocardial oxygen availability.

In the early years, usually saphenous veins were used as the bypass conduit. However, these tend to degenerate with time. Nowadays, the internal mammary artery, usually the left, is frequently used

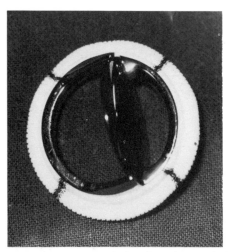

Figure 17.23 A mechanical cardiac valve prosthesis

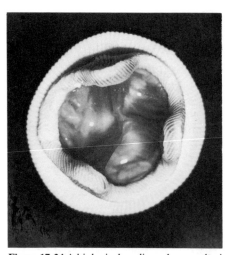

Figure 17.24 A biological cardiac valve prosthesis

because of its high long-term patency and lack of a tendency to degenerate. Since most patients now need multiple grafts, the use of saphenous vein is inevitable for some of them, but the internal mammary is used to bypass the most important artery.

On admission to the surgical ward, all patients for coronary bypass operations will have been investigated already by coronary angiography. Before operation these angiograms must again be reviewed and must, therefore, be available.

The history of such patients must be detailed in the nature of the symptoms, the exact drug dosages and previous myocardial infarctions. Examination is not usually rewarding, but attention to the legs may show vein varicosities which will alter the surgical approach.

Beta-blocker drugs are usually given so that the patient arrives for surgery with a therapeutic blood level. This and a well sedated patient are essential if a myocardial infarct is to be avoided in the immediate preoperative period.

Beta-blocker drugs may cause problems with the level of serum potassium during or immediately after the operation. Because of impaired tissue uptake, the level may rise, leading to cardiac depression. Frequent (say 0.5 hourly during operation and 2-hourly for 12 h afterwards) measurements of the serum potassium are needed.

Potassium problems apart, however, the patient who has had coronary grafting usually presents fewer problems than with any other form of cardiac surgery. Most patients are discharged taking only aspirin, 300 mg daily, and dipyridamole, 100 mg t.d.s. These drugs have an antiplatelet effect and may help to maintain the patency of the grafts.

Urgent coronary grafting is performed on patients experiencing severe and worsening angina in an effort to prevent a myocardial infarction. Salvage operations are also performed on patients suffering mechanical complications of infarcts, such as repair of infarct defects of the ventricular septum, leaking mitral valves or ventricular aneurysms. The risks of these operations are much higher than those of operations for uncomplicated angina.

Postoperative cardiac care

A successful repair of a cardiac lesion often leads to an immediate improvement in heart function. However, there may be a temporary cardiac deterioration and, in addition, the surgery causes problems potentially with every other organ system. The postoperative care is, therefore, complex and usually consists of vigilance rather than action. When treatment is needed, however, it is usually given urgently.

The patient leaving the operating theatre is usually wheeled to the surgical intensive care ward on his bed. The head is mostly raised about 15° and the bed usually has a sheepskin or ripple mattress device to prevent pressure sores. The time between operation and arrival in the ward is very dangerous: most of the surgical team are tired and the prudent house surgeon will stay with his patient during this period and undertake no duties apart from close observation.

The following devices are attached to the patient during the operation and immediately afterwards (Figure 17.25).

1. Endotracheal tube. Most patients are mechanically ventilated for a few hours via this tube which has an air cuff to prevent leakage. The usual practice is for the anaesthetist to adjust the

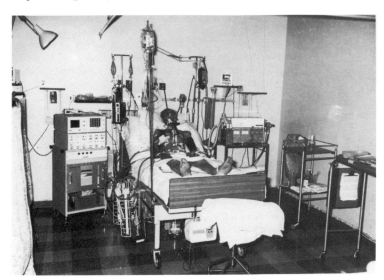

Figure 17.25 Showing a patient in the intensive care ward immediately on return from open heart surgery

amount of air in this and it is then left untouched. However, if the volume of the cuff is changed, then the minimum volume of air necessary to create occlusion should be used. This volume will vary from person to person – too little will allow a leakage of air around the tube; too much will cause pressure ulcers of the trachea.

2. Indwelling arterial catheter for pressure measuring and blood sampling.
3. Central venous pressure catheter and a method of measuring left atrial pressure.
4. Urinary catheter which is attached by a closed system to a measuring device which can accurately read volumes of under 30 ml.
5. Electrocardiogram.
6. A large venous cannula for rapid administration of fluid is necessary.
7. Skin temperature measuring probe.
8. Nasogastric tube (optional).
9. Blood drainage tubes from the chest. These are attached to an underwater seal and suction as already described.

The observations of bodily functions outlined are recorded on a chart, or series of small charts, so that changes occurring over time can be detected. The nursing staff usually record all observations and every unit has its own system of identification of various measurements. One of the first duties of the house surgeon on the intensive care ward is to write down details of when he has to be informed of changes. These details usually consist of prescribing a lowest and highest acceptable limit for all the commonly performed recordings. This manoeuvre avoids giving busy nurses the additional worry of deciding when to call the doctor.

The administration of drugs on the intensive care ward must always be by the intravenous route; there can be no certainty that any other form of administration will allow the drugs to work.

Care of the alimentary system

Nearly all patients have a paralytic ileus after cardiac or major thoracic surgery. A nasogastric tube is left on continuous free drainage and intravenous fluids given. In most units, 5% dextrose is given (usually 500 ml/m² of body surface area/24 h). This rather limited volume will not overload the circulation and will not create electrolyte problems. Oral fluids and removal of the nasogastric tube are permitted when bowel sounds return.

Care of the central nervous system

All patients after cardiac surgery suffer pain and apprehension. These symptoms may be controlled by the use of frequent small intravenous doses of a narcotic. Papaveretum, 5 mg i.v. (or morphine

sulphate 2.5 mg) every few minutes, until pain is controlled and then as necessary, is highly effective, providing analgesia and sedation. Diamorphine is a useful drug if the patient is allergic to papaveretum.

Some patients after cardiac surgery may suffer microembolism to the brain. Those microemboli are usually composed of air from the cardiac chambers. Calcium from damaged valves, fat, thrombus and other debris may also embolize to the brain. The result will be cerebral damage and the amount of this will vary according to the quantity and site of embolization.

Every patient, therefore, is at risk and needs to be assessed immediately after operation. Early recovery of consciousness and ability to move all four limbs on command, usually means that cerebral damage is slight at the most. Failure to recover consciousness fully or to move as commanded usually means cerebral damage and early action must be taken to avoid further problems from cerebral oedema. Dexamethasone, 8 mg i.v., immediately followed by 4 mg 8-hourly for 3 days, is effective. Mannitol given in a 200 ml dosage will also reduce cerebral oedema but is less effective than dexamethasone.

The agitation of a patient at this time may be due to arterial hypoxaemia and any restless patient should have blood oxygen tensions measured and corrected if necessary.

Most patients are, however, simply frightened as they wake up after cardiac surgery. A good response is usual after being told the time of day, the operation's success and where they are. A patient cannot speak and may appear unconscious, yet be conscious of all stimuli and suffering from violent emotion. Nurses and doctors must remember this and ensure their behaviour and talk help the patient during this difficult time.

In the days after a cardiac operation some patients will have agitation, nightmares or depression. Some become paranoid for a while. All of these symptoms may be due to hypoxia and this should always be ruled out before giving some powerful drug. Failure to treat hypoxia may lead to an 'unexpected' cardiac arrest.

Care of the respiratory system

In most cardiac diseases the lungs are affected. Many adults have a background of chronic lung disease. Lung function usually deteriorates for a while after cardiopulmonary bypass.

Consequently, there is always some impairment of respiratory function after cardiac surgery. In its most mild form, this impairment can be corrected by oxygen given through a face mask. More serious derangements need oxygen-enriched mechanical ventilation for a variable length of time.

The need for treatment can be assessed clinically by judgement of the patient's ventilation and by his colour. These observations are frequently misleading, however, and ideally the pressure of carbon dioxide and oxygen in the arterial blood should be measured frequently. These measurements are best performed by the medical or nursing staff in a side laboratory attached to the intensive care ward, using one of several commercially available machines.

Ventilation may be needed for 'stiff' lungs as well as impaired lung function, for the additional work involved in inflating such lungs may be exhausting to the patient.

Most units use a volume-controlled ventilator which delivers oxygen-enriched air via an endotracheal tube. The routine care of this is left to the anaesthetists but all staff should understand the principles of the ventilator in case of mechanical breakdown or power failure. Oxygen toxicity may occur if the concentration exceeds 50% and rarely should higher concentrations be necessary. All air from the ventilator should be humidified (see p. 448).

On return of the patient to the ward following operation, a chest radiograph should be taken, if possible with a few degrees of head-up tilt. Portable radiographs of this type give limited information about the heart but three major surgical problems of the lungs are detectable. These are: (1) pneumothorax, (2) haemothorax, (3) malposition of the endotracheal tube in one of the major bronchi. Each will cause severe hypoxia and should be treated immediately.

The patient is usually left on the ventilator until he has recovered from the anaesthetic. If he is then completely stable, spontaneous respiration should be allowed, leading to removal of the endotracheal tube in a few hours or minutes. If, however, there is cardiovascular instability, bleeding or any other major problem, or the blood-gas results are poor, mechanical ventilation should continue until these problems have been corrected.

Care of the chest drainage tubes

Bleeding occurs after every cardiac operation and cardiopulmonary bypass causes some impairment of the clotting mechanism. However, the major cause of haemorrhage is surgical trauma, even in the presence of a bleeding tendency, and attention to haemostasis during the operation will have a major influence on postoperative bleeding.

Even with the greatest care, some patients will bleed excessively after surgery. Blood loss is regarded as excessive if more than 500 ml are lost in 1 h or more than 300 ml/h for 3 consecutive hours. In these circumstances, it is wise to return the patient to theatre for exploration and surgical control of the bleeding points. Such a policy may be inconvenient

in the short term. However, the early termination of bleeding is necessary to avoid many problems. If bleeding continues for a long period, cardiac tamponade may occur at any time and, in all cases, a large amount of blood will be infused. This is undesirable for the patient and the blood bank. In addition, the late return to theatre may have to be hurried because of the patient's poor condition and that return is usually in the small hours of the morning. A planned early organized return to the theatre will avoid all these problems. The use of routine laboratory tests for blood clotting is not good practice since time may be wasted.

If, however, a second operation shows no surgically caused bleeding, then clotting studies are undertaken. This situation usually arises in infected repeat operations or cyanosed cases, but may appear unpredictably in an otherwise straightforward patient. Usually, it is possible to identify and correct a specific clotting deficit, but often many deficits are present, particularly if a large volume of blood has already been transfused. Haematological opinion favours the use of specific components of blood as treatment, but many surgeons prefer to use whole fresh blood taken from donors less than 4 h previously. Fresh blood reliably stops bleeding due to impaired coagulation and the only drawbacks to its use are logistical.

Microfilters are used whenever bank blood is given. Considerable evidence has accumulated which shows that blood of more than 12 h after collection contains particulate debris which can damage the lungs. Filters remove this debris and help to prevent lung damage. The use of filters is not necessary when fresh blood is being used because no debris is present. In a bleeding problem, blood should be infused according to the state of the circulatory system (see below) and the amount of blood being lost. Obsessive attention to the 'blood balance', however, ignores the dynamic changes in the circulation system and should not be allowed to obscure the treatment of the whole patient.

Most routine cases will lose 300–600 ml of blood in the first 24 h. After that time, the drainage is usually about 10–20 ml/h and the drains may be removed.

Care of the circulatory system

The function of the heart is to create a cardiac output and a satisfactory cardiac output will lead to adequate perfusion of all the body tissues, permitting normal metabolic activity.

A fall in cardiac output leads to impairment of perfusion and, therefore, a reduction in metabolic activity of some tissues. This clinical state is known as 'shock' or more recently 'low cardiac output syndrome'. The latter term is ugly, but precise. 'Shock' is widely used, but in the minds of many doctors is linked with low blood pressure rather than low cardiac output.

In nearly every cardiac surgical case, the cardiac output is assessed indirectly by recording the perfusion and metabolic activity of various tissues. In order of importance, the indirect indices of cardiac output are:

1. Urinary output (minimum 0.5 ml/kg body weight/ h. This is an index of visceral perfusion and function.
2. Skin temperature. The site of measurement is usually the big toe and this index is very useful in children.
3. The arterial blood pressure. This is important only when it falls outside wide limits, e.g. below 80 mmHg and above 120 mmHg. The presence of a normal blood pressure in an anuric, cold-skinned patient is compatible with shock.
4. The presence of metabolic acidosis which is caused by anaerobic respiration of underperfused muscle. Acidosis is a late sign of low cardiac output.

A large part of the care of the circulatory system lies in the frequent measurement of these indirect indices of cardiac output. Direct measurement of cardiac output by some form of dye or thermodilution is increasingly used.

It is very important to understand why the arterial blood pressure is given less importance in present thinking. The normal physiological response to a lowered cardiac output is for vasoconstriction to occur in all tissues apart from the cerebral and coronary circulations. This vasoconstriction maintains the blood pressure even though the cardiac output is low and the perfusion of the tissues poor. Thus, low output syndrome may be present with an *elevated* blood pressure but poor urinary output and a falling skin temperature. Conversely, a patient with a blood pressure of 85 mmHg systolic and warm skin and a good urinary output does not have low output syndrome. Excessive attention to the level of the blood pressure diverts the mind from consideration of the cardiac output.

Causes of low cardiac output

The cardiac output may be inadequate, either because the heart does not fill properly or because it fails as a pump. Table 17.2 outlines the main causes in each of these two groups. A single causative factor is uncommon except very early in the disturbance. Since treatment is influenced by the cause of the low output, the ability to distinguish between hypovolaemia and cardiogenic low output is essential. The most useful observation is the measurement of the central venous pressure.

Table 17.2 Causes of low cardiac output in cardiac surgery

A. Failure of the heart to fill – hypovolaemia
  1. True hypovolaemia:
    (a) Haemorrhage
    (b) Loss of plasma
    (c) Loss of fluid and electrolytes
    (d) Pulmonary embolism
  2. Relative hypovolaemia:
    (a) Vasodilatation of septicaemia
    (b) Vasodilatation of spinal injuries
    (c) Pharmacological vasodilatation

B. Failure of the heart as a pump
  1. Myocardial causes:
    (a) Acidosis
    (b) Electrolyte disturbances
    (c) Hypoxia/necrosis
    (d) Toxic depression
  2. Endocardial/valve causes:
    (a) Sudden regurgitation of aortic valve, e.g. endocarditis
    (b) Sudden regurgitation of mitral valve, e.g. ruptured papillary muscle
  3. Pericardial causes
    (a) Tamponade

Measurement of the central venous pressure (CVP) (Figure 17.26)

The level of pressure in the right atrium and great intrathoracic veins cannot be accurately assessed clinically.

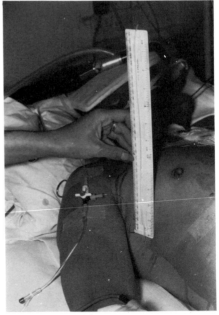

Figure 17.26 Showing measurement of the central venous pressure at the bedside

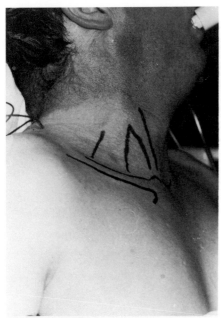

Figure 17.27 Position of the clavicular and sternal heads of the right sternomastoid muscle before insertion of an internal jugular cannula for measuring central venous pressure

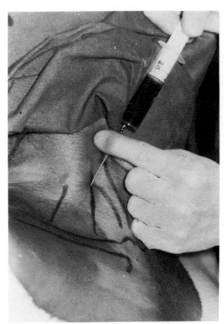

Figure 17.28 The actual cannulation during this procedure

A catheter is passed under aseptic conditions into one of these chambers. The site of insertion may be the basilic vein in the forearm, the subclavian or the internal jugular vein. Many surgeons insert a CVP catheter during operation into the left brachio-cephalic vein, but clearly this route is not always available. For reasons of simplicity and safety, the internal jugular technique is preferred and will be described in detail.

The insertion is carried out under local or general anaesthesia with the patient 15° head down and with the head half turned to the left. If general anaesthesia is used, marking of the sternal and clavicular heads of the right sternomastoid muscle (Figure 17.27) before induction will help identify these structures later.

The point of insertion of the catheter is at the apex of the triangle formed by the converging heads of the right sternomastoid muscle (Figure 17.28). A needle inserted at this point and passed downwards towards the right nipple and backwards at 30° will enter the internal jugular vein 3–4 cm from the skin. The needle is held in the right hand and the left is placed on the right common carotid artery, dis-placing it medially away from danger.

When venous blood enters the needle and attached syringe, the syringe is removed and a guide wire passed through the needle into the lumen of the vein (Figure 17.29). The needle is then slid up the

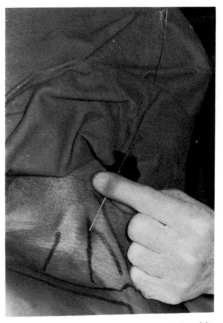

Figure 17.29 A guide wire insertion during this procedure

wire out of the patient, and discarded. The catheter is then threaded onto the wire (Figure 17.30) and passed into the superior vena cava and right atrium over the guide wire, which is then removed.

The catheter is now attached to a disposable three-way tap (Figure 17.31) and then via an

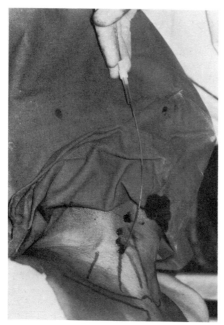

Figure 17.30 The CVP cannula being passed *over* the guide wire

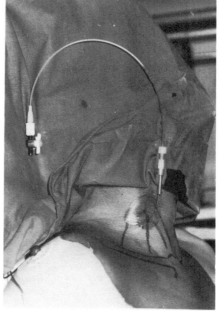

Figure 17.31 CVP cannula attached to three-way tap and intravenous infusion set

infusion set to 500 ml of 5% dextrose solution. This infusion is adjusted to run very slowly so as to prevent blood clotting in the catheter. A sterile disposable manometer lead is then attached to the third arm of the three-way tap. This manometer line is fixed to a simple ruler with graduations in centimetres.

The CVP is then measured either electronically or by adjusting the three-way tap so as to fill up the side arm with fluid from the infusion. The ruler is held vertically with its base at the level of the right anterior axillary fold (see Figure 17.26). A further turn of the three-way tap will allow the fluid in the side arm to fall to a level equal in centimetres of water to the CVP. Finally, the three-way tap is adjusted so that the system can again function as a drip with the side arm excluded.

Complications of central venous cannulation

Injury to the common carotid artery

If this artery is pushed medially with the fingers of the left hand, damage is unlikely. Should a puncture occur, the needle is withdrawn and firm pressure applied for 5 min. If the insertion of the CVP line is being performed prior to heparinization, as in open heart surgery, many surgeons would postpone the surgery for 24 h to avoid haemorrhage.

Air embolism

This complication cannot happen if the patient is placed in the head-down position described.

Pneumothorax

This is a common complication by the subclavian route, but may be completely avoided in internal jugular cannulation by never allowing the needle to penetrate the tissues by more than 4 cm.

Misplacement of the catheter

Using the route and the technique described, the only common misplacement is for the catheter to pass into the inferior vena cava. Partial removal of the catheter will remedy the problem.

Interpretation of the central venous pressure measurement

The normal CVP lies between 5 and 10 cmH$_2$O. Under most circumstances, a reading of 10 cm or more will indicate a satisfactory blood volume and a reading of less than 5 cm will indicate hypovolaemia.

However, certain major exceptions occur and should always be considered.

1. The catheter may be blocked and a false reading be made. A normally functioning CVP will show

a respiratory (slow) and a cardiac (fast) variation in the pressure column.

2. Hypovolaemia is accompanied by a varying degree of venospasm which may maintain a 'normal' CVP in the presence of hypovolaemia. If this is suspected, a volume 'challenge' to the circulation is made; 250 ml of blood, plasma or electrolyte solution are rapidly infused into the patient. The response of the CVP to this volume will indicate whether hypovolaemia is present or not. A rapid increase to, say 15–20 cmH$_2$O rules out hypovolaemia. If no changes in the CVP occurs, hypovolaemia is probably present.

3. In diseased hearts with gross elevation of left-sided pressures, the CVP may not reflect the left atrial pressure. Under these circumstances, an indirect left atrial pressure measurement is needed. The Swan-Ganz catheter is used and is passed into the pulmonary arteries via the right heart. The catheter is then advanced until it jams in a peripheral pulmonary artery of small calibre. The pressure recorded at the tip will accurately reflect the left atrial pressure.

Treatment of low output syndrome

Figure 17.32 shows the suggested course of actions once the syndrome has been diagnosed. Certain points need emphasis. There is usually more than one cause of low output present. Hypovolaemia should be treated first and then all other possible causes systematically searched for and treated, if present.

Myocardial causes

Inotropic stimulation of the heart in myocardial failure carries costs and benefits. The usual drugs used are isoprenaline, adrenaline and dopamine. Each is given intravenously into the CVP line. All inotropic agents will increase cardiac output by making the myocardium contract more vigorously. This increased contraction will, however, increase myocardial oxygen demands. Up to a point, this demand can be met by improved coronary blood flow as a result of the improved cardiac output. This point is reached when the pulse rate rises to 110/min

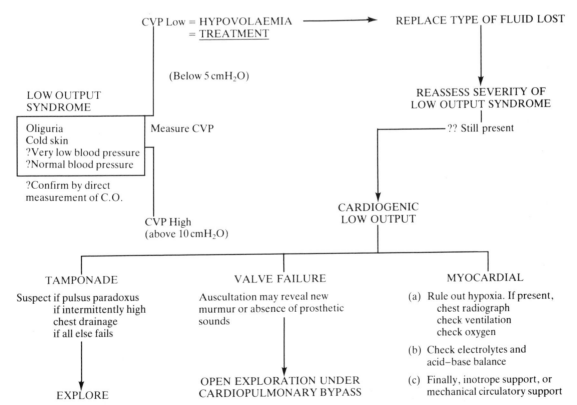

Figure 17.32 Stages of management of low output syndrome in cardiac surgery

or the systolic blood pressure to 120 mmHg. After that, myocardial damage will be caused by inotropic drugs. Should signs of low output persist, some other manoeuvre must be performed.

1. Adrenaline, isoprenaline: usually 2 mg of the drug are diluted in 500 ml of normal saline and given into the CVP line at 10–40 drops/min.
2. Dopamine: this drug is given by central infusion also. At doses of 4 µg/kg/min, there appears to be an improved cardiac output and renal vasodilatation. At 8 µg/kg/min, only the cardiac output is affected.

Acidosis

This is measured by the deviation from the normal bicarbonate level of 24 mmol/l of plasma. A deficit is corrected by giving sodium bicarbonate in the following schedule.

mmol $NaHCO_3$ required = Base deficit × 0.33 body weight/kg.

A 4.2% sodium bicarbonate solution is available on most intensive care wards and contains 0.5 mmol $NaHCO_3$/ml.

Reduction of cardiac 'afterload'

Physiological studies of the failing heart show that an increase of cardiac output can be achieved at no oxygen cost if the arterial resistance against which the heart is working can be reduced. This may be achieved by the use of arteriolar dilating agents, such as nitroglycerine by the intravenous route. This drug has a very short half-life when given intravenously and acts mainly on arterioles. Given in cautious doses, the drug lowers peripheral resistance and thereby increases cardiac output. Ideally, the cardiac output should be directly measured, but this is not necessary providing that only sufficient nitroglycerine is given to reduce the arterial blood pressure slightly. Clearly, however, the drug is inappropriate where the systolic blood pressure is below 80 mmHg systolic.

Mechanical support of the failing heart

Short-term mechanical support is available to support the failing myocardium. A 30-ml or 40-ml balloon is inserted into the descending thoracic aorta via a femoral artery. This balloon is then inflated and deflated with gas in time with the heart beat. Deflation occurs just before the aortic valve opens during cardiac systole, thereby reducing the systolic pressure and reducing the work of the heart. When diastole occurs, the balloon inflates, thus raising the diastolic pressure and improving the perfusion of all tissues including the heart.

The timing is clearly critical and is governed by electronic sensing of the electrical activity of the heart.

By following a rational approach to the management of low output syndrome, most cases can be accurately identified and treated. However, a small number of patients will fail to respond to treatment. Under these circumstances, surgical exploration of the pericardium should be performed. The diagnosis of tamponade can be very difficult and the ultimate diagnostic test is exploration. No patient should die with this highly remediable cause of low output neither diagnosed nor treated. If the patient does not have tamponade on exploration, little difference will have been made to the gloomy outlook.

Endocarditis following cardiac surgery

Transient episodes of bacteraemia are common during cardiac surgical operations and the intensive care which follows. Colonization and the development of endocarditis following these episodes are serious events, carrying a high mortality. The clinical features of endocarditis occurring with surgery may occur rapidly or may take up to a year to develop. The chances of endocarditis developing and persisting are particularly great if a foreign body, such as a prosthetic valve or patch, is inserted at the time of the operation.

Prevention

The patient who is to undergo surgery should be examined carefully to exclude foci of infection. If these are found, postponement of the operation may be justified. As part of the preoperative investigation, pathogens are looked for in the sputum and urine and are treated if present.

The routine use of prophylactic antibiotics is now universal in cardiac surgery. Commencing with an initial dose at the time of the premedication, they are continued for at least 2 days. The actual types and combinations of antibiotics are determined by the conditions under which each unit works. However, antibiotic policies should be agreed with bacteriological advice and maintained until the need for change arises.

At surgery, contamination can be reduced by restriction of movement within the operating theatre. In the intensive care ward, contamination will be minimized by careful nursing and medical procedures. Endotracheal suction is always performed by a no-touch technique using sterile, single-use, disposable catheters. All intravenous injections, whether into the patient or through drips, are given through well sterilized sites. Early removal of all indwelling foreign bodies, such as drips, venous and arterial cannulae, urinary catheters and endotracheal tubes, will further reduce the opportunity of contamination.

Daily bacteriological examination of sputum, urine and any discharges, together with culture of the tips of the removed central venous and arterial lines, is performed.

Everyday the dressings which cover the entry site of indwelling cannulae should be replaced with sterile dressings after the site has been cleaned with an iodine-containing antiseptic ointment (povidone).

Detection

Early recognition of infection is necessary for effective treatment. Many cardiac surgical units perform daily blood culture monitoring whilst the patient is in intensive care. Further cultures of the blood are taken whenever the clinical condition of the patient suggests. The most common indication for these is the persistence of a mild pyrexia for more than 3 days after surgery.

At the same time as the bacteriological culture examinations, the level of the white cell count should be determined and the trends of change noted.

Drug treatment after cardiac surgery

Digoxin

As in the preoperative period, this drug is required mainly for the control of atrial fibrillation. The usual adult dose after digitalization is 0.25 mg/day by mouth. Doses should be omitted if the pulse rate falls below 70/min.

Diuretics

Most patients will benefit by a short course of diuretics in the early postoperative period. Frusemide 40 mg daily is usually given. However, longer treatment is necessary if there is evidence of increased left atrial pressure (dilated upper lobe veins) on the chest radiograph or if peripheral oedema persists. Frusemide, in particular, causes increased potassium loss in the urine, leading to a lowered serum concentration. This low level will often cause ventricular extrasystoles and will exacerbate digitalis toxicity. Oral potassium tablets will help to avoid this depletion.

Anticoagulants

Most types of prosthetic valve require at least short-term anticoagulation to reduce the incidence of thromboembolism. Because of temporary disturbance of clotting function following bypass, anticoagulants are not needed before the second postoperative day. Usually, coumarin-type oral anticoagulants are used and a very much smaller initial dose is needed than in the non-surgical patient. Thereafter repeated monitoring of the effect of the drug is necessary, beginning with three times weekly, but eventually lengthening to once every 6 weeks.

Antiplatelet agents

Many surgeons use these drugs in an effort to reduce thromboembolism from prosthetic valves and to maintain patency of vein grafts. Commonly soluble aspirin, 300 mg daily, is given except to patients with a history of peptic ulceration or dyspepsia. Dipyridamole, 100 mg t.d.s., also has an antiplatelet effect and the two drugs are often used together.

Convalescence after cardiac surgery

The recovery after successful cardiac surgery is rapid and most patients are fit to leave hospital by the sixth or seventh postoperative day. However, the preoperative condition of the patient may have been so poor that a longer stay in hospital is necessary. This is particularly true in patients who have had mitral valve surgery after many years of illness.

Before patients leave hospital, they should have shown the ability to climb at least 20 stairs unaided. This increases their morale and lessens their feelings of dependence on the hospital. In addition, their return home allows them to live normally by going upstairs to bed. This, in turn, reduces the tendency of loving relatives to treat such patients as cardiac invalids.

For the same reasons, patients on discharge should be instructed on taking exercise. This usually begins with 5 min slow walking each day and progresses slowly to a limit determined by the age, sex and disease of each individual. An active approach to rehabilitation will improve the quality of life of all patients.

Depending on the nature of each patient's occupation, work can be resumed 6–16 weeks following surgery. In some patients who have had mitral valve disease for many years before surgery is performed, the full benefits of the operation may not be felt for perhaps 2 years and the return to work may be very slow.

Arrhythmias after cardiac surgery

Surgeons involved in the care of patients after cardiac surgery should have the ability to diagnose and treat the commonly occurring types of arrhythmia. In theory, any rhythm apart from normal sinus rhythm is an arrhythmia. However, the practical necessities of dealing with patients with heart disturbances restrict the term arrhythmia to those abnormalities of the cardiac rhythm which create serious disturbances in the circulation, either immediately or after some time. In most, urgent diagnosis and action are called for.

The use of cardioplegia during open heart surgery is associated with an increased incidence of supraventricular arrhythmia, possibly as a result of inadequate right atrial cooling.

Diagnosis

Since all patients are connected to an ECG oscilloscope, the temptation is to diagnose the nature of the arrhythmia from the visual trace. Experience shows that this is very inaccurate and a paper recording should always be made.

Sinus tachycardia

Sinus rhythm of more than 110/min in an adult, or 130 in a child, perhaps 150 in a neonate, is pathological. The three major causes of this are: (a) hypoxia; (b) hypovolaemia; and (c) cardiac tamponade. Extreme emotional stress may cause tachycardia, but should not be assumed until the other more serious causes have been excluded.

Sinus bradycardia (Figure 17.33)

This is uncommon after surgery unless beta-blocking drugs have been used.

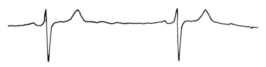

Figure 17.33 Diagram of an electrocardiogram showing sinus bradycardia

Treatment is not usually necessary until the rate falls below 50/min. Atrial pacing is the best treatment, but isoprenaline may be given as a very dilute solution into a central vein (2 mg isoprenaline in 500 ml normal saline).

Heart block (Figure 17.34)

Damage to the AV bundle during surgery may create heart block. Temporary pacing will enable most cases to maintain an adequate output whilst recovery occurs. Permanent pacing is needed for those who do not recover within 7 days.

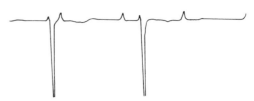

Figure 17.34 Diagram of an electrocardiogram showing complete heart block

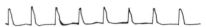

Figure 17.35 Diagram of an electrocardiogram showing atrial fibrillation

Atrial fibrillation (Figure 17.35)

Long established atrial fibrillation with a ventricular rate of between 70 and 110/min is not regarded as an arrhythmia. In the postoperative period maintenance treatment with digoxin should be continued.

Sometimes the ventricular rate becomes very fast in a patient who appears to be adequately digitalized. After excluding the causes of tachycardia given above, the rate can usually be controlled either by an extra dose of digoxin or the addition of a small dose, e.g. 5 mg i.v. of acebutolol, a beta-blocker.

The sudden onset of rapid atrial fibrillation in a patient previously in sinus rhythm can lead to low output syndrome. Once the diagnosis is established and hypoxia excluded, either rapid full intravenous digitalization or a synchronized direct current defibrillation is performed. The latter is more rapidly effective.

Ventricular extrasystoles and ventricular tachycardia (Figure 17.36)

These are life-threatening arrhythmias because they may lead, without warning, to ventricular fibrillation and cardiac arrest.

On the electrocardiogram, the ventricular extrasystole shows as a widened slurred QRS complex. The cause of these arrhythmias is ventricular irritability and this is usually a consequence of

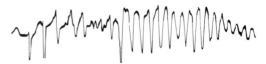

Figure 17.36 Diagram of an electrocardiogram showing ventricular extrasystoles progressing to ventricular fibrillation

temporary ventricular damage incurred at the time of surgery and a low serum potassium. Nearly all ventricular extrasystoles will respond to elevation of the serum potassium level.

During and after cardiac surgery, the level of the serum potassium is measured frequently. The safe level is between 4.5 and 5.0 mmol/l. Hyperkalaemia will lead to ventricular depression. One of the major features of modern postoperative cardiac care is the attention given to serum potassium estimations.

All the factors governing the level of serum potassium are not well understood. However, one of the most important of these is the urinary loss of potassium, which after surgery is closely linked with the volume of urine passed. By frequent (say 2-hourly) measurements of serum potassium and the amount of urine passed it is possible to gauge a patient's potassium requirement. However, the construction of the matrix shown in Table 17.3 involves a good deal of guesswork and may be grossly inaccurate. In an unstable situation, therefore, it may be necessary to measure the serum potassium at intervals of 30 min.

Table 17.3 Matrix to determine patient's potassium requirement

Urine volume per hour (ml)	Serum potassium level (mmol)		
	Below 3.5	3.5–4.5	Above 4.5
30	10	5	0
30–100	20	10	5
100	20	20	10

Very unstable – frequent measurements needed
A guide to the amount of potassium needed each hour: 1 g KCl = 14 mmol K$^+$ (approx.)

Potassium chloride must always be given intravenously by a *central route*. Injection into a peripheral vein will cause necrosis and skin loss.

A useful interim measure is possible whilst waiting for a laboratory result. The effect of 2 mmol KCl injected centrally will be enough to control temporarily most extrasystoles. Should the measurement eventually show a normal serum potassium level, no great harm will ensue from such a small dose.

In a minority of cases, attention to the level of serum potassium will not abolish ventricular extrasystoles or tachycardia. Intravenous lignocaine therapy should be given if the serum potassium is above 4.5 mmol/l. Initially, 1 mg/kg body weight of lignocaine is given as a rapid injection and this is followed by an intravenous infusion at such a rate as to control the abnormality.

Supraventricular tachycardias (Figure 17.37)

These tachycardias are associated with a normal QRS complex on the ECG but precise identification may be very difficult and an experienced cardiological opinion should be sought. The usual cause is atrial flutter with a varying degree of atrioventricular block. Treatment may consist of direct current counter shock or digitalization.

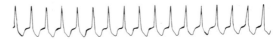

Figure 17.37 Diagram of an electrocardiogram showing supraventricular tachycardia, treated with practolol

Hyperkalaemia

Elevation of the serum potassium level above 5–5 mmol/l frequently occurs after cardiac surgery. The usual causes are:

1. Excessive administration of potassium chloride.
2. Haemolysis created by mechanical damage in the heart–lung circuit.
3. Continuation of some beta-blocking drugs up to the time of surgery. Non-cardioselective beta-blockers may inhibit the peripheral utilization of potassium.

At levels of 5.5–6.5 mmol/l treatment with intravenous frusemide, 40 mg i.v., will cause a rapid decrease of serum potassium to normal levels. If the level rises above 6.5 mmol/l, soluble insulin (10 units) and 10 g of glucose given intravenously will be effective rapidly (20 ml of 50% dextrose and 10 units soluble insulin can be accommodated in a 20 ml syringe). After 30 min, the serum potassium is again measured and the treatment repeated as necessary.

Arterial cannulation

During cardiac operations and in the intensive care ward afterwards, an arterial catheter permits continuous pressure monitoring and gives a convenient way of obtaining samples of arterial blood.

Hazards are present when an arterial line is placed and afterwards and can be greatly reduced by the use of correct techniques.

Insertion of an arterial catheter

Choice of artery

Since damage to the artery may occur which leads to its occlusion, a peripherally situated vessel is always chosen if available. In the upper limb the radial

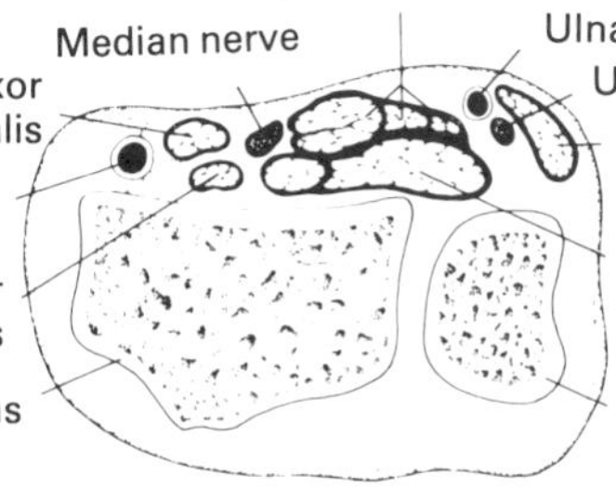

Tendons of flexor
digitorum sublimis

Median nerve

Tendon of flexor
carpi radialis

Radial artery

Tendon of flexor
pollicis longus

Radius

Ulnar artery

Ulnar nerve

Flexor carpi ulnaris

Tendons of flexor
digitorum profundus

Ulna

Figure 17.38 Diagram of a cross-section of the wrist, showing the relationships of the radial and ulnar arteries

artery at the wrist is usually used (Figure 17.38) and in the foot the dorsalis pedis.

Usually the radial artery on the non-dominant side is used. An adequate alternative circulation to the hand via the ulnar artery must be demonstrated before proceeding (Allen's test). This involves digital pressure on the radial and ulnar vessels at the wrist, causing the hand to blanch (Figure 17.39). Release of the ulnar artery whilst maintaining pressure on the radial will demonstrate an adequate alternative circulation if flushing occurs. This test is clearly necessary before cannulating a radial artery which may turn out to be the only arterial supply to the hand.

Percutaneous cannulation

An infiltration of 2 ml of 0.5% lignocaine by a no-touch technique before the operator scrubs and puts on sterile gloves will provide anaesthesia and some arterial dilatation. An assistant supports the wrist and hand in a moderately dorsiflexed position with the forearm supinated. The wrist and forearm are then prepared with 0.5% chlorhexidine in spirit. A plastic cannula is mounted on a 5 ml syringe filled with normal saline.

The artery is located by touch and the cannula on its needle advanced through the skin. As the artery is approached, a pulsation may be detected through the needle and the syringe barrel is gently withdrawn as the needle is advanced into the lumen of the artery (Figure 17.40). A jet of red blood will enter the syringe when the lumen is entered. Holding the syringe and needle absolutely still with the left hand, the cannula is advanced into the arterial lumen until the hub is next to the skin entry point. The needle and attached syringe are removed.

The cannula bleeds arterial blood and a three-way tap and flushing system are now attached (Figure 17.41) and blood in the cannula is washed away by flushing the system with normal saline. The cannula is retained in position by tying a thick linen ligature around the level on the hub. The ligature is then firmly attached to the arm by adhesive strapping (Figure 17.42).

Arterial cut-down

The operator infiltrates the wrist with local anaesthetic before scrubbing and donning sterile gown and gloves. The wrist is held in the position already

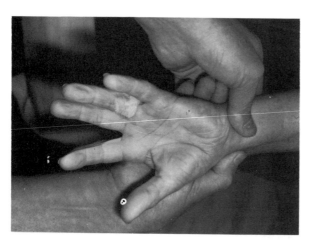

Figure 17.39 Allen's test

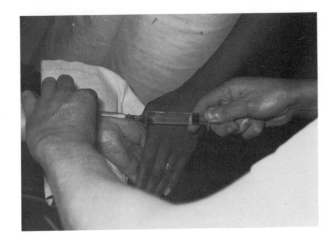

Figure 17.40 Radial artery cannulation

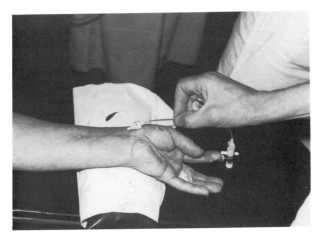

Figure 17.41 Connection of the three-way tap and flushing system

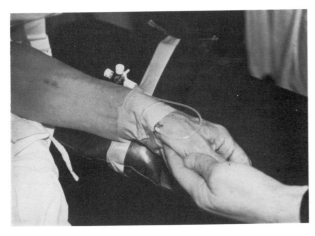

Figure 17.42 Method of fixation of the arterial cannula

described and then the area is painted with chlorhexidine in spirit and towelled.

A 2 cm transverse incision is made over the radial artery approximately 2 cm proximal to the base of the thenar eminence at the level of the proximal skin crease.

Using artery forceps the soft tissues above the artery are separated and the artery exposed. The haemostat is then used to pass non-absorbable ligatures around the artery above and below the site of insertion of the cannula. The distal ligature is tied, the proximal one is not tied but held in a pair of artery forceps.

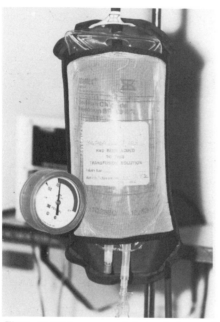

Figure 17.43 The pressure infusion device attached to the arterial cannula in order to maintain patency

Using fine pointed scissors a small transverse cut is made in the artery between the two ligatures. Bleeding is controlled by traction on the proximal, untied ligature.

The same cannula already described but without its accompanying needle is attached to a filled syringe of saline. The cannula is advanced along the lumen of the artery and flushed. Both ligatures are then tied. Two sutures close the skin incision and then the cannula is secured as already described.

Care of the arterial cannula

The cannula must be flushed continually with a small volume of normal saline in order to keep it patent. A 0.5 litre flexible bag of normal saline is placed in a pressure bag (Figure 17.43) and the pressure increased to around 300 mmHg.

The infusion set leading from the saline is attached to a device which allows 3 ml of fluid per hour into the cannula. At the same time, the device allows constant recordings of arterial pressure to be made. Such devices are commercially available and a commonly used one is shown in Figure 17.44.

This system avoids the need for repeated injections from a syringe to maintain the patency of the cannula. In addition to being more efficient in this respect, the introduction of small arterial emboli is avoided. Such emboli can block small side branches of the radial artery which supply small areas of the skin of the forearm and may cause areas of skin necrosis.

Insertion of a balloon flotation catheter (e.g. Swan-Ganz)

Surgeons are increasingly aware of the need to understand the level of left-sided filling pressures in order to maximize cardiac action. In some cases, a

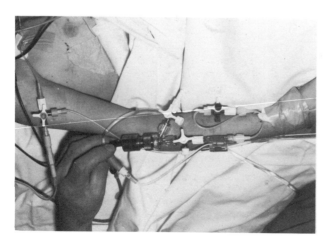

Figure 17.44 A device which permits the constant infusion of a very small volume of fluid into the arterial cannula

direct left atrial pressure line is inserted during operation. (However, the use of a balloon flotation catheter inserted through the internal jugular vein and advanced into a distal pulmonary arteriole provides just as reliable information, and has the additional advantage that the catheter may be inserted clinically.

The usual route of insertion is by the internal jugular vein, as for central venous cannulation. The catheter is attached to a pressure monitor and advanced into the right atrium with the balloon deflated. On entering the right atrium, the pressure tracing will show characteristic 'a' and 'v' waves. The balloon is then inflated and the catheter advanced. In most cases, the catheter will then pass into the right ventricle with its characteristic pressure curve. Further advancement of the catheter leads to the pulmonary artery. The catheter is then finally inserted with the balloon inflated to the point where it occludes a small pulmonary arteriole and then the pressure tracing again becomes atrial in character, reflecting the left atrial pressure.

Not infrequently, the catheter fails to pass from the right atrium into the ventricle and instead goes into the inferior vena cava. The balloon should be deflated and the catheter pulled back so that its tip lies in the right atrium again. The whole procedure of balloon inflation and catheter advancement is then repeated until success is achieved.

The step which is very dangerous and should never be done is to advance the catheter tip into the pulmonary arterial tree into a 'wedge' position with the balloon deflated. If the balloon is subsequently inflated, rupture of the pulmonary arteriole will occur and lead to bleeding within the lung and even into the tracheobronchial tree. Fatal haemorrhage has been recorded.

Pulmonary bleeding may rarely occur despite strict adherence to all the rules. Most patients who sustain this complication are elderly and often suffer with mitral valve disease. Caution should be exercised in these cases and the dangers weighed against the need for information.

Those patients who have undergone tricuspid valve surgery, whether repair or replacement, are amongst the most difficult in whom to place a balloon flotation catheter and often the procedure has to be abandoned. The difficulties and dangers associated with the measurement of indirect left atrial pressure are sufficiently great to lead to the prudent surgeon inserting a direct left atrial pressure line during surgery, especially in patients with mitral or tricuspid valve disease.

Measurement of pulmonary artery pressure

In subjects with a normal pulmonary vascular resistance, the mean left atrial pressure is about equal to the diastolic pressure within the pulmonary artery. In patients undergoing aortic or coronary artery operation, the measurement of the diastolic pulmonary artery pressure gives useful information without the dangers of left atrial cannulation or of the balloon flotation catheter. The pulmonary artery pressure cannula is inserted during operation into the right ventricle and advanced into the main pulmonary artery. The cannula is removed before the chest drains – usually at 18–24 h after surgery. In its routine use in every suitable case for 8 years, we have encountered one case of bleeding which was due to the cannula being inserted by the infundibulum rather than the main chamber of the right ventricle.

Removal of arterial cannulae

The strapping around the cannula is removed and the cannula is pulled out of the artery. Firm digital pressure for 5 min (as measured on a clock) will be sufficient to control the bleeding which follows.

Pain relief after cardiothoracic operations

Pain always occurs after any surgical operation and its relief is a major part of postoperative care. Unfortunately, the relief is frequently only partial and the patient suffers extreme discomfort for a number of days afterwards. Several reasons account for this deplorable situation:

1. The intensity of pain after an operation is only truly understood by those who have experienced surgery personally.
2. Failure to realize that individuals have different pain thresholds.
3. The reluctance to administer sufficient drugs because of worries concerning respiratory depression.
4. Techniques of administration not allowing drugs to work fully and quickly.
5. Attitudes amongst some nursing and medical staff regarding the 'improving' qualities of some discomfort after surgery.

Adequate relief of pain will not only ensure a high patient morale but also promote a smooth postoperative recovery. In no field of surgery is this more true than in cardiothoracic surgery. Good relief of pain after a chest operation will allow a patient to breathe and cough more adequately, thus avoiding respiratory complications. Inadequate pain relief will cause inadequate depth of respirations and coughing, leading to poor removal of bronchial secretions. This in turn leads to small airway obstruction and subsequent collapse and infection.

Thus the house surgeon's duty to his patient is to ensure adequate pain relief for moral and practical reasons. How can pain relief be safely and effectively achieved? First, a powerful drug must be used. The morphine derivatives are probably the best and these drugs are titrated into each patient by using small (say 5 mg in an adult) doses intravenously every 5 min until pain is relieved. Our experience over 15 years has shown that pain relief always occurs before significant respiratory depression and no patient managed in this way has ever developed respiratory failure. The intravenous route is ideal because it allows the drug to work quickly and effectively and removes doubts as to whether absorption has occurred.

Most patients managed in this way have no pain whatsoever. In addition, there is a degree of mild euphoria which is a bonus to most patients just after an operation. Measurement of blood gas levels will show a slight elevation of the P_{CO_2} to around 6 kPa.

In those few cases where morphine is poorly tolerated causing nausea or vomiting, another morphine derivative such as diamorphine, is usually effective.

In practice, intravenous administration of morphine can be achieved by repeated injections into a suitably cleaned rubber fitting on the drip tubing which all patients have after cardiothoracic surgery. Later, repeated injections may be made into an indwelling cannula (butterfly needle). Thus the repeated injection technique can easily be taught to nursing staff.

In the past few years postoperative analgesia has been provided by the use of epidural analgesia. However, this technique demands a high degree of expertise in the surgeon's colleagues and is time-consuming to initiate. This technique can never provide a complete substitute for adequate parenteral analgesia which is applicable to all groups of patients.

Bronchoscopy

The flexible fibreoptic bronchoscope is now in wide use by physicians for the diagnosis of pulmonary disease. This instrument has two main drawbacks, however: it does not permit the operator to assess the amount of rigidity in the trachea and bronchial tree and the ability to remove secretions and foreign bodies is at present very limited.

All thoracic surgeons use the rigid bronchoscope as a final preoperative test before pulmonary surgery. Rigid bronchoscopy for the removal of viscid bronchial secretions is widely practised, and is particularly valuable in the tired patient who has had major surgery of any kind.

The accumulation of secretions in the bronchial tree will lead to bronchial obstruction and atelectasis. This in turn leads to impairment of lung function and bronchopneumonia. Clearly prevention of accumulation is very important and relies mainly on physiotherapy and adequate analgesia. However, these measures may partially or wholly fail and then the patient begins to present a characteristic picture. The breathing becomes more rapid and shallow and rattles are heard in the chest. The skin becomes sweaty and the patient often becomes exhausted and irrational from hypoxia. Further encouragement to cough is clearly useless at this stage and will exhaust the patient even further.

By removal of the secretions in the large airways bronchoscopy will allow better ventilation and give the patient some rest, after which he will cough more effectively. Bronchoscopy for toilet purposes after major surgery is extremely valuable but often used reluctantly at a late stage when bronchopneumonia is present. Earlier and more frequent use would prevent many 'postoperative chests'.

Delay in bronchoscoping a patient because of undue attention to the measured levels of blood gases is not advisable. Exhaustion and an ineffective cough in the presence of increasing accumulation of secretions indicate the need for early bronchoscopy and suction under local anaesthesia. All surgeons in training should familiarize themselves with the technique.

Technique

Most patients are so distressed that a benzocaine lozenge is not tolerated. Surface anaesthesia to the mouth, pharynx and larynx is provided by a spray containing 10 ml of 4% lignocaine. This is best applied by gently inserting a laryngoscope and spraying the pharynx and larynx under vision. A further 2 ml of 4% lignocaine may be instilled into the trachea by an injection through the cricothyroid membrane (Figure 17.45).

Figure 17.46 shows the ideal position of the patient, with his neck extended. The operator stands behind him on a stool. Before inserting the bronchoscope, the operator checks that the light is working and that the suction apparatus is attached to a wide-bore suction tube. For his own protection the surgeon should wear gloves and eye protection of some sort. The bronchoscope is held in the right hand with the beak forward. The patient's upper jaw is held by the index and middle fingers of the left hand passed into the patient's mouth. The bronchoscope is passed into the pharynx and the uvula visualized. The operator then directs the instrument into the lower pharynx until the epiglottis is seen. In order to achieve this, the right hand must be gently pulled back, using the fingers of the left hand as a fulcrum. Once the epiglottis is located, the bronchoscope beak is passed beyond it and the vocal cords visualized. The instrument is then turned through 90° in its long axis and passed through the cords and

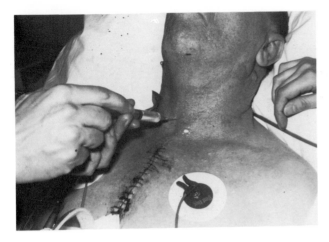

Figure 17.45 Therapeutic bronchoscopy:
injection of local anaesthetic into the trachea
via the cricothyroid membrane

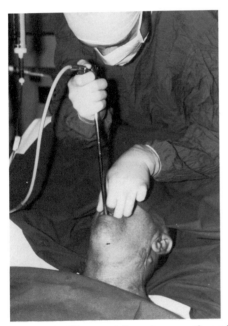

Figure 17.46 Therapeutic bronchoscopy: the position of
the patient and surgeon

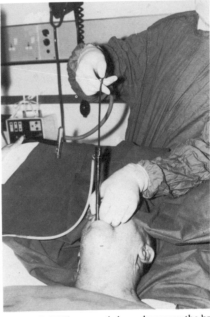

Figure 17.47 Therapeutic bronchoscopy: the bronchoscope
being inserted and suction applied

into the trachea. Suction of secretions then begins
(Figure 17.47). Attention must be paid to both sides
and more secretions will be mobilized if a physiotherapist encourages deep respirations and applies
vibration at the end of expiration.

The procedure is very well tolerated by this group

of ill patients. The secret is to apply topical
anaesthesia at least 5 min before attempting to
introduce the bronchoscope. General anaesthesia is
undesirable because of its dangers in such patients
and because the removal of secretions is less
efficient.

18

Management of gastrointestinal cases

D. H. Johnston

Most abdominal operations carry a risk of complications which at worst may be life-threatening and at best may cause distress and a prolonged stay in hospital. One of the foremost responsibilities of all members of the surgical team is to anticipate and, where possible, avoid such problems. By attention to detail, thinking ahead and good communication, each member of the surgical team can contribute to this process.

Symptoms of alimentary tract disease

Diseases of the gastrointestinal tract may give rise to a wide variety of presenting symptoms and signs. A careful history and physical examination are essential in diagnosis and to avoid over-investigation.

Dysphagia

Difficulty in swallowing is one of the most serious alimentary symptoms. Progressive dysphagia to solids and then to semi-solid or liquid food suggests an underlying carcinoma of the oesophagus or gastric cardia. Very gradual onset may be due to development of a peptic stricture secondary to gastro-oesophageal reflux disease or due to achalasia. Sudden complete dysphagia may be due to impaction of a bolus of food in the lower oesophagus or to a foreign body.

Anorexia and weight loss

Loss of appetite is a non-specific symptom which may occur in a variety of diseases. It is also a frequent presenting feature of gastric carcinoma.

Weight loss in a patient who professes to be eating normally may be an early clue to an underlying malignancy. Weight loss may occasionally be due to malabsorption.

Dyspepsia

Epigastric discomfort related to or relieved by food may occur in a number of conditions including cholelithiasis, peptic ulceration and gastric malignancy. Duodenal ulceration typically gives rise to burning discomfort in the upper epigastrium radiating to the back. Symptoms occur some hours after eating and during the night and are relieved by milky foods or antacids. Gallstones can cause a cramping pain in the epigastrium and right hypochrondrium which may radiate to the right side of the back or the right shoulder. It may be associated with fatty foods and often occurs soon after eating. There is marked nausea and it may be partially relieved by vomiting.

Abdominal pain

Pain arising from the gastrointestinal tract is perceived as a dull ill-defined discomfort. Its location is related to the embryological origin of the affected segment of gut. Pain from the upper gastrointestinal tract is referred to the epigastric area, while pain arising from the colon is located below the umbilicus. Pain in the periumbilical area may arise from the distal small intestine. Colicky pain which waxes and wanes and prompts the sufferer to move restlessly frequently accompanies intestinal obstruction. Local tenderness irritated by movement or coughing suggests inflammation of the parietal peritoneum. This type of pain is more accurately localized and prompts the sufferer to lie still.

Altered bowel habit

In adulthood most individuals have a regularly established pattern of bowel frequency and, unless there is a marked change in the diet, it is generally constant. Alteration in bowel habit may be due to a variety of systemic conditions, or to diseases of the gastrointestinal tract. Infective agents such as *Salmonella* or *Shigella* species can be detected by culture and microscopy of fresh stool samples. Chronic diarrhoea may suggest inflammatory bowel disease. Carcinoma of the proximal colon often causes looseness of stools. Abuse of proprietary laxatives is occasionally encountered.

Decreased frequency and increased solidity of the stool can be due to various medications, dehydration, immobility or medical conditions such as hypothyroidism. They are also frequent symptoms in patients with colonic carcinoma.

Dark stools may be due to gastrointestinal tract bleeding or medications such as ferrous sulphate or bismuth salts. Pale stools may occur in obstructive jaundice and in malabsorptive conditions.

Vomiting

Vomiting accompanied by abdominal pain may suggest biliary colic or intestinal obstruction. Copious vomiting of large volumes may occur in gastric outlet obstruction. Dark coloration of the vomitus (coffee ground vomiting) may suggest gastric bleeding, which should be confirmed by chemical testing.

Upper gastrointestinal bleeding

Intermittent chronic bleeding may occur from an occult carcinoma situated in the gastric fundus. The stool should be tested for faecal occult blood. More severe bleeding may lead to passage of melaena – loose black sticky stools with a tarry appearance and a characteristic odour. Brisk haemorrhage can lead to the passage of burgundy-coloured or even bright red blood per rectum. Haematemesis suggests heavy upper gastrointestinal tract haemorrhage.

Rectal bleeding

Passage of bright red blood after defaecation may be due to haemorrhoids or an anal fissure. Discovery of haemorrhoids does not obviate the need for further investigations to exclude other pathology. Bleeding may also be due to a polyp, cancer or diverticular disease. Bleeding due to angiodysplasia most often arises in the proximal colon and is difficult to localize.

Signs of alimentary tract disease

General signs of alimentary tract disease

The facies may suggest weight loss, anaemia or the discoloration due to jaundice. Angular stomatitis or smooth atrophic glossitis is seen in anaemia. Aphthous mouth ulcers occur in inflammatory bowel disease and circumoral pigmentation may suggest the rare Peutz–Jeghers syndrome. Pigmentation of the axillae and limb flexures (acanthosis nigricans) can accompany gastric and other malignancies. Metastatic skin deposits can occur from alimentary tract tumours. The skin at the umbilicus is occasionally involved (Sister Joseph's nodule).

The hands may reveal palmar erythema (liver disease), koilonychia (anaemia) or finger clubbing (inflammatory bowel disease). The lymph node areas should be carefully examined. Virchow's node in the left supraclavicular fossa is often involved by metastatic carcinoma.

Abdominal signs

The patient should be examined lying supine with his hands by his sides and a single pillow beneath his head.

Inspection may reveal abdominal distension or a visible mass. Peristalsis may be visible with intestinal obstruction or excessive epigastric pulsation with an aneurysmal abdominal aorta. Decreased respiratory movement (splinting) suggests peritonism. Surgical scars suggest the possibility of adhesions or recurrent pathology. Skin excoriation suggests itching, perhaps due to liver disease. Venous dilation in the flanks may be due to obstruction of the inferior vena cava. Dilated veins distributed radially around the umbilicus indicate portal vein thrombosis (caput medusae).

Palpation and percussion are intended to reveal abdominal masses, visceral enlargement or areas of tenderness. The abdominal viscera are normally soft and not individually palpable, though faecal material in the colon may be readily palpable, and on deep palpation can usually be indented. Aortic pulsation is usually palpable in the epigastrium, particularly during held expiration. Resistance to palpation (guarding) due to increased tone of the abdominal wall musculature occurs in response to peritoneal inflammation. Generalized peritonitis due to a perforated duodenal ulcer can cause a board-like abdominal rigidity. In acute pancreatitis, the abdomen is frequently soft, though extremely tender. Local pain due to peritoneal inflammation is aggravated by movement, coughing, percussion or sudden withdrawal of a steady pressure (rebound tenderness).

Riedel's lobe of the liver projecting below the costal margin is a normal anatomical variant. Hepatic metastases may be palpable below the right costal margin or in the epigastrium. A distended gallbladder will be palpable in the right upper quadrant.

Renal masses arise in the flanks and descend on inspiration. A much enlarged spleen may be felt below the left costal margin. It descends on deep inspiration and is dull to percussion. A non-tender mass may be neoplastic whilst a tender mass suggests an inflammatory cause, e.g. Crohn's disease.

Auscultation of bowel sounds is used to assess bowel motility. Bowel sounds increase with gastrointestinal bleeding and intestinal obstruction, and decrease due to paralytic ileus in peritonitis. It is necessary to listen for several minutes; normal bowel motility is quiescent at times.

Abdominal examination is not considered complete without a rectal examination.

Preparing for planned abdominal surgery

An unnecessarily long preoperative stay heightens anxiety, carries an increased risk of wound infection by hospital acquired pathogens and thromboembolic complications. Before meeting the patient the house surgeon should know what treatment is proposed and read any relevant correspondence. This can avoid embarrassing confusion, is reassuring to the patient and helps an expedient evaluation. Information about previous illness and treatment can often be ascertained in greater detail from the patient's records. The admitting doctor should be satisfied that the diagnosis is correct, the proposed operation necessary (and desired by the patient) and that the patient is fit to have it performed.

Preoperative investigations

All patients should have their temperature, pulse rate, blood pressure and weight recorded on admision, and a sample of urine should be tested for glucose and protein. The need for additional investigations is determined by the patient's general health, the illness and the proposed surgery.

Cardiorespiratory investigations

Most anaesthetists prefer to see a preoperative chest radiograph and ECG in patients over the age of 40 years. Preoperative chest physiotherapy and sputum culture are advisable in patients with chronic respiratory disease and heavy smokers (see Chapters 11 and 31).

Haematological investigations

Many chronic abdominal conditions may lead to anaemia due to blood loss, malabsorption or vitamin deficiency. If there is suspected liver disease, clotting parameters should be checked. Patients from Africa and the Caribbean should be tested for sickle cell anaemia. Unanticipated bleeding may occur during any laparotomy and blood should be grouped. For major procedures several units of cross-matched blood should be available in the theatre before the operation.

Biochemical and serological studies

Urea and electrolytes should be checked in elderly patients or if there is a history of renal or cardiovascular disease, diabetes, vomiting or diarrhoea. Serum protein and albumin may help identify patients with malnutrition. Liver enzyme assays are indicated in suspected liver disease and screening for hepatitis B surface antigens in patients who have had previous jaundice.

Obtaining consent for surgery

It is a legal requirement to obtain fully informed consent from a patient prior to surgery or in the case of a child from the parent or legal guardian. It is advisable for the surgeon who will perform the operation to see the patient and to discuss the treatment. A consent form signed after anaesthetic premedication is not legally valid. It is a sensible safeguard to mark the operation site if there is any possibility that the wrong incision could be made.

Prophylactic antibiotics

The healthy stomach and small intestine contain few bacteria; however many diseases cause extensive colonization. Patients with gastric carcinoma have decreased acid production and extensive bacterial colonization of the stomach. Similarly, inflammatory and obstructive conditions of the small intestine carry increased risks of sepsis. The colon contains vast numbers of pathogenic bacteria. Any antibiotic regimen for colonic surgery must cover a very wide spectrum. One well tried regimen consists of ampicillin with metronidazole and *either* gentamicin *or* a broad-spectrum cephalosporin intravenously for 48 h beginning at induction of anaesthesia.

Bowel preparation

Apart from an overnight fast prior to surgery, bowel preparation is not essential for most elective gastric or small intestinal procedures. Administration of an oral laxative is advisable if barium from recent contrast studies may still be retained within the bowel as dense concretions can otherwise develop. Physical preparation of the colon for elective colonic surgery can be achieved by administration of oral sodium picosulphate (Picolax) for 24 h prior to surgery. A suitable regimen is described in Chapter 20.

Prophylaxis of deep vein thrombosis

Abdominal procedures carry a high risk of thromboembolic complications. The risks are greatest in obese patients, and those who develop postoperative sepsis or are slow to regain mobility. The following preventive measures are recommended:

1. In the weeks before surgery:
   (a) Stop smoking.
   (b) Weight reduction, if obese.
   (c) Oestrogen-containing oral contraceptive agents also increase the risk of thromboembolism and should be discontinued for several weeks prior to elective surgery.
   (d) Correction of any dehydration.
2. At the time of operation:
   (a) Anticoagulation with subcutaneous heparin, 5000 units 8-hourly beginning prior to surgery and continuing until the patient has regained mobility.
   (b) This may be combined with graduated compression (TED) stockings or other mechanical methods.
3. After the operation:
   (a) Continuation of antithrombotic measures until the patient is fully ambulant.
   (b) Active exercise of calf muscles.
   (c) Early mobilization.

Surgical management

Choosing an incision

Incisions should be adequate to allow the chosen procedure to be performed safely. It is unwise to cause extra risk to a patient by struggling to perform an operation through a small incision. The use of

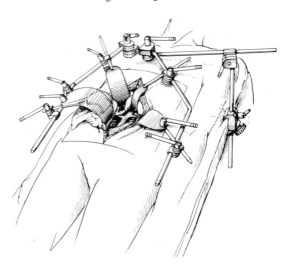

Figure 18.1 'Omnitract' fixed frame retractor

precision engineered fixed retractor frames with interchangeable retractor blades can improve exposure for many procedures (Figure 18.1).

The midline incision

The modern approach to most major abdominal procedures is by a vertical (midline) incision. This has the advantage that it can easily be extended either upwards or downwards if exposure proves difficult. It can be rapidly closed by the single layer mass suture technique and heals well with a low incidence of complications.

The paramedian incision

This is an alternative to the midline incision and remains popular with some surgeons. It is more time consuming to open and to suture than the midline incision, but offers good exposure and heals well. A paramedian incision which offers excellent access for one procedure may not always be the optimal incision for another abdominal procedure, should the patient be unfortunate enough to require further surgery.

The grid iron incision

This is the incision of choice for the removal of an acutely inflamed appendix in a young person. It is not advocated in patients over the age of 50 years as it does not allow satisfactory laparotomy and there is an increased probability of a concomitant pathology or a mistaken diagnosis.

Table 18.1 Characteristics of suture materials

Suture material	Characteristics	Possible applications
Chromic catgut	Rapidly absorbed Low tensile strength	Suture of urothelium, common bile duct
Vicryl	Slowly reabsorbed	Gastric and small intestinal anastomoses. Ligatures
Dexon	Slowly reabsorbed	Gastric and small intestinal anastomoses. Ligatures
Braided silk	Non-absorbable Knots well	Colonic and oesophageal anastomoses
Braided nylon (Nurolon) Monofilament nylon	Non-absorbable Non-absorbable High tensile strength Recoil memory	Colonic and oesophageal anastomoses Wound closure Hernia repair
Monofilament polypropylene (Prolene)	Non-absorbable High tensile strength Recoil memory	Wound closure Hernia repair
Monofilament polydioxanone sulphate (PDS)	High tensile strength Very slowly reabsorbed	Wound closure

Ligatures and sutures

Traditionally the most widely used materials have been chromic catgut and silk. Chromic catgut loses tensile strength rapidly and is reabsorbed over a number of weeks. It is suitable for suturing rapidly healing epithelia such as gastric mucosa and for bile ducts and the urinary tract where non-absorbable material might form a nidus for stone formation. Where healing may be slow and sustained strength is required, a non-absorbable material should be used. Examples include the seromuscular layers of the rectum or oesophagus. Traditionally braided silk sutures have been most widely used. Newer materials can also be classified as absorbable and non-absorbable, and a selection of suitable materials is now available for most purposes (see Table 18.1).

Avoiding adhesions

Postoperative adhesions cause considerable morbidity. The factors which predispose to the development of adhesions are not understood. Talc powder from surgical gloves can give rise to adhesion formation and, if gloves packaged with powdered talc are used, they should be washed before use.

Avoiding sepsis

Postoperative intra-abdominal sepsis may develop when contaminating bacteria are left in the peritoneal cavity in sufficient numbers to overwhelm natural defences. In most cases the bacteria have originated from a hollow viscus opened during the procedure. Skin organisms rarely cause postoperative intra-abdominal sepsis unless a prosthetic device has been implanted.

Patients undergoing surgery on the gastrointestinal tract require broad-spectrum intravenous antibiotic therapy. Mechanical cleansing of the peritoneal cavity by irrigation with a solution of broad-spectrum antibiotic (e.g. tetracycline, 1 mg/ml) in warmed saline diminishes the risk. Necrotic material such as pedicles of ligatured tissue can form a focus for development of sepsis.

Drainage of the peritoneal cavity

Few aspects of surgery provoke such controversy as the indications for peritoneal drainage. The only type of surgical drains currently in widespread use are sealed tubular drainage systems, often connected to a suction vessel. There is uncertainty about the value of peritoneal drainage in many situations. They allow drainage of blood which accumulates during the first few hours after surgery. Clots will not be removed though with retraction exuded serum may be drained away. The lumen of a tube drain affords a recess in which an anaerobic environment can develop, promoting the risk of sepsis. Most drains soon become walled off, effectively draining only a small local area. Positioning of drains near anastomoses may increase the risk of anastomotic leakage. Drainage of the gallbladder bed after cholecystectomy may draw attention to potentially serious leakage of bile from the denuded liver surface. Drainage is not necessary after surgery for acute appendicitis unless complicated by abscess formation.

Postoperative management

The care of patients after abdominal surgery depends upon the magnitude and nature of the operation which has been performed. Some procedures, e.g. herniorrhaphy, are simple and straightforward and the patient may return to his home the same evening. Other procedures involve extensive excision or reconstruction and the patient will require intensive monitoring and diligent postoperative care.

Food and drink

Patients should be allowed to eat and drink as soon as it is safe to do so. Even after minor procedures it is advisable not to eat and drink for the first few hours as the delayed effects of anaesthetic agents may cause nausea and vomiting. After more major procedures it is necessary to allow the intestinal tract to rest and recover for a variable period. Gastric suture lines may disrupt or bleed if the stomach should become overdistended and decompression by a nasogastric tube is necessary. Administration of oral fluid before the intestine has regained its normal propulsive activity will lead to distension, discomfort, nausea and vomiting. Oral fluid intake should resume gradually with intake of 30–50 ml of clear fluids hourly for the first 12 h. If this is well tolerated, the amount of fluid can be gradually increased. When the patient has tolerated 120 ml/h for 12 h or so and feels hungry, it is safe to begin to take soft solids such as custard, soups or ice-cream.

Intravenous fluids

The purpose of postoperative intravenous fluid administration is to prevent dehydration until the patient is able to drink normally. Most patients return from theatre haemodynamically stable and with an intravenous infusion running. In uncomplicated cases this can be stopped after 24–48 h as normal peristalsis returns. In complicated cases recovery may take many days and maintenance of fluid and electrolyte balance requires considerable skill and attention. Loss of intestinal secretions due to gastric aspiration, intestinal obstruction or external fistulae should be separately recorded to permit appropriate replacement (Table 18.2).

Unless there is renal dysfunction, urine output serves as a rough guide to the adequacy of fluid replacement. A urine output in excess of 30 ml/h is considered satisfactory. The osmotic diuresis which accompanies glycosuria can cause a misleadingly high urine output despite developing hypovolaemia and dehydration. If the urine output falls and the urine becomes concentrated, the general fluid balance of the patient should be re-evaluated. Correction of the underlying deficit will normally restore urine output. Use of diuretics under these circumstances is inappropriate. If prolonged intravenous fluid administration is necessary serum electrolytes should be checked regularly.

Nasogastric aspiration

Nasogastric tubes (Figure 18.2) are exceedingly unpleasant for the patient and predispose to respiratory infection. After many abdominal operations nasogastric decompression is not necessary and patients should not be subjected to the distress of prolonged nasogastric intubation unless it is clearly indicated. Initially nasogastric tubes should be aspirated at regular intervals and left on free drainage between aspirations. It is safe to allow patients with nasogastric tubes to take a small quantity of water by mouth. This helps to ease discomfort by moistening the oropharynx and poses no risk to the patient.

As gastric emptying resumes oral fluids may be increased to 60 ml/h, the tube can be aspirated 4-hourly and spigoted between aspirations. When the aspirate is consistently less than the oral intake, the tube can be safely removed.

Table 18.2 Electrolyte content of gastrointestinal secretions

Secretion	Na^+ (mEq/l)	K^+ (mEq/l)	Cl^- (mEq/l)	HCO_3^- (mEq/l)	Volume (ml/day)
Saliva	4–8	20–30	12–18	30	800–2000
Gastric	50–115	10–30	30–120	0	500–4000
Duodenal	130–140	10	70–90	0	500–2000
Bile	140–160	10	120–160	30–50	250–800
Pancreas	130–160	5	50–80	90–125	200–700
Ileum	100–140	5	50–130	20–30	500–6000

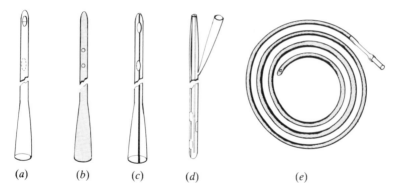

(a)   (b)   (c)   (d)   (e)

Figure 18.2 Nasogastric tubes: (a) Plastic; (b) Ryle; (c) Levin; (d) Salem; (e) Portex

Management of abdominal drains

Surgeons differ greatly in their management of abdominal drains. Many surgeons like to have drains shortened on the third or fourth day and then removed the following day. Others remove all drains at 24 or 48 h without apparent detriment. The policy observed should be that approved by the surgeon responsible for the patients, and the junior surgeon is best advised to acquaint himself with the preferred practice of his senior colleagues and adhere to it.

Management of the wound

Most wounds are covered with an absorbent dressing which is left undisturbed unless there is a particular indication to inspect it, such as an unexplained fever or a discharge from the wound. Some surgeons leave abdominal incisions completely uncovered without apparent detriment. If there is an intestinal stoma it is wise to isolate the wound with a watertight dressing or an aerosol spray of 'plastic' polymer materials. Expensive dressings should be avoided as should unnecessary interference with clean dressings. Skin sutures are removed on the tenth to twelfth postoperative day. Self-absorbing subcuticular sutures are increasingly used.

Mobilization

Most patients can begin to mobilize on the first postoperative day. Initially this may amount to little more than assisted transfer into a bedside chair for a brief period. Thereafter a progressive increase should be encouraged. Intravenous drips can be disconnected temporarily to assist mobilization. Elderly patients in particular should be encouraged to be self-caring as soon as possible, a process which may require considerable patience and compassion.

Peptic ulceration

Peptic ulcer disease includes both duodenal and gastric ulceration. Damage to the epithelial lining of the stomach or duodenum may be due to loss of protection of the mucosa, to the action of gastric acid, digestive enzymes or bile salts. A significant proportion of patients with duodenal ulceration produce excessive amounts of gastric acid, whereas only a small proportion of gastric ulcer patients have hyperacidity. Refluxing bile salts or other agents may play a greater role in the gastric ulceration.

The management of these conditions has undergone a dramatic change during the last decade as a result of the advent of the H_2-receptor blocking class of drugs and medical treatment of *Helicobacter pylori* infection. Operation is often not needed.

Duodenal ulcers are more common than gastric ulcers and occur predominantly in young to middle-aged men. The commonest symptom is a burning epigastric discomfort in the mid or upper epigastrium, sometimes with radiation to the back. It is associated with a sensation of hunger. Nocturnal symptoms are common and eating milky foods generally affords relief. Symptoms are episodic and worsened by psychological stress. Smoking, strong alcoholic spirits and aspirin are aggravating factors. The diagnosis is most easily established by gastroscopy, performed when the patient has symptoms. Contrast studies are less helpful.

General management of peptic ulceration

Patients should be advised of the relationship between stress and peptic ulceration, to eat regular meals and avoid strong alcoholic spirits. Aspirin is absolutely contraindicated. Smokers should be strongly advised to stop. Care is required in prescribing non-steroidal anti-inflammatory drugs. Regular use of antacid preparations such as aluminium hydroxide helps ulcer healing and relieves dyspeptic symptoms. H$_2$-receptor blocking drugs such as cimetidine and ranitidine should be given in full doses for an initial course of 6–12 weeks. Elective surgery is reserved for patients with chronic intractable symptoms which have failed to respond to conservative treatment. The aim of surgical procedures is to diminish gastric acid secretion by dividing the vagal innervation or by removing part of the stomach. If a truncal vagotomy is performed a pyloroplasty or gastrojejunostomy is also necessary to help gastric emptying. After truncal vagotomy a proportion of patients suffer from post-vagotomy diarrhoea. Accelerated gastric emptying can lead to the rapid transit of gastric contents causing dumping syndromes. 'Early' dumping syndrome is associated with symptoms of faintness, sweating, palpitations and a sensation of abdominal bloating, occurring soon after eating. In the late dumping syndrome, rapid transit of gastric content into the small intestine promotes an excessive insulin response causing hypoglycaemia.

Highly selective vagotomy is now widely advocated as the optimal elective procedure. Small vagal filaments are divided close to the stomach, preserving the supply to the antropyloric area. It is unnecessary to perform a drainage procedure and the risk of post-vagotomy diarrhoea and dumping syndromes is largely avoided.

Perforation of a duodenal ulcer causes sudden peritonitis. It can usually be confirmed by the appearance of free intraperitoneal gas below the diaphragm on an erect chest radiograph. Occasionally limited leakage leads to tracking of gastric content through the right paracolic gutter into the right iliac fossa. In patients on long-term therapy with corticosteroids, typical features of peritonitis may be absent and the diagnosis of perforation seriously delayed. Occult perforation of a peptic ulcer may also occur in intensive care patients.

Surgical treatment is the closure of the perforation by oversuture with omentum followed by peritoneal lavage to remove gastric contents. A definitive procedure should be considered if the patient has a long-standing history of medically treated peptic ulceration. Erosion into a blood vessel (e.g. posterior gastroduodenal artery) may result in severe gastrointestinal haemorrhage. Urgent surgical intervention may be necessary and early surgery should be considered if there have been previous episodes of haemorrhage. Truncal vagotomy and pyloroplasty is the most commonly performed procedure in this situation.

Inflammatory bowel disease

Mucosal ulcerative colitis and Crohn's disease are idiopathic inflammatory bowel diseases which often affect young people. Crohn's disease has increased considerably in incidence over the last 20 years and the two diseases are now almost equal in incidence (3.5 per 100 000). Ulcerative colitis primarily affects the colon and rectum. Crohn's disease most frequently involves the terminal segment of the ileum, though any part of the gastrointestinal tract may be involved. Both tend to be chronic and their response to treatment is unpredictable. Their management requires good collaboration between gastroenterologists and surgeons as many patients will be under combined care.

Crohn's disease

Crohn's disease may affect any part of the gastrointestinal tract. It most often affects young adults but can occur in children and the elderly. Affected intestine shows transmural inflammatory changes with intense fibrosis. Inflammation is patchy with confluent linear ulcers and deep fissures. There is thickening of the wall of the intestine and the mesentery may appear inflamed and encroach around the intestine (Figure 18.3).

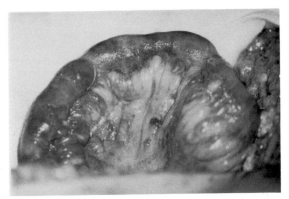

Figure 18.3 Typical appearance of terminal ileal Crohn's disease

Lymph nodes in the mesentery appear inflamed. The terminal ileum is frequently involved but there may be 'skip lesions' separated by long intervals of macroscopically normal intestine. Affected intestine may form an inflammatory mass adherent to other viscera or the abdominal wall. Deep fissures penetrating the bowel wall may form abscesses or fistulae with the abdominal wall or adjacent organs. Colorectal lesions are common.

Clinical presentation and diagnosis

The onset is insidious and symptoms have usually been present for several years before diagnosis.

Recurrent abdominal pain may be due to intermittent intestinal obstruction associated with fibrosis, stricturing or oedema. Localized pain in the right iliac fossa is due to peritoneal inflammation. Symptoms follow a chronic course of exacerbations and remissions. Diarrhoea develops due to malabsorption of fats and bile salts in the diseased terminal ileum and bacterial colonization of the small intestine. Weight loss is marked and children may show growth retardation. In 30% of cases the disease is restricted to the small intestine and in 20–35% the colon is primarily affected. Perianal inflammation is common, with fistula formation and the development of painful oedematous skin tags. Extraintestinal manifestations include arthritis or spondylitis (20%), skin lesions including pyoderma gangrenosum and erythema nodosum (5%), involvement of the eyes by iritis or uveitis (3%), and hepatic involvement. Occasionally the presenting feature may be pneumaturia and urinary tract infection due to an ileovesical fistula.

The diagnosis is confirmed by radiological and endoscopic investigations. Small bowel contrast studies may show a characteristic pattern of irregular narrowing with deep fissures in affected segments. Colonoscopic appearances with biopsy of affected areas may show the diagnostic granulomas. Blood tests may show anaemia, leucocytosis, high sedimentation rate and a low serum folate.

Treatment

Long-term treatment with sulphasalazine may help to control the disease without serious side effects. Corticosteroid therapy or azathioprine may also help to suppress the disease, though the long-term side effects need to be considered. Surgery has a well defined role to play in the management of some forms of Crohn's disease. Disease in the terminal ileal region can be resected in most cases and some patients will have no further need for medical treatment or surgery. Management of recurrent or widespread disease can be difficult and the indications for surgery are strict and conservative. Alleviating local complications of the disease such as abscess or stricture formation may require surgical intervention and though further intestinal resections may be necessary, every effort must be made to conserve functional intestine.

Ulcerative colitis

Ulcerative colitis is a chronic inflammatory condition which primarily affects the mucosal layer of the colon and rectum. Symptoms may begin at any age, most often in early adulthood. Affected colon appears congested and the bowel is shortened. The mucosa shows patchy ulceration, is friable and bleeds on contact. Islands of normal mucosa between the ulcers can become enlarged and polypoid in appearance (inflammatory pseudopolyps.)

These changes may affect the distal colon and rectum and extend proximally for a variable distance or involve the entire colon.

Presentation and diagnosis

Intermittent abdominal pain and chronic bloody diarrhoea are the principal symptoms. Weight loss is common and fever may occur during exacerbations. Extraintestinal manifestations include joint pains, arthropathy, skin changes and iritis. On sigmoidoscopy the rectum may contain mucus, pus or blood and the mucosa is friable or ulcerated and bleeds on contact. A double contrast barium enema may show the smooth shortened bowel with loss of the normal haustrations. Inflammatory pseudopolyps may give a typical 'cobblestoned' appearance. Colonoscopic examination with multiple biopsies from different parts of the colon is useful to define the extent of the disease.

Fulminating exacerbations can be life-threatening and may require emergency colectomy. In a severe fulminating attack the colon becomes greatly distended (toxic megacolon) and may perforate.

Carcinoma of the colon is an important long-term risk. After 10–12 years the cancer risk is approximately 20% and it increases thereafter. Endoscopic surveillance is necessary with periodic mucosal biopsies to try to identify early dysplastic changes. Prophylactic proctocolectomy is advocated for patients who have had colitis for more than 10 years.

Treatment

Medical treatment can often control the symptoms for considerable periods of time. Corticosteroids are the mainstay of treatment, by enema and systemically. Sulphadiazine (Salazopyrin) may be useful. In difficult cases total bowel rest with parenteral nutrition may help a severe episode to settle. If medical treatment fails surgery is considered. In the past the most widely performed procedure has been a total proctocolectomy with formation of a permanent ileostomy. Subtotal colectomy with ileorectal anastomosis has been advocated but there is a substantial risk of carcinoma in the rectal stump. Nowadays the procedure of choice for young fit patients is a total proctocolectomy with formation of an ileal pouch neorectum from several loops of the terminal ileum. This procedure is not always successful but avoids the need for an ileostomy and the risk of malignancy. When emergency colectomy is required a safe option is to excise the colon, construct an end colostomy and exteriorize the distal end of the bowel as a mucous fistula.

Abdominal malignancy

Intra-abdominal malignancies arising from the gastrointestinal tract are a major cause of mortality in developed nations. Surgery is the mainstay of treatment for this group of diseases which comprise a substantial proportion of the workload of most general surgeons.

Oesophageal cancer (see p. 231)

The incidence of oesophageal cancer shows marked geographical variation and is more than 20 times more common in Northern China, Iran and parts of Africa than in Europe or North America. It occurs in the elderly, is commoner in men, and is increasing in incidence in most parts of the world. Chronic irritation of the oesophageal lining plays an important role and smoking and consumption of alcohol are risk factors. Most cases are sporadic though several predisposing conditions and a hereditary variant are recognized. Corrosive damage to the oesophagus by caustic agents causes a 100-fold increase in risk. Achalasia carries approximately a 10% risk of carcinoma, and there is an association with chronic iron deficiency anaemia and oesophageal webs (the Plummer–Vinson syndrome). The presence of columnar cell lining (Barrett's oesophagus) also carries a substantial risk of malignancy.

Most are squamous carcinomas, though in 5–10% of cases an adenocarcinoma may develop, usually in the lower third. Overall, 50% of tumours arise in the middle third of the oesophagus and about 30% in the lower third. Macroscopically they may appear polypoid, ulcerating or diffusely infiltrating. Direct spread occurs both circumferentially and longitudinally and microscopic spread may extend a considerable distance from the limits of macroscopic involvement. Lymphatic spread occurs readily.

Presentation and diagnosis

Dysphagia is the principal symptom, but unfortunately many patients present late with advanced tumours. The patients are often debilitated and suffering from advanced malnutrition, factors which contribute to the very poor prognosis. The diagnosis can be established by a contrast swallow showing the characteristic irregular stricture with 'shouldered' borders, or by endoscopy and biopsy.

Attempted curative treatment

This may take the form of radical radiotherapy or surgical resection. Usually an abdominal laparotomy with mobilization of the stomach and often a pyloric drainage procedure are performed initially.

The oesophagus is then resected through a right thoracotomy and an anastomosis performed at the level of the aortic arch. A three-stage oesophagectomy with a cervical oesophagogastric anastomosis is an alternative. Operative mortality is between 10% and 20%.

Radical radiotherapy for squamous tumours of the middle third has achieved encouraging results in some studies, though it also carries an appreciable mortality rate and a significant proportion of patients are unable to complete treatment. Long-term survival after either form of treatment is less than 15%.

Palliation

Surgical removal of the primary tumour is the best form of palliation of dysphagia. The technique of blunt transhiatal oesophagectomy is gaining popularity in some centres. The oesophagus is mobilized entirely by blunt dissection through the opened oesophageal hiatus of the diaphragm below and from a cervical incision above. The mobilized stomach is then drawn up and anastomosed to the cervical oesophagus. This technique avoids the morbidity associated with thoracotomy and also the risk of the (usually fatal) complication of intrathoracic anastomotic leakage.

Where attempted surgical removal of the primary tumour is not feasible, palliation of dysphagia may be possible by intubation of the stricture. Endoscopic insertion of an Atkinson tube is the safest option, but the quality of life achieved leaves much to be desired and tubes are prone to reflux (causing bronchopneumonia and aspiration pneumonitis) and to blockage and migration.

Techniques are being developed to palliate symptoms by endoluminal ablation of the tumour using endoscopically guided laser energy.

Gastric cancer

Gastric cancer is a disease of advancing years. The incidence has been declining for several decades. In many parts of the world there appears to be an increased incidence in coal mining areas, and smoking is also a risk factor. Chronic atrophic gastritis associated with pernicious anaemia carries a six-fold increased risk of cancer, particularly of the gastric fundus.

A small ulcerating gastric cancer can be mistaken for a benign ulcer and careful endoscopic follow-up with multiple biopsies is advocated for all gastric ulcers. Malignant degeneration of a benign gastric ulcer is uncommon. There is an increased incidence of gastric cancer in the gastric stump after partial gastrectomy.

Tumours may be polypoidal in shape and encroach into the gastric lumen, or may have a flat ulcerated appearance. Occasionally they show extensive diffuse submucosal infiltration (linitis plastica carcinoma). Lymphatic spread increases with the depth of invasion of the primary tumour but may be present even with the most superficial tumours. Haematogenous spread is variable, with a propensity to form multiple liver metastases which are seldom amenable to resection. Mucin-producing 'signet ring cell' tumours can spread in the peritoneal cavity giving rise to metastases in the ovary (Krukenberg tumours).

Presenting symptoms and diagnosis

Anorexia, dyspeptic symptoms and weight loss are the most frequent initial features. There may be anaemia due to occult bleeding from the tumour. Tumours near the cardia or pylorus may cause obstructive symptoms with dysphagia or vomiting.

Surgical treatment

In most cases surgery is palliative as the disease has reached an incurable stage. The usual symptoms requiring palliation are pain, obstructive symptoms and bleeding. Resection of the primary tumour offers the best palliation and distal lesions can be treated by a distal or subtotal gastrectomy with restorative gastrojejunal anastomosis. An obstructing lesion which cannot be resected can sometimes be bypassed by constructing a high gastrojejunostomy. Symptoms due to obstructing lesions of the cardia can be managed by palliative intubation if they are not resectable.

Curative procedures are limited to a minority of patients with lesions confined to the stomach and neighbouring lymph nodes. A radical total gastrectomy including the spleen, omentum and draining lymph nodes *en bloc* achieves a 5-year survival of approximately 25%.

Colorectal cancer

In Europe, North American and Australasia, colorectal cancer is the greatest cause of cancer mortality in non-smokers. The incidence increases with advancing years. A diet high in meat and low in fibre is associated with an increased risk. In approximately 10% of cases heredity plays a major role.

Familial adenomatous polyposis of the colon is one form of hereditary colonic cancer. Affected individuals develop hundreds or thousands or adenomatous colonic polyps and as the risk of colorectal cancer is almost inevitable, prophylactic surgical removal of the colon and rectum is advocated. The accompanying congenital hypertrophy of the retinal pigment epithelium can be useful in early identification of family members at risk.

Excessive proliferation of the epithelial lining initially gives rise to a premalignant adenomatous polyp. At this stage most adenomatous polyps can be curatively removed by endoscopic techniques. If not removed, most polyps will develop advancing dysplasia and ultimately give rise to an invasive malignancy (Figure 18.4).

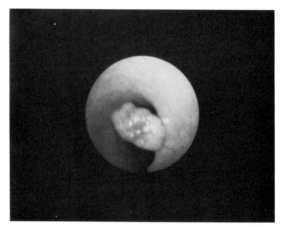

Figure 18.4 Colonoscopic appearance of a pedunculated adenomatous polyp

Table 18.3 Survival and Dukes' pathological staging system for colorectal cancer

Dukes' stage	Corrected 5-year survival
A. Tumour confined to mucosa	95%
B. Tumour invading muscle	68%
C. Lymph node metastases	34%

Where distant metastases are apparent at the time of surgery, the patient is often said to be Dukes' stage D, irrespective of the pathological invasion at the site of the primary tumour. In this case the 5-year survival is less than 10%.

Dukes' pathological staging system is summarized in Table 18.3. Factors which influence prognosis are the degree of cellular differentiation, the amount of lymphocyte infiltration, ability to metastasize to nearby lymph nodes, and the extent of fibrotic stromal reaction (the greater the fibrosis, the worse the outlook).

Presenting symptoms and diagnosis

The most common symptom is an alteration of previously regular bowel habit. Rectal bleeding may occur due to more distal lesions or a chronic iron deficiency anaemia may develop due to bleeding from an otherwise occult tumour often in the caecum. There is often weight loss and the mass may be palpable. Less frequent presentations include abdominal swelling due to malignant ascites or symptoms due to distant metastases.

In 50% of cases, tumours are situated in the sigmoid colon or rectum. Unless there is obstruction, the entire colon should be examined by barium enema or colonoscopy as multiple primary neoplasms may occur.

Surgical treatment

Surgical excision of the segment of colon containing the tumour and its chain of draining lymph nodes is the mainstay of treatment. The extent of the resection is dictated by the anatomy of the blood supply to the colon. Where possible bowel continuity is restored by primary re-anastomosis. Circular stapling instruments may facilitate restorative anastomosis of the distal rectum and occasionally achieve a successful anastomosis which would be technically difficult by direct suture. For some tumours which lie in the lowest part of the rectum, abdominoperineal excision of the rectum and anal canal is necessary, with formation of a permanent end colostomy. Formation of a temporary defunctioning proximal stoma is occasionally indicated to ensure safe healing of an anastomosis. This may be considered in patients with connective tissue disorders or high-dose steroid therapy, if preoperative preparation of the colon has not been satisfactory or the anastomosis has been technically particularly difficult. Defunctioning terminal loop ileostomy has gained popularity in some centres as an alternative to defunctioning loop colostomy. After 6 weeks the patency of the anastomosis can be checked by a limited contrast enema and the defunctioning stoma closed.

Tumours of the colon and rectum have a propensity to metastasize to the liver. Occasionally such metastases may be solitary or limited to one part of the liver, and resection or destruction of these lesions may improve survival. Intraoperative ultrasonography is useful in the detection of such lesions (Figure 18.5).

Emergency abdominal surgery

One of the most challenging and rewarding aspects of the general surgeon's duties is the management of patients with abdominal emergencies. Many of these conditions are life-threatening and develop without warning in previously healthy individuals.

Early acute appendicitis

Lower right-sided abdominal pain leading to a suspected diagnosis of acute appendicitis is a frequent reason for emergency admission to most general surgical wards. The many possible causes include benign, self-limiting conditions as well as rapidly progressing diseases which may develop life-threatening complications. The diagnosis of acute appendicitis requires considerable clinical skill and judgement and is achieved by taking a good history and carefully assessing the physical signs. The earliest symptom of acute appendicitis is often anorexia. In a typical case this will be followed after a variable period by vague intermittent mid-abdominal discomfort and some degree of nausea. Vomiting may occur. At some stage the patient notices a pain in the right iliac fossa, which gradually worsens, may begin to spread and is exacerbated by coughing and movement. Typically the pain is maximal at a point one-third of the way up a line drawn between the anterior superior iliac spine and the umbilicus (McBurney's point). On examination there may be signs of systemic toxicity with a flushed appearance and sometimes (particularly in children) a circumoral pallor. The tongue may be slightly furred and there may be a fever and tachycardia. On abdominal examination tenderness may be localized to the region around McBurney's point or it may be more diffuse. There are signs of peritoneal irritation. Pressure away from the area of maximal

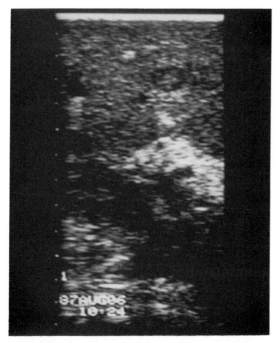

Figure 18.5 Intraoperative ultrasound appearance of a 1.5 cm diameter liver metastasis

tenderness, for instance in the left iliac fossa, may cause pain in the right iliac fossa (Rovsing's sign). If the fingers pressing gently over the tender area are suddenly removed the pain increases markedly, a phenomenon known as rebound tenderness.

It must be stressed that though this is a common presentation of acute appendicitis, it is by no means the only one. The appendix may lie behind the caecum or a long appendix lying in the pelvis may only be inflamed in its distal portion. In the elderly early symptoms and signs may be absent and the condition presents with abdominal distension, vomiting and generalized tenderness due to a developing peritonitis. When the findings are inconclusive the patient should be kept under observation and re-examined at intervals. If there is steady improvement then conservative management can be continued, but if tenderness is persistent or progressive, surgery is indicated. If the clinical findings suggest acute appendicitis surgery should be performed promptly. Perforation of the appendix was once of grave significance, though nowadays most cases can be successfully treated. There is an increased risk that perforation may occur if the appendix contains a solid faecal concretion, and great care should be taken to ensure that such a faecolith should not be left within the peritoneal cavity. Systemic antibiotics are indicated if there is substantial local sepsis and many surgeons routinely administer a suppository of metronidazole preoperatively. Peritoneal lavage with antibiotic solution decreases the risks of postoperative sepsis.

Late appendicitis

Some patients only arrive at hospital after many days of abdominal symptoms; by this time a tender mass is palpable in the right iliac fossa. A localized appendix abscess of this type can be conservatively managed by the Ochsner–Sherren regimen. The patient's temperature and pulse rate are recorded 4-hourly. The size of the mass is determined each day and its outline drawn on the anterior abdominal wall with a skin pencil. Though the patient may often be able to absorb some oral fluids, there is a risk of dehydration aggravated by pyrexia and intravenous fluids should be given to restore fluid balance. Intravenous antibiotics are given in full doses (metronidazole 500 mg 8-hourly with ampicillin 500 mg 6-hourly and either gentamicin 80 mg 8-hourly or a broad-spectrum cephalosporin such as cefuroxime 750 mg 8-hourly). Pain relief can usually be achieved without need for opiates. Purgatives are absolutely contraindicated. In most cases steady improvement will be apparent after the first 24 h which will be maintained until the patient has completely recovered. An elective appendicectomy should be performed approximately 3 months later.

If the mass enlarges or the patient's condition deteriorates, surgical intervention may be necessary. In most cases external drainage of an abscess is the only procedure possible.

Acute mesenteric adenitis

This self-limiting condition occurs mainly in children and teenagers. The symptoms are due to inflammatory swelling of lymph nodes in the ileocaecal area, secondary to viral infection. The condition can mimic the principal features of acute appendicitis. Pyrexia is common and there may be a history of shift of pain from the central abdomen to the right iliac fossa with some signs of local peritoneal irritation.

Meckel's diverticulitis

This diverticulum situated on the antimesenteric border of the ileum 60 cm from the ileocaecal valve is a remnant of the embryonic yolk sac and is present in about 2% of the population. Acute inflammation of a Meckel's diverticulum may be indistinguishable from acute appendicitis. In some cases the apex is attached to the umbilicus by a fibrous cord (the obliterated vitello-intestinal duct) which may cause a band obstruction or volvulus. Meckel's diverticulum may contain ectopic gastric mucosa and peptic ulceration may lead to haemorrhage or perforation.

Solitary caecal diverticulum

Right-sided colonic diverticula tend to be solitary and to cause symptoms in the fourth decade. They are situated within a few centimetres of the ileocaecal valve and can become acutely inflamed. The caecal wall contains a mass which feels like a caecal carcinoma.

Gynaecological causes of right iliac fossa pain

Acute salpingitis (inflammation of a fallopian tube) may cause pain in the right iliac fossa. A history of vaginal discharge together with slight urinary frequency or dysuria may suggest the diagnosis. Alimentary symptoms are less than in acute appendicitis. Maximal discomfort is lower than McBurney's point, extending to the suprapubic area. Vaginal examination may elicit tenderness in both vaginal fornices and excitation tenderness of the cervix uteri. Speculum examination and culture of vaginal swabs may also be helpful. Treatment with high-dose broad-spectrum intravenous antibiotics should not await bacteriological confirmation.

Torsion of an ovarian or fimbrial cyst may cause a sudden onset of severe pain spreading into the thigh or lower back, with vomiting or retching.

Rupture of a graafian follicle at ovulation may cause some bleeding around the ovary with local pain. Symptoms typically occur at mid-cycle (Mittelschmertz). Ectopic pregnancy of the right fallopian tube can cause severe colicky pains in the suprapubic area and right iliac fossa. There may be a history of unprotected intercourse with a subsequently missed menstrual period. Pregnancy tests are usually negative as the pregnancy is seldom viable when symptoms develop and vaginal bleeding usually occurs. Ectopic pregnancy can occur after tubal ligation. Ultrasound scanning of the pelvis is useful in diagnosis. Intraperitoneal rupture of the ectopic pregnancy can cause fatal haemorrhage.

Intestinal obstruction

Intestinal obstruction may be the result of vascular occlusion, mechanical or neuromuscular factors. These latter two types may constitute the initial presentation of disease, e.g. carcinoma of the colon or strangulated hernia, or they may develop after an abdominal operation, e.g. paralytic ileus.

Obstruction of the small bowel leads to loss of alimentary secretions either due to vomiting or accumulation within the lumen of the intestine. Up to 6 litres of salt-rich fluid a day are secreted into the small intestine and normally this fluid is subsequently almost entirely reabsorbed in the colon and rectum. Strangulation of the intestine due to obstruction to its arterial blood supply or venous drainage may lead to loss of viability with necrosis, gangrene and perforation of the affected intestine.

The cause of the obstruction may be due to extrinsic compression, e.g. a band adhesion, an abnormality such as a tumour in the wall of the intestine itself, or may be due to an obstructing foreign body such as a swallowed object or a gallstone in the lumen. The predominant clinical features are abdominal distension, vomiting, abdominal pain and in some cases cessation of passage of flatus. Proximal small intestinal obstruction causes recurrent colicky pains often terminated by vomiting. In a distal obstruction distension will be pronounced.

Bowel sounds are highly variable. A rush of high-pitched tinkling sounds may coincide with an episode of abdominal colic and precede vomiting. Thereafter no sounds may be audible for many minutes. With developing peritoneal irritation due to strangulation of the intestine the bowel may become atonic and the bowel sounds ominously quiet. On examination local tenderness may suggest

developing strangulation. Local tenderness over part of a previous surgical incision may suggest that the obstruction is due to adhesions to the old healed wound. It is essential that the hernial orifices should be carefully examined as incarceration in a hernia is one of the commonest causes of obstruction.

Plain erect and supine abdominal radiographs generally confirm the clinical diagnosis, showing the typical pattern of multiple luminal gas/fluid levels on the erect image. The nature of the distended bowel can be determined from the pattern of markings on the bowel wall on the supine image. The plicae semilunares or valvulae coniventes of the small intestine run across the entire width of the bowel and are parallel and close together whereas the haustra of the colon are further apart and do not traverse the radiological image of the bowel. Occasionally a foreign body may be apparent on the radiograph or gas within the biliary tree may suggest gallstone ileus due to erosion of a gallstone from the gallbladder into the intestine, with subsequent obstruction of the terminal ileum.

A white cell count may be useful as intestinal infarction is usually associated with a marked neutrophilia and a rising white count may warn of developing intestinal ischaemia. A very high white count may suggest mesenteric vascular occlusion. Urea and electrolytes may suggest gross dehydration and the serum amylase may be moderately elevated, particularly if there is intestinal infarction or strangulation. The treatment of intestinal obstruction consists of resuscitation of the patient followed by surgical relief of the obstruction.

Differentiation between small intestinal obstruction and large intestinal obstruction has important implications for management since the probable causes of the obstruction differ between the two conditions. In a patient with large bowel obstruction a period of resuscitation is generally possible and, unless there are signs of impending strangulation or the colon is very grossly distended, it is usually safe to delay surgery until a limited contrast enema study has provided the diagnosis. If there is marked tenderness, a high white cell count or a caecal diameter of greater than 10 cm, it is unwise to postpone surgery. In the case of a small intestinal obstruction, preoperative investigation by contrast studies will not aid diagnosis and surgery should not be delayed to obtain such investigations.

Obstruction due to adhesions and fibrous bands

One of the commonest causes of small intestinal obstruction is constriction of the intestine or its mesentery by a fibrous band. Three-quarters are due to adhesions forming after previous abdominal surgery. A fibrous band may compress the intestine or trap a loop together with its mesentery. This type of obstruction carries a high risk of strangulation. Sometimes the adhesion may form a pivotal point about which a loop of intestine may be twisted causing an intestinal volvulus.

Strangulated external hernia

Strangulated external herniae are responsible for approximately one-third of cases of small intestinal obstruction. The diagnosis should provide little difficulty and is suggested when a previously reducible hernia becomes tender and irreducible. Strangulation occurs more frequently in femoral or umbilical herniae than in inguinal herniae. The veins are occluded by pressure at an early stage and cause swelling of the incarcerated intestine. Venous thrombosis eventually develops followed by venous gangrene of the intestinal wall. After surgical release the colour of the intestine may return to normal and peristalsis may occur. If the colour fails to return to normal and there is no peristaltic activity, the affected segment should be resected. Richter's hernia is an abdominal hernia in which a portion of the circumference of the gut is imprisoned, so reducing but not obliterating the lumen of the intestine. This type of hernia most often occurs in the femoral region and may be difficult to diagnose as signs of obstruction may be equivocal, despite advancing necrosis of the part of the intestinal wall imprisoned in the hernial sac.

Strangulation due to incarceration of intestine in an internal hernia is rare and usually diagnosed at laparotomy. Internal herniae may occur around the duodenojejunal flexure (paraduodenal), in peritoneal folds around the ileocaecal valve, or through the foramen of Winslow.

Colonic obstruction due to tumours

Because many colonic carcinomas grow in an annular fashion, they are a frequent cause of large intestinal obstruction. Onset is usually insidious with some history of altered bowel habit. There is usually gross abdominal distension and a cessation of passage of flatus. Vomiting may not be marked, particularly if the ileocaecal valve remains closed in the face of increasing intracolonic pressure (closed loop obstruction). This can lead to gross distension of the closed loop with ultimate rupture of the caecum. If the ileocaecal valve opens, vomiting may be more marked and the risk of colonic rupture is less. Plain abdominal radiographs show gross distension of the large bowel and there is usually a large fluid level in the caecum on the erect view. A

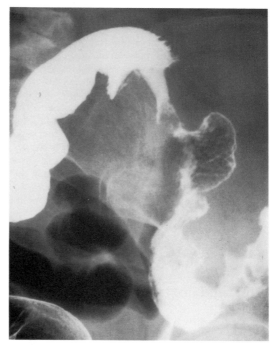

Figure 18.6 Barium enema appearance of a stenosing annular carcinoma of the sigmoid colon ('apple-core' lesion)

limited contrast enema may establish the diagnosis (Figure 18.6).

The patient should be adequately resuscitated with intravenous fluids prior to surgery and a definitive resection should be attempted. For tumours of the ascending and transverse colon a right hemicolectomy extended to include excision of the obstructed segment is the procedure of choice. The terminal ileum can then be anastomosed to the collapsed colon distal to the site of the obstruction. For lesions in the descending colon and sigmoid, the distension of the bowel with liquid faeces makes surgery technically difficult and potentially hazardous. When the condition of the patient permits, a definitive resection of the tumour should be performed. The distal colonic stump can be closed and the proximal colon taken out as an end colostomy as advocated by Hartmann. For many years it was considered unsafe to perform a restorative anastomosis under these circumstances, but with modern anastomotic techniques this can be achieved safely in an increasing proportion of patients. The technique of intraoperative irrigation of the obstructed colon as described in Chapter 20 can be very useful under these circumstances to decompress the distended colon and permit restorative anastomosis to be safely performed.

Minimal surgery for colonic obstruction

Definitive surgical management of colonic obstruction requires considerable surgical expertise. There are circumstances under which it may be unwise to attempt these major procedures but emergency surgery to decompress the obstructed colon is necessary as a life-saving emergency procedure. Under these circumstances decompression of the colon by formation of a defunctioning transverse loop colostomy may save the life of the patient, and definitive surgery can be peformed later under safer circumstances. A laparotomy should be performed to allow decompression of the colon, an assessment of the cause of obstruction, and construction of a defunctioning stoma. The distended colon is often near to rupture and should be handled with great care. It is advisable to decompress the colon before attempting to construct a stoma. The overdistended and friable colonic wall may tear easily and be unable to hold a pursestring or stay sutures. It is safer to decompress the colon by inserting a large (20–24 French gauge) Foley catheter with a 20 ml balloon through a small incision on the anti-mesenteric border of the terminal ileum about 10 cm proximal to the ileocaecal valve (Figure 18.7). Thereafter a transverse loop colostomy can be constructed.

Paralytic ileus and pseudo-obstruction of the colon

The intestine may become distended without being mechanically obstructed. Paralytic ileus develops when normal peristaltic motility is interrupted and the intestine becomes atonic and distended. This occurs to some extent after most abdominal procedures and also as a secondary phenomenon in other abdominal conditions such as pancreatitis. Pseudo-obstruction of the colon (Ogilvie's syndrome) is a variant of adynamic ileus occurring in patients with another major illness such as orthopaedic trauma or myocardial infarction. It may develop after non-abdominal surgery. Enormous distension of the colon (particularly the caecum) may develop and there is a substantial risk of perforation. Colonoscopic decompression is the treatment of choice.

Mesenteric vascular occlusion

Acute ischaemia of the intestine causes a sudden onset of severe abdominal pain, followed shortly by development of peripheral circulatory failure. The peripheral blood white count is usually extremely

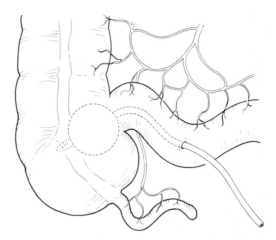

Figure 18.7 A safe technique for decompression of the obstructed colon. After the Foley catheter has been removed, the incision on the antimesenteric border of the terminal ileum is sutured

high which may be a clue to the diagnosis. Acute mesenteric ischaemia may be due to a mesenteric embolus, but most cases are due to atheromatous disease of the mesenteric vessels. A similar clinical picture may be caused by venous obstruction. Intensive resuscitative measures may be necessary, and administration of high-dose broad-spectrum antibiotics. Systemic heparinization is frequently advocated despite the risk of haemorrhage from the infarct. A short segment of affected intestine may be successfully resected. Unfortunately there is often an extensive necrosis of much of the small intestine and the mortality of this condition is extremely high.

Peritonitis and massive abdominal sepsis

The diagnosis of generalized peritonitis is generally not a difficult one. Provided that the underlying cause is not acute pancreatitis, a brief period of intensive resuscitation followed by laparotomy is indicated. Peritonitis due to a perforated peptic ulcer causes extreme peritoneal irritation and frequently board-like rigidity. The threat of residual sepsis is not serious provided that surgical treatment is prompt and adequate. Peritonitis due to leakage of bile into the peritoneal cavity is more insidious and bacterial contamination can be considerable. The most severe form of generalized peritonitis is due to contamination by faecal material. This is associated with extreme systemic toxicity, with evidence of rapidly advancing peripheral circulatory failure. Attempts to restore the peripheral circulation by administration of intravenous fluids are unlikely to prove successful. Under these circumstances a prolonged attempt to restore the patient's blood pressure prior to surgery will not be met with a successful outcome. Excessive administration of fluid will aggravate postoperative respiratory complications. The sooner the faeces are removed from the peritoneal cavity, the greater the chance of survival. Even with expeditious surgery, the mortality rate for this condition is extremely high and if the patient survives the first 24 h, shock lung and some degree of renal failure are to be expected.

Management of peritonitis

The patient should be seen by an experienced surgeon as soon as possible. Resuscitation by intravenous infusion should begin immediately. Vital signs should be monitored at 15 min intervals. Oxygen 50% by mask and broad-spectrum intravenous antibiotics should be given. Blood samples should be sent for urea and electrolytes, amylase, full blood count and cross match. A urinary catheter and a nasogastric tube should be passed. Plain chest and abdominal radiographs and an ECG should be obtained.

The aims of surgery are to deal with the cause of the peritonitis and to cleanse the peritoneal cavity. As a rule the fastest procedure which will reliably prevent further peritoneal contamination is the procedure of choice. Thorough cleansing of the peritoneal cavity can be achieved by washing the peritoneal cavity with up to 15 litres of warmed normal saline. The last few litres should contain a broad-spectrum antibiotic (e.g. tetracycline, 1 mg/ml).

Complications of abdominal surgery

The complications which may occur after abdominal surgery fall into three groups:

1. Those which may follow any operation, e.g. deep venous thrombosis, pulmonary embolism, or pulmonary atelectasis.
2. Complications that may result from laparotomy and a wide range of intra-abdominal procedures.
3. Those peculiar to specific operations.

Postoperative nausea and vomiting

Most modern anaesthetic agents do not cause much nausea, but some patients may still experience unpleasant nausea and vomiting. Opiate analgesics make many people nauseated and an anti-emetic (prochlorperazine, 12.5 mg) should also be given by intramuscular injection. Some antibiotics, anti-inflammatory drugs and aspirin may irritate the gastric lining.

During recovery from postoperative ileus, nausea suggests that the patient is taking too much oral fluid too soon. Vomiting may also be an early sign of a developing early postoperative intestinal obstruction.

Wound dehiscence

This very distressing complication is fortunately rare. A number of predisposing factors are recognized:

1. Obesity.
2. Advanced age.
3. Causes of impaired wound healing such as connective tissue disease, long-term corticosteroid therapy.
4. Malnutrition.
5. Postoperative abdominal distension due to a variety of causes such as prolonged paralytic ileus.
6. Wound infection.
7. Violent coughing.
8. Postoperative pancreatitis.

Dehiscence occasionally occurs in an otherwise young and fit patient and in these cases is usually attributed to failure of suture material. Monofilament suture of polymer materials such as nylon or polypropylene may be greatly weakened if the suture is crushed in forceps or the jaws of a needle holder during the suturing of the wound.

In some cases only the deeper layer of the wound gives way throughout part of its length. A discharge of bloodstained serous fluid between the remaining skin sutures will often follow. Intestine or omentum may become visible between gaping wound sutures.

Management

The patient should be reassured, consent to repair the defect obtained, and sedation given. A moist abdominal pack should be placed over extruding viscera and surgical repair of the defect undertaken as soon as feasible.

Postoperative peritonitis and abdominal sepsis

Peritonitis may have been present before surgery, may arise due to contamination of the peritoneum at the time of surgery or leakage from a suture line or anastomosis afterwards. Diagnosis of postoperative peritonitis is not always easy. Postoperative pancreatitis must be excluded.

Clinical features

Pain may be difficult to evaluate in a patient who has had major surgery and who may be receiving opiate analgesics. The patient often appears ill and worried. Tachycardia and pyrexia are common. Vomiting may occur. The urine output may decline and renal function may deteriorate.

Management

Further surgery should be undertaken if there is evidence of mechanical obstruction, if bile or intestinal contents are freely entering the peritoneal cavity or there are good reasons for believing that this is happening. In the latter case failure to operate will result in a steady downhill course with progressive renal and circulatory failure. Surgery should also be considered when the general condition of the patient continues to deteriorate during conservative management.

Conservative management

1. Maintain circulating volume and fluid and electrolyte balance. There is a risk of renal failure due to the generalized effects of massive sepsis. Urea and electrolytes should be checked at least once a day. Urine should be checked for glucose.
2. High-dose broad-spectrum antibiotics should be given. Blood cultures should be performed periodically as a resistant organism may predominate and emerge to give rise to septicaemia.
3. Temperature, pulse and respirations should be closely monitored. A spiking temperature will often be apparent if an abscess has developed.
4. If breathlessness and cyanosis develop, oxygen should be given, a chest radiograph performed and arterial blood gases measured. There is a substantial risk of shock lung.
5. Pain relief should be administered, e.g. pethidine 50 mg intramuscularly with prochlorperazine. Care should be taken to avoid respiratory depression if there is dyspnoea. If necessary the effects of pethidine can be reversed by giving naloxone.
6. Nasogastric aspiration to keep the stomach empty and avoid the risk of vomiting and inhalation pneumonitis.
7. H_2-receptor antagonists should be given intravenously to diminish the risk of acute duodenal ulceration or gastric erosions.

Bacteraemic shock (see also p. 21)

Bacteraemic (septic or endotoxaemic) shock is a syndrome characterized by peripheral vasodilatation coinciding with hypotension and variable systemic signs of septicaemia. In the early stages of the syndrome there is a hyperdynamic state with an increase in cardiac output due to increased cardiac motility and peripheral vasodilatation. The patient has warm extremities and hypotension, unique to this syndrome. Paradoxically, oxygen consumption is diminished due to mitochondrial dysfunction and acidosis is apparent. Subsequently myocardial depression develops and there is a decreased cardiac output. If allowed to progress multisystem failure will develop, with concomitant shock lung and renal failure.

Management

Careful monitoring with hourly recording of urine output, blood pressure, pulse and temperature are necessary. Central venous pressure should be monitored and a Swan–Ganz catheter to monitor intracardiac pressures is valuable. The source of the infection should be determined and if possible eliminated, and blood cultures should be performed. Broad-spectrum antibiotics should be given intravenously.

The use of inotropic agents in the early hyperdynamic stage is controversial. The use of steroids is also controversial, but many surgeons prescribe short-term high-dose prednisolone. Post-mortem analysis of patients who have died after prolonged septic shock frequently shows evidence of adrenal lipid depletion, suggesting that adrenal insufficiency may have developed at some stage during the course of the illness. If there is reason to suspect adrenal insufficiency, intravenous hydrocortisone, 100 mg 8-hourly, may be considered. Special attention must be paid to maintenance of fluid, electrolyte and acid–base balance, and renal function.

Shock lung

Shock lung (also known as the *adult respiratory distress syndrome* and *non-cardiogenic pulmonary oedema*) is an acute respiratory disorder which can develop in a number of clinical settings. It may be associated with endotoxic shock, DIC, trauma and overhydration. The radiographic appearance is that of widespread patchy opacification. The lungs become rapidly congested with interstitial fluid. Clinical deterioration can be rapid and precedes the radiographic changes. High flow rate oxygen must be administered, preferably in an intensive care unit. Central venous pressure should be monitored to warn of potential fluid overload. Arterial blood gases need to be monitored regularly. Elective ventilation should be considered early before it becomes necessary due to exhaustion.

The mortality is high and recovery slow. Inotropic drugs may be needed to support the heart, and other organs, e.g. kidneys, may fail.

Residual abscesses

The cardinal feature is an intermittent high pyrexia. The temperature often rises rapidly in the evening. The patient may not feel particularly ill and there may be few localizing signs. Ultrasonic scanning or computed tomography may be useful in localizing the site of the abscess if there are no localizing signs.

Pelvic abscess

A pelvic abscess in the pouch of Douglas can complicate a variety of abdominal diseases and operations. After a few days a swinging pyrexia appears. There may be a mucous discharge per rectum or urinary frequency due to irritation of the bladder or rectum. Rectal examination reveals a tender mass anterior to the rectum.

Treatment

The abscess may discharge spontaneously into the rectum. If not it should be drained. Under general anaesthesia sinus forceps are inserted through a large proctoscope and plunged through the bulging rectal wall into the abscess.

Subphrenic abscess

Localizing signs are often minimal. Hiccups may occur due to peritoneal irritation or there may be some shoulder tip discomfort. The diagnosis is suspected when a spiking evening pyrexia develops and there is no other evidence of sepsis. Screening of the diaphragm reveals a high immobile diaphragm on one side.

Treatment

Surgical drainage is the treatment of choice, though smaller abscesses may be drained by ultrasound guided aspiration. The precise location of the abscess should be determined in order to choose the optimal extraperitoneal approach. A large-bore drainage tube should be inserted and left for 7–10 days. Sinogram radiographs can be taken to assess healing before the drains are removed.

Intestinal fistula

A faecal fistula arising from the large bowel may develop due to leakage from a suture line or anastomosis. If this develops early in the postoperative period there is a substantial risk of peritonitis. A simple fistula without peritoneal contamination can be managed much like a colostomy. Provided that there is no distal obstruction it will usually close up spontaneously after some weeks.

Small intestinal fistulae may lead to a substantial loss of fluid and electrolytes and the irritant digestive enzymes cause skin excoriation.

Conservative management

Nothing is given by mouth and the stomach is drained by a nasogastric tube. The patient's nutritional state is maintained by intravenous nutrition. Loss of fluid and electrolyte from the fistula itself and as a result of the gastric drainage may be substantial and particular care is required to replace them. It may take many weeks for the fistula to seal off. If there is distal obstruction, conservative management will be unsuccessful. Contrast studies can identify the level of the fistula. If conservative management fails and the condition of the patient permits, resection of the fistulated segment may be attempted.

Laparoscopic surgery

While gynaecologists have used the laparoscope for several decades, it is only recently that general surgeons have begun to exploit the operative potential of this instrument. At the present time (1991) the operation most frequently performed by this minimally invasive technique is laparoscopic cholecystectomy, but other intra-abdominal and intrathoracic procedures will almost become commonplace in the next few years.

For laparoscopic cholecystectomy, it may be necessary to have an ultrasound scan or intravenous cholangiogram carried out the day before. As the patient will leave hospital 2 or 3 days after operation, it is important to inform the family doctor beforehand about the line of treatment proposed.

19

Management of biliary and pancreatic cases

T. K. Choi and J. Wong

Gallstone colic

Gallstone colic arises when a stone impacts in the neck of the gallbladder, in the cystic duct, or in the bile duct. The pain can begin gradually or very suddenly and is felt as repeated spasms, usually in the right hypochondrium, or less often in the epigastrium, with radiation to the interscapular region. It may, on occasion, be referred to the right shoulder. It may last only a few minutes or may go on for many hours. The most suitable drug for relieving pain and biliary colic is pethidine hydrochloride which should be given in doses of 50 or 100 mg. An initial dose of 50 mg should be given intravenously for rapid action; if found insufficient, a further 50 mg may be given. This can be repeated 4-hourly, but if the pain returns 1–2 h after the first injection the dose may be repeated at that time.

Acute cholecystitis

Diagnosis

Clinical

The onset may be quite sudden or may be preceded by a history of chronic gallbladder disease. The upper abdominal pain is often sharp but continuous, and there may be a superimposed element of biliary colic. Gradual fading of the pain may signify either resolution of the condition or the development of a quiet perforation of the gallbladder. Tenderness is usual in the right hypochondrium and there is often enough rigidity to prevent palpation of an enlarged gallbladder. Tachycardia is moderate and the temperature is commonly about 38°C. If the temperature rises to 39.5°C, empyema should be suspected. Leucocytosis is usually present but can be absent in the elderly. If jaundice develops, a stone may be present in the bile duct, but jaundice may rarely be due to a localized inflammatory mass compressing the bile duct.

The most important conditions to be differentiated are perforated peptic ulcer, acute pancreatitis, appendicitis and intestinal obstruction. The condition may also resemble myocardial infarction, pneumonia and diaphragmatic pleurisy.

Ultrasonography

A plain film of the abdomen is useful to exclude gas under the diaphragm from a perforated viscus. Only about 15% of the gallstones are radio-opaque. Ultrasound of the gallbladder is very useful in demonstrating gallstones in almost all cases. Other pertinent ultrasound findings are oedema, thickening of the gallbladder wall and collections of fluid around the gallbladder. In the rare situation when ultrasound is not diagnostic but cholecystitis is strongly suspected on clinical grounds, ^{99m}Tc-labelled dimethyl-acetanilide-iminodiacetic acid (^{99m}Tc-IDA) scanning can be performed. The gallbladder is not visualized in acute cholecystitis.

Conservative or surgical treatment

Acute cholecystitis nearly always subsides spontaneously, but occasionally a patient's condition so deteriorates that operation becomes essential. The advocates of early surgery believe that it is the logical treatment for an acute process because it eliminates the possibility of later complications such as gangrene of the gallbladder and perforation, while it also reduces the duration of the illness and hospitalization. Those who prefer conservative management believe that definitive surgery can be carried out more safely at a later stage after the acute process has subsided.

Indications for urgent laparotomy

If conservative treatment is adopted, urgent laparotomy may be indicated in several situations. Laparotomy should be carried out at once if there is evidence of empyema of the gallbladder or peritonitis from rupture of the gallbladder. These patients usually have persistent tachycardia, fever, pain and rising leucocytosis. A tender mass may be palpable in the right hypochondrium.

In an occasional patient the acute symptoms subside but mucocele of the gallbladder develops. Mucocele is recognized by the presence of a large, relatively non-tender gallbladder swelling in the absence of fever or leucocytosis. It is impractical to persist with conservative management and cholecystectomy should be carried out.

Management of acute cholecystitis

1. Bed rest.
2. Nothing by mouth.
3. Intravenous fluids.
4. Broad-spectrum antibiotic therapy, e.g. cefuroxime or cephradine.
5. Analgesics if pain is severe.

Acute cholangitis

Acute cholangitis occurs as the result of bacterial infection of the bile ducts usually preceded by biliary obstruction. Obstructions are in most cases caused by stones or benign strictures. The incidence of acute cholangitis accompanying malignant biliary obstruction is on the rise because increasing numbers of endoscopic or percutaneous transhepatic investigative and therapeutic procedures are being done for malignant obstruction.

Diagnosis

Clinical

The classic symptom complex described for acute cholangitis is fever, right upper quadrant pain and jaundice. One or two components of the complex may be absent in patients having mild cholangitis; on the other hand, patients having severe cholangitis may be mentally confused and in shock. A history of previous biliary tract diseases or operations is frequently present.

Laboratory investigations

On admission into hospital a set of blood tests including complete blood count, liver function tests, serum albumin, electrolytes and urea should be

performed. Elevations in serum direct and total bilirubin, alkaline phosphatase and gamma-glutamyl-transpeptidase indicate obstructive jaundice. Severe cholangitis is usually accompanied by elevations of liver parenchymal enzymes, glutamic oxalacetic transaminase (SGOT) and glutamic pyruvic transaminase (SGPT). The elevations of SGOT and SGPT do not reach the levels seen in hepatitis, and usually drop to near normal levels in a few days as cholangitis subsides.

Ultrasonography

Ultrasonography of the liver, bile ducts, gallbladder and pancreas is most informative. The biliary system is grossly dilated. Stones in the gallbladder and bile ducts may be detected. Liver abscesses which occur in late severe cholangitis can be seen as space-occupying lesions in the liver.

Radiology

Endoscopic retrograde cholangiopancreatography (ERCP) and percutaneous transhepatic cholangiography (PTC) are done after the resolution of cholangitis. These procedures can aggravate cholangitis because injection of contrast material further increases the pressure in the biliary system. If performed in the acute stage, these procedures should be followed by immediate drainage. Drainage is effected by a percutaneous transhepatic catheter if PTC is done, and nasobiliary catheter or endoscopic papillotomy if ERCP is done.

Management of acute cholangitis

1. Bed rest.
2. Nothing by mouth.
3. Intravenous fluids.
4. Broad-spectrum antibiotics, e.g. cefoperazone, cefotaxime, or an aminoglycoside.
5. Hourly measurement of vital signs.
6. CVP monitoring.
7. Foley catheter inserted to measure hourly urine output.
8. Measurement of intake and output.

Management of patients with obstructive jaundice

The management of patients with obstructive jaundice depends on whether there is coexisting cholangitis. If cholangitis is present, management as depicted in the section on acute cholangitis is promptly instituted. If cholangitis is absent, the patient is investigated before operation or other forms of intervention. Ancillary aids to diagnosis, particularly liver function tests, ultrasonography and cholangiography are fully utilized. The patient is questioned carefully about recent drug ingestion.

Diagnostic aids in jaundice

Clinical

The past history of relevance includes previous biliary surgery, exposure to icterogenic drugs, alcohol, viral hepatitis and haemolytic anaemia. Any clinical features typical of viral hepatitis, stone in the bile duct or cancer of the head of the pancreas should be noted. Whereas a fluctuating jaundice is characteristically that caused by a stone in the bile duct, a progressively deepening jaundice is typical of carcinoma.

Laboratory investigations other than liver function tests

The following tests could be carried out: haemoglobin, red blood cell count and morphology, white blood cell count and differential count, and prothrombin and activated partial thromboplastin time. In prehepatic haemolytic jaundice, spherocytosis and reticulocytosis are common. Leucopenia with relative or absolute lymphocytosis is usual in viral hepatitis, whereas polymorphonuclear leucocytosis is a feature of cholangitis. Anaemia is common in cirrhosis and is usually microcytic, although it may be macrocytic, and megaloblastic marrow change is sometimes seen. Hypersplenism is reflected as neutropenia and thrombocytopenia. Coagulation defects are also found in jaundice associated with cirrhosis. The deficiencies are usually multiple and can involve prothrombin, fibrinogen, factor V and factor VII. Fibrinogen deficiency is rather uncommon, but fibrinolysins have been demonstrated. The prothrombin time estimation is of value in differential diagnosis; if elevated, a good response to intravenous vitamin K is evidence of posthepatic jaundice, whereas the absence of a response favours hepatic jaundice with the implication of there being impaired synthesis of prothrombin by the hepatocyte. The presence of hepatitis A and B viral antigens and antibodies is also tested. Antimitochondrial antibodies are found in the great majority of patients with primary biliary cirrhosis. Smooth muscle antibodies and antinuclear factor are found in patients with chronic active hepatitis. Alpha-fetoprotein is found in the serum of patients with hepatocellular carcinoma.

Liver function tests

As the parenchymal cell has many different functions, and each liver function test measures only one aspect of liver function, it follows that a number of tests are required. It should be remembered that the liver has a high functional reserve and patchy lesions of the liver may show no abnormality in the function tests until 80% of the liver has been destroyed. All tests are of value only if the clinician appreciates both the normal and pathological range for each individual test and the various possibilities for error in the laboratory methods used. Furthermore the discriminatory value of some of the tests, particularly the liver enzymes, is poor. The following tests and groups of tests have been found to be the most useful:

Serum bilirubin

The total serum bilirubin is an objective index of the depth and progress of jaundice, and so it is valuable to repeat this observation every 3 or 4 days. The normal mean total bilirubin is approximately 6 mmol/l with an upper limit of 20 mmol/l. In jaundice a fall in the level is a favourable sign, whereas a sudden rise should be viewed with concern. Partition of serum bilirubin into the direct and indirect fractions is often done, but the direct van den Bergh reaction is given by both the mono- and diglucuronides of bilirubin which regurgitate into the blood in both hepatic and posthepatic jaundice. Thus, estimation of these fractions is of no value in the differentiation of hepatic from posthepatic jaundice. However, the indirect fraction is high in prehepatic jaundice.

Serum alkaline phosphatase

This is a mixture of several phosphatases originating from bone, intestinal mucosa and liver. Thus it reflects activity of hepatic and extrahepatic conditions, and high values are found in rickets, osteomalacia, hyperparathyroidism, Paget's disease and in the last trimester of pregnancy, in addition to the high values traditionally found in posthepatic jaundice. The level of serum alkaline phosphatase is the result of bony, intestinal and hepatobiliary phosphatase activity, together with the ability of the liver to excrete these phosphatases in the bile. Serum alkaline phosphatase estimation is normally considered with other tests for diagnostic purposes, but has a limited value because of the phosphatase activity in serum being due to a series of isoenzymes.

Aminotransferase (transaminases)

Alanine aminotransferase (formerly glutamic pyruvic transaminase, SGPT) is especially abundant in the liver cells, although it occurs elsewhere in the heart, skeletal muscle, etc., but an elevation in the activity of this enzyme is one of the most useful tests to distinguish between hepatic cellular damage and posthepatic obstruction as a cause of jaundice. The activity of aspartate aminotransferase (formerly glutamic oxalacetic transaminase, SGOT) is also widely carried out in investigation of liver function and in the diagnosis of jaundice. Very high values (normal range 10–40 IU/l) are found in viral hepatitis and in hepatocellular necrosis. Particularly high activity of SGOT and SGPT is found in the early phases of viral hepatitis. Levels of SGPT are regarded as more specific for liver damage than SGOT as SGPT is so much more abundant in liver tissue.

Gamma-glutamyl transpeptidase

This enzyme is found in the mucosal cells of the bile ducts and the serum level is elevated in obstructive jaundice.

Other enzymes

One of the isoenzymes of lactic dehydrogenase is found extensively in the liver and blood levels of this enzyme are raised in hepatocellular damage. The high level of this enzyme and alanine amino-transferase would be an important diagnostic combination suggesting hepatic jaundice. Increased levels of 5'-nucleotidase and leucine aminopeptidase are also found in hepatocellular damage. On the other hand, in jaundice due to hepatocellular disease, the serum level of pseudocholinesterase activity falls. Pseudocholinesterase is an alpha-globulin synthesized by the liver cells in a manner parallel to that of albumin synthesis.

Single readings of any enzyme level are of little help in deciding the nature of hepatic disease. Rising or falling values are more useful indicators of the nature and progress of the condition.

Ultrasonography

Abdominal ultrasonography is routinely done in patients with suspected obstructive jaundice. The liver, bile ducts, gallbladder and pancreas are systematically examined. The biliary system is dilated in obstructive jaundice. The entire biliary system including the gallbladder is dilated if obstruction is at the lower common bile duct. Only the intrahepatic bile ducts are dilated if obstruction is at the hilar region. The liver is inspected for space-occupying lesions. The hilar region and the pancreas are inspected for mass lesions which may be the cause of obstruction.

Radiography

A good soft tissue radiograph will show an enlarged liver or spleen and will also demonstrate any radio-opaque gallstones. Barium meal examination may disclose oesophageal varices, an alimentary

tract cancer if the jaundice is metastatic in origin, or a widening of the duodenal loop if there is a cancer of the head of the pancreas. Suitable films of the second part of the duodenum may show an ampullary carcinoma.

Endoscopic retrograde cholangiopancreatography (ERCP)

ERCP is a well developed technique whereby the bile and pancreatic ducts are cannulated by a catheter introduced through a side-viewing duo-denoscope and visualized radiographically after injection of contrast (Figure 19.1). This is one of the most useful techniques in investigating a jaundiced patient. Stones and benign or malignant strictures of the bile ducts are clearly demonstrated. Obstruction of the pancreatic duct is diagnostic of pancreatic cancer. Bile, pancreatic juice and duodenal washings can be obtained for cytology. A brush cytology of the bile duct can also be performed. ERCP cannot delineate the upper part of the biliary tract if obstruction is complete. In expert hands, ERCP can be successfully performed in 90% of the attempts. The complication rate of ERCP is low.

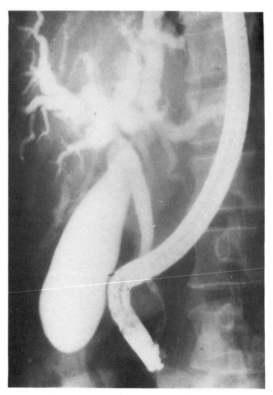

Figure 19.1 ERCP of a patient with obstructive jaundice caused by a malignant hilar tumour. The intrahepatic ducts are dilated

The common complications are duodenal perforation and cholangitis due to introduction of bacteria into an obstructed system. If the system is already infected, ERCP may precipitate septic shock.

Cephalosporin or aminoglycoside antibiotic prophylaxis should be routinely given before ERCP.

Percutaneous transhepatic cholangiography (PTC)

PTC provides a clear picture of the part of the biliary tract proximal to the obstruction. The bile ducts of the right and left lobes may not communicate because of obstruction by a hilar tumour. In this situation, separate punctures should be performed to visualize the bile ducts in both lobes. The success rate of PTC is more than 90% in patients with dilated intrahepatic ducts. The complications most commonly encountered are bleeding and bile leakage. Any clotting deficiencies should be corrected before PTC. PTC should not be performed on patients having moderate to severe ascites.

Percutaneous liver biopsy

This examination is rarely used as a diagnostic measure in jaundice, but occasionally proves of value in differentiating intrahepatic cholestasis from posthepatic jaundice. Liver biopsy should not be carried out if there is evidence of a bleeding diathesis in the patient, if the prothrombin time is prolonged or if it does not return to normal or near-normal after parenteral vitamin K or if the platelet count is below 50 000/mm^3. After liver biopsy the patient should lie quietly in bed for 24 h and a careful record must be kept of the pulse and blood pressure. Minor local symptoms are not uncommon after liver biopsy near the site of the skin puncture but usually disappear after several hours.

Non-operative treatment of obstructive jaundice

In the past, patients with obstructive jaundice were almost always treated surgically. Recently, techniques of percutaneous or endoscopic drainage of the biliary system have been developed. The role of these techniques in the management of obstructive jaundice is discussed below.

Percutaneous transhepatic or endoscopic biliary drainage as definitive therapeutic procedure

This is mainly indicated for patients with malignant biliary obstruction who have limited life expectancy because of advanced staging and whose site of obstruction is not favourable for surgical bypass. An endoprosthesis of about 2–3.5 mm in diameter is inserted by percutaneous transhepatic or endoscopic approach. However, these tubes can be blocked by debris and sludge. An experienced endoscopist or radiologist is necessary for these approaches.

Preoperative percutaneous transhepatic or endoscopic biliary drainage

Surgery in jaundiced patients carries a mortality of about 20%. The recognized risk factors are old age, malnutrition, ongoing biliary infection, malignancy and high serum urea. Some of these risk factors can be corrected. Preoperative percutaneous transhepatic or endoscopic biliary drainage may allow the biliary infection to subside. While the bilirubin is dropping, malnutrition and high serum urea can be corrected. Liver function may also improve. In spite of all these benefits, preoperative biliary drainage has not been shown to reduce the operative mortality or morbidity. More controlled studies are needed.

Preoperative preparation for biliary surgery
Correction of coagulation abnormalities

In posthepatic jaundice, the absence of bile salts from the alimentary canal decreases the absorption of the fat-soluble vitamins, including vitamin K. The shortage of vitamin K impairs the synthesis of prothrombin by the liver. This results in a tendency to bleed. Formerly this made biliary surgery in obstructive jaundice very hazardous. Any increased bleeding tendency can be estimated preoperatively by the prothrombin time. If this is elevated, vitamin K should be given in the form of K$_1$ intravenously. A dose of 20 mg is followed by a rapid return to a normal prothrombin time within 12–24 h if the liver is normal. If the first observation of prothrombin time shows an elevation, a further test should always be carried out after giving vitamin K to ensure that conditions have indeed returned to normal before operation. Vitamin K$_1$ in a dose of 10–20 mg should be given daily intravenously or intramuscularly until operation takes place. It is usually unnecessary to continue the administration of vitamin K postoperatively. When there is severe hepatocellular damage, the parenteral administration of vitamin K$_1$ will not bring the prothrombin time back to normal, as prothrombin cannot be made by badly damaged liver cells. The only other source of prothrombin in these circumstances (to permit safe operation) is fresh plasma frozen after separation from the red cells. Prothrombin activity is retained in these plasma fractions for several months. Stored whole blood contains little or no prothrombin.

Prevention of renal failure

Jaundiced patients undergoing surgery have an increased tendency to develop renal impairment due to renal tubular damage and hepatorenal syndrome. It is important to keep the patient well hydrated before operation. Use of nephrotoxic antibiotics should be avoided. Mannitol 50 g daily should be given as a continuous intravenous infusion for its osmotic diuretic effect.

Preoperative biliary drainage

As mentioned in the section on management of obstructive jaundice (see p. 275) no benefit has been demonstrated for preoperative external biliary drainage on the management of patients with obstructive jaundice. Trials are currently being done on the use of preoperative internal biliary drainage.

Postoperative complications
Bleeding

This may come from the liver bed or cystic artery. Careful preparation of jaundiced patients with vitamin K and careful haemostatic technique during the operation should prevent bleeding.

Leakage of bile

This can arise from the gallbladder, cystic duct or bile duct, or from the liver. Bile leakage is usually first manifested by the drainage of green-coloured fluid from the abdominal drain. If there are no signs of peritonism and if fever and tachycardia are absent, the patient can be observed. The point of leakage usually seals up spontaneously if the leaked bile is adequately drained and if there is no biliary obstruction. If the patient has undergone common duct exploration, a cholangiogram is performed to see if the T-tube has dislodged (see Management of the T-tube below). If the leaked bile is not adequately drained, localized subhepatic abscess, generalized peritonitis or fistula formation may occur. A sudden escape of bile may lead to generalized peritonitis and shock. The affected patient is given intravenous fluid therapy and urgent laparotomy is performed to drain bile from the peritoneum and deal with the site of leakage to prevent further extravasation.

Jaundice

Jaundice which appears rapidly after operation may well be due to operative injury to the bile duct. On the other hand, it may be due to a cholangitis which had been present preoperatively but had flared up as a result of the operative manoeuvres. Jaundice may also be due to the use of old blood for transfusion or, rarely, to a mismatched transfusion. If jaundice is due to haemolysis, then renal shutdown is very likely, followed by tubular necrosis – a very serious complication for a jaundiced patient after biliary tract surgery, in some cases necessitating the use of renal dialysis. Jaundice which either occurs or becomes worse postoperatively may be due to pathology in the bile duct such as retained stones or a missed carcinoma. Finally, drugs given in the perioperative period and anaesthetic agents may cause jaundice.

Pancreatitis

This complication may occur after biliary tract operations, particularly when there has been manipulation near the lower end of the duct, which facilitates regurgitation of infected bile up the pancreatic ducts (see p. 283).

Laparoscopic cholecystectomy
See p. 273

Drainage after biliary tract procedures
Drainage tubes

A tube draining the gallbladder bed is shortened on the third day, and removed on the fourth or fifth day, unless there is undue discharge of bile or blood in which event the tube should be left *in situ*. Persistent blood or bile drainage requires investigation into the cause. If the amount is subsiding, the drain is left until the drainage ceases or becomes minimal and then it is removed.

Management of the T-tube
Selection of appropriate T-tube

A soft flexible tube of suitable size is usually chosen. It should lie freely in the bile duct, which is closed round it by absorbable sutures sufficiently tight to prevent bile leakage. There is no need for the short limbs of the T-tube to be longer than 1.0–1.5 cm. Generally a V is cut out of the T-tube on the wall of the tube opposite the long limb (of the T-tube) and a gutter removed from the length of the short limbs, involving one-third to a half of the circumference of

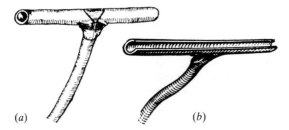

Figure 19.2 (*a*) If a V is cut out of the tube, as shown, the tube is more easily withdrawn; (*b*) half of the circumference can be cut away for easy withdrawal and improved drainage of bile

the tube (Figure 19.2). This improves drainage down the bile duct, past the T-tube, and also facilitates removal of the tube. The T-tube is brought out directly through the abdominal wall, and a certain amount of slack should be left within the abdomen so that there is no danger of the tube being pulled out of the bile duct by a sudden movement of the patient. The T-tube is also secured by a stitch to the skin, tying the stitch firmly around the tube in criss-cross fashion, but not kinking or otherwise obstructing it.

Management of a T-tube in the bile duct

Bile usually drains freely in the early postoperative days because of oedema in the distal end of the bile duct and spasm of the sphincter, consequent upon passage of instruments during operation. This temporary obstruction normally subsides during the first week. A postoperative cholangiogram is performed between the 8th and 10th day. If the cholangiogram is normal (no filling defects in the bile ducts and free passage of contrast into the duodenum) and if the patient is not jaundiced, the tube may be clamped with a screw clamp for 24h. The clamp should be opened if the patient has any abdominal pain. If no pain occurs, the tube can be removed.

Removal of the tube

After cutting the skin suture attached to the tube, the T-tube may be removed by a steady pull. If it cannot be extracted with moderate tension, a haemostat may be applied to the tube, close to the abdominal wall, and the patient permitted to walk about. This often allows the tube to come away; if it fails to do so, the manoeuvre should be repeated on the following day. After removal of the T-tube there may be a small amount of biliary discharge for the first 24 or 36h, but often there is little or no discharge and the drainage tract heals rapidly.

Contraindications to the removal of the T-tube

1. Jaundice.
2. Fever.
3. Recurrence of pain after clamping the tube.
4. Leakage of bile around the tube after clamping.
5. Abnormal T-tube cholangiogram.

Complications associated with choledochotomy

As there is a tendency for the sphincter of Oddi to be held closed postoperatively, biliary pressure rises if free drainage is not possible through the T-tube. Leakage will occur through the divided small ducts in the gallbladder bed, around the choledochotomy opening when there is a T-tube in position, and even through the small stitch holes in the bile duct used for closing the incision in the bile duct. A drain should thus always be used to drain the subhepatic region.

Occluded T-tube

In the early postoperative period the tube may become blocked by blood clot or by biliary mud. Gentle syringe irrigation with isotonic sterile saline will usually restore patency. When a T-tube has been retained in the common duct for a longer period, it sometimes happens that the lumen becomes occluded by encrustation. Again, saline irrigation should be employed rather than chemical solvents which are not recommended.

Dislodgement of T-tube from the duct

This can occur if a stuporous, confused or restless patient pulls the tube out completely, or if the tube is caught by the patient's clothes or bedding while he is turning in bed or attempting to sit up. Much more often, and with greater resulting peril, the T-end of the tube can be dragged out of the bile duct into the peritoneal cavity by some apparently innocent movement of the patient in bed. The particular danger of this form of dislodgement is that it is not marked by any symptom or sign other than the cessation of bile drainage from the tube. This may pass unnoticed until bile peritonitis supervenes, or the dressing becomes yellow and saturated by a copious escape of bile along the side of the tube. Bile peritonitis is sinister but often difficult to diagnose. The shorter the lapse of time between operation and the extrusion of the tube, the more serious are the consequences. If the tube is dislodged before the fourth day, the abdomen must be reopened, the bile sucked out of the peritoneal cavity and a new T-tube inserted. If dislodgement occurs on or after the fourth day, whether reinsertion should be done is guided by clinical findings. Reoperation is performed if fever and tachycardia occur or if abdominal pain is experienced. The patient is carefully observed if there is no evidence of bile peritonitis. The drain and the dislodged T-tube should be left *in situ* until all drainage subsides.

Retained stone in the common bile duct

A stone demonstrated on cholangiography may be removed by a steerable Dormia-type basket under fluoroscopic guidance. This is done about 6 weeks postoperatively through a matured T-tube tract. If the tract is not wide enough, dilatation is performed by stenting the tract with catheters of progressively larger diameter. Alternatively, a choledochofibre-scope can be used. The scope is passed into the biliary system through the matured T-tube tract and the stone is ensnared and removed under direct vision.

The management of bleeding varices

The rate of blood loss in patients with bleeding oesophageal varices can be variable. At one end of the spectrum the patients may be asymptomatic except for one or two episodes of melaena. At the other end of the spectrum, hypovolaemic shock and coma may ensue from massive exsanguinating bleeding. Liver cirrhosis is usually the cause of portal hypertension in bleeding varices and patients commonly have physical signs of chronic liver disease and liver failure. An urgent gastroscopy is performed after gastric washout to confirm variceal bleeding and to see if there is concurrent bleeding from gastric or duodenal sources.

It is essential to replace the blood volume lost and to stop the bleeding. Further difficulties may arise from aspiration of vomited blood into the lung, or from the alimentary breakdown of blood into ammonia (and other products) with the later development of hepatic coma.

Early on the patient may not have lost much blood and blood transfusion may not appear to be urgent. However, alarming haemorrhage may come on at any time, so that 3 or 4 units (2000 ml) of compatible blood should be available at immediate notice during a bleeding phase. When blood is taken for cross-matching, specimens should also be obtained for the determination of liver function, blood ammonia, coagulation profile, blood and platelet counts.

Resuscitation of shock and hypovolaemia is the same for bleeding varices as for bleeding from other gastrointestinal sources. The volume of blood to be transfused is deduced from the usual clinical indices of pulse, blood pressure, haemoglobin, mixed venous haematocrit, CVP and repeated assessment of the patient's general condition.

A comatosed patient is best nursed on his side and, if systemic blood pressure is very low, the foot of the bed should be raised on blocks until resuscitation has raised the blood pressure. All sedation is potentially dangerous, but the patient must be given as much physical and mental rest as possible. Morphine should be avoided as an adequate dose may result in the patient going into coma. Paraldehyde or choral hydrate can be given by tube and are safe drugs, but it will be found necessary in some cases to give a small dose of phenobarbitone or diazepam. Barbiturates and diazepam, however, should be given with the greatest care in this condition. The measures available for treatment of continuing or recurrent bleeding are as follows:

Balloon tamponade

Balloon tamponade is usually the first treatment instituted, although some recommend a trial of drugs such as pitressin before balloon tamponade. The three-channel Sengstaken-Blakemore tube (Figure 19.3) is commonly used. A four-channel version, which has additional suction holes proximal to the oesophageal balloon, is also available. One lumen of the Sengstaken-Blakemore tube is to insufflate the gastric balloon. The second lumen is for oesophageal balloon insufflation and the third lumen communicates with suction holes at the tip of the tube for gastric aspiration.

The balloons are first tested for leakage and checked that the ports connected to various channels are correctly labelled. Local anaesthetic lozenges are given to the patient while the tube is being prepared and the pharynx and nose are sprayed with a local anaesthetic just before tube insertion. The tube should be well lubricated and can be passed orally or through the nose. The patient's eyes are covered so that he does not see the details of the procedure which might disturb him. The tube is inserted and the patient is asked to swallow when the tube reaches the pharynx. Once in the oesophagus, the tube should be pushed in with gentle steady pressure until a good length of it is in the stomach as indicated by the markings on the side. To ensure that the tip of the tube is in the stomach, the port connected to the suction holes in the tip is aspirated for blood and stomach contents. The gastric balloon is inflated with 20 ml of water which is coloured with an ampoule of methylene blue and 20 ml of radiographic contrast. The contrast is added so that the position of the balloon

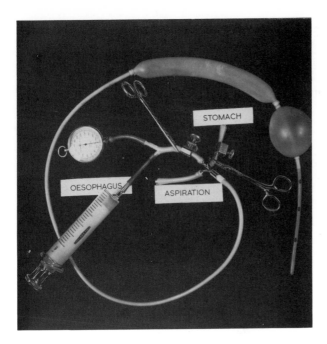

Figure 19.3 The Sengstaken triple-lumen tube for oesophageal tamponade, together with the necessary fittings for its successful use in compressing bleeding gastro-oesophageal varices

can be checked radiologically. The reason for colouring the water is that if the gastric balloon ruptured, the gastric aspirate will be coloured blue and, when recognized, the tube should be removed to prevent the upward migration of the oesophageal balloon. The tube is then pulled back until the gastric balloon is felt to impinge on the cardia, and the tube is fixed to the patient's cheek with adhesive strapping. An abdominal radiograph is taken. If the position of the gastric balloon is correct, the oesophageal balloon is inflated by connecting its port to a sphygmomanometer. Air is pumped in until a pressure of 25–30 mmHg is reached. Screw clamps should be applied to the balloon ports to prevent air or water leakage.

Balloon tamponade is effective in stopping bleeding in about 80% of the patients. If it is difficult to maintain traction by strapping, the tube should be connected to a 0.5 kg weight by a string looping over a pulley. The direction of the pull should parallel the bridge of the nose. The stomach is aspirated intermittently to ascertain whether the bleeding is stopped. Saliva and other secretions are removed by suction as often as necessary to prevent aspiration.

The oesophageal balloon is deflated after 18–24 h. The tube is left in position. If bleeding recurs, the balloon is again inflated. Other bleeding control measures are added. Repeated tamponade is not recommended because of the possibility of development of pressure necrosis at the lower oesophagus. The tube is removed if there is no further haemorrhage during the next 24 h.

Intravenous vasopressin (Pitressin)

This has been shown to bring about a pronounced lowering of the portal venous pressure without lowering the systemic pressure. Twenty units of vasopressin are given intravenously over a 10 min period in 100 ml of 5% dextrose solution. Alternatively, a constant infusion of 40 units per hour can be given. Vasopressin should not be used in patients with a history of myocardial ischaemia, although in extreme cases when very active bleeding is going on, its careful use may be indicated even in such a desperate situation. If vasopressin is to be successful, it presumably acts by lowering the portal pressure in the region of the bleeding point in the oesophageal varix, thus allowing haemostasis to occur. Unfortunately, recurrence of bleeding is common and repeated dosage of vasopressin eventually fails to control the situation. Terlipressin (Glypressin) has a similar action to vasopressin on the portal venous pressure, but without cardiac side effects.

Sclerotherapy

Injection sclerotherapy is used by some doctors as the first-line treatment while there is active bleeding. Some endoscopists prefer to perform the procedure immediately after bleeding is controlled by balloon tamponade. Injection can be performed through either a rigid oesophagoscope or a flexible gastroscope. About 4–5 ml of 5% ethanolamine oleate is given intravaricely or paravaricely to each column of varix up to a maximum of 20 ml per session. Combined with balloon tamponade the success rate of bleeding control is about 90%. Injection can be continued at 2–4 week intervals until all varices are ablated to prevent rebleeding.

Surgery

Surgery is reserved for patients whose bleeding is not controlled by the above measures. Devascularization plus oesophageal transection is usually performed. For patients who have undergone repeated injection sclerotherapy, oesophageal transection may not be safe. Portasystemic shunting is performed in this situation. Transgastric variceal plication is performed in high risk patients of the Child C category.

Hepatic coma

This condition is a neuropsychiatric disturbance with certain characteristic features – an often disordered consciousness, altered personality, noise delirium, flapping tremor, rigidity, increased reflexes and many other neurological disturbances. Although patients may suddenly emerge from a deep coma and survive unexpectedly, hepatic coma should always be regarded as a grave condition with a grim prognosis.

Precipitating factors

Common among these is upper gastrointestinal haemorrhage in a patient with cirrhosis and portal hypertension. Here, the effect is due to ammonia or other products of bacterial breakdown of blood in the intestine, acting on a cirrhotic liver whose oxygen supply is further impaired by the anoxia following the haemorrhage. Other precipitating factors are sepsis, an alcoholic bout, a surgical operation or the use of diuretics which may be related to a fall in serum potassium.

Treatment of hepatic coma

1. No protein: calories are supplied by glucose drinks in the pre-comatose state or by 20% glucose given in an intracaval drip if the patient is in coma. Full vitamin supplements are given parenterally, especially vitamins B and K. After recovery from coma, protein may be recommenced but only in small amounts until the limit of the patient's tolerance is found. This may be between 25 and 50 g daily.

2. Blood transfusion: the haemoglobin level should be maintained above 10 g/dl to enable an adequate supply of oxygen to reach the failing liver.

3. Neomycin and lactulose: 6 g neomycin are given daily in divided doses. The purpose of neomycin is to decrease the formation of ammonia and other nitrogenous products during bacterial decomposition of blood and other protein in the gut. The bacterial flora of the colon may also be modified by giving lactulose to alter the pH of the gut. An osmotic diarrhoea is also produced.

4. Purges: purgation with magnesium sulphate and the use of enemas are very important in clearing the bowel of protein.

5. Other therapy: glutamic acid, arginine, ornithine and choline have all been recommended in hepatic coma. None has proved to be of any real value. Corticosteroids may be used in acute coma associated with viral hepatitis.

6. Fluid and electrolyte balance must be maintained in the usual way. An accurate fluid chart is essential with daily serum electrolytes and acid–base estimations.

7. Avoid thiazide diuretics, paracentesis, morphine, barbiturates and all sedation as far as is possible.

Acute pancreatitis
Diagnosis
Clinical

It is important to establish the diagnosis of acute pancreatitis from other acute abdominal conditions as conservative management is the treatment of choice in pancreatitis, while emergency operation is required in certain of the conditions which can be confused clinically with pancreatitis, such as perforated peptic ulcer, intestinal obstruction, acute cholecystitis, acute appendicitis and mesenteric thrombosis. In many instances abdominal pain like that of pancreatitis is associated with nausea and vomiting, and there may also be tenderness and abdominal rigidity. However, chemical and radiological aids to diagnosis are available to reinforce the clinical diagnosis, which can be difficult to establish in some cases of acute pancreatitis.

Laboratory investigations

The following blood tests should be obtained: serum amylase, complete blood picture, platelet count, serum electrolytes, calcium, urea, lactic dehydrogenase, glucose, albumin, liver function tests and arterial blood gases. These tests supply information on the condition of the patients and some are also predictive of the severity of pancreatitis.

Serum amylase can be elevated in a number of acute abdominal conditions: perforated peptic ulcer, intestinal obstruction, acute cholecystitis and mesenteric thrombosis. However, the elevation is seldom as high as that seen in acute pancreatitis. The upper limit of normal varies in different laboratories, but an elevation of more than five times the upper limit is considered diagnostic of acute pancreatitis. The highest levels are recorded usually within a few hours of the onset of the disease and these high levels usually return to near-normal levels within 48 h of onset of symptoms. Therefore, if blood is not taken soon enough after the onset of pancreatitis, the peak level may be missed and near normal levels may be obtained. Serum lipase or urinary amylase:creatinine clearance ratio are also diagnostic but the sensitivity of these tests is not higher than amylase.

Radiography

A plain radiograph of the abdomen may show one or two gas-filled coils of distended jejunum in the upper abdomen. This appearance has been called the 'sentinel loop' and is thought to be pathognomonic of acute pancreatitis. The 'colon cut-off' sign is sometimes seen affecting the transverse colon in acute pancreatitis. A gastrografin meal on occasion shows widening of the C-curve of the duodenum and displacement of the stomach by an inflamed, swollen pancreas. Pleural effusion, usually on the left side, may be present on chest radiography. Pleural effusion is associated with more severe pancreatitis.

Ultrasonography

Ultrasonography of the upper abdomen should be routinely performed during the acute phase of pancreatitis. The liver, gallbladder, bile ducts, pancreas and peripancreatic regions are systematically examined. Gallstone, which is a cause of acute pancreatitis, may be detected. Bile duct dilatation is indicative of biliary obstruction by impacted stone or swollen pancreas. The pancreas may be swollen and fluid collections may be found. These collections are usually located in the lesser sac and in front of the kidneys.

Computed tomography

Computed tomography (CT) is indicated if the condition of the patient does not improve within a few days or deteriorates. It should also be performed if pancreatic abscess is suspected. The finding of free gas within fluid collections or contrast rim enhancement around fluid collections is diagnostic of pancreatic abscess (Figure 19.4).

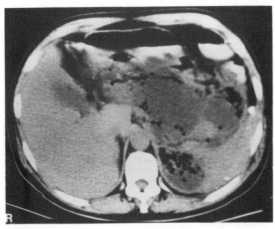

Figure 19.4 CT scan of a patient with a pancreatic abscess; gas is present within the peripancreatic fluid collection signifying an abscess

Abdominal paracentesis

If there is some doubt with regard to the diagnosis of acute pancreatitis, abdominal paracentesis may prove a valuable investigation, and possibly may spare the patient an operation which would not benefit him if the diagnosis is, in fact, pancreatitis. The following is a safe method of carrying out diagnostic paracentesis.

Technique

A fine lumbar puncture needle is used – one that will just admit No. 6/0 polythene tubing. The needle, its stylet and 45 cm (18 in) of the polythene tubing are first sterilized. The needle, with stylet in place, is introduced through the anaesthetized skin of the right iliac fossa at a point 3 cm (1.2 in) below the umbilicus and just lateral to the sheath of the rectus abdominis. The needle is steadily advanced and a characteristic sensation is felt as it enters the peritoneal cavity. The needle is advanced no further. The stylet is removed and aspiration attempted. If fluid is not obtained, the polythene tubing is threaded through the lumen of the needle and the needle is then withdrawn, leaving the tubing in place. Aspiration is performed with the patient in several positions. Unless all the intraperitoneal fluid is trapped in the lesser sac, a specimen will be obtained.

The peritoneal exudate in acute haemorrhagic necrosis of the pancreas is prune-juice coloured and its amylase content is extremely high, a reading of many thousands being obtained.

In the commoner, milder types of pancreatitis only a little fluid is present, and this is pale and serous in character, with no bacteria seen in the smear. The amylase concentration, however, is very high. Where there is gangrene of the bowel in the various conditions with strangulation, the peritoneal aspirate may be bloodstained and foul smelling, and may contain many intestinal bacteria and can have a high amylase content.

Management of acute pancreatitis

Nasogastric aspiration

Nasogastric aspiration should always be used. Continuous suction removes the gastric hydrochloric acid as soon as it has been secreted and so prevents it from entering the duodenum, thus suppressing the hormonal stimulation of the exocrine secretion of the pancreas. In addition to this important therapeutic function, nasogastric suction also brings relief from the persistent and very characteristic nausea and vomiting associated with pancreatitis, and so helps to alleviate the considerable pain found in this condition.

Relief of pain

Pethidine hydrochloride is the most appropriate drug to use in a dosage of 50–100 mg according to the degree of pain and the clinical condition of the patient. Morphine is contraindicated because it increases spasm of the involuntary muscle of the sphincter of Oddi and so, by impeding drainage from the pancreatic duct, results in increased pressure in pancreatic ducts and acini. Epidural anaesthesia and splanchnic block have been recommended for the relief of severe pain, but these procedures are very rarely required.

Oxygen therapy

Oxygen is given by mask or nasal prongs if the Pao_2 is less than 70 mmHg. Low arterial blood oxygenation is associated with severe pancreatitis and hypoxia may also aggravate pancreatitis. Patients who become progressively more dyspnoeic or hypoxic in spite of oxygen administration are intubated and assisted with respirators.

Supportive intravenous therapy

In acute pancreatitis there is often widespread intraperitoneal or retroperitoneal inflammatory exudation resulting in lowered blood volume and hypovolaemic shock. There is an urgent need to restore an adequate blood volume as soon as possible. Physiological saline is the most appropriate solution. The choice of fluid to be used and the amount required are judged from blood volume estimations, if these are available, or by changes in haematocrit and observations of pulse rate, CVP and blood pressure. Shock is the principal cause of

death in the first 48 h. In older patients, fluid replacement is best monitored by Swan–Ganz catheter measurement of pulmonary artery wedge pressure.

A careful daily and cumulative fluid balance chart should be kept with appropriate allowance made for insensible loss. Daily serum electrolyte estimations are made, together with acid–base studies, as metabolic acidosis can readily develop in the course of the illness. Full water replacement is given by the intravenous route, calories are given as glucose, and sodium, potassium and chloride are given in appropriate amounts to keep the serum levels within normal limits and to keep pace with any losses. Hypokalaemia can develop in the more severe cases and is treated by potassium chloride intravenously – given with care and only if the urinary flow is adequate. Calcium deficiency is uncommon but, if it occurs, is treated by calcium gluconate given intravenously. If renal anuria develops, the full conservative management of anuria is instituted. If this is insufficient, dialysis may be required.

Drugs

Anticholinergic drugs such as atropine and propantheline bromide were widely used in the past, but have not been shown to decrease the mortality or morbidity of pancreatitis. Aprotinin (which inactivates pancreatic enzymes) and glucagon (which suppresses pancreatic secretion) have also been used but no improvement in morbidity or survival has been demonstrated. Somatostatin is a potent inhibitor of pancreatic enzyme secretion. Initial studies indicate that its use may decrease the incidence of local complications of acute pancreatitis. Confirmation is needed.

An antibiotic should always be prescribed in acute pancreatitis as a prophylactic against the infection of the necrotic retroperitoneal tissues and also against bronchopneumonia, so often the terminal event in severe pancreatitis. A broad-spectrum antibiotic such as cefoperazone should be given for 3–5 days.

Recovery phase

The majority of patients recover spontaneously after several days of conservative treatment. As recovery proceeds, nasogastric suction and intravenous fluid can be replaced by cautious oral feeding, and antibiotics and other drugs can be stopped. Early dietary requirements are met by a bland diet of high calorie content; large meals are forbidden, to avoid major exocrine pancreatic activity. Although acute pancreatitis can be an isolated incident, it is regrettably the case that recurrences are quite common.

Indications for surgery

If a positive diagnosis of pancreatitis has been made, there is no need for laparotomy if the patient continues to improve on a conservative regimen. Patients having severe pancreatitis have a higher chance of developing complications which require surgical intervention. Severity of pancreatitis can be predicted using schemes such as those developed by Ranson or Imrie. These schemes usually use a combination of biochemical and clinical criteria to predict severity. Leucocytosis ($>15\,000/mm^3$), elevated serum SGOT ($>200\,IU/l$), lactate dehydrogenase ($>600\,IU/l$), urea ($>16\,mmol/l$), glucose ($>10\,mmol/l$), depressed serum albumin ($<32\,mmol/l$), calcium ($<2\,mmol/l$), Pao_2 ($<60\,mmHg$), old age (>55 years) and requirement of massive volume of fluid for initial resuscitation are found to be associated with severe pancreatitis.

The most common indications for immediate laparotomy are uncertain diagnosis and pancreatic abscess formation. If the diagnosis of acute pancreatitis is equivocal, if other acute abdominal conditions requiring surgical intervention such as perforated peptic ulcer and appendicitis are suspected, urgent laparotomy should be performed. Pancreatic abscess formation is suspected if fever and leucocytosis continue. An epigastric mass or fullness may then develop. Pancreatic abscesses are surgically drained. The patient is put on a 2-week course of potent antibiotics. Broad-spectrum antibiotics are used initially. The antibiotics may be changed depending on the result of bacterial culture and sensitivity tests of the abscess contents. If untreated, sepsis, shock, multiorgan failure and death almost certainly ensue.

Severe pancreatitis accompanied by the formation of pancreatic phlegmon can give rise to similar physical and laboratory findings. The danger of draining a sterile pancreatic phlegmon is contamination which may lead to abscess formation. If the diagnosis of pancreatic abscess is uncertain computed tomography should be performed.

Computed tomography and, if necessary, guided aspiration, can differentiate between a phlegmon and an abscess. Computed tomography is also used to monitor the resolution of abscess after treatment is started.

Intra-abdominal haemorrhage, massive upper gastrointestinal haemorrhage, massive pancreatic necrosis and biliary obstruction are other complications requiring urgent laparotomy. If a patient survives a very severe attack of acute pancreatitis, late unexpected metastatic abscesses may develop in the retroperitoneum, mediastinum or pelvis. Watch must be kept for same.

Pancreatic pseudocyst is a complication which also requires surgical treatment but operation is usually performed 4–6 weeks after formation of the pseudocyst. Ultrasound and CT may detect small cysts and the radiologist may aspirate these. Many collections, especially the smaller ones, are spontaneously resorbed. Larger ones may persist and increase in size. Patients with a protracted course and prolonged elevation of serum amylase have a higher tendency to develop pseudocyst. Internal surgical drainage, e.g. cystgastrostomy, is usually performed after the cyst wall has matured, a process which usually takes 4–6 weeks. An undrained pseudocyst is liable to become infected. Rupture, haemorrhage into the cyst and gastrointestinal obstruction may also occur.

Investigations after acute pancreatitis

Abdominal ultrasonography is performed on patients who did not have the examination during the acute stage and on patients in whom the initial ultrasound failed to detect gallstones. In the latter patients, ultrasonography performed after resolution of pancreatitis may reveal stones. If gallstones are not found and no other cause of pancreatitis is evident, ERCP is performed. ERCP can identify the occasional patient with stones present only in the bile ducts. Other uncommon causes of pancreatitis such as pancreatic divisum, ampullary neoplasm, pancreatic neoplasm and choledochal pancreatic sphincteric stricture can also be identified.

Chronic pancreatitis

After repeated attacks of pancreatitis, fibrosis of the gland occurs with the loss of exocrine-secreting tissue. By far the most common cause of chronic pancreatitis is alcoholism.

Diagnosis
Clinical

Pain is the most common complaint. The pain may be continuous or intermittent and accentuated by meals. The pain may be so severe that the patient is incapacitated and dependent on narcotics for relief. Another symptom, steatorrhoea, is the result of defects in fat absorption. In the absence of pancreatic lipase, the stools become bulky, foul smelling and loose. Globules of fats are seen floating on the surface. Islet cells are also damaged by chronic pancreatitis leading to diabetes mellitus which often occurs before the onset of steatorrhoea.

Pancreatic function tests
Glucose tolerance test

Abnormal values in the test are found in over 50% of patients with chronic pancreatitis, especially those with pancreatic steatorrhoea. The test is therefore of value in the differential diagnosis of steatorrhoea.

Faecal fat measurement

Lundh test meal

1. Patient fasts from 22.00 hours the previous evening.
2. A radio-opaque weighted nasogastric tube is passed (intramuscular metaclopramide hydrochloride 10 mg may be given).
3. Patient is screened. Tube should be in second part of the duodenum.
4. Fasting specimen is put in universal container and placed in the freezer compartment of the fridge.
5. Test meal containing 6% fat, 5% protein, 15% carbohydrate is given

   $$\left.\begin{array}{l} 18\,\text{g Corn oil} \\ 15\,\text{g Casilan} \\ 40\,\text{g Glucose} \end{array}\right\} \text{ in } 300\,\text{ml water}$$

6. Connect to suction pump at 3 lb pressure for collection of specimens over 2 h. Place suction receptacle on ice and store all specimens on ice.

It may be necessary to change the position of the patient if a specimen is difficult to obtain. Fasting and post-stimulation samples are analysed for amylase and trypsin, both of which are reduced in chronic pancreatitis.

The response to the challenge of the meal is age-dependent. In a young adult the volume of juice aspirated may be increased ten fold. Changes in trypsin output are more helpful than those for amylase. The normal concentration of trypsin is 10–30 IU/l; it may increase three-fold after stimulation. Normal amylase content is 10–200 IU/l.

Radiography

Plain abdominal radiograph may show pancreatic calcifications. The appearance of the pancreatogram obtained by ERCP is characteristic. The duct is dilated with one or more strictures along its course. The secondary and tertiary branches are also dilated.

Treatment

Steatorrhoea is treated by pancreatic enzyme replacement. This is usually given in divided doses accompanying meals. Cimetidine may be added in resistant cases. This drug reduces the acidity and volume of gastric and duodenal secretions, enhancing the digestive action of enzyme substitutes.

Diabetes mellitus may be difficult to manage because these patients are sensitive to insulin. A small dose may cause prolonged hypoglycaemia.

Pain is the only symptom which requires surgical treatment and this is done only when control by analgesics has failed and the patient is debilitated. Pancreatic duct drainage, usually pancreatojejunostomy, is performed when the pancreatic duct is markedly dilated. Whipple's operation is the procedure of choice if the duct is not markedly dilated and pancreatitis is confined mainly to the pancreatic head. The incidence of diabetes mellitus is very high after any form of pancreatic resection. Procedures blocking the coeliac ganglion are either not effective or only temporarily so.

Cancer of the pancreas

Adenocarcinoma is the most common cancer of the exocrine pancreas. Cystadenocarcinoma accounts for only about 1% of pancreatic neoplasms but is of importance because the prognosis is good after surgical excision. Pancreatic adenocarcinomas tend to occur at the head while cystadenocarcinomas tend to occur at the tail.

The first manifestation of carcinoma of the head of the pancreas is usually obstructive jaundice. The jaundice is not accompanied by pain or infection. The section on management of obstructive jaundice should be referred to (see p. 275). If a mass is found at the pancreas, confirmation of malignancy can be made by arteriography, ERCP or CT-guided aspiration cytology. Serum carcinoembryonic antigen and CA 19–9 measurements are also helpful. The staging of carcinoma is best done by CT. The liver is screened for metastases. The liver hilum, the areas around the superior mesenteric vessels, and aorta are common sites for lymph node metastases.

Cancer confined to the head of the pancreas should be resected by a Whipple's operation. The regional lymph nodes are removed *en bloc* because occult metastases may be present. If at operation the tumour is found to be not resectable because of extensive invasion of surrounding tissues, portal vein invasion, or lymph node or liver metastasis, a double bypass procedure is performed. A double bypass consists of a biliary-enteric bypass, usually a cholecystojejunostomy or choledochojejunostomy to bypass the biliary obstruction and a gastrojejunostomy to bypass the duodenal obstruction. If gastrojejunostomy is not performed, about 20% of the patients will have symptoms of duodenal obstruction before death.

Cancer of the body and tail of the pancreas are usually silent until an advanced stage is reached. Epigastric pain radiating to the back, abdominal distension from malignant ascites, discovery of abdominal masses, general malaise and weight loss are the common presenting symptoms. Treatment is usually for palliation of symptoms.

20

Management of anorectal cases

R. J. Nicholls

Patients with anorectal lesions are usually in pain, often anxious and frequently embarrassed by the examination. The doctor should be reassuring and explain clearly exactly what he is doing.

Anorectal examination

Anorectal examination is best carried out with the patient in the left lateral position. The four essential features are: long axis of patient's trunk at 45° to long axis of couch, feet level with far edge of couch, buttocks raised on sandbag, and buttocks extending about 10 cm beyond the near edge of the couch (Figure 20.1). With the patient in this position the examiner avoids leaning across the couch and the

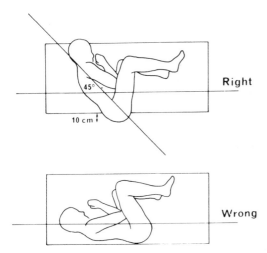

Figure 20.1 Position for sigmoidoscopy. Plan view of patient on examination couch, with buttocks projecting 10 cm beyond the edge on the examiner's side (top)

patient's legs during sigmoidoscopy. The knee–elbow and lithotomy positions favoured by some are less comfortable for the patient and may require special tables. The order of examination should be inspection, palpation, sigmoidoscopy and procto-scopy.

Inspection

The buttocks are held apart to reveal the anus and perineum. The perianal skin should be examined for dermatitis, excoriation, ulceration, warts, scars, carcinoma and fissure. A fissure lies in the midline and particular attention should be paid to the inspection of these areas by deliberate parting of the anal verge. Fissure is diagnosed on inspection and on no other part of the examination.

Palpation

Digital examination per rectum is poorly taught to medical students. It is, however, a most important part of the general examination. The gloved lubricated finger is placed at the anal verge and gently inserted through the anal canal into the rectum. At this stage a method of examination should be carried through. The rectal mucosa is systematically examined for benign and malignant tumours. This is possible to at least 10 cm from the anal verge in most cases. The posterior tissues are felt for masses. Then attention is turned to the prostate or cervix uteri and the peritoneal cavity above this level. Pathology here includes gynaecolo-gical masses, abnormalities in the sigmoid colon, pelvic abscess and peritoneal secondaries. Finally an assessment of the anal sphincter should be made with an assessment of resting tone and voluntary contraction.

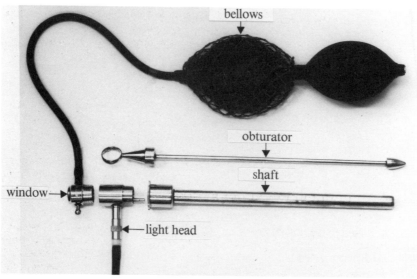

Figure 20.2 Rigid sigmoidoscope, with bellows and obturator

Sigmoidoscopy

Rigid sigmoidoscopy

Rigid sigmoidoscopy is obligatory in any patient with symptoms of large bowel or anal disease. Instruments can be divided into those with proximal and those with distal lighting. The former are more satisfactory as the bulb does not get coated with faeces. Lloyd Davies' pattern is very satisfactory for general work (Figure 20.2). It is made in two diameters (14 and 19 mm) and the larger comes in three lengths (20, 25 and 30 cm). A fibreoptic light is preferable to a battery pack where there is access to a power point.

In some units the bowel is routinely prepared by a disposable phosphate (Fletcher's) enema but this may remove signs of disease, for example blood and mucus, and prevent an assessment of the faeces and the chance to take a faecal specimen for microbiological examination. Sigmoidoscopy in the unprepared bowel is therefore preferable and only about 10% of examinations are obscured by faeces. Under this circumstance a phosphate enema can be given.

The instrument is lubricated and passed gently into the anal canal towards the patient's umbilicus (Figure 20.3a). A fall of resistance indicates that the tip has entered the rectum, the obturator is removed and the eyepiece, light and bellows are attached. The examination is always carried out under direct vision without blind advancement with just sufficient air insufflated to keep the rectal wall apart. The instrument is angled backwards along the sacral curve (Figure 20.3b), past the valves of Houston until the rectosigmoid junction is reached at about 15 cm from the anal verge. It is then advanced

anteriorly and to the left (Figure 20.3c) into the sigmoid colon. Passage through the rectosigmoid junction may cause discomfort and force must never be used. It is possible to enter the sigmoid in about 50–80% of cases, depending on sex, but attempts to do so should be abandoned if pain is produced. The instrument should be withdrawn slowly, inspecting all parts of the bowel wall and taking care to

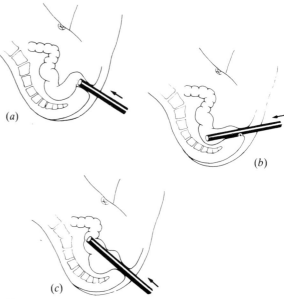

Figure 20.3 Sigmoidoscopy. The sequence of angles through which the instrument is advanced under direct vision and with the help of air insufflation

examine behind folds where lesions such as polyps may be hidden.

The normal mucous membrane is pale pink with visible submucosal vessels (vascular pattern). Loss of the vascular pattern is the most sensitive sign of inflammation. The following should be looked for: abnormal faeces, blood, pus or mucus in the lumen, focal mucosal lesions, e.g. polyp, carcinoma or solitary ulcer, and diffuse lesions, e.g. inflammation. The total distance the sigmoidoscope has been passed must be recorded as well as the distance of any abnormality from the anal verge, its site and extent, both proximal and circumferential.

Biopsy

A biopsy of a suspected carcinoma should be taken from the edge of the lesion using large cusp forceps (e.g. Patterson's pattern). A partial biopsy of a polyp should be avoided first because the pathologist may have insufficient material to examine for invasion through the muscularis mucosae (the criterion of malignancy), and secondly since it may be difficult subsequently to find the lesion for complete removal. Polyps should therefore be removed by complete excision biopsy. In diffuse proctitis a site below the peritoneal reflection, i.e. below about 10 cm, should be chosen to minimize the consequences of any perforation.

After taking a biopsy the site must be inspected for bleeding and a biopsy is contraindicated in patients on anticoagulants or with clotting disorders. Bleeding can usually be controlled by the local application of topical adrenaline solution (1:1000) soaked on a swab passed up the sigmoidoscope. A barium enema should not be performed within 10 days of a biopsy owing to the risk of perforation.

Flexible sigmoidoscopy

A modified short colonoscope (60 cm in length) is available for examination of the left colon in the outpatient department. About four times the number of neoplasms are seen when compared with rigid sigmoidoscopy and flexible sigmoidoscopy is therefore useful in selected cases where more proximal disease is suspected.

The instrument consists of a fibreoptic shaft and head with eyepiece and drive wheels (Figure 20.4). There is a single channel down the shaft for suction, air or water injection and taking biopsies. Lighting and air supply are provided by a combined air/light source unit and suction by a separate suction unit, although a standard suction pump is adequate.

The skilled exponent can perform flexible sigmoidoscopy without any preparation. This saves time and avoids the problems that can occur with an enema. These include faintness in old people and failure to retain the enema in patients with a weak sphincter.

Examination is carried out without sedation with the patient in the left lateral position. Preparation of the bowel with two phosphate enemas is satisfactory in 80% of patients. The lubricated instrument is gently inserted through the anus with the help of the examiner's right index finger. The instrument is

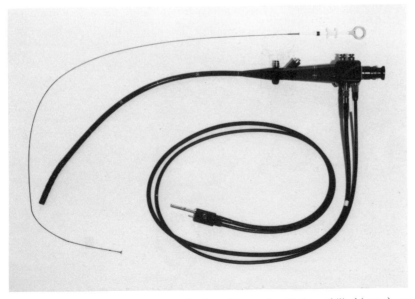

Figure 20.4 Flexible short colonoscope (or sigmoidoscope), with the umbilical (outer) carrying the light, suction and water flush services

advanced under direct vision, using a combination of rotation of the shaft and angulation of the tip by operating the drive wheels, the former best controlled by the right hand, the latter by the left. The lumen should be kept in view and it may be necessary to withdraw the instrument from time to time to achieve this. Insufflation of air should be just sufficient to obtain an adequate luminal view. The problems of negotiating angles and flexures and of loop formation are similar to those with full colonoscopy. Being 60 cm long the instrument is potentially able to reach the splenic flexure (in practice perhaps 30–40% of examinations do so) but it should not be forcibly advanced if pain or resistance are encountered. The physical signs are similar to those seen on rigid sigmoidoscopy and, as with rigid sigmoidoscopy, further investigation of the colon is indicated if more proximal disease is suspected. Lesions are biopsied with standard flexible endoscope biopsy forceps; the specimen is very small.

Proctoscopy

The proctoscope (Figure 20.5) is designed to examine the lower rectum and anal canal only. An ordinary tubular instrument is satisfactory for general work but the Graeme Anderson pattern with an oblique end is useful for inspecting the side wall of the anal canal, e.g. when examining the internal opening of an anal fistula. Lighting is supplied by a fitted fibreoptic light attachment or by an adjustable Anglepoise-type light behind the examiner's head.

The instrument is inserted to the full distance in the direction of the umbilicus and the obturator is withdrawn. Any stool or mucus is swabbed away and the mucosa of the lower rectum examined. It is then slowly withdrawn. This will reveal in turn the anorectal junction (marked by the point at which the mucosa closes at the tip of the proctoscope), the normal anal cushions and the dentate line. The proctoscope is reinserted and the examination repeated with the patient straining downwards. Haemorrhoids are seen as enlargements of the normal anal cushions in the anterior, left lateral and right posterior positions. Internal openings of fistula tracks, anal polyps, fissures and ulceration may also be identified by proctoscopy.

Colonoscopy

Colonoscopy is a more sensitive method of examining the large bowel than contrast radiography. However it requires more medical time to perform. Diagnostic colonoscopy is indicated when large bowel symptoms (especially bleeding) are present despite a normal barium enema or where the barium enema is equivocal. Other uses for colonoscopy include removal of polyps and surveillance of the large bowel in cases with colitis or after treatment for neoplasia.

Recording of findings

The results of the anal examination are conveniently recorded on a rubber stamp diagram (Figure 20.6). The outer circle represents the anal margin, the

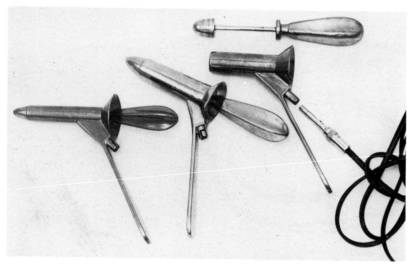

Figure 20.5 Tubular proctoscopes, with interchangeable illumination. The longest one shown is that normally used for the examination of adults

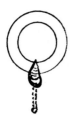

Figure 20.6 Facsimile record of the findings in a case of a chronic posterior fissure with a short direct fistula

inner the anorectal junction. Lesions can be shown graphically and the same system can be used for recording operative procedures. If the circles represent a clock face, the position of any lesion can be given with reference to the midline anterior point of 12 o'clock.

Surgical management of minor anorectal cases

Outpatient operations

No particular bowel preparation is required. Procedures above the dentate line (e.g. injection or rubber band ligation of haemorrhoids) do not require anaesthesia. Operations below this level do so and local anaesthesia is satisfactory for most. For these, the skin should be cleaned with aqueous chlorhexidine or povidone-iodine (Betadine). Under no circumstances should a spirit-based solution be used. The left lateral position is most comfortable for both patient and surgeon.

Local anaesthesia

For small perianal lesions local infiltration of about 5 ml of lignocaine (1%) is sufficient. If more extensive anaesthesia is required' (e.g. for sphincterotomy), 5–10 ml of lignocaine are injected into each ischiorectal fossa using a long spinal needle. This blocks the inferior haemorrhoidal nerves producing relaxation of the lower sphincter and perianal anaesthesia. A further 1–2 ml of anaesthetic can be placed around a local lesion. Bleeding is reduced if lignocaine containing adrenaline (1:200 000) is used. The maximum permitted doses of lignocaine without and with adrenaline are 4 mg/kg and 7 mg/kg body weight respectively.

Inpatient operations

The rectum should be emptied by a phosphate enema given 1–2 h beforehand unless the anal lesion is very painful when no preparation should be given. General anaesthesia is quick and reliable but some surgeons prefer spinal or caudal block. If either is contraindicated, local anaesthesia is sufficient for many procedures. The anal region can be shaved at the start of the operation and the skin prepared as above. Shaving on the ward is not necessary; it can

be done when the patient is anaesthetized before preparation of the skin. The lithotomy position is used by most surgeons in this country, but the jack-knife or left lateral position gives better access for pilonidal sinus.

Postoperative care

Outpatient operations

A mild laxative should be prescribed. Wounds should be dressed with gauze soaked in Eusol or Milton's (2.5%) solution and overlaid by a gauze pad (20 × 10 cm). The dressing is held in place by disposable underpants or adhesive tape. Over the next few days this is changed at home twice daily after a bath and the wound is then reviewed in the outpatient department.

Inpatient operations

General

Normal feeding is resumed on recovery from the anaesthetic and mobilization started as soon as possible, depending on the degree of discomfort of the wound. A limited number of opiate injections (e.g. papaveretum) should be prescribed and constipating analgesics (e.g. codeine) avoided. Analgesia is not usually necessary after perianal operations on the rectum, e.g. local removal of rectal neoplasms.

Bowels

After most anal operations, patients should receive an aperient (e.g. Milpar, 15 ml b.d.) from the first postoperative day until the bowels are open (usually within 3–4 days). A bulk laxative for 1–2 weeks helps to maintain a soft stool. After a pelvic floor repair for incontinence higher doses of aperient (e.g. magnesium sulphate, 20 ml t.d.s.) are given for a few days to produce diarrhoea, thus avoiding straining which might damage the repair.

Wound

At the end of the operation a gauze dressing soaked in Eusol solution is laid onto the wound. Packing or drains placed in the anal canal are painful and unnecessary. The dressing is overlaid with a gauze pad which is held in place by a T-bandage (see Figure 6.12, p. 69). The T-bandage is tied to produce some pressure on the dressing. The dressing is removed after a warm bath on the first postoperative day. Closed wounds, e.g. after sphincterotomy, usually require no more than twice daily baths at home applying surface gauze dressings for a week.

Large open wounds should be irrigated and dressed with Eusol-soaked gauze. Some large fistula wounds may require redressing under anaesthetic on one or two occasions. With deep wounds, the dressing should be tucked into the apex of the cavity with sinus forceps. The wound should not be forcibly packed. During irrigation, the patient lies in the left lateral position on a waterproof sheet draped into a bucket. A reservoir containing normal saline on an infusion stand is connected by tubing to a nozzle. This is introduced into the wound and the flow of liquid controlled by a tap on the nozzle. Debris and pus are washed from the wound in this manner. Irrigations and twice-daily dressings should be continued until the wound is small enough for the patient to be managed at home.

Complications

The common complications after anal operations are bleeding, urinary retention and faecal impaction.

Bleeding

Reactionary bleeding occurs during the first few hours postoperatively and the dressing should be checked during this time. Bleeding from a small vessel at a wound edge may be stopped by pressure or by the application of gauze soaked in topical adrenaline solution (1:1000), a method which can also be applied to rectal wounds via a proctoscope or sigmoidoscope. If local measures fail the patient should be taken back to the operating theatre to secure haemostasis under direct vision.

Secondary haemorrhage occurs in 2–5% of cases with open wounds, usually on the ninth to tenth postoperative day and can be brisk. The pulse and blood pressure should be monitored and blood taken for cross-matching. The foot of the bed is elevated, the patient sedated and an intravenous infusion started if there is evidence of shock. Local pressure is then applied to the bleeding site. With bleeding from within the anal canal this can be achieved by two methods. A large balloon catheter (30 F gauge, 30 ml balloon) is inserted into the rectum and the balloon inflated. Traction is applied to the catheter to bring the balloon against the bleeding site and the catheter is strapped under tension to the thigh. Alternatively, a large rubber tube with a thick coat of paraffin gauze wrapped around it is inserted into the anal canal via a proctoscope. The proctoscope is withdrawn, leaving the tube in place with the gauze surround pressing against the bleeding site. The tube is transfixed with a safety pin on the outside and held in place by gauze dressings and adhesive strapping. It is removed after 24–48 h, after which it is most unusual for bleeding to recur. This method is more reliable since, with the first, the catheter is liable to slip out of the anus. If these measures fail, the patient should be examined under anaesthetic and control of bleeding directly established.

Urinary retention

Retention is more likely if there is pre-existing bladder outflow obstruction or where the anal wound is large. The patient should be catheterized and the catheter removed after 1–2 days (p. 309). The advice of a urological surgeon should be sought if retention recurs. Retention may occur when there is faecal impaction.

Faecal impaction

Impaction is uncommon if aperients are given, but is a likely sequel to confining the bowels. It often presents as the frequent passage of small amounts of liquid faeces. The diagnosis is made by digital examination per rectum. Olive oil retention enemas and aperients should be given. Occasionally disimpaction under general anaesthetic is necessary.

Digital examination

It is unnecessary to perform digital examination in the early postoperative period unless there is an indication, e.g. suspected faecal impaction or bridging of wounds. After haemorrhoidectomy this can be done on the first outpatient visit provided the bowels are working satisfactorily, the aim being to establish that there is no stricture. After fistula operations digital examination should be performed to ensure that bridging of the wound is not taking place. This can be done a few days after the operation to be repeated if necessary at regular intervals (e.g. every 2 days) until the wound is healing satisfactorily. Analgesics may be necessary shortly after operation.

Major rectal cases

Preoperative preparation

Investigations

These include: haemoglobin, blood for cross-match (3–4 units), urea and electrolytes, ECG, chest radiograph, barium enema examination, with or without an intravenous urogram if a growth is possibly involving the urinary tract.

Bowel preparation (also used for colonic resections)

It is important to obtain physical clearance of the bowel. Many surgeons have changed from traditional methods of bowel preparation to using Picolax (sodium citric acid 12 g, magnesium oxide 3.5 g). This is a powerful osmotic laxative which eliminates the need for enemas thus saving nursing time. A suitable regime is shown below:

Preoperative days 4 and 3: low residue diet
Preoperative days 2 and 1: liquid only diet
Day of admission: 1 sachet Picolax in morning, repeated in afternoon

All methods are contraindicated in complete intestinal obstruction and with partial obstruction castor oil should not be used, as there is a danger of perforation as a result of induced gut contraction. For patients with obstruction or those found to have unsatisfactory preparation at operation, on-table lavage can be carried out. An appendicectomy is performed and a large calibre (30 F) Foley catheter is brought through the anterior abdominal wall and inserted into the caecum and retained in place by inflation of the balloon and insertion of a pursestring suture on the bowel. After removal of the operative specimen, the divided colon is then intubated by wide bore corrugated anaesthetic tubing which is draped over the patient's side into a bucket. The Foley catheter is connected to a giving set and normal saline is infused until the bowel is clean. The anaesthetic tubing is removed and the operation is completed. The Foley catheter is left as an intubated caecostomy for 10 days postoperatively after which it is removed.

Antibacterial agents

The postoperative wound infection rate is reduced by intravenous antibacterial agents; giving them for 24 h during and around the time of surgery is as effective as any other regimen. Any combination of agents should include metronidazole (Flagyl) which is active against anaerobic bacteria. Metronidazole (500 mg i.v.) is given on induction of anaesthesia and repeated at 8 and 16 h postoperatively. Many surgeons add an antibiotic such as an aminoglycoside (e.g. tobramycin, gentamicin) or a cephalosporin to metronidazole giving it at the same frequency and for the same duration. Antibiotics are given for no more than 24 h in the non-infected case. A full 5–7 day course should be given where sepsis or toxicity is already present, e.g. diverticular abscess, colonic abscess.

Stomas

Preoperative counselling and site marking are important (see p. 295).

Sexual function

A high proportion of male patients (20–50%) having rectal operations for carcinoma become impotent or have failure of ejaculation owing to operative damage to autonomic nerves. They should be warned in advance about this possibility. Impotence after intersphincteric excision of the rectum as used in inflammatory bowel disease is very uncommon since pelvic nerves are avoided by the close rectal dissection.

Postoperative management

The postoperative care of patients having major rectal surgery is similar to that following any abdominal operation. Almost all will have an intravenous infusion and urinary catheter and many an abdominal or perineal drain. A nasogastric tube is not needed routinely since in most cases bowel function recovers satisfactorily without it. Occasionally a nasogastric tube has to be passed postoperatively, e.g. if paralytic ileus develops.

The first few hours

The house surgeon should check the following:

1. Pulse (rate, volume).
2. Blood pressure.
3. Respiration.
4. Urine (output, colour).
5. Stoma (colour, viability).
6. Drains (patency, volume drained).
7. Dressings (blood).

After operation on the rectum there is often temporary bloodstaining of urine. It is most important to inspect the colour and assess the viability of the stoma. Drains and dressings should be checked for blood loss and soaked dressings should be changed.

The first few days

The house surgeon should attend to the following:
1. Mobilization.
2. Oral fluids.
3. Urinary catheter.
4. Wounds.
5. Intravenous fluids.

The patient should be mobilized and given energetic chest physiotherapy. Recovery of normal bowel motility is indicated by the passage of flatus and the appearance of gut sounds along with a soft, non-distended abdomen. Oral fluids can then be started and the intravenous infusion removed when oral intake is well established.

The urinary catheter should be left on open drainage for at least 5–6 days until the patient is reasonably mobile. In patients with a large perineal wound or preoperative symptoms of prostatic obstruction it should be left longer. The catheter is removed in the morning and the patient encouraged to pass urine. If, after several hours, there are symptoms or signs of retention the catheter should be re-inserted and left for a few more days before withdrawing it again. If retention occurs on the second occasion a urological opinion should be obtained. The frequent passage of small volumes of urine with an enlarged bladder indicates incomplete emptying and is an indication to re-insert the catheter.

Urinary continence may be disturbed after rectal operations but is usually regained during the first few postoperative weeks. The urologist should advise if symptoms persist.

Perineal wound

At operation the perineal wound can be left open or closed by primary suture.

Open perineal wound

The pack or drain is removed at 48 h and the wound is dressed twice daily. It is irrigated and a finger is inserted daily to check for pockets or loculi. The edge of a large gauze dressing is tucked into the wound gently to hold the wound surfaces apart. On no account should small pieces of gauze or cotton wool be used as they may easily become lost within the wound.

Where the posterior vaginal wall has been excised, the perineal wound is in effect open, even if the skin has been sutured. The wound is drained by a suction or corrugated drain brought out through the posterior vaginal wall. This is removed on the second to third day and the skin sutures on the 14th day.

Closed perineal wound

Primary suture is now widely practised, both after intersphincteric excision of the rectum where a small wound is produced and after rectal excision for cancer. It is contraindicated where there has been gross contamination of the wound. Suction drainage is provided by a vacuum drain or sump suction system, the drain being brought out to the side and away from the wound suture line. This should be checked daily to ensure it is not blocked and a note made of the volume of blood draining in the previous 24 h. A satisfactory system using a three-channel sump drain is shown in Figure 20.7. The

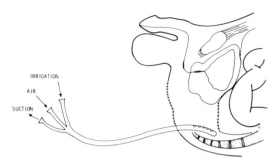

Figure 20.7 Three-way catheter providing drainage for the presacral space after excision of the rectum

removed on the fifth postoperative day, and the sutures on day 10–14.

The management of the abdominal wound is described on p. 262.

wound can be irrigated by a slow infusion of normal saline down one channel. The drain should be removed on the fifth postoperative day, and the sutures on day 10–14.

The management of the abdominal wound is described on p. 262.

Anastomosis

There is no special management of a colorectal or coloanal anastomosis. Early digital examination can be damaging and should be avoided. It may be desirable, however, to know whether the anastomosis has healed satisfactorily. Radiological and digital examination of colorectal anastomoses are unlikely to cause harm beyond the tenth postoperative day. A water-soluble contrast medium (e.g. gastrografin) should be used. A coloanal or ileoanal anastomosis should be assessed at about 2 weeks by digital examination and very gentle sigmoidoscopy or proctoscopy.

Stomas

Life for patients with intestinal stomas has improved in the past 20 years for two chief reasons. First, the development of disposable adhesive appliances has made daily management easier, and secondly the availability of specially trained stoma therapists has helped both the practical and psychological difficulties of the patient. The stoma therapist should counsel the patient *before* operation, and her advice and assistance afterwards are invaluable.

There has been a tendency for the number of stomas to fall with the increasing application of sphincter-preserving operations.

Stoma care nurses

Stoma care nurses are now employed in many general hospitals and all patients should, if possible, be seen preoperatively. In collaboration with the medical team she will be able to help with the following:

Preoperative counselling

Explanation, reassurance and advice to the patient are essential. A stoma is compatible with a normal life. The help of ileostomy or colostomy associations is also available and members are ready to meet patients.

Siting of the stoma

The success of the stoma depends greatly on its site and this should be decided preoperatively. The stoma should be well away from skin creases, scars, including the umbilicus, and previous surgical wounds and bony prominences. It must be visible to the patient and easily accessible for fitting appliances. The site should be marked preoperatively with waterproof ink with the patient standing and a disposable appliance fitted immediately. The patient can then spend several hours finding out whether the site is satisfactory. He can try sitting, bending, walking, etc. to get the feel of the appliance. An unsatisfactory position can be changed.

Appliances

All stoma appliances consist of a bag and a flange which attaches to the skin surrounding the stoma. These are inseparable in a one-piece appliance but can be detached from each other in a two-piece appliance. With the former, the flange is backed by a non-irritant adhesive and is penetrated in its middle by a hole which fits round the stoma. The hole may be bounded by a polyethylene ring or gasket between bag and flange onto which a belt can be fitted. In some one-piece models there is a ring of karaya gum on the skin side of the gasket. Bags are available in gasket sizes ranging from 25 to 100 mm diameter. With a two-piece appliance, the separable flange is usually backed by a sheet of Stomahesive (see below) in which a hole can be cut with scissors to the size of the stoma. A protruding polythene ring on the flange forms a joint with a slightly larger ring on the bag. The bag can thus be removed without disturbing the flange.

Disposable bags have largely replaced non-disposable appliances made of rubber or latex, but these may be preferred by some patients.

Appliances may be drainable or non-drainable, both being available as one- or two-piece units. A drainable appliance (Figure 20.8) must be used for an ileostomy where the stool is fluid whereas for a sigmoid colostomy producing solid faeces a non-drainable bag is more suitable (Figure 20.9).

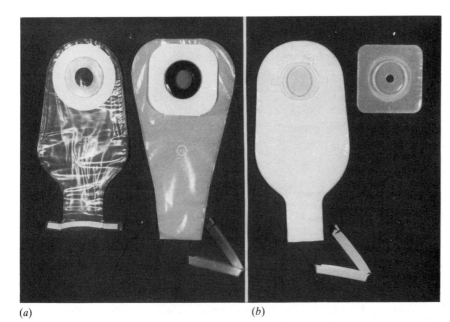

(a)   *(b)*

Figure 20.8 Draining types of disposable ileostomy bags: (*a*) sticking directly to the skin; and (*b*) having a separate adhesive flange

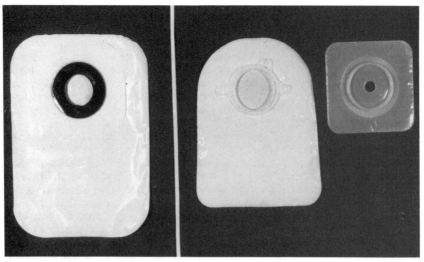

Figure 20.9 Colostomy bags

Plastic caps with belt attachments or adhesive covers are available for patients who have adopted the natural method of colostomy evacuation or use irrigation.

Accessories

A variety of accessories are available (Figure 20.10). Karaya and Stomahesive paste are useful in filling small defects between stoma and flange, especially where there is irregularity of skin contour. Several barrier creams to protect the skin are marketed and deodorants can be obtained. Gas in the bag may cause unsightly bulging or lead to detachment of the flange. It can be released by puncturing the bag with a needle and covering the site with a charcoal filter which allows gas to continue to escape while trapping its odoriferous elements. Adhesive sheeting (Stomahesive, Hollister) is incorporated into the flange of some appliances but can also be obtained separately. The sheets are 10 cm square and are made of material consisting of sodium carboxymethyl cellulose polyisobutylene, gelatin and pectin. The substance is non-reactive to skin and can stick to moist surfaces; it can be moulded to skin contour and easily cut with scissors.

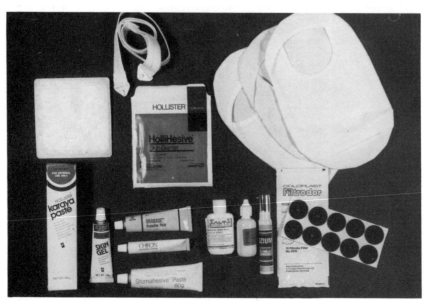

Figure 20.10 Accessories for stoma care, including cover bags (top right) to hide disposable bag, waist belt for greater security (top), skin barrier mini-blankets (centre), karaya paste (bottom left) and odour filter (bottom right)

Ileostomy

An ileostomy may be permanent or temporary. A permanent ileostomy results after proctocolectomy where the anal sphincter mechanism has been removed and is therefore an end ileostomy. A temporary ileostomy is usually fashioned as a loop. Either should be constructed to form a spout about 2–3 cm long to allow the effluent to pass directly into the bag. The postoperative management is similar for both.

Physiology

The daily output is about 500 ml and volumes over 1000 ml are abnormally large. The effluent contains proteolytic enzymes which will digest skin. The electrolyte composition is very variable among different individuals but average concentrations are as follows: Na, 110–120 mmol/l; K, 6–12 mmol/1; Cl, 40–70 mmol/l; and HCO, 30–40 mmol/l.

Management

A permanent ileostomy should be sited in the right iliac fossa just medial to the outer border of the rectus abdominis, away from the umbilicus and the anterior superior iliac spine (Figure 20.11). At the end of the operation, a one-piece translucent drainable bag of the correct size is applied, taking care that it is properly fixed. This may be satisfactory for several days and the absence of any leakage in the early postoperative period gives confidence to the patient.

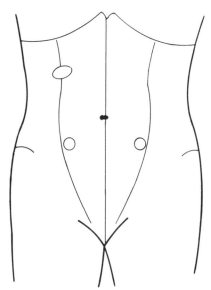

Figure 20.11 Sites for ileostomy (lower) just medial to lateral border of rectus muscle, and for a transverse colostomy (upper right)

In the first 1–2 days, the stoma should be inspected through the translucent bag for necrosis, bleeding and retraction. Most ileostomies act within 48 h and for the first few days may produce volumes of over 1000 ml/24 h. This high output gradually settles but water and electrolyte balance must be maintained until it does so. Mucocutaneous sutures (even if absorbable) should be removed after the tenth day.

The patient will discover by experimentation which appliance is most satisfactory. With time, the ileostomy becomes smaller and a smaller appliance will be necessary. The aim is to change the flange as infrequently as possible, and most ileostomists do so every 4–5 days. The bag should be emptied when half-full, since it can detach the flange if it becomes too heavy.

Complications of ileostomy

Skin problems

Skin problems may arise from too vigorous cleansing, allergy or contact of effluent with the skin, due either to leakage or to an appliance too large for the stoma. Secondary fungal infection may occur.

Allergy

The skin may be allergic to substances within the adhesive although this is uncommon. Allergy should be suspected if the area of involved skin corresponds with the area of the appliance in contact. The appliance should be removed, the skin gently cleaned and Stomahesive or a karaya sheet should be placed on the skin before reapplying the bag. Steroid creams may be necessary.

Leakage

There are several causes of leakage including: poorly fitting appliance; irregular skin contour; retraction of the stoma; ulceration of the stoma; lack of tuition; and lack of manual dexterity.

The first two are common problems which may be solved simply by changing the size of the appliance or overcoming skin irregularities with karaya paste or Stomahesive. Retraction will require refashioning and resiting of the ileostomy may be necessary if contour difficulties are insurmountable. Ulceration at the mucocutaneous junction may cause bleeding and discharge which can lift the flange from the skin. It is usually caused by local pressure of the appliance which should be changed.

Ileostomy dysfunction

This term refers to excessive output from the ileostomy which may produce water and electrolyte (especially sodium) depletion and increases the likelihood of calculus formation (renal, biliary). A persistently high output (>1000 ml/24 h) may be due to: subacute small bowel obstruction; non-obstructing small bowel disease; pancreatic disease; drugs; diet.

Mechanical obstruction may be caused by adhesions, strictures (e.g. ischaemic, Crohn's disease), food bolus or stenosis of the stoma. Non-obstructing small bowel disease includes inflammation (e.g. Crohn's disease) and the short bowel syndrome. Common drugs producing diarrhoea include laxatives and antibiotics, and certain foods, e.g. vegetables especially onions, fruits and alcohol may be responsible. Often, no cause is found when symptomatic treatment should be tried. Bulk laxatives thicken the stool but increase sodium and water output. Codeine, loperamide and diphenoxylate with atropine (Lomotil) may slow transit and reduce volume.

Other complications

Prolapse occasionally occurs and may require refashioning. Parastomal hernia is uncommon. Lateral space obstruction, also rare, occurs when small bowel loops pass between the terminal ileum and parietal wall and become obstructed. Many surgeons close this space in an attempt to avoid this complication. Stenosis may be due to ischaemia or recurrent Crohn's disease of the terminal ileum. It may be manageable by dilatation but refashioning is often necessary.

Colostomy

A colostomy may be permanent or temporary. The two commonest types are: (1) a permanent end colostomy, and (2) a temporary loop colostomy. A permanent colostomy results after excision of the rectum and anal canal, usually for cancer, and is formed by the sigmoid colon. A temporary loop colostomy is used to defunction the distal bowel and is usually sited in the proximal transverse colon or in the sigmoid colon.

Physiology

The effluent from a transverse colon colostomy resembles that from an ileostomy, being fluid and discharging more or less continuously. It contains proteolytic enzymes and can therefore damage skin and excessive output may cause water and electrolyte depletion. A colostomy in the left side of the colon usually produces 1–3 actions of formed faeces/24 h.

Management

The practice of delayed opening of a colostomy has now been superseded by immediate opening at the end of the operation, the edge of the bowel being sutured to the skin directly after closing the main incision (mucocutaneous suture).

Permanent end colostomy

An end colostomy in the sigmoid colon should be sited in the left iliac fossa about halfway between the umbilicus and anterior superior iliac spine centred just medial to the outer border of the rectus abdominis muscle (see Figure 20.11). As with an ileostomy, the appliance should be translucent to enable the stoma to be inspected postoperatively for viability and retraction. It should also be drainable as the effluent is usually liquid in the early postoperative period. A viable stoma will bleed when pricked with a needle. Occasionally some necrosis occurs and its proximal extent can be assessed by introducing a paediatric sigmoidoscope gently into the stoma. If the distal 1–2 cm only are affected the patient should be kept under careful observation. If more is necrotic, revision of the stoma is necessary. Digital examination should not be performed in the early postoperative period. The colostomy usually acts within 3–5 days, producing some flatus before faeces appear. Some oedema of the stoma is common during the first week but this settles spontaneously.

Long-term management

There are three methods of long-term management.

Natural method

Occasionally the colostomy can be relied upon to act at a predictable time each day, often in response to a stimulus, such as tea. Between actions a covering such as a plastic cap supported by a belt may be all that is required to maintain cleanliness. Dietary adjustments and antimotility drugs, e.g. codeine, loperamide or Lomotil, may help to establish this method.

Appliance method

More often, however, the action is not predictable and many patients find a permanent appliance satisfactory. One- or two-piece non-drainable bags are most commonly used, being disposed and changed after each action. One-piece appliances may be applied to a Stomahesive base which stays in place for several days.

Irrigation method

The distal colon is emptied by irrigation every 24–48 h. Advantages include freedom from an appliance between irrigations, and perhaps some saving in time and cost. Irrigation should start 2–4 weeks postoperatively under the supervision of a stoma therapist. Kits are commercially available (Hollister, Coloplast) including a short plastic cone, and long plastic sleeve backed by an adhesive flange which fits around the stoma. With the cones now available perforation is no longer a hazard. The technique is as follows: the patient sits on the lavatory and connects the cone to a plastic reservoir suspended at the level of his head. The cone is gently inserted into the stoma and 750–1000 ml of water at room temperature are run in from the reservoir. A sleeve is then applied to the stoma and its open end is directed into the lavatory bowl. The colon acts after 10–30 min. The sleeve is then folded and clipped, enabling the patient to walk around carrying on normal activities during which time a little more effluent is evacuated. The sleeve can then be removed, the stoma cleaned and an adhesive stoma seal applied.

Complications

Severe skin problems are less likely than with ileostomy but allergy and maceration by moisture resulting from leakage may occur. The remedies are similar to those given for ileostomy. The commonest late complications are paracolostomy hernia, prolapse and stenosis. Hernia is very common and repair is often followed by recurrence. Usually, however, symptoms are minimal and no specific treatment is required. An abdominal support may be necessary if bulging is causing discomfort. Occasionally strangulation occurs when operation is obligatory. Stenosis and prolapse may require refashioning of the stoma.

Temporary loop colostomy

The site for a sigmoid loop colostomy is identical to that for an end colostomy. A transverse loop colostomy should be made through the rectus abdominis muscle away from the costal margin and the abdominal wound (see Figure 20.11). The loop is supported by a rod placed through the mesentery adjacent to the bowel. It can be made of non-absorbable (e.g. glass, rubber tubing, plastic) or of absorbable material (e.g. fibrin (Ethicon)). A non-absorbable rod should be removed at about 1 week postoperatively.

A transverse colostomy requires a permanent appliance which should be drainable in view of the liquid effluent. A larger appliance than is necessary for an end stoma is required and the problems in management are more akin to those of an ileostomy than to a left-sided colostomy.

Complications

These include those seen with ileostomy and left-sided colostomy.

Some anal procedures
Thrombosed perianal varix (perianal haematoma)

This common condition follows rupture or thrombosis of a perianal vein usually after straining at stool. Painful, tender perineal swelling is produced, resolving gradually over a few days. If seen within 48 h, evacuation or excision of the haematoma results in dramatic relief. The operation is carried out under local anaesthesia with the patient in the left lateral position. The overlying skin is incised and the clot released. The wound is trimmed flat and the resulting defect left to heal by granulation (Figure 20.12). Alternatively, the lesion may be completely excised and the resulting wound closed by primary suture.

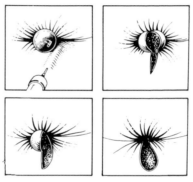

Figure 20.12 Excision of an anal haematoma. The drawings show the successive stages from the superficial injection of lignocaine to the splitting of the swelling into two portions and their excision. Adequate external drainage by a pear-shaped wound is effective

More extensive thromboses of the perianal veins are best treated conservatively, including bed rest, local application of lead lotion and a mild aperient to keep the stool soft.

Fissure

Anal pain is usually associated with defaecation but may be present most of the day. The diagnosis is made on inspection.

All chronic fissures should be treated by operation. Some acute fissures may heal with conservative treatment, including softening of the stool and application of local anaesthetic gel. An anal dilator does not appear to increase the chance of healing and is therefore not necessary. If conservative treatment fails in 3 weeks or so, operation should be carried out.

Both lateral sphincterotomy and anal stretch are adequate operative treatments for fissure.

Lateral sphincterotomy

The operation involves division of the lower half of the internal sphincter and can be performed by the open or closed method.

Open method (Figure 20.13)

An anal retractor is inserted and its blades opened to expose the anal canal laterally. A short circumferential incision is made in the intersphincteric groove which is easily palpable and the lower border of the internal sphincter is identified. Scissor blades are inserted on each side of the internal sphincter

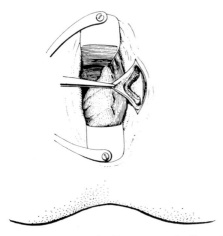

Figure 20.13 Lateral sphincterotomy for fissure-in-ano. The lower internal sphincter is divided between the anal margin and the level of the anal valves

which is divided to the level of the dentate line. The external sphincter is not touched in this operation. Local pressure is applied for a few minutes to secure haemostasis and the wound closed and dressed. Any skin tag or papilla should be removed at the same time.

Closed method

A tenotomy knife is inserted through the skin into the space between the internal and external sphincter. The blade is turned towards the internal sphincter which is divided below the dentate line by a series of sawing actions of the knife.

Anal stretch

The anus is gently stretched by both index fingers until both middle fingers can be inserted as well. The stretch lasts several minutes and should not be forced.

Haemorrhoids

Always exclude other causes of rectal bleeding. Over 90% of haemorrhoids are managed by conservative methods and less than 10% by haemorrhoidectomy. The choice depends on the stage of haemorrhoid and preference of the surgeon. Symptomless haemorrhoids should not be treated.

Symptoms of haemorrhoids spontaneously come and go. When mild, reassurance of the patient (after full examination) and avoidance of constipation by increasing dietary fibre are all that is required.

Injection

This is indicated when there is bleeding with little prolapse. A solution of phenol (5%) in arachis oil is slowly injected into each primary haemorrhoid, 3–5 ml being placed in the submucosa at the level of the upper anal canal (Figure 20.14). The aim is to cause sclerosis around the supplying vessels. A correctly given injection causes the mucosa to swell with submucosal vessels remaining visible. If the mucosa turns white the injection is too superficial,

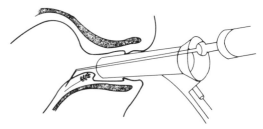

Figure 20.14 Injecting haemorrhoids – submucous, perivascular injection with an angled needle under direct vision

and if there is no swelling it is too deep. Pain results if the injection is placed too low and other structures, e.g. the prostate, may be damaged if it is too deep. Ten per cent of cases complain of pain, and occasionally mucosal ulceration with bleeding, haematuria or haematospermia occur. If injection into the prostate is suspected antibiotics should be given. After the injection a mild aperient should be taken for 48 h. Injection should be repeated only if symptoms persist.

Rubber band ligation

The aim is to apply a rubber band to occlude the feeding vessel of the haemorrhoid. The method is indicated in prolapsing haemorrhoids. A proctoscope is inserted and the mucosa above the haemorrhoid is grasped with tissue forceps. The mucosa is drawn down within the rubber band applicator and provided no discomfort is produced the band is released. After banding, pain or discomfort occurs in 25% of cases and is usually due to the application of the band too low in the anal canal. The band should be removed if marked pain occurs immediately after application. The patient is usually able to continue normal work after banding but he should be warned about the possibility of secondary haemorrhage (5% of cases).

Haemorrhoidectomy

This is indicated in large prolapsing haemorrhoids with an extensive external component. In the Milligan–Morgan operation the posterior, left lateral and right anterior haemorrhoids are grasped with artery forceps and removed in that order. A V-shaped incision lateral to the haemorrhoid is made with scissors and after dissection lateral to the external venous plexus the internal sphincter is identified. The haemorrhoid is then dissected from the internal sphincter and its pedicle transfixed or ligated. At the end of the operation there will be three pear-shaped anal wounds and it is important that there are adequate mucocutaneous bridges between them. There is no need to place dressings or drains in the anal canal; the wound should simply be covered with moist gauze.

Acute strangulated haemorrhoids

There is usually a considerable degree of external venous thrombosis and reduction of the mass is often impossible. The condition can be managed conservatively or by haemorrhoidectomy. Conservative management consists of analgesics (e.g. morphine), aperients and measures to reduce the swelling including elevation of the foot of the bed, and local applications of lead lotions and ice packs.

Draining of abscess

A radial incision is made over the most fluctuant part of the abscess. Pus is collected for bacteriological culture and the cavity gently explored with a finger to break down loculi. The skin edges are trimmed to form an open wound permitting drainage. On inserting an anal speculum, the internal opening of a fistula track may be apparent. This should, however, not be dealt with in the acute stage. The wound is dressed with Eusol-soaked gauze held in place with a T-bandage. A second examination under anaesthetic 7–10 days later may be necessary to establish whether a fistula is present.

21

The urinary tract

D. F. Badenoch

Trauma to the urinary tract

Urological trauma is fortunately uncommon, but when it does occur it is frequently in addition to other visceral injuries.

Renal trauma

Classification and pathology

Injury to the kidney in the UK remains rare. It is helpful to classify this by cause:

1. Blunt injuries (the commonest) which may result from road traffic accidents, fights, falls or contact sports.
2. Penetrating injuries resulting from gunshot, knife or impaling injury.
3. Accelerating/decelerating injuries, usually from road traffic accidents, involving avulsion of the renal pedicle.
4. Iatrogenic injuries may rarely occur during colectomy, but also renal biopsy and percutaneous renal surgery may lead to renal vascular damage or by extension produce a significant cortical laceration or even perforation of the renal pelvis.

It must be remembered that a pathological kidney is more readily traumatized and so may present following a relatively minor insult; this is particularly the case in polycystic kidneys, but may also be so in hydronephrotic, ectopic and horseshoe kidneys. The pathological effects of blunt trauma may include:

1. Minor renal trauma (85%) with renal parenchymal contusion, superficial cortical laceration or subcapsular haematoma.

2. Major renal trauma (15%) which includes deep corticomedullary lacerations, perinephric haematomas and lacerations of the renal pelvis.
3. Vascular injury (<1%) which includes avulsion of the renal pedicle and thrombosis of renal artery or vein.

Symptoms and signs

The clinical features of blunt renal trauma will vary according to the severity, but loin pain and haematuria are almost invariable. Haematuria is usually gross but on occasion may only be microscopic, and if there is hypovolaemic shock anuria may hide this. Examination may reveal loin tenderness, a loin mass and flank bruising. Associated injuries frequently complicate the clinical picture and as in abdominal trauma in general, repeated examination of all systems must be carefully undertaken.

Management

An intravenous urogram (IVU) should be performed as early as possible after resuscitation. Its purpose is to confirm or deny the diagnosis, define the type of injury and to assess the contralateral kidney. On the control film there may be a fractured 10th, 11th or 12th rib or transverse process, loss of psoas outline, loss of renal outline and elevation of the ipsilateral diaphragm. After contrast there may be seen distortion of the collecting system, clot within the collecting system or ureter, the outline of a laceration with extravasation of contrast and, more rarely, failure to opacify at all. The absence of opacification may be due to renal artery avulsion or intimal damage with thrombosis, a clot filling the collecting systems, or hypovolaemic shock (Figure 21.1).

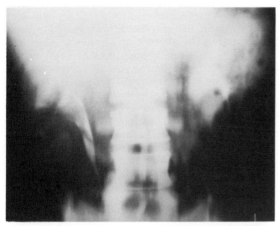

Figure 21.1 Intravenous urogram showing large clot filling the right renal pelvis and upper ureter from a laceration of the right kidney as a result of blunt trauma

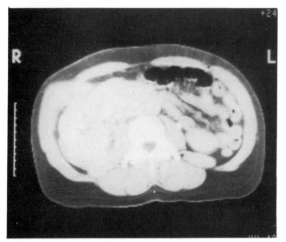

Figure 21.2 CT scan of abdomen showing right kidney surrounded by large perinephric haematoma

An emergency computed tomographic (CT) scan (Figure 21.2) has been advocated where this is feasible to more accurately define the extent of the injury and to carefully assess progress by repeated scanning, but at present this is not generally available.

Renal angiography is only performed where there is failure to visualize the whole or part of the kidney on IVU, where there is persisting gross haematuria or prior to exploration to assess vascular damage and vascular anatomy. Renal ultrasound may be useful in distinguishing clot in the renal pelvis from perinephric haematoma.

Further management

The vast majority of blunt injuries to the kidney may be managed conservatively. A minimum of 2 units of blood should be cross-matched and baseline values of haemoglobin, serum creatinine, urea and electrolytes estimated. As well as a large-bore intravenous cannula, a CVP line is helpful to assess blood loss and tranfusion needs. Bed rest, analgesia and careful monitoring of vital signs and urine output are mandatory. Where available, serial CT scans may be helpful to assess progress.

Indications for urgent operation

In closed injury, operation is only undertaken for continuing haemorrhage as evidenced by increasing flank mass and/or general signs of haemorrhagic shock despite rapid blood transfusion. Ideally, an angiogram should have been performed and if this displays haemorrhage from a renal artery branch, radiological embolization should be attempted. A transperitoneal abdominal approach to the kidney should be made so that other abdominal viscera are carefully inspected. This approach also allows the rapid control of both renal artery and vein. Nephrectomy should only be undertaken as a last resort. All penetrating renal injuries should be explored and 80% of these will also have damage to other viscera.

Follow-up and sequelae

Fortunately, delayed rupture of a subcapsular haematoma is a rare event. The length of hospital stay will be determined by the severity of injury and no didactic number of days in hospital can be advised.

In major injury serial CT scan can be a useful adjunct to inform the clinician of progress.

The majority of damaged kidneys fortunately heal with preservation of function. An IVU (Figure 21.3) or ultrasound with DMSA isotope renogram should

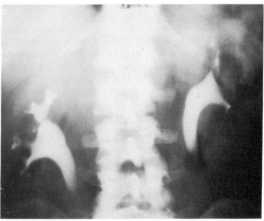

Figure 21.3 IVU at 3 months showing good function in the right kidney with no evidence of obstruction or dysfunction

be performed about 3 months after injury. Rarely, closed trauma may be complicated by the development of a urinoma or abscess in the early stages or later by atrophy, the development of hydronephrosis or a pseudocyst. Hypertension is a recognized sequel and the patient should be advised to have regular blood pressure checks by his family doctor.

Bladder and urethral trauma

Trauma to the urinary bladder may be due to external trauma by:

1. Direct compression of a full bladder in a road traffic accident or following a fall or kick which may frequently be in association with excess alcohol intake.
2. In association with pelvic fractures. In 15% this will be in combination with urethral trauma.

Iatrogenic bladder injury may follow gynaecological surgery, colorectal surgery, urological surgery (during transurethral resection of bladder tumours or even endoscopic bladder biopsy) or be a sequel to radiotherapy, notably for carcinoma of the cervix.

Traumatic bladder rupture

Intraperitoneal rupture typically follows a story of direct violence to a full bladder resulting in a longitudinal tear in the midline. Lower abdominal pain associated with tenderness and eventually features of general peritonitis are typical. The diagnosis is further made by IVU which will show intraperitoneal extravasation of contrast. Occasionally, the diagnosis may be delayed in a drunk patient in whom auto-peritoneal dialysis has occurred. Treatment is by open exploration through a lower midline incision, closure of the bladder with two layers of a non-absorbable suture and urethral catheter drainage for 10–14 days.

Extraperitoneal rupture of the bladder is associated with pelvic fractures and is usually the result of a road traffic accident or crush injury. The general problems of pelvic fracture, blood loss and other associated injuries frequently predominate. Clinical suspicion of the associated bladder rupture in all complex pelvic fractures is the key to diagnosis. Haematuria or, if associated with a urethral injury, anuria with blood at the penile external meatus are common findings, but not invariable. An IVU may display extravasation of contrast from the bladder, but is not invariable and if there is suspicion then endoscopic assessment – preferably by flexible fibreoptic cystoscopy under urethral lignocaine anaesthesia – is best performed since this can be carried out with the patient supine and without need for a general anaesthetic.

A voiding cystogram is another means of making the diagnosis but may be difficult to satisfactorily perform. In the absence of a urethral injury and where there is a small fresh rupture (<1 cm) without appreciable extravasation, it is permissible to perform urethral catheter drainage for 14 days and then check endoscopically that healing has occurred. In all other circumstances, open exploration should be performed and the bladder repaired. The retroperitoneal space is drained and the bladder drained by urethral or suprapubic catheter for 10–14 days.

Male urethral trauma

There is perhaps no subject in urology that has engendered as much heat and controversy – how best to manage posterior urethral ruptures – yet since the problem is rare, no trial of treatment has been performed and inevitably comparison of results is, to say the least, difficult. Two broad categories of injury exist: bulbar urethral injury and posterior membranous urethral ruptures.

Bulbar urethral injury is a result of a compression of the bulbar urethra against the symphysis, brought about either by a fall astride (bicycle bar, manhole cover or classically ship's rigging) or a direct blow (sport or assault). The story should give rise to suspicion of the injury. There may be blood at the tip of the penis or on the underpants, and later the butterfly perineal haematoma defined by the attachment of Colle's and Scarpa's fascia is classic. Generally, there is retention of urine. The haematoma, if present, should be drained; one attempt at urethral catheterization by an expert may be made using a soft size 12 Fr catheter. Should this fail, suprapubic catheterization is at once performed. The urethra is later examined by urethrogram using water-soluble contrast and at around 14 days from injury, urethroscopic assessment performed with placement of a Silastic urethral catheter across the rupture. This is left for a further 10–14 days.

Posterior membranous urethral ruptures are more complex. They may result from a road traffic accident, a fall from a height or crush injury and almost invariably are associated with pelvic ring fractures, either with a 'butterfly' type of fracture of the middle segment of the pelvic ring or a more severe disruption of the pelvic ring (Figure 21.4) frequently in association with gross displacement of the urethra due to distraction forces on its attachments. Awareness of the possibility of pelvic ring disruption is vital to making the diagnosis; again the passage of blood per urethram and retention are common features, *but not invariable*.

The immediate management is secondary to general resuscitation as frequently this forms only part of a multiple injury. Formal suprapubic cystotomy should be performed to allow urinary

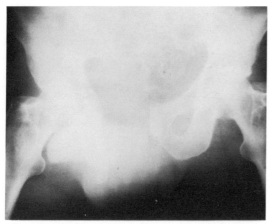

Figure 21.4 Severe disruption of the pelvic ring associated with posterior urethral injury

drainage – being particuarly careful not to decompress the pelvic haematoma. As soon as the general condition of the patient allows (3–14 days), the fracture is reduced and fixed by external fixation devices. This often reduces the soft tissue displacement of the urethra. Studies are then made by means of ascending and descending urethrograms (via suprapubic catheter) made with water-soluble contrast media. If there is a short gap or baffle, it may then be possible to endoscopically negotiate the problem using a Sachse Urethrotome from below aided by a flexible or rigid telescope introduced through the bladder neck via the suprapubic tract. If this is not possible, then open urethroplasty is necessary. Major urethral stricture may result even more than 20 years after injury.

Renal and ureteric stones

Nowhere in urology have there been such dramatic changes as in the management of upper urinary tract stones. Over the past decade the advent of percutaneous surgical techniques and subsequently of external shock wave lithotripsy have radically altered the options available. The line of management of upper urinary tract stones remains: (1) diagnosis; (2) conservative treatment; (3) surgical treatment; (4) look for the underlying cause.

Ureteric/renal colic

Diagnosis and conservative treatment

The correct diagnosis of renal/ureteric colic can usually be made from the history: severe loin pain radiating to the ipsilateral iliac fossa and testis or labium majus, associated with nausea and reflex vomiting. Generally, apart from mild loin tenderness, uncomplicated cases will lack physical signs, but a thorough examination must be made to exclude other intra-abdominal crises, in particular acute intraperitoneal problems, pancreatitis or even, rarely, a leaking abdominal aortic aneurysm. On occasion, bowel sounds may be scanty or absent due to a reflex paralytic ileus. On urinalysis, the presence of microscopic haematuria will add weight to the diagnosis. Provided no allergy to iodine exists, an intravenous urogram should be performed within 12 h of onset since some 10% of urinary stones are radiolucent and others may overly bone on the radiograph, particularly the sacrum; thus a plain urinary tract radiograph alone is inadequate. Renal ultrasound may on occasion have to suffice in the presence of iodine allergy, but at times the affected renal pelvis and calyces may not be dilated so that a false negative ultrasound may lead to an incorrect diagnosis and, where dilatation does exist, the level of obstruction may not be apparent.

The most effective initial analgesic is probably still pethidine, but subsequently the use of non-steroidal anti-inflammatory drugs is to be preferred (diclofenac sodium or indomethacin) since these are not narcotics and may be given by suppository. Adequate hydration rather than overhydration is to be encouraged. Subsequent management will depend on the size of the stone, site of the stone, the presence or development of complications and the progress of conservative management. The common areas of hold-up or impaction of ureteric stones are at the pelvi-ureteric junction, the pelvic brim or above the vesico-ureteric junction. Since 95% of stones of 5 mm diameter or less will pass spontaneously, despite all the advances in stone management that have occurred, these should still be left to be given a chance to pass naturally.

Surgery for ureteric stones

The indications for surgery may be grouped as:

1. Urgent: complete obstruction of a solitary kidney or bilateral complete obstruction (which may rarely, but typically occur with uric acid lithiasis), evidence of infection above an impacted stone (the patient will typically have pyrexia, continuous loin pain and may be markedly tender in the affected loin), or very rarely perforation of the ureter.
2. Early surgery should be undertaken when it is obvious that the stone is not going to pass, i.e. where there is a stone greater than 1 cm diameter or the patient has persisting, unremitting bouts of ureteric colic.
3. Subsequent surgery may be required where there has been failure of the stone to pass naturally over an agreed but arbitrary time period such as 6 weeks.

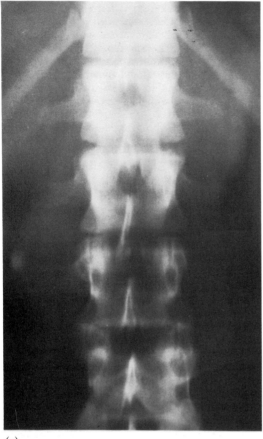

(a)

(b)

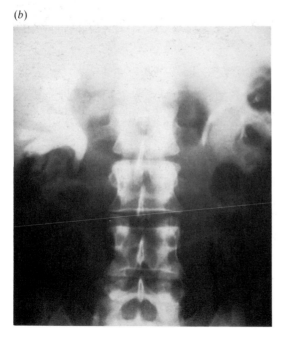

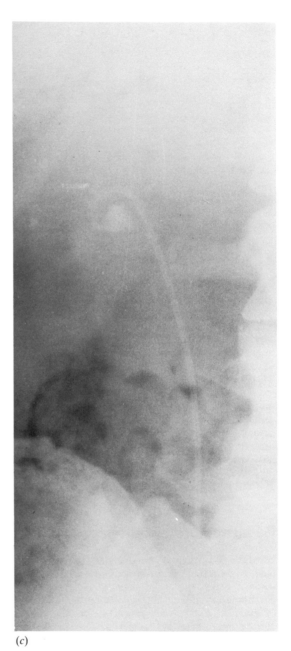

(c)

Figure 21.5 (a) Stone at right pelvi-ureteric junction; (b) obstruction due to stone at right pelvi-ureteric junction; (c) stone pushed back into renal collecting system with a double J stent inserted

Methods of ureteric stone removal

The method chosen will depend very much on the availability of a lithotripter or of modern ureteric endoscopy and the expertise to perform such manoeuvres. Certainly no operation should ever be performed on the ureter or kidney without a prior radiographic examination being made on the day of (and preferably en route to) theatre to confirm the presence and exact site of the stone.

Where urgent surgery is required for complete obstruction or infection above an impacted stone, it is now best to decompress the affected kidney by performing a needle nephrostomy under ultrasound guidance. This can be performed under local anaesthesia with sedation and, using modern needle nephrostomy sets, can be undertaken with relatively little risk to the affected kidney. This should firstly decompress the kidney and secondly, where there is an infection, allow purulent urine to be sent off for microbiological studies so that the subsequent antibiotic treatment may be changed on a rational basis as appropriate. It will allow an acutely ill patient to improve so that further strategy as to how to best remove the stone can be decided and carried out under optimum conditions.

The treatment will not only depend upon the available options but also on the position of the stone.

Upper third and middle third ureteric stones

Upper third and middle third ureteric stones may be treated in the same way. Ideally, the stone should be flushed back up into the renal pelvis as follows: a ureteric catheter is introduced by cystoscopy under image intensifier control to the level of the stone. The catheter should have a terminal hole such as the Pollack catheter and the stone is then flushed up into the renal pelvis by injecting 5–10 ml of saline via this catheter. Immediately this is done a guide wire is passed through the catheter and a double-J ureteric stent of correct proportions is placed between the renal pelvis and bladder in order to decompress the urinary tract and make it less possible for the stone to drop back into the ureter (Figures 21.5a, b, c). Ideally, under the same anaesthetic, the patient should then undergo lithotripsy. On occasion the stone will not move up from its position, but a guide wire and double-J stent may be passed beyond the stone to lie between the renal pelvis and bladder. This provides sufficient fluid/stone interface for lithotripsy to be carried out with the stone remaining in the ureter. However, results of lithotripsy on ureteric stone *in situ* are less satisfactory than where these have been moved back into the kidney. Should the stone be impacted and a guide wire and double-J ureteric stent cannot be

passed beyond the stone, the best option remains that of open removal. For upper third ureteric stones, the ureter is approached via an abdominal incision made from the tip of the 12th rib, whereas for middle third ureteric stones a transverse extraperitoneal approach is appropriate. The ureter is always drained following this procedure via a tube drain down to the ureterotomy. This should not be removed until 5 days after surgery to ensure that any urinary leakage may satisfactorily drain to the exterior.

Lower third ureteric stones

These can now be satisfactorily treated *in situ* by lithotripsy with increasingly good results. It is probable that the passage of a ureteric stent past the stone will enhance fragmentation and subsequent drainage. If lithotripsy is not readily available then endoscopic retrieval of the stone may be undertaken. Modern rigid ureteroscopes have developed rapidly in design since their first introduction a few years ago. They are now of smaller calibre, more flexible and less traumatic to the ureter; however, they should never be used by the inexpert and the patient must always be warned that open ureterolithotomy may be required. After retrograde passage of a guide wire to the renal pelvis past the

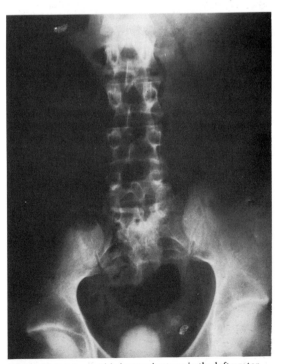

Figure 21.6 A lower third ureteric stone in the left ureter shown on X-ray with the stone beside being removed by ureteroscopic basketry

stone, the ureteric orifice is dilated. This can be performed by passing an olivary type metal dilator, by hydrostatic dilatation or using a graduated single dilator of the 'Nottingham' type. The ureteroscope may then be passed to the level of the stone. If the stone is seen to be mobile and small (i.e. of a similar calibre to the ureteroscope), it may be trapped by a basket passed through the operating channel of the ureteroscope and retrieved (Figure 21.6). However, if the stone is seen to be mobile and large then some form of fragmentation will be necessary. Several novel methods have recently been developed. At the present time, the best method is undoubtedly using a pulsed dye laser, but unfortunately this is not generally available. The electrohydraulic probe is generally felt to be a dangerous means of performing this and the ultrasound generated drill should also be extremely carefully used. Although ureteroscopic stone removal for lower third ureteric stones has quite definitely expanded the success of basket retrieval of stones, it should be used with extreme care and caution. If the stone is impacted then an open procedure to remove the ureteric stone is to be preferred. Through a Pfannensteil or Abernethy extraperitoneal approach the lower end of the ureter is identified, necessitating the division of the superior vesical pedicle on that side, and following retrieval of the stone a tube drain should be left down to the level of the ureterostomy for a minimum of 5 days.

Haematuria

Haematuria remains perhaps the most important urological symptom. Its presence must alert any clinician to fully investigate the urinary tract. The fact that the patient may be on anticoagulants is not sufficient to ignore this important symptom as this may merely accelerate the presence of such an important matter. If there is doubt as to haematuria existing then a fresh specimen of urine should be examined microscopically as well as 'stick' tested. Nowadays, with so many routine medical examinations being carried out, the presence of microscopic haematuria is a common finding. Again such findings should not be ignored and certainly, if the patient has more than one specimen of urine with microscopic haematuria and is over the age of 40 years, he or she should be fully investigated despite the lack of symptoms. After thorough abdominal examination and pelvic examination, the patient's urine should be examined cytologically. It is important that a fresh specimen of urine (not a first voided specimen in the morning) is centrifuged down and examined rapidly for abnormal transitional cells using the Papanicolaou stain. A sample of urine should also be cultured and an urgent intravenous urogram performed. In the case of iodine allergy, ultrasound of the urinary tract should be adequate. Further management will obviously depend on the radiographic or ultrasound findings, but even should these be entirely negative, a cystoscopy should be carried out. With the advent of modern purpose-built flexible cystoscopes, this can be accomplished in a 20-min period under local anaesthesia on an outpatient basis without the need for starvation or sedation, let alone general anaesthesia.

Urethral catheterization

The proper use of the urethral catheter is the most important single factor in successful management of the bladder and prostatic cases: misuse can cause damage.

In the male a brusque forcing of the catheter may bruise the urethra and cause copious bleeding, while cruder effort will tear a false passage and result in

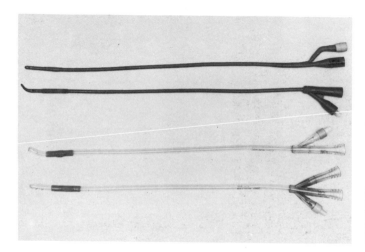

Figure 21.7 Various types of urethral catheter: (*a*) simple latex with Foley balloon; (*b*) Tiemann with balloon; (*c*) Simplastic coudé tip with balloon; (*d*) Simplastic irrigating catheter with balloon

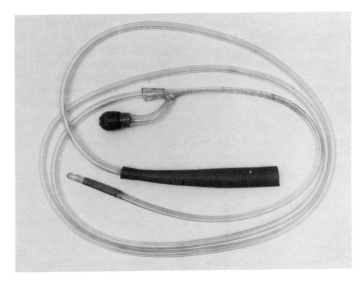

Figure 21.8 Gibbon catheter with Foley bag

failure to enter the bladder. Both misdemeanours may lead to a stricture. This mechanical disaster is equalled only by the introduction of infection. The bladder is especially liable to infection if it has been a long time distended. Imperfect aseptic technique is inexcusable.

Types of catheter

The introduction of the plastic catheter has brought many advantages (Figure 21.7). The old-fashioned red-rubber catheters were irritant to the urethra and strength was obtained at the expense of internal diameter.

Gibbon catheter

The modern Gibbon catheter, constructed of polyvinyl chloride, is relatively small, has a wide bore in relation to its external diameter, and causes minimal irritation (Figure 21.8). In our opinion it is ideal for the relief of long-standing urinary retention. To facilitate introduction the catheter is stiffened by a plastic stylet which is subsequently withdrawn by holding the entire length of tubing straight and exerting a steady pull.

Tiemann neoplex catheter

Where a Gibbon catheter cannot be introduced a Tiemann neoplex catheter is recommended (Figure 21.7). This catheter has a slightly curved extremity which is tapered. Plastic catheters of the Porges or neoplex variety have the advantage of being relatively rigid so that they may be used to negotiate a urethra rendered narrow by prostatic disease or urethral stricture.

Foley catheter

The latex Foley catheter (Figure 21.9) is of softer material and has an inflatable bag near its end so that on distension (with water) the latter is held

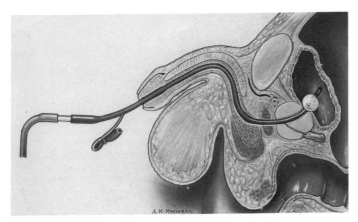

Figure 21.9 Foley's balloon-ended self-retaining catheter in place

within the internal meatus. The bag capacity varies from 5 to 30 ml and is clearly marked on each catheter. The disadvantages of the Foley catheter are that its lumen is relatively small and, despite the thickness of its wall (in which the inflation channel is fully incorporated), it remains only semi-rigid. It cannot therefore be used to overcome serious urethral obstruction. In such a case it is better to use a Tiemann balloon catheter made of neoplex. Metal introducers should not be used in the conscious patient. By nature of its softness the latex Foley catheter will collapse if firm suction is applied so its use is not recommended if much bleeding and clot obstruction are likely. Uneven distension of the balloon with consequent angulation of the tip may sometimes interfere with drainage, but nevertheless this type of catheter is extremely valuable, especially in female cases, and is widely used. A combination of Gibbon catheter and Foley balloon is available (Figure 21.8).

Plastic catheters

Advances in plastic engineering have led to a wide range of firm, yet supple catheters. The ratio of bore to wall thickness has steadily increased, a fine irrigating channel can be incorporated in the wall as in the Kinder catheter, or a Foley retaining balloon may be incorporated in addition as in the Hamilton Stewart catheter. Most varieties of catheter are also manufactured with a coudé tip to aid passage past the prostatic urethra. The modern plastic catheter has the advantage of causing minimal urethral irritation.

Sizes of catheters

Catheters and bougies are calibrated according to two main scales. The widely used French (or Charrière) scale is a direct indication of the external circumference in millimetres. For simple drainage in cases of adult urinary retention an 18 Fr catheter should be used. This permits free drainage of the urethral secretions but prevents meatal stenosis, and is comfortable for the patient.

Sterilization of catheters

The immense advantage enjoyed by the modern catheter is its method of sterilization. Plastic catheters are packed in a series of sealed envelopes at the factory and then submitted to sterilization by gamma irradiation. There is thus no handling between manufacture and time of use. The outer envelope is cut by an assistant and the inner envelope containing the catheter shaken out on to the dressing trolley. After cutting or tearing this inner envelope the catheter itself is made to protrude and is then introduced into the urethra from within the evelope, being at no time touched by the house surgeon's hands.

Catheterization for retention

In cases of acute (painful) retention of urine or where difficulty in catheterization is expected there is every reason to relieve the patient's anxiety and discomfort by suitable sedation. If the patient is much distressed give an injection of diazepam, 10 mg i.v. (dosage for men of average build). In the male the glans penis should be carefully cleansed, the foreskin being withdrawn and all smegma wiped away. Aqueous chlorhexidine (strength 1%) is preferred for this purpose. Holding the penis in the left hand the anterior urethra is anaesthetized and lubricated by injecting a gel of 1% lignocaine and 0.25% chlorhexidine via the external meatus (Figure 21.10).

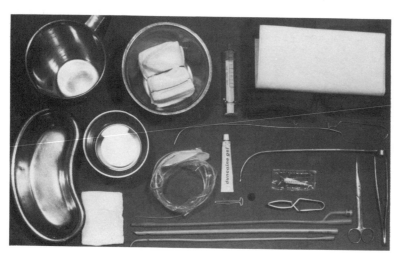

Figure 21.10 Catheterization trolley. On the left are receptacles and gallipots containing swabs and chlorhexidine. A variety of catheters are at the bottom; above them is a tube of local anaesthetic, penile clip, spigot, metal urethral bougie and catheter introducer. On the right are sterile glove packet (top) scissors and forceps for no-touch technique.

After the lubricant has been injected it should be massaged well down the urethra for a few moments before a penile clamp is applied. The latter should be left in place for 2 min to allow the anaesthetic to act and the house surgeon should use the time to wash his hands again. In some units the use of sterile disposable gloves has become routine and there is much to recommend this practice. The penis is then wrapped in a sterile swab and held in the left hand, while the tip of the catheter, lubricated and held vertically in the envelope in the right hand, is gently introduced down the urethra. As the bulb of the urethra is reached the penis should be rotated down into the line of the patient's body and the catheter further introduced towards the bladder. This man-oeuvre is only necessary with the more rigid catheters. If a stylet is present it should now be removed and a sample of the urine collected in a sterile bottle for laboratory analysis.

In difficult cases it is often helpful to place a sandbag under the patient's buttocks so that the curvature of the bulbous urethra is diminished. Once the catheter has been introduced into the bladder and a specimen of urine taken it should immediately be connected to the drainage bag or bottle. In cases of acute retention due to prostatic hypertrophy or stricture and where there is no bleeding, the use of a uri-bag with the Gibbon-type catheter is advised. This has but one junction so that the risk of introducing infection is minimized. The bag is light, may be hooked on to the side of the bed and is easily handled by the nursing staff during bed making. Moreover, on account of its lightness the ambulant patient can carry the bag about with him so that his activity is in no way curtailed. It is important, however, that it should be carried well below the level of the bladder.

Securing the catheter

The usual Gibbon catheter has two flaps attached to the tubing, some 20 cm (8 in) from its tip. These flaps are secured to the shaft of the penis by strapping, or in the female to the inner side of the thigh (Figure 21.11).

If a small catheter of the Foley type has been used the balloon should immediately be distended to the requisite volume, thus rendering it self-retaining. At this stage it is imperative to replace the prepuce over the glans penis otherwise paraphimosis may de-velop. A small protective dressing of ribbon gauze or lint smeared with flavine emulsion is then applied to the external meatus.

Methods of securing other indwelling catheters rely mainly on the use of adhesive strapping applied longitudinally along the exposed portion of the catheter and continued proximally over the shaft of the penis: the surface of the catheter should be cleansed of lubricant and carefully dried and the

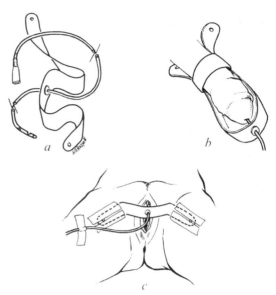

Figure 21.11 (*a*) Gibbon's catheter; (*b*) in use in the male; (*c*) in use in the female

pubis shaved. Three 15 cm lengths of 1.25 cm (½ in) adhesive tape will suffice (with some overlapping) to enclose the circumference of the catheter. A further 20 cm (8 in) length of 1 cm strapping wound spirally upwards around the catheter and continued on to the penis will complete the fixation. Tight cir-cumferential strapping around the penis should be avoided as it is likely to lead to oedema.

Collecting apparatus

Bacteriological studies have demonstrated that infection may readily occur via the lumen of the drainage tube attached to the catheter. A closed system of drainage such as that provided by the Gibbon catheter connected with a uri-bag or ending under a measured quantity of antiseptic solution in a sterile bottle is thus to be recommended (Figure 21.12). When a separate drainage tube has to be

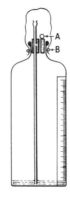

Figure 21.12 The Bristol pattern of infection-preventing urine-collecting bottle. A, Tablet of formagene; B, rubber band

attached to an ordinary catheter the choice may lie between rubber or transparent plastic tubing. Rubber tubing is heavier and may drag on the catheter, but has the advantage of being more easily 'milked' to free the system of debris or clots. The tubing should of course be sterile and a glass connection of suitable size will be required to link it with the catheter. Care should be taken to ensure that the lumen of the latter is adequate and small-bore glass nozzles are to be avoided. Plastic tubing can usually be directly inserted into the end of the catheter, and in some types of collecting apparatus the end of the tubing is shaped for this purpose. This equipment also incorporates a plastic 'trap' at its distal end to avoid bacterial contamination when changing the collecting bags (Figures 21.13 and 21.14).

Sterile disposable collecting bags for urine vary in their efficiency and cost. The following features are important:

1. They should preferably be made of transparent material so that the quality and quantity of drainage can readily be observed.
2. The incorporation of a printed scale to register the approximate amount is an advantage.

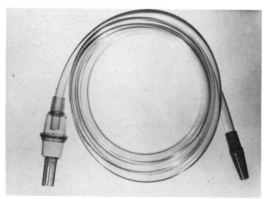

Figure 21.13 Bard Davol drainage tube with 'trap'

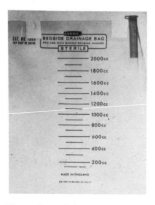

Figure 21.14 Disposable drainage bag

3. They should be so constructed as to avoid seams which may leak when the bag becomes distended.
4. Provision should be made for a carrying handle which can either be used by the patient (if ambulant) or attached to the side of the bed.
5. The junction of the collecting tubing with the bag should be reinforced or capable of support in such a way to avoid angulation with consequent obstruction of drainage.
6. An adequate length of collecting tubing of sufficient calibre should be attached.

Catheterization at operation

Since the great majority of prostatectomies and of operations for bladder tumour are performed per urethram, bladder drainage in these circumstances is effected by catheters of the Foley type. If bleeding is likely to be heavy an irrigating catheter should be used. After prostatic surgery it is sometimes difficult to negotiate the catheter over the lip of the bladder neck; in these circumstances the use of a Maryfield introducer is recommended; alternatively, a catheter of the coudé type should be used.

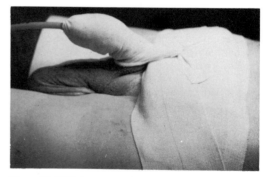

Figure 21.15 Tubegauz penile dressing and catheter

If open surgery has been performed, a simple whistle-tip catheter may be secured by passing a nylon suture through its eye and bringing the ends out through the bladder and anterior abdominal wall where they may be secured either by knotting over a metal bar or by pinching in an MSA button. This permits accurate positioning of the catheter before the prostatic capsule or bladder incision is closed. In either case Tubegauz No. 12 forms a simple and effective penile dressing (Figure 21.15).

Failed catheterization

When catheterization fails to relieve retention the bladder must be drained suprapubically. As a temporary measure suprapubic aspiration may be

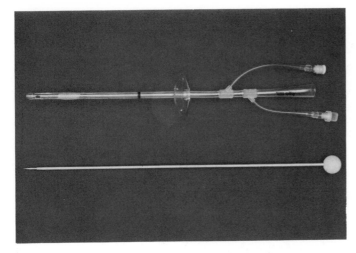

Figure 21.16 Argyle suprapubic catheter

performed (see p. 318) or a fine catheter introduced by the Supracath or Argle technique (Figure 21.16).

Suprapubic catheterization

Suprapubic stab cystotomy

If it is thought that temporary suprapubic drainage is required for only a few days, then suprapubic stab drainage should be carried out. An intradermal weal of 1% xylocaine is raised in the midline two finger-breadths above the pubis. The intended track through the abdominal wall into the distended bladder is then infiltrated with the same anaesthetic agent and after making a small incision through the skin a 12 Fr Argyle trocar-catheter is introduced firmly and steadily through the abdominal wall and into the bladder. The trocar is then withdrawn and the retaining balloon inflated. This is an extremely effective method of relieving painful retention of urine.

Formal suprapubic cystotomy

Owing to improvement in the quality of urethral catheters, and to the better control of infection by chemotherapy, the need for permanent suprapubic cystotomy drainage has nowadays greatly diminished. In most cases where corrective surgery is excluded by senility or intercurrent disease, continuous drainage with an indwelling urethral catheter of the latex Foley type is generally to be preferred. When, however, catheterization is impracticable for mechanical reasons, or fails to provide free drainage on account of debris or clot in the bladder, formal suprapubic drainage may be called for.

Technique

The procedure, which should be carried out in the operating theatre, consists of the introduction of a large self-retaining catheter, at least 32 Fr, of the De Pezzer or Malecot type (Figure 21.17). These catheters are nowadays made of latex rubber which retains its resilience and is less irritant than the old-fashioned red-rubber variety. Encrustation is minimal and the risk of the material perishing and the expanded head breaking off in the bladder when the catheter is changed has all but been eliminated.

Formal suprapubic cystotomy should always be carried out well away from the symphysis pubis and preferably at a point at least half-way between the latter and the umbilicus. If a retaining belt is going to be worn it will 'sit' more comfortably at this level, while if drainage is only to be temporary the obliquity of the track will encourage more rapid closure after the catheter is withdrawn.

The formal operation may be performed under either general or local anaesthesia, infiltrating 1% lignocaine subcutaneously and into the abdominal wall at the above-mentioned site. The bladder is distended. A 4-cm vertical incision is then made through the skin and between the rectus muscles. The peritoneum is swept cranially with a swab, the recti being gently retracted laterally. Two catgut stay stitches are inserted into the bladder wall and, using a scalpel, a small stab incision is made between

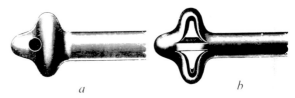

Figure 21.17 (a) De Pezzer catheter; (b) Malecot catheter

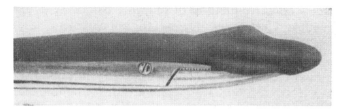

Figure 21.18 Method of stretching a De Pezzer catheter with a haemostat

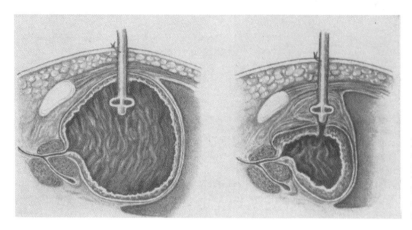

Figure 21.19 Unless the expanded end of the catheter is pushed well into the bladder it will be dragged out as the bladder contracts, for the catheter is fixed to the skin by a stitch

them. Excess bladder fluid is sucked away and a 22 or 24 gauge Foley catheter introduced. If a Malecot or De Pezzer catheter is used it should be introduced by placing the tip of a long haemostat into the lumen of the catheter via one of the drainage openings and pulling the catheter up tightly so as to reduce the calibre of the expanded end (Figure 21.18).

Care should be taken to advance the catheter sufficiently within the cavity of the bladder to avoid extrusion as the latter contracts (Figure 21.19). On the other hand, the expanded end should not be allowed to dangle like the clapper of a bell, as intermittent contact with the sensitive trigone may cause considerable discomfort.

The stay stitches may then be crossed and tied to ensure a snug fit for the emerging tube. A few interrupted stitches complete the closure of the small abdominal incision; a skin stitch may help secure the tube.

Changing the tube

When permanent suprapubic drainage has been established it becomes necessary to change the tube from time to time. If latex catheters are used an interval of between 3 and 4 weeks is usually sufficient and a gentle wash-out with sterile saline (using a 50 ml disposable syringe) should be given through the new catheter to ensure that drainage is satisfactory.

To remove the tube a blunt-ended introducer is inserted into the lumen and advanced as far as it will go. The catheter is pulled up tightly over the introducer so as to straighten out the expanded end and then withdrawn from the bladder. A sterile replacement should be immediately available and is introduced in similar manner.

Difficulty may sometimes occur when the previous catheter has fallen out and the fistulous track has contracted. In such an event gentle dilatation with graduated uterine dilators (Hegar's) will often facilitate reintroduction.

It must be emphasized that nowadays permanent suprapubic cystostomy is seldom justified.

Instrumentation of urethral stricture

Method

The secret of success in relieving acute retention due to urethral stricture is gentleness. After appropriate sedation and anaesthetization of the urethra a small sound or bougie (12 Fr) should be cautiously introduced down the urethra using an aseptic technique. If after careful manipulation this fails to negotiate the stricture, filiform bougies should be tried. The possession of a set of graduated screw-on bougies offers an incalculable advantage in such circumstances, since if a small filiform can be induced to pass, further 'followers' of increasing size can be attached in sequence and the stricture thus enlarged (Figure 21.20).

Should a filiform bougie fail to negotiate the stricture the method of 'faggoting' should be tried, several filiforms being introduced to the face of the

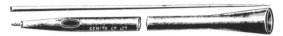

Figure 21.20 Philips' catheter. The guide is inserted through the stricture, after which the catheter is screwed on to the guide

stricture so that one may be induced to pass through the stretched face of the obstruction. Once a fine bougie has entered the bladder urine will trickle alongside it and it is often wise at this stage to leave the instrument indwelling for the time being. As the oedema subsides the flow will usually increase and in 48 h further dilatation may be attempted with a greater prospect of success.

Meatal stenosis

Narrowing of the external meatus may be either congenital or acquired, when it may result from the forcible instrumentation of the small meatus or from indwelling catheterization using too large a catheter. The condition will generally yield to regular dilatation, and once a reasonable size has been achieved the patient can be provided with a dilator and taught how to use it himself: the tapering plastic sheaths in which disposable intravenous needles are supplied, or plastic catheter spigots are ideal for the purpose. Should a meatal stenosis require immediate treatment, as for the relief of acute retention, a 6 mm incision should be made in a downward direction either with the tip of a pair of scissors or with a small scalpel.

Management of clot retention

Bleeding into the bladder of such severity as to cause clot retention may occur with vesical tumour, in benign prostatic hypertrophy, after irradiation, or as a complication of surgery to the lower tract although the use of an irrigating catheter has much reduced its incidence in the last circumstance.

Aspiration and wash-out

If an indwelling catheter is already in place (failing which a wide-bore plastic catheter should be passed), suction applied with a glass Wardill syringe (Figure 21.21) or plastic bladder syringe will often suffice to clear the obstruction. Once the obstructing

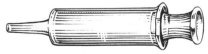

Figure 21.21 Wardill's all-glass bladder syringe

clot has been evacuated the bladder should be washed out with sterile normal saline until all clots have been removed and the fluid is returned clear. It is wise then to leave the catheter *in situ* until all evidence of further bleeding has ceased.

Ellick's evacuator

Should suction with a syringe fail the patient must be taken to theatre and more forceful irrigation and suction applied using an evacuating cannula or catheter attached to Ellick's evacuator. In resistant cases the secret of success often lies in introducing the cannula and then rapidly and repeatedly withdrawing the obturator until the clot follows through.

Suprapubic drainage

When catheterization and evacuation fail the bladder must be drained suprapubically.

Acute retention of urine

Paramount among the commoner urological emergencies requiring immediate attention is acute urinary retention. The combination of a painfully distended bladder with inability to void distinguishes the condition from:

1. Chronic retention in which the distension, though often greater, is painless and associated with ineffectual frequency or overflow incontinence.
2. Oliguria or anuria when little or no urine is passed but the bladder remains empty.

Except in unconscious patients or in traumatic cases with severe shock, acute retention is unlikely to be overlooked. Even in such circumstances routine clinical examination should immediately reveal the distended viscus. Uncertainty may yet occasionally arise on account of obesity, abdominal distension from other causes or where the bladder has become displaced, as following previous surgical excision of the rectum. In a majority of cases, however, the condition is self-evident and some idea of the more usual causes (excluding postoperative retention) may be gleaned from Table 21.1.

Careful attention to the history, antecedent urinary symptoms or disease and recent use of drugs, e.g. alcohol, antispasmodics or sympathomimetics, as well as to the age of the patient and the circumstances in which retention has occurred, will often suggest the cause. Further evidence must be sought by clinical methods, always including rectal examination. The information thus gained will in most cases reveal the diagnosis and indicate the appropriate means of relief.

Table 21.1 Analysis of 300 consecutive cases of acute retention in a general hospital

	No. of cases
Benign prostatic hyperplasia	193
Malignant disease of the prostate	39
Urethral stricture	23
Phimosis	14
Vesical tumour (clot retention)	9
Inflammation (cyst-prostatitis)	4
Impacted urethral calculus	3
Rupture of urethra	2
Papilloma of urethra	1
Spinal injury	4
Neurological disease	4
Miscellaneous (drugs, constipation, etc.)	4

As will be seen from Table 21.1 a majority of cases stem from some form of prostatic obstruction which, even where drugs or neurological disorders are implicated, often coexists as an essential component. Stricture has nowadays become less common because of the better treatment of urethral inflammation and trauma. Among the elderly uncircumcised, however, inflammatory phimosis (particularly in diabetics) remains a not unusual cause of obstruction.

Management of acute retention

Irrespective of the cause, the presence of a painfully distended bladder calls for early relief. Except in obvious cases of hysteria and occasionally others where no obstructive cause is immediately apparent, attempts to induce voluntary voiding are generally a waste of time. Traditional remedies such as sedation or sitting in a hot bath are rarely effective and even if successful seldom bring more than temporary relief. Similar objections apply to the use of parasympatheticomimetic drugs such as carbachol which, in addition to carrying certain risks, may only increase discomfort.

It should be clearly recognized that with few exceptions the onset of retention reflects the presence of an underlying obstructive lesion for which admission to hospital and further investigations will be required. The practice of relieving the condition by catheterization in the casualty department and then discharging the patient to await events is only mentioned to be condemned.

Outside hospital

Nowadays, except in isolated areas, transfer to hospital is generally practicable within a few hours and it is unlikely that the patient will come to any harm during this period if adequately sedated. Such a course is strongly to be recommended as avoiding the risk of infection, etc. contingent on an immediate attempt to decompress the bladder in unfavourable surroundings. In adverse circumstances, however, the latter may have to be considered, the choice lying between catheterization and suprapubic aspiration. Briefly, the factors influencing a decision will be (1) the presumed nature of the obstruction, (2) the availability of suitable equipment (catheters, aspirating needles, etc.) and (3) the period likely to elapse before hospitilization can be effected. Generally speaking catheterization is to be preferred and is more readily accepted by the patient as a logical method of relief. The risk of infection can be reduced by appropraite chemotherapy and when, as for example at sea, some delay can be foreseen before further assistance is obtainable, the catheter should be left indwelling. Continued or repeated suprapubic aspiration, on the other hand, is fraught with the hazard of extravasation and can only be condoned as a short-term expedient or as a forced alternative where attempts at urethral instrumentation have failed. In the latter case, if circumstances permit, the deliberate performance of open cystostomy drainage may well prove preferable (see p. 315).

Inside hospital

On arrival at hospital management becomes more clearly defined. All cases with acute retention should be admitted forthwith and any thought of relieving the condition in the casualty department must be rigorously excluded. Once in bed and following suitable sedation the conditions are favourable for an attempt at catheterization. Strict attention to asepsis is obligatory. Unless there is good reason to believe that the cause is purely temporary (e.g. drugs, alcoholic excess) the catheter should be left indwelling while further investigations are being undertaken.

If catheterization fails, preparation should be made for a further attempt under general anaesthesia. Suprapubic aspiration as an alternative has little or no place in hospital practice save when an anaesthetic is precluded or in occasional cases of acute urethral inflammation.

Subsequent investigation

Once the distended bladder has been relieved the emergency is over. Continued catheter drainage affords an opportunity for further study and the planning of definitive treatment. Three factors affect the latter:

1. The nature of the obstruction.
2. The condition of the remainder of the urinary tract (including renal function).
3. The overall clinical status of the patient.

The pattern of investigation should thus be arranged accordingly. The essential urological investigations include:

1. Laboratory analysis of the urine, including bacteriology and sensitivities.
2. Haemoglobin estimation, blood grouping and saving of the serum for cross-matching.
3. Estimation of blood urea, creatinine, serum acid and alkaline phosphatase (bearing in mind that raised values of acid phosphatase may follow recent palpation of the prostate or urethral instrumentation).

With regard to other systems, simultaneous investigation and restorative therapy should be carried out as indicated. It is unnecessary to carry out intravenous urography in every case of acute urinary retention. If there is a clear cut history of increasing prostatism and physical examination and blood values are normal, the expense of this examination may be saved. In such a case the chances of intravenous urography revealing any serious pathology are so remote as to make the examination unjustified.

Chronic retention of urine

This may be defined as the presence of a palpable bladder following micturition (which represents 800 ml or more of urine) and is caused by a decompensated bladder. Although as in the acute variety benign prostatic enlargement remains the commonest cause, the relative frequency both of urethral stricture and prostate cancer is somewhat increased and the possibility of a neurogenic dysfunction must be considered. Chronic retention occurs in two different groups of patients.

Group 1

These patients are without upper tract back pressure and may have obstructive symptoms such as hesitancy, poor urinary stream or stuttering stream, or prolonged stream with terminal dribbling. As well as this, they may have overflow incontinence and the hallmark is the presence of a palpable bladder on examination. As for acute retention, in addition to laboratory studies, ultrasound study of the upper urinary tract and bladder is performed firstly to confirm the presence of a large residual and also to examine the state of the upper urinary tract. Provided the patient is able to void and his blood urea and creatinine remain within normal limits, he should be admitted for prostatic surgery as soon as is possible.

Group 2

In these patients there is evidence of upper urinary tract back pressure. The patient may present with uraemia or even coma with thirst, malaise, anaemia and the presence of a palpable bladder. The blood urea will be found to be greater than 14 mmol/l and the patient should be catheterized. In the past the need for slow decompression has been overstressed and the potential hazards of haemorrhage from the urinary tract are more than counterbalanced by the benefits of unobstructed drainage and early mobility. Nevertheless, great care should be taken in these patients, particularly those in coma or pre-coma. There may result a period of rapid diuresis following catheter drainage which will be due to the relief of long-standing obstruction at the kidney level. At first this may be quite appropriate in that excess fluid and sodium which has been retained will then be lost, but there may follow a period of prolonged sodium and water diuresis. The patient should be very carefully monitored by means of strict fluid balance, daily or more frequent creatinine, urea, haemoglobin, haematocrit and electrolyte studies, daily weighing and the measurement of urinary electrolytes. Once the blood urea and creatinine have fallen, either to below 14 mmol/l or 150 μl/l respectively, or to a level plateau, then prostatic surgery is performed. It may well be that a severe anaemia may become evident requiring preoperative transfusion.

Urinary tract infections
Acute pyelonephritis

Acute pyelonephritis is an infectious inflammatory condition involving both the pelvis and the parenchyma of the kidney and may affect one or, occasionally, both kidneys. Typically, the responsible organism is an *E. coli*; however, species of *Proteus*, *Klebsiella*, enterococci, *Streptococcus faecalis* and *Pseudomonas* may more rarely cause such infections. Where *Proteus* is the causative organism, it is especially important since these produce urease, an enzyme that splits urea into ammonium ions favouring the precipitation of phosphates to form triple phosphate (Struvite) stones. Such renal infections typically ascend from the urethra and lower urinary tract, though haematogenous infections of the kidney may occur. Since lower urinary tract infections are much more common in women and girls, it is not surprising that such episodes of acute pyelonephritis are far more common in the female sex.

Typically the symptoms of acute pyelonephritis are those of a constant ache in the loin, urinary frequency, nocturia, urgency and dysuria and, frequently, awareness of a high fever together with shaking chills. On examination, the patient may appear quite unwell with a high temperature exceeding 38.5°C; tachycardia and percussion over the affected kidney may cause discomfort. Laboratory findings typically show a leucocytosis of the blood and urinalysis generally reveals opaque urine which on microscopy shows a heavy pyuria and proteinuria on stick testing. Frequently there is microscopic or even gross haematuria. The urine should be cultured and if the patient has a high temperature, it is sensible to perform blood cultures since bacteraemia may ensue. An intravenous urogram should be carried out. Generally this is normal; however with severely infected and oedematous kidneys this may show as enlargement on the nephrogram with poor outline on the pyelogram due to compression of the collecting system.

Where there is evidence of a severe infection or complications such as bacteraemia, hospitalization will be needed. After taking urine and blood specimens for microbiology, initial treatment with an intravenous antibiotic such as amoxycillin, cefuroxime or even an aminoglycoside such as gentamicin or one of the modern quinolones (such as lomefloxacillin or ciprofloxacin) is preferable.

Renal abscess

A renal abscess is, nowadays, fortunately rare. Formerly the most common pathogenesis was by means of haematogenous spread of *Staphylococcus aureus*; however, more recently coliform organisms have become a more common cause, frequently in association with anaerobes. Clinically, the picture is similar to that of acute pyelonephritis, but once developed there may be a palpable mass together with inflammation and oedema of the overlying skin. An intravenous urogram may display a space-occupying lesion with compression and distortion of the pelvicalyceal system. Ultrasonography may be confusing and usually a CT scan is required

and in order to both make the diagnosis and treat the condition, percutaneous needle aspiration under CT control has been shown to be of great benefit.

Guided by the microbiological finding, a prolonged course of systemic antibiotic should be given where *Staphylococcus aureus* is the causative organism. This will usually consist of flucloxacillin or vancomycin, whereas if a coliform is found to be the causative organism then antibiotics as for acute pyelonephritis are more appropriate.

Pyonephrosis

Pyonephrosis, which is the presence of pus filling the collecting system·of the kidney, may be a sequel to any obstruction to the renal pelvis or ureter. It can thus be caused by a ureteric stone, a ureteric stricture or, more commonly pelvi-ureteric junction obstruction, a sloughed papilla in papillary necrosis or, more rarely, an intramural tumour or extrinsic compression of the ureter. The story may be very similar to that of acute pyelonephritis, but the presence of a flank mass which may be in association with overlying skin inflammation must alert the clinician to the possibility. Diagnosis is usually made by a combination of intravenous urogram and ultrasound. The intravenous urogram frequently shows a non-functioning kidney with renal enlargement and ultrasound confirms a dilated collecting system with material within.

Formerly, it was necessary to perform an urgent nephrectomy in order to prevent development of septicaemia and its sequelae. However, with the advent of needle nephrostomy this is now the initial treatment of choice and can be performed under local anaesthetic by ultrasound control. Once the kidney is decompressed then, if the cause of the obstruction is not evident, antegrade urography through the nephrostomy can be performed when the patient's septic condition has been improved. Subsequent management will depend on the cause found.

22

Endocrine disease

J. R. Farndon

Many endocrine diseases requiring surgical treatment are rare and their investigation (biochemical and radiological) and perioperative care is often complex and specialized. There is, therefore, good reason to suggest that patients with these conditions should be treated in units with appropriate skills and experience. In this way the team of physician, surgeon, biochemist, radiologist and pathologist increase their exposure to rare conditions and hopefully improve the quality of patient care given. Important surgical management will be described for adrenal, pancreatic, thyroid and parathyroid disease.

The adrenal glands

Most tumours (benign or malignant) of the adrenal gland retain functional activity and therefore declare themselves by excess production of the appropriate hormone from either cortex or medulla. Cortical tumours produce an excess of glucocorticoid – cortisol – *Cushing's syndrome*, or mineralocorticoid – aldosterone – *Conn's syndrome*. More rarely tumours produce an excess of oestrogen or androgen and these are often malignant, especially in children. Conn's tumours are rarely malignant, but Cushing's tumours may present with metastases. Tumours of the adrenal medulla (*phaeochromocytoma*) produce an excess of noradrenaline and/or adrenaline and 10% can be bilateral and 10% malignant.

Cushing's syndrome

This describes the clinical disorder produced by supraphysiological levels of corticosteroids in the circulation whether endogenously produced or administered to the patient (Table 22.1).

The syndrome affects women four times more commonly than men and the characteristic clinical features and signs are shown in Table 22.2.

The diagnosis of Cushing's syndrome is established when plasma cortisol levels are elevated and

Table 22.1 Causes of Cushing's syndrome

ACTH-dependent causes
1. Pituitary-dependent: increased ACTH produces bilateral adrenocortical hyperplasia
2. Ectopic ACTH syndrome: ACTH production by malignant or benign tumours of non-endocrine nature
3. Iatrogenic: treatment with ACTH or its synthetic analogues

Non-ACTH dependent causes
1. Adenomas or carcinomas of the adrenal cortex.
2. Iatrogenic: treatment with supraphysiological doses of steroids

Table 22.2 Features/signs/symptoms of Cushing's syndrome

Ostoporosis	Plethoric facies
pathological fractures	Moon face
vertebral collapse	Thin skin
loss of height	Acne
kyphosis	Greasy skin
Protuberant abdomen	Hirsuties
Striae	Easy bruising
Buffalo hump	Oedema
Truncal obesity	Hypertension
Thin arms and legs – proximal	Oligomenorrhoea
myopathy	Amenorrhoea
Thirst	Impotence in males
Polyuria	
Glycosuria	
Nocturia	

Table 22.3 Tests to distinguish between pituitary disease, ectopic ACTH production and adrenal adenomas

	Pituitary disease	Ectopic ACTH	Adrenal adenoma
Dexamethasone suppression:			
Low dose	Absent	Absent	Absent
High dose	Usually present	Usually absent	Absent
Insulin tolerance test	Absent	Absent	Absent
Response to metyrapone	Exaggerated	Usually absent	Absent
Plasma ACTH	Detectable – normal or high	Usually very high	Not detectable

there is loss of the normal circadian rhythm of production (nadir usually late evening and early morning hours). Other measurements and stimulation tests which help distinguish between pituitary disease, ectopic ACTH production and adrenal adenomas or carcinomas are shown in Table 22.3.

Conn's syndrome

This is a rare cause of hypertension and will be due to cortical adenoma in 60–70% of patients with the syndrome. In the others, bilateral cortical hyperplasia exists. Females are affected 2–3 times more often than males and the main symptoms and signs are shown in Table 22.4.

Table 22.4 Symptoms and signs of Conn's syndrome

Renal	Polydipsia, polyuria and nocturia
Neuromuscular	Muscle weakness, paralysis, tetany, paraesthesiae
Hypertension	May be severe – headaches, cardiomegaly and retinopathy

Diagnosis is suspected when a patient with hypertension is found to have hypokalaemia. It is confirmed by finding: hypokalaemia (<3.5 mmol/l); raised bicarbonate and a plasma sodium over 140 mmol/l; hyperkaluria (>10 mmol/day in face of hypokalaemia); elevated plasma aldosterone; and decreased plasma renin.

Phaeochromocytoma

The clinical features are the result of increased catecholamine production and can mimic many other conditions, e.g. anxiety, hysteria, hyperthyroidism, hypoglycaemia or diabetes and hypertension.

The hypertension may be sustained or paroxysmal so the recording of a normal blood pressure between 'attacks' does not preclude the diagnosis. The tumour can occur during pregnancy and cause both fetal and maternal death. Therefore, this diagnosis should be considered before ascribing the hypertension to eclampsia. The first intimation of the presence of this tumour may be severe hypertension and cardiac arrhythmias occurring at times of stress, e.g. anaesthetic administration for coincident disease – hernias or fracture manipulations are favourites!

Hyperglycaemia may be present as a direct effect of the excess of catecholamines.

Symptoms include tachycardia, tremors, sweating, blanching or sudden pallor, headaches, nausea and vomiting, mental symptoms sometimes including a feeling of impending doom, precordial or abdominal pain, diarrhoea and weight loss. It can be seen how the tumour can mimic so many other conditions.

The diagnosis can be made by measuring plasma catecholamine levels directly (adrenaline, noradrenaline and dopamine). They may be elevated non-specifically in anxiety states. Over production from tumours, however, is autonomous and cannot be suppressed. Non-specific elevation may be suppressed by giving a ganglion blocking agent such as pentolinium.

Diagnosis is usually made by measurement of urinary catecholamines – free amines or metabolites or breakdown products such as metadrenaline and normetadrenaline and their conjugates and, more usually 4-hydroxy-3-methoxymandelic acid (HMMA). Different laboratories use different methods and readers should consult their hospital laboratory for the 'in-house' test or determination and the normal ranges, which may vary slightly.

Preoperative localization of adrenal tumours

Adrenal adenomas or carcinomas producing Cushing's syndrome or catecholamine excess may be large enough to be detected by non-invasive and relatively cheap means such as ultrasound. The technique is operator-dependent.

Computed axial tomography (CT) is able to detect lesions as small as 1 cm in diameter (Figure 22.1) and again this is a non-invasive, although more expensive, test. It is unusual for Cushing's tumours or phaeochromocytomas to declare themselves symptomatically, clinically or biochemically at this size and CT scanning will, therefore, localize most of these tumours. The examination will also demonstrate that the contralateral adrenal appears normal (10% of phaeochromocytomas may be bilateral or extra-adrenal).

Tumours producing Conn's syndrome are often less than 1 cm in diameter and may not be readily seen on ultrasound or CT scans due to their limited resolution – especially if the patient is thin.

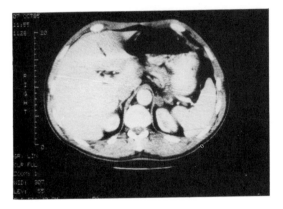

Figure 22.1 CT scan showing a 1 cm left-sided adrenal adenoma producing Conn's syndrome. The adenoma is seen immediately anterior to the kidney and lateral to the aorta

Radioisotope scans may be used with specific agents for each tumour: iodocholesterol for the Conn's tumour and Cushing's adenoma and meta-iodobenzylguanidine for phaeochromocytomas. These tests would only be used if the other procedures were negative or equivocal.

If localization is negative and the clinical and biochemical diagnosis still strongly held, then more invasive procedures can be used such as arteriography and/or venous catheterization for venography or venous sampling for specific hormones. The former carries the risk of adrenal infarction. The latter is technically difficult and aims to detect differential levels of hormone from each adrenal. If these investigations are used where a phaeochromocytoma is suspected, then blockade (see below) needs to be instituted beforehand.

The value of magnetic resonance imaging remains to be evaluated for adrenal tumours.

Once diagnosis is confirmed and the lesion lateralized, then preoperative preparation precedes operative intervention.

Preoperative preparation

Cushing's syndrome may be produced by autonomous functioning adrenal adenomas or carcinomas, pituitary driven disease (pituitary tumours producing ACTH – Cushing's disease) or by ACTH production from other tumours (ectopic ACTH syndrome, commonly from oat cell carcinoma of the lung).

Whatever the cause, excess cortisol production can be blocked using *metyrapone*, a competitive inhibitor of 11 β-hydroxylase enzymes within the adrenal cortex. This can produce symptomatic relief before surgery, e.g. muscle strength may be improved and this will reduce morbidity such as chest infections. In inoperable carcinoma producing Cushing's syndrome long-term relief can be obtained for the rest of the patient's life. The dose ranges from 0.25 to 6.0 g per day, tailored to cortisol production. Total blockade will require cortisol replacement. It may aggravate hirsutism and acne and may cause nausea.

Mitotane (*o,p'*-DDD) inhibits biosynthesis of corticosteroids and destroys adrenocortical cells secreting cortisol without interfering with aldosterone production. It is used mainly in the treatment of adrenocortical carcinoma associated with Cushing's syndrome.

Patients with Conn's syndrome frequently complain of muscle weakness due to hypokalaemia and their hypertension is often severe. Preoperative treatment with *spironolactone* for 3 weeks allows replacement and correction of the potassium deficit and decreases the risk of arrhythmia. Correction of hypokalaemia usually improves muscle strength and corrects the hypertension making the surgery safer. A dose of 200–400 mg per day for a short period of time should not be associated with troublesome side effects. Long-term therapy causes nausea and gynaecomastia.

Excess catecholamine production from phaeochromocytomas makes surgery, any form of stress or invasive radiological procedures particularly dangerous. Sudden surges of amines can precipitate fatal arrhythmias or paroxysms of hypertension which may lead to a cerebrovascular accident or acute, severe heart failure. Once the diagnosis is made, effective blockade should be instituted:

1. *Alpha-adrenergic blockade*: phenoxybenzamine is used in a dose of 10 mg t.d.s. and the dose increased until mild orthostatic hypotension is noted. Blood volume will expand and may create anaemia which can be corrected preoperatively. Residual tachycardia after correction of anaemia may be due to unopposed α-adrenergic effects.
2. *Beta-adrenergic blockade*: propranolol is used in increasing dosage from 10 mg t.d.s. until tachycardia is controlled. Beta-blockade will be

required if the tumour secretes predominantly adrenaline. It is said to be safer to institute alpha- before beta-blockade to avoid the consequences of unopposed agonist, pressor alpha effects.

As well as restoring blood pressure to normal, blockade allows the patient to feel better, often restores euglycaemia and reduces the incidence of ventricular extrasystoles. Such preoperative prep- aration carried out over a period of up to 4 weeks has substantially reduced the operative mortality.

Operative procedure

Functioning endocrine adrenal tumours are usually unilateral and will have been accurately localized preoperatively. Surgical exploration can then be directed to the abnormal gland. For tumours up to about 5 cm in diameter the posterior approach is preferred, excising the 12th rib. Neither pleura nor peritoneum should be breached and recovery can be speedy with discharge in 3–4 days, for example, after resection of a small Conn's tumour.

For tumours greater than 5 cm diameter or if there is a risk of malignancy, the lateral approach is used taking the 11th or 10th rib. It is still possible to stay outside the peritoneum but more likely to be transpleural especially on the right. A chest drain will be required.

The anterior transperitoneal approach should be avoided if possible, especially in Cushing's syn- drome where prolonged ileus and reduced mobility increase the risk of deep vein thrombosis and pulmonary embolism. The anterior approach should be reserved for patients with bilateral tumours, one of which may be bigger than 5 cm diameter, or if malignancy is anticipated, e.g. a phaeochromo- cytoma with suspected deposits within the para- aortic nodes. If haemostasis is careful there should be no need for a wound drain. It is important to remember the increased risk of sepsis in patients with Cushing's syndrome. If the pleura has been breached it is repaired on wound closure and no more than a Redivac drain need be placed if the lung is fully expanded at the conclusion of the operation. If the pleural space has been purposely crossed, for example, to remove a large right-sided tumour, an underwater seal drain must be placed (see p. 221). Chest drains will be removed once the patient is breathing spontaneously and once haemopneumo- thorax is resolved.

Postoperative care

Once unilateral lesions are removed there is no need for continued blockade and there will be no need for replacement therapy except in patients with Cushing's syndrome. Adrenal medullary function is not missed after bilateral adrenalectomy and Conn's syndrome is not associated with mineralocorticoid suppression in the opposite adrenal.

Bilateral adrenalectomy is, of course, an indi- cation for immediate and life-long steroid replace- ment therapy. Glucocorticoid replacement is with hydrocortisone 20–30 mg per day orally – say 20 mg each morning and 10 mg in the evening. An optimum dose is determined by clinical response. There is no real advantage in the use of a synthetic, more potent glucocorticoid such as prednisolone. It offers no advantage and has less mineralocorticoid effect. Fludrocortisone will almost certainly be required with hydrocortisone and in adults the requirements will vary from 50 to 300 µg per day.

Table 22.5 Equivalent doses of glucocorticoids

Drug	Equivalent anti-inflammatory dose (mg)
Betamethasone	0.75
Cortisone acetate	25.0
Dexamethasone	0.75
Hydrocortisone	20.0
Methylprednisolone	4.0
Prednisolone	5.0
Prednisone	5.0
Triamcinolone	4.0

Response is best monitored by attainment of normal serum potassium concentrations. If other steroid therapy is encountered, the equivalent doses are shown in Table 22.5.

Acute adrenocortical insufficiency

Hydrocortisone is given intravenously (as sodium phosphate or succinate) in doses of 100 mg every 6–8 h in sodium chloride intravenous infusion (0.9%).

Corticosteroid cover for adrenalectomy, hypophysectomy or operations on patients on long-term steroid replacement therapy

Adrenal suppression can be profound and pro- longed in both adrenals in pituitary driven Cushing's disease or in the contralateral adrenal in Cushing's syndrome due to adenoma or carcinoma. Normal secretion of glucocorticoid is not possible after bilateral adrenalectomy and cannot be anticipated in those on long-term steroid treatment, unless this has been stopped for more than 6 months.

In a normal person, major stress rarely leads to the production of more than 300 mg cortisol in 24 h. Once the stress resolves production rapidly falls to the normal level of 20–30 mg each day. Replacement attempts to mimic these responses, with an added bonus for caution!

Suggested operative steroid regimen

Day of surgery: 100 mg hydrocortisone
                       (sodium phosphate or
                       succinate). i.m. or i.v. with
                       premedication. Thereafter
                       100 mg every 8 h
Postoperative day 1:   100 mg hydrocortisone t.d.s.
                       i.v.
Postoperative day 2:   50 mg hydrocortisone t.d.s.
                       i.v.
Postoperative day 3:   25 mg hydrocortisone t.d.s.
                       i.v.
Postoperative day 4:   As day 3 but orally
Postoperative day 5:   20 mg orally in the morning,
                       10 mg orally in the evening.
                       Introduce mineralocorticoid as
                       required

Assessment of hypothalamo-pituitary-adrenal (HPA) axis

The above regimen must be used if there is established adrenal suppression. It can be used empirically if suppression is suspected. The only certain way to ensure the state of the HPA axis is to test its integrity (Table 22.6).

Prednisolone, prednisone and cortisone all produce appreciable cross-reactivities in radioimmuno-assays and must be stopped for 24 h before cortisol measurements are made.

Pancreatic endocrine disease

The pancreas contains many types of endocrine cells each capable of producing individual hormones and specific syndromes if one cell type produces a tumour (Table 22.7). Remember the G cell ($\rightarrow$ Gastrin $\rightarrow$ Gastrinoma) does not normally reside in the pancreas but the majority of gastrinomas are found within the gland!

Endocrine tumours of the pancreas are very rare, perhaps one patient presenting per million population per year. An index of suspicion should be maintained for their existence may be declared by specific symptoms, signs and biochemistry as shown in Table 22.8.

Diagnosis

The diagnosis of pancreatic endocrine tumours may be simple or very complex. A casualty officer may see a patient with the initial 'attack' of hypoglycaemia and its associated symptoms: confusion, disorientation, pallor, faintness, coma and hypotension. Blood may be drawn and a rapid determination of a blood sugar level may provide the diagnosis. Administration of glucose (orally or intravenously) restores the patient to normal. Blood from the same sample could subsequently be assayed for insulin. If other causes of hypoglycaemia are excluded (e.g. secondary due to alcoholism or factitious by self-administration of oral hypoglycaemic agents or insulin), then the insulin will be found to be inappropriately high for the ambient glucose level. The combination of hypoglycaemia, symptoms and reversal by glucose administration is sometimes called 'Whipple's triad' – diagnostic of an *insulinoma*.

Table 22.6 Tests for HPA axis integrity

Test	Cortisol levels
Baseline functional assessment:	09.00 h plasma cortisol level (190–720 nM/l) Urinary free cortisol excretion (100–370 nM/24 h)
Dynamic tests:	
1. Short tetracosactrin test:	250 µg i.m. between 08.00 and 09.00 h. Cortisol levels measured 30 min before and 60 min after. Normal response: peak to at least 550 µM/l
2. Long tetracosactrin test: use if (1) negative	1 mg depot tetracosactrin i.m. at 09.00 h. Samples taken before and at 1, 4, 6, 8 and 24 h
3. Insulin stress test (IST): If (2) is not normal, then IST is the best discriminator. It can be dangerous	Induce hypoglycaemia by injection of 0.15 u/kg of soluble insulin (Actrapid). Blood glucose should be <2.2 mmol/l with symptoms

Table 22.7 Pancreatic endocrine cells and their tumours

Cell type	Hormone	Tumour
Alpha	Glucagon	Glucagonoma
Beta	Insulin	Insulinoma
Delta	Somatostatin	Somatostatinoma
F, D_2 or PP	Pancreatic polypeptide	hPP apudoma
Enterochromaffin	Serotonin	Carcinoid

Table 22.8 Index of suspicion for tumours of the pancreas

	Symptoms	Diagnosis
Obvious	Hypoglycaemia	Insulinoma
	Fulminating peptic ulcer	Gastrinoma
Less obvious	Diabetes, anaemia, rash	Glucagonoma
	Diarrhoea, hypokalaemia, hypochlorhydria	Vipoma
Impossible!	?Asymptomatic	hPP apudoma
		Somatostatinoma

The diagnosis may be suspected, but may not present so dramatically, in which case the abnormality may be precipitated by a prolonged fast of up to 72 h and, more rarely, abnormal insulin levels can be provoked by a stimulation test, e.g. by injecting calcium (2 mg ionic calcium/kg body weight). Normal subjects show no response, but those harbouring an insulinoma show increased insulin output.

A classic history of peptic ulcer disease, often fulminant with repeated episodes of perforation or bleeding, is suggestive of excess acid production possibly driven by gastrin excess from a pancreatic tumour. Excess acid secretion (even that driven by a gastrinoma) may be effectively and unwittingly reduced by H_2-receptor blockade or omeprazole (see later).

The combination of signs and symptoms which are produced by a glucagonoma or a vipoma must be remembered and investigated if the index of suspicion is present. Measurement of fasting levels of the hormone may confirm the diagnosis.

Localization procedures

Once the biochemical diagnosis of the endocrine tumour is confirmed, it has been customary to attempt to localize the tumour within the pancreas. Some gastrinomas can produce their effects when only 2 mm in diameter and, even with the pancreas fully mobilized, it might be impossible to feel or locate the tumour. There is no place for 'blind' distal pancreatectomy.

The situation is much improved recently, however, by the use of peroperative ultrasound – the intraoperative examination of the pancreas directly by the surgeon working with the radiologist. This has allowed the detection of tumours as small as 2 mm in diameter even when placed ectopically, for example, in the duodenal wall.

Other techniques which may be used preoperatively, or if previous surgery has failed to locate the tumour, include: CT scan, ultrasound, arteriography, selective venous sampling with hormonal assays and pancreatic parenchymography.

CT scan

Non-invasive but probably better if used with synchronous contrast injection – dynamic CT scan. It is still not the best localizing modality for small pancreatic tumours.

Ultrasound

Totally non-invasive, but limited by its ability to resolve small tumours in the retroperitoneal pancreas overlaid by the gas-containing stomach.

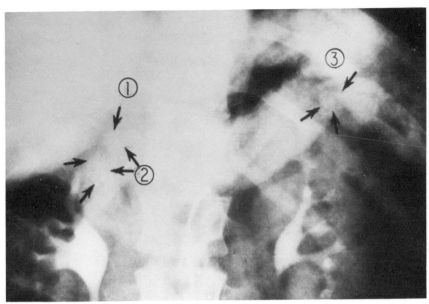

Figure 22.2 Coeliac axis arteriogram showing three endocrine tumours within the pancreas (labelled 1, 2 and 3)

Arteriography

Invasive, but may show tumour blushes, especially with multiple tumours (Figure 22.2).

Selective venous sampling

Percutaneous transhepatic cannulation of the portal and splenic veins for hormone assays for whichever

tumour is suspected. An invasive, costly and not too specific or sensitive a test (Figure 22.3).

Pancreatic parenchymography

This is the combination of ERCP (p. 278) and digital subtraction imaging. The ERCP requires parenchymal filling and this often produces mild

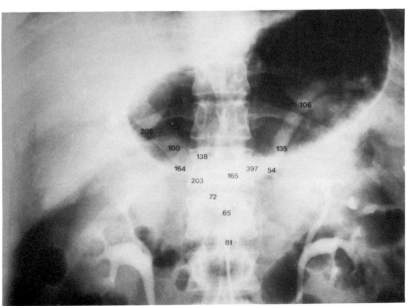

Figure 22.3 Splenic and portal vein insulin concentrations taken during selective venous sampling, demonstrating a sudden increase in concentrations in the body of the gland just left of the vertebral column (397 units). The catheter is in the aorta. The catheter has been removed from the portal system

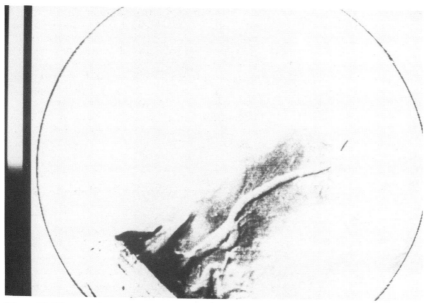

Figure 22.4 Pancreatic parenchymogram in a patient who had had a previous 'blind' distal pancreatectomy elsewhere. The tumour lies deep in the head above the main pancreatic duct and is seen as a filling defect in the parenchyma

pancreatitis. The pancreatic parenchyma is demonstrated with the ductal system and endocrine tumours are shown as negative or 'cold' areas within the gland. The advantage of this procedure is that it demonstrates the relationship between the tumour and the pancreatic duct – a particularly important observation, especially if tumour enucleation is to be carried out with its attendant risk of pancreatic fistula (Figure 22.4).

Preoperative preparation

As with hyperfunctioning adrenal tumours it is often possible to block excess pancreatic endocrine secretion with specific therapy.

Insulinomas

Diazoxide is a benzothiadiazine analogue which can be used in severe hypertension but which reverses hypoglycaemia due to excess endogenous insulin secretion. It is used at a dose of 5 mg/kg up to 1 g per day. It may cause anorexia, nausea, vomiting, hypotension, oedema, arrhythmias, extrapyramidal effects and hypertrichosis during prolonged treatment.

Streptozotocin is a cytotoxic, specific beta-cell poison which may be used in the treatment of malignant insulinomas – 50% may respond. It is infused intravenously at a dose of 2–4 g on alternate days for four treatments repeated monthly; 90% of vipomas respond to this drug.

Gastrinomas

Current medications used to treat peptic ulcer disease reduce gastric acid output very effectively. Unwittingly the use of such drugs as cimetidine, ranitidine and famotidine may treat peptic ulcer disease due to *undiagnosed* gastrinomas. Omeprazole is a substituted benzimidazole which inhibits the secretion of gastric acid by interacting with the enzyme H^+, K^+-ATPase – believed to be the proton pump of the parietal cell. Omeprazole is a potent and long acting antisecretory drug for use in patients with a gastrinoma. Its safety and efficacy in long-term use remain to be assessed.

Surgical treatment

Pancreatic endocrine tumours can produce effects when less than 1 cm in diameter. Exploration is carried out more effectively if preoperative localization procedures have been positive. Even with the pancreas fully mobilized it may be difficult to palpate the tumour and there is little to be gained from blind resections since endocrine tumours do not occur in higher proportions in the body and tail of the gland (the easier parts to remove).

Resections can be enucleation, various distal pancreatectomies, total pancreatectomy or a Whipple procedure. Splenectomy need not be a part of the procedure – this organ can survive on short gastric vessels even if the splenic artery and vein have to be divided.

Intraoperative monitoring of blood glucose is essential during surgery for insulinomas – the detection of a reactive hyperglycaemia is taken by some to be indicative of effective surgery.

The operative procedure is determined by the site of the tumour, whether multiple or not, the size of the lesion and whether the lesion is felt to be malignant. Some advocate total pancreatectomy for the treatment of gastrinomas because of their malignant potential, especially if they occur in a familial setting as part of the multiple endocrine neoplasia type I (MEN I) syndrome – parathyroid, pituitary, pancreatic and adrenocortical adenomas. In this condition the pancreatic tumours are multiple, may be producing differing hormones and recur asynchronously.

The small tumour in the head could be treated by enucleation. The tumour close to the hilum of the spleen would be more easily removed by distal pancreatectomy. Care must be taken in the identification of the pancreatic duct so that it may be securely ligated or oversewn to reduce the chance of fistula formation. Enucleation of a large tumour in the head of the gland has a greater risk of producing a fistula from the main duct or one of its larger branches.

Postoperative care and complications

Major pancreatic resections may require blood transfusion. A secondary haemorrhage in the postoperative period should not be overlooked.

There should be little or no endocrine disturbance and once the source of gastrin has been removed then antacid therapy can be discontinued. It is better to ensure biochemical normality before finally stopping H_2-receptor blocking drugs. Diazoxide should be stopped after removal of an insulinoma. The 'normal' islets will be hypoplastic as a consequence of the excess insulin and glucose intolerance may be seen in the first 2–3 days after surgery. One or two small doses of insulin might be needed if the hyperglycaemia reaches 15–20 mmol/l.

Table 22.9 Signs and symptoms of lesser sac collection

Signs	Symptoms
Epigastric mass	Malaise
± Ileus	Abdominal fullness
Persistent nasogastric aspirates	Nausea and vomiting
Pyrexia (swinging if infected)	Fever

± Wound changes – redness with a discharge
± Fluid rich in amylase

A significant problem may be the lesser sac collection with or without ductal damage. Pancreatic juice nearly always 'finds its way' to the surface through sugical wound or drain site to establish a fistula. The collection may or may not be infected. Percutaneous drainage under CT or ultrasound guidance is an option which may obviate re-exploration. Small fistulae should close spontaneously provided there is no infection or proximal duct obstruction. The signs and symptoms of a collection are shown in Table 22.9.

Thyroid and parathyroid surgery

The indications for thyroid surgery are shown in Table 22.10. The indications and extent of surgery for each of these conditions is outwith the brief of

Table 22.10 Indications for thyroid surgery

Benign conditions	Malignant
Thyrotoxicosis	Follicular cell origin:
Symptomatic unilobular or multilobular disease	Papillary carcinoma
	Follicular carcinoma
Cyst	Anaplastic carcinoma
Solitary nodule, e.g. adenoma	Parafollicular cell origin: Medullary carcinoma
Multinodular goitre	Mesodermal and mixed origin:
Teratoma including struma ovarii	Lymphoma
	Fibrosarcoma

this chapter, but specific mention should be made of diagnostic tests which help provide information to determine operative strategy.

Thyroid function tests

Measurement of thyroid stimulating hormone (TSH), serum thyroxine and sometimes triiodothyronine will allow documentation of thyroid status, i.e. hypo-, eu- or hyperthyroid. Occasionally measurement of free T_3 and use of a TRH stimulation test of TSH is required to confirm a clinical suspicion of thyrotoxicosis. Thyroid antibodies help confirm the clinical diagnosis of Graves' disease or thyroiditis.

Isotope studies

^{99m}Tc (technetium) or, less commonly, ^{131}I (iodine) uptake tests give two sorts of information. They measure avidity of uptake which gives an indication of function. The pattern of uptake within the gland demonstrates the presence of multiple or single sites of disease. Areas of minimal uptake are called 'cold'

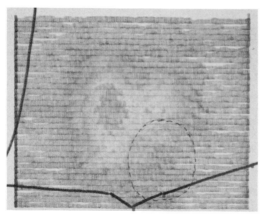

Figure 22.5 Thyroid scan demonstrating a cold nodule in the left thyroid lobe, which in this instance was a thyroid cyst

and are associated with poorly functioning adenomas, cysts, thyroiditis or a thyroid carcinoma. Up to 10% of cold nodules may be carcinomas (Figure 22.5).

Ultrasonography

Ultrasonography may help distinguish solid from cystic lesions and may demonstrate multifocal disease when only a single swelling was apparent clinically.

Fine needle biopsy

This is the most important test and should allow definitive diagnosis. In experienced hands it has very few complications – haemorrhage, nerve damage and tumour seeding occur in insignificant numbers. The experienced cytologist should be able to diagnose benign and malignant conditions with the exception of the distinction between follicular adenoma and follicular carcinoma.

Preoperative preparation of patients with thyrotoxicosis

As in other endocrine conditions preoperative control of hyperfunction is essential in thyrotoxicosis. Surgery in the patient with uncontrolled disease could possibly lead to a thyroid storm or crisis or to malignant hyperpyrexia.

Carbimazole is one of the most commonly used antithyroid drugs. The initial dose is 10–15 mg every 6 h. Once control is achieved the dose may be reduced until the patient is euthyroid, but if a commitment is made to surgical treatment it is better that the full blocking dose is maintained and thyroxine replacement instituted. There is no convincing evidence that the addition of iodine or iodides helps in the preparation. It was said to reduce vascularity.

More patients are being controlled perioperatively with β-adrenergic receptor blockers, e.g. propranolol. These agents reduce the heart rate, cardiac output, sweating, tremor and anxiety of hyperthyroidism but have no effect on thyroid hormone production or circulating hormone concentrations. Some acute phase proteins, which increase after surgery, bind propranolol and thereby reduce its efficacy in the postoperative period. Since the half-life of thyroxine is measured in hours it is essential, therefore, to continue propranolol for at least 5 days postoperatively to prevent thyroid storm.

Complications of thyroid and parathyroid surgery

These are essentially the same whether surgery is undertaken for thyroid or parathyroid disease. The more substantial the surgery the more likely are complications. For example, total thyroidectomy is more likely to be associated with problems than is exploration of the neck in hyperparathyroidism or partial lobectomy for benign thyroid disease.

Haemorrhage

With modern techniques of diathermy and ligature (silver clips and ties) blood loss should be minimal in any thyroid/parathyroid surgery. Drains need hardly ever be placed and the risk of secondary haemorrhage should be minimal. Patients are often discharged home by the second or third postoperative day. It remains traditional nursing/ward practice to keep equipment beside the patient's bed in case of secondary haemorrhage. Haematoma compressing the airway can be frightening for patients and doctors and requires emergency treatment – opening the wound on the ward and preparing theatre as soon as possible. A single bleeding point is rarely found on re-exploration and all that can be done is evacuation of haematoma, irrigation of the wound and closure with drainage.

Hypocalcaemia

Inadvertent damage to the parathyroids or their purposeful excision in thyroid cancer will result in hypoparathyroidism and hypocalcaemia. The patient will complain of muscle cramps and frequent premonitory signs or symptoms are perioral tingling and cramps or abnormal sensation in the fingers and hands. Chvostek's and Trousseau's signs may be positive. The diagnosis is confirmed by measurement of serum calcium – ionized fraction if possible.

Table 22.11 Treatment regimes for mild hypocalcaemia

Calcium supplements (tablets)	Vitamin D
Calcium gluconate (600 mg): 1.35 mmol Ca^{2+}	Calciferol (high strength): 250 µg
Calcium lactate (300 mg): 1.0 mmol Ca^{2+}	1 α-Hydroxycholecalciferol: 250 ng or 1 µg
Calcium lactate gluconate (3.08 g) equivalent to calcium gluconate (4.5 g): 10 mmol Ca^{2+}	1,25-Dihydroxycholecalciferol: 250 or 500 ng

Secondary hypoplasia or atrophy occurs in the 'normal' parathyroid glands if there is an adenoma producing excess parathyroid hormone (PTH). Removal of the adenoma with biopsy of one other gland for comparative histology is often sufficient to produce hypocalcaemia until the other parathyroids 'recover' or return to normal. The hypocalcaemia may be profound especially if there is bone disease – osteitis fibrosa cystica (hungry bone syndrome). Normocalcaemia may only be achieved by calcium and vitamin D supplements. In extreme cases calcium may have to be given intravenously. It is best given as a dilute infusion of calcium gluconate. The 10% solution is very hypertonic and extravasation outside a vein can produce severe tissue reactions and even skin loss; 10 or 20 ml of 10% calcium gluconate may be needed every 4–6 h. Too aggressive a biopsy policy in the surgery of hyperparathyroidism results in a higher incidence of hypocalcaemia.

Mild but symptomatic hypocalcaemia can be treated effectively by oral calcium supplements and vitamin D (Table 22.11).

Nerve damage

Superior laryngeal nerve

The superior laryngeal nerve arises from the nodose ganglion of the vagus and through its internal branch supplies sensory fibres to the supraglottic mucosa of the larynx and through its external branch supplies motor fibres to the cricothyroid muscle. The external branch runs close to the superior thyroid vessels making it vulnerable during thyroid surgery (Figure 22.6). Paresis of the cricothyroid causes a reduction in average pitch and a reduced voice range. This can be a serious deficit in singers or professional speakers. The nerve can be damaged in some patients but this will often be a neuropraxia and recovery can be anticipated.

Recurrent laryngeal nerve

Permanent damage to this branch of the vagus nerve has more significant consequences. It provides sensory fibres to the infraglottic mucosa of the larynx and motor fibres to all the intrinsic muscles of the larynx except cricothyroid. Damage to the nerve (Figure 22.6) produces hoarseness and even if this is due to neuropraxia it may take many weeks to recover. Bilateral recurrent nerve damage produces an incompetent unprotected larynx with stridor. Tracheostomy is required.

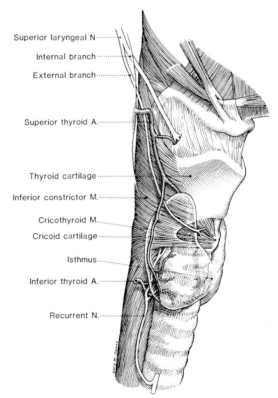

Figure 22.6 Demonstrates the important relationships between arteries and nerves close to the thyroid gland. The external branch of the superior laryngeal nerve is vulnerable during ligature of the superior thyroid artery. Damage to it results in paresis of the cricothyroid muscle. The recurrent nerve usually lies deep to the inferior thyroid artery as it ascends in the neck in the tracheoesophageal groove to disappear beneath the inferior constrictor. It is vulnerable during ligature of the inferior thyroid artery or dissection on the posterior surface of the thyroid lobes, e.g. in parathyroidectomy

Some patients have partial or total cord paresis *before* any neck surgery and preoperative cord assessment demonstrates this. It is usual practice to ask an ENT colleague to carry out indirect laryngoscopy to assess vocal cord movements. Normal cord movement seen on extubation after completion of surgery is no guarantee of maintained normal recurrent nerve function which could be subsequently compromised, for example by haematoma formation or drain pressure.

Nerve damage during neck surgery provides a fertile ground for the growth of patient aggrievement and the even more prolific development of medicolegal wrangles! An uninformed or disinformed patient is a very unhappy patient. Be sure to describe these potential hazards to your patient preoperatively and enter the fact in the notes.

Long-term complications

After thyroid surgery the most important long-term consequence is hypothyroidism. After subtotal thyroidectomy for Graves' disease as many as 70% of patients may be rendered euthyroid. There appears to be no good correlation with the subsequent development of hypothyroidism and potential markers such as the presence of thyroid antibodies or remnant size. The patient and his or her medical practitioner must be warned of this possibility developing later on if the patient is not to be followed in a specialist clinic.

Features peculiar to patients with hyperparathyroidism

The surgery of this endocrine problem is slightly different from most of the others from two points of view. First, there is little or no need to correct or control the biochemical abnormality before surgery and, second, there is no reason to try to localize the abnormal parathyroid gland before first time neck exploration. The only indication for biochemical control or amendment is in the rare situation of 'hypercalcaemic crisis'. 'The only localization before first time neck exploration is the location of a good and experienced parathyroid surgeon. A good thyroid surgeon is not enough and much mischief will be done by the 'let's look and see' surgeon' – Aphorisms of Fuller Albright (1948). There is no excuse for this surgery being carried out by the inexperienced surgeon – it will result in an unacceptable rate of failed explorations.

Hypercalcaemic crisis

The development of this situation occasionally occurs as a consequence of primary hyperparathyroidism rather than disseminated skeletal meta-static disease. Markedly raised serum calcium (>4 mmol/l) results in confusion or coma, nausea, vomiting and impaired urine output. Confusion and vomiting worsen dehydration and increase serum calcium concentrations further – a truly vicious circle.

The mainstay of correction is vigorous rehydration with eventual exhibition of frusemide to aid renal clearance of calcium. Intravenous phosphate can be dangerous especially if renal function is impaired. Steroids are of little value in this situation. Other drugs are more effective in the treatment of hypercalcaemia of malignancy and include calcitonin, diphosphonates and the antimetabolite mithramycin. It is unusual to need these other agents as rehydration with continued forced diuresis with frusemide usually controls the situation.

If the diagnosis of hyperparathyroidism can be obtained rapidly (for example, classic features in the bones on skeletal survey or an inappropriate PTH level in a rapid assay) there is every indication for a 'semi-urgent' parathyroidectomy once the hypercalcaemia is reduced.

Postoperative care

Complications as discussed above can occur after parathyroidectomy. Perturbations in serum calcium are more common and the most likely is a period of temporary hypocalcaemia requiring either intravenous or oral calcium and vitamin D supplements as described above.

Persistent and recurrent hyperparathyroidism

Recurrent hyperparathyroidism is rare and is designated: recurrent hypercalcaemia after at least 1 year of normocalcaemia and the finding of a diseased parathyroid gland at the site of a previously biopsy proven normal gland – maybe only 1% of all recurrent hypercalcaemia.

Persistent hypercalcaemia will be due to an inadequate or failed exploration with errors possible in surgical hands, e.g. too limited an exploration, or in pathology hands, e.g. error in frozen section diagnosis. A third possibility not infrequently encountered is an error in the initial diagnosis. Possible causes of hypercalcaemia which may have been overlooked are:

1. Familial hypocalciuric hypercalcaemia.
2. Granulomatous disease, e.g. sarcoidosis.
3. Drug related, e.g. thiazide diuretics.
4. Occult or overt malignancy with or without metastases.
5. Thyrotoxicosis.

If the diagnosis of hyperparathyroidism is confirmed, then before localization procedures are

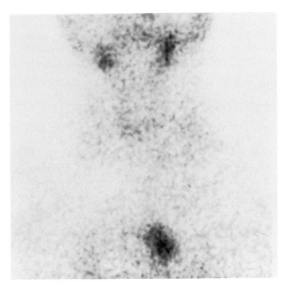

Figure 22.7 Thallium technetium subtraction scan demonstrating marked thallium uptake by a parathyroid adenoma in the anterior mediastinum. Other uptake is seen in the submandibular glands, but not in the parathyroid tissue in the neck

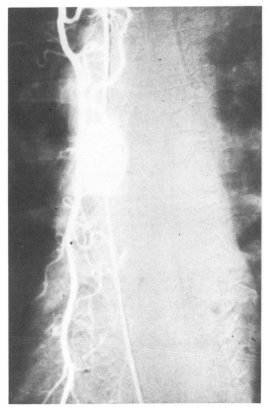

Figure 22.9 Selective arteriogram showing an ectopic mediastinal parathyroid adenoma fed by the internal mammary artery

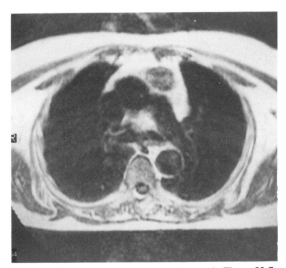

Figure 22.8 MRI scan of the same patient as in Figure 22.7 showing marked resonance in the mediastinal tumour

carried out it must be ascertained that symptoms warrant surgical treatment, which is associated with a slightly increased morbidity and mortality. In the majority of patients the abnormal gland will still be in the neck; 15% may have an adenoma within the mediastinum. Previous operation notes and pathology reports must be obtained as these sometimes provide clues to the whereabouts of the missed gland. The following localization procedures may be used:

1. Ultrasound of neck.
2. Thallium/technetium subtraction scan (Figure 22.7).
3. CT scan.
4. MRI scan (Figure 22.8).
5. Arteriography (Figure 22.9).
6. Venography with selective venous sampling.

The latter two techniques might only be used if other less invasive techniques have proved negative.

It must be acknowledged that re-exploration is technically more demanding and associated with an increased morbidity – especially risk of recurrent nerve injury. It is essential in this situation that vocal cord function is assessed both pre- and postoperatively.

Hypocalcaemia is more likely to occur after re-exploration especially if the previous surgery excised or biopsied multiple glands.

23

The breast

R. W. Blamey

This chapter on the breast deals with diagnostic procedures, with some of the minor operations on the breast which may be performed by junior surgical staff, and with procedures used in the treatment of advanced disease. These various procedures will be introduced with a description of the indications for their use. Lastly, mention will be made of breast cancer screening and the techniques necessary for this.

The referral clinic

The commonest reason for referral to a breast clinic is for investigation of a true or supposed breast lump.

The history is largely irrelevant, for whether a lump is discovered or not depends on the physical examination. The patient is asked whether she has had a previous operation on the breast since this could distort the physical signs, and whether she has a first degree relative who has been diagnosed with breast cancer, since this will reflect on whether she should be regularly screened in the future.

Examination

Experience in examination of the breast is essential and trainee surgeons should ensure that they regularly attend a busy breast clinic for some while.

The patient is seated on the edge of the couch facing the examiner. Inspection is initially made with the arms hanging by the side and is for:

1. Lump.
2. Tether–of skin or nipple (Figure 23.1).
3. Inflammation–of skin or nipple.

The patient is asked to slowly raise her arms and place them above her head; then she is asked to

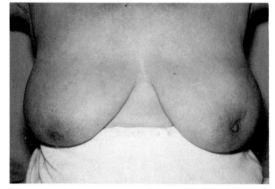

Figure 23.1 Malignant tether of the nipple. Nipple and areola are tethered and this is irregular

indicate where she feels the lump and to repeat the movement of raising her arms: the examiner concentrates on the area indicated.

Benign inpulling of the nipple is often seen and takes the form of either a line across the nipple (Figure 23.2) or inpulling of a few ducts in the centre of the nipple. These are correctable by flattening the nipple with the fingers. If the patient has not attended to the toilet of the inpulled nipple then inspissated exfoliated tissue will give inflammation of the pit and may stimulate nipple discharge. Malignant inpulling usually involves the areola as well and is often eccentric in appearance as seen in Figure 23.1.

The patient lies on the couch for palpation with the upper body propped up to around 30° with pillows, arms by the side. Palpation is with the flat of the fingers, not digging the tips in: the examiner should not press too hard. Work around the breast through all four quadrants, then the areola, then the axillary tail. Palpation is repeated with the arms placed above the head and then sitting up with the

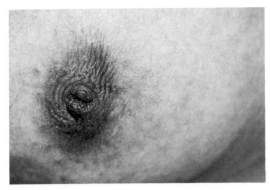

Figure 23.2 Benign inpulling across the nipple: this condition is often seen

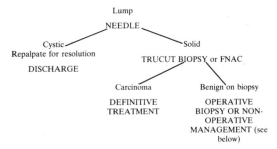

Figure 23.3 The path of investigation of a breast lump

arms by the side. If no lump is found the woman is asked to hold her finger over the lump and the examiner feels directly the finger is removed.

The decisions are:

1. A lump is present.
2. There is no abnormality.
3. There is no definite lump but the breast does not feel entirely normal.

The first group require further investigation (see below). In the second group, where the examiner is confident that no lump is present, the patient should be discharged and not asked to return to the clinic. The third category should be kept to a minimum, for it essentially means that whilst the examiner believes no lump to be present, he or she is unsure often due to general lumpiness; either the patient should be re-examined at a different phase of her cycle in 6 weeks when the breast may be less 'lumpy', or she should have a mammogram and be discharged. If a patient is re-seen at 6 weeks the examiner must make up his or her mind as to whether the breast is normal or abnormal and not keep re-calling the woman.

Investigation of a breast lump
(Figure 23.3)

Cysts are very uncommon below the age of 35 years and after the menopause, but are the commonest reason for a lump between these ages.

A 23 gauge (blue) needle on a 10 ml syringe is pushed into the lump and an attempt at aspiration made. If the lump proves to be a cyst it is emptied and the breast repalpated. As long as the lump has completely resolved there is no need for the patient to re-attend. In the uncommon situation of a lump still being palpable, investigation as for a solid lump is required.

If the original lump proves to be solid rather than cystic then the investigator proceeds to a tissue diagnosis. This may be by fine needle aspiration cytology (FNAC) or by using a Trucut biopsy needle (Travenol Laboratories).

Cytology

Although cytology appears simple to obtain from the breast, a period of training is required to obtain reasonable samples. Even with a good sample only a few pathologists have trained in the reading of breast cytology, the problems being that 100% specificity is needed (i.e. no false positives for cancer) and that benign cells from a fibroadenoma may appear malignant to a reader trained on uterine cervical cytology.

A 23 gauge needle and 10 ml syringe are used. The needle is advanced to the lump and then suction applied to the syringe using the thumb and finger: the needle is then pushed to and fro through the lump 10–15 times. The syringe is disconnected from the needle before withdrawing the needle through the skin to avoid sucking the cells up into the barrel. The cells are expressed onto a slide and smeared between two slides. The specimens are air dried or fixed depending on the local practice (Figure 23.4).

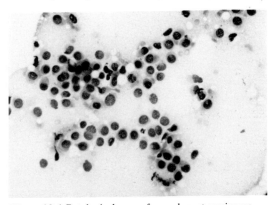

Figure 23.4 Cytological smear from a breast carcinoma

Trucut needle biopsy

A Trucut needle (Figure 23.5) is designed to take a specimen for histological evaluation. Local anaes-

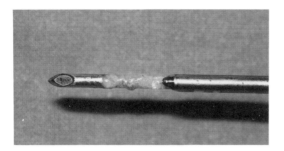

Figure 23.5 Trucut needle with needle advanced. The biopsy specimen lies in the slot

thetic containing adrenaline is infiltrated into the skin and the lump. A small skin incision is made with a sharp pointed scalpel blade (No. 11) and the closed needle pushed through this and advanced to the lump. The inner needle is pushed into the lump and the outer sheath closed over it, cutting a specimen which is retained by a slot in the inner needle. The closed needle is withdrawn.

Carcinomas tend to give a good specimen, the tissue cutting easily. Benign tissue is much tougher and gives a poor specimen. Small fibroadenomas will often be pushed away by the needle rather than biopsied. Therefore in the diagnosis of a breast lump a positive Trucut finding of cancer means that definitive surgery is required; a negative finding is usually disregarded.

Imaging a breast lump

This may be by radiograph mammography (Figure 23.6) or by ultrasound. Description of these is

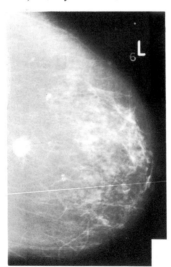

Figure 23.6 A mammogram (lateral oblique view of breast) showing a breast cancer

outside the scope of this book. However, it should be appreciated that 15–20% of palpable breast cancers are not visible on mammography. The finding of a lump on physical examination means that a diagnosis must be obtained (as above) even in the face of a normal mammogram. Palpation remains the paramount investigation for the symptomatic woman. The mammogram should not be viewed before palpation or the examiner may be influenced in making the decision as to whether a lump is felt or not.

Surgical excision biopsy

If a palpable lump has not proved to be a cyst or a breast cancer by needling techniques, then many surgeons would remove it. This leads to a number of unnecessary operations and is a policy which is being modified.

The younger a woman is, the more likely that a lump is a fibroadenoma and breast cancer is very rare in women under 25 years. Several units recommend leaving a lump which feels like a fibroadenoma, under this age, without operation. Our policy is to take one FNAC as an extra precaution and to leave the lump as long as this shows no malignant cells and the patient does not wish it to be removed.

This policy can be used in managing lumps in older women but as the age increases so does the cancer risk; more care has to be taken to ensure that the lump is benign before leaving it. The criteria used are summarized in Table 23.1.

Operative biopsy of a breast lump

Breast biopsy under local anaesthetic can be uncomfortable and bleeding may be a problem; unless the lump is at the periphery of the breast, general anaesthetic is preferred.

Day case biopsy is suitable. A number of rather indefinite edged lesions, thought to constitute a definite lump in the clinic, may not be palpable on the day of admission. The operating surgeon must examine the breast and, if uncertain that a lump is present, call for a re-evaluation by a senior member of the breast team; juniors should not feel obliged to operate unless they themselves are convinced that a lump is present.

The planned operation for a discrete lump is excision; that for a larger indefinite area is incision biopsy, taking a generous sized thin slice from the centre of the mass. After skin incision a lump is not as easy to locate as beforehand, so it is worth placing an 18 or 21 gauge needle in the lump prior to incising the skin.

Table 23.1 Criteria which have to be satisfied before deciding that a lump is benign and may be left *in situ*

Age (years)	Imaging used	FNAC
≤25	Ultrasound	×1 – no suspicious cells seen
26–35	Ultrasound	×2 – benign epithelial cells only
>35	Ultrasound and mammogram	×2 – benign epithelial cells only

FNAC, fine needle aspiration cytology. In *all* cases the lump must feel firm, smooth and fully mobile and on imaging must appear as benign image.

For the best cosmetic result the skin around the edge of the areola is marked in ink and a skin incision made just avoiding the pigment in order to avoid the rare complication of tattooing. Lumps 3–4 cm from the areola can be reached through such an incision by dissecting subcutaneously with large straight blunt scissors. The plane between subcutaneous fat and breast fat is readily identified. If the lump is further from the areola, or is deep in the breast, the incision is made over the lump. A circumferential incision parallel to the areola edge is to be preferred.

Once over the lump the superficial fascia is pushed aside and the deeper layers over the lump are reached. The inexperienced surgeon may again be caught unawares. The lump feels as though it is directly under the superficial fascia and the surgeon may try to seize it with tissue forceps. A smooth lump, however, such as a fibroadenoma lies deeper among the connective and epithelial tissue of the breast and simply slips from the tissue forceps leaving the surgeon holding the wrong piece. The preferred approach is to incise the breast tissue vertically with a scalpel until the lump itself is reached.

If there is no clearly defined lump at operation then incision is made to the centre of the mass and a piece of tissue about 0.5 cm wide and encompassing the breadth of the main mass is cut out with a scalpel (incision biopsy).

If there is a clear rounded lump – for example, a fibroadenoma – the surgeon dissects close to this with a scalpel or sharp scissors until enough of the surface is exposed to seize the lump with tissue forceps, after which dissection close to the surface is completed.

Diathermy haemostasis is carried out throughout and a lengthy inspection of the cavity is required. A suction drain is placed in all but the smallest and driest wounds and the skin is closed with interrupted 4/0 polypropylene (Prolene) sutures (which are replaced by adhesive sutures on the fourth day) or by subcuticular 4/0 polyglycolic acid (Dexon). Usually the drain can be removed in 1–2 days.

Minor breast operations

Nipple biopsy

Soreness of the nipple, accompanied by obvious inflammation and especially if the nipple is raw and granulating, may well be caused by Paget's disease of the nipple – *in situ* carcinoma.

If there is any suspicion of this, even only a good history of recurrent inflammation without clinical signs at the time of examination, nipple biopsy should be undertaken. This is easily done in the clinic. Local anaesthesia with adrenaline is used. A pointed No. 11 scalpel blade is held in the fingers and two parallel cuts about 1 mm apart are made from the periphery to the centre of the nipple. The piece between the two cuts is lifted with a small hypodermic needle and then removed by cutting underneath. One small skin stitch is inserted.

Nipple discharge

If a lump is present in the woman complaining of nipple discharge, the management becomes that of a breast lump. Otherwise a multiduct discharge, especially if bilateral, is not a cause for alarm.

About 5% of single duct discharges are caused by intraduct cancers. The presence of blood in the discharge does not aid the differentiation of malignant from benign causes. Until recently single duct discharge was treated by microdochectomy (excision of the involved duct) but the management now advocated is to carry out a magnified, retroareolar mammogram. If the mammogram shows a significant anomaly, microdochectomy is undertaken; if not, the patient is seen again in 1 year; if the discharge persists a further mammogram is taken and if again normal she is not followed up further.

Microdochectomy

This operation may be carried out under local anaesthetic although many patients prefer general anaesthesia day case surgery. On the day of admission the patient is examined to ensure that discharge can still be expressed and this is again checked in the anaesthetic room.

The surgeon may prefer to wear a magnifying hood. The duct is identified and a lacrymal probe is placed in it and advanced as far as it will easily pass (usually about 3 cm). A silk suture is then placed at the nipple and the probe tied in firmly. The skin over the probe is infiltrated with 1 in 80 000 adrenaline solution and an incision made over the length of the probe. The skin edges are each held back with a suture.

The duct is freed along its length as far as possible – multiple divisions finally making this difficult. If discharge is coming from the divisions then each of these is further followed for 1–2 cm as they are encountered. The duct may lead to a lesion: a localized area of cystic disease or a small solid carcinoma *in situ*. Otherwise, once the duct has been freed it is opened and a papilloma may be found. The skin is closed with 4/0 polypropylene sutures after careful haemostasis, leaving a suction drain if a solid area was excised.

Mamillary fistula and periareola abscess

Duct ectasia – dilated ducts under the nipple with inspissated secretions, periductal fibrosis and inflammation – is a common condition in women in the 40–60 age group.

The static secretion within these ducts is prone to infection by anaerobes. Once infection is present it is difficult to clear, as in similar conditions with static material in other organs. The infection results in small abscesses presenting at the edge of the areola. These may discharge, sometimes leaving a fistula (Figure 23.7) or may present as an indefinite lump at the areola edge.

If presenting acutely or as a lump, the abscess is incised and if possible the fistula found. A probe is

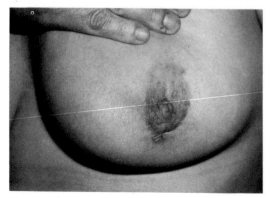

Figure 23.7 A mamillary fistula

passed up to the duct through the nipple and an incision made up to the nipple; the wound is then left to granulate. On recurrence the best operation is to excise the central ducts (Hadfield's procedure, mammodochectomy).

Excision of the central ducts

The lower edge of the areola is carefully marked with a pen and an accurate cut made around the lower circumference. Nipple and areola are raised from the breast, cutting deep to the venous plexus. The under surface of the nipple is inspected and any duct ends seen are removed. With a long scalpel a cut is made straight down into the breast tissue in a circle directly under the areola edge to a depth of 2 cm. The subareolar block of tissue is excised. The subcutaneous dissection around the areola is extended for about 2 cm and the deep tissue is inspected and the ducts are ligated where seen. The deep tissue is apposed under the nipple by catgut sutures. If necessary the nipple is everted by a subcutaneous suture around the base. Skin closure is with several polypropylene sutures. Before closure a suction drain is placed in the wound.

Is sepsis has been evident shortly before operation, antibiotic cover with flucloxacillin and metronidazole should be given.

Breast cancer
Primary breast cancer

Breast cancer usually presents as a palpable lump 2–3 cm in diameter but around 20% of cases are first seen with locally advanced tumours. There are several ways of treating the primary cancer. After full discussion with the patient to determine what operation she favours, a treatment plan is drawn up. The house surgeon has an important role in coordinating the roles of the radiologist, pathologist, radiotherapist and oncologist in the overall therapeutic endeavour.

Breast conservation by excision of the primary tumour, followed by whole breast irradiation with a boost to the tumour site, is inceasingly being undertaken (Figure 23.8). The majority of units report good results. However recurrence within the irradiated breast may be as high as 20% in those women surviving for 10 years after surgery. In some centres lumpectomy is combined with clearance of axillary nodes.

The indications for more extensive surgery are not fully worked out, but women with tumours which are large, multicentric or poorly differentiated should probably undergo mastectomy. The commonest procedure for these cases currently is simple mastectomy, sometimes with a clearance of the

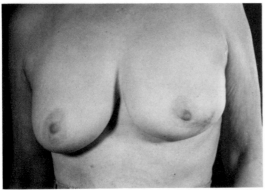

Figure 23.8 Breast cancer treated with breast conservation by wide excision and whole breast irradiation

lower part of the axilla. The draining lymph nodes are not removed extensively nor irradiated since oedema of the arm can result and the majority of cases will never require such treatments if left. Subcutaneous mastectomy or mastectomy with the use of a tissue expander can be undertaken to give more acceptable cosmetic result (Figure 23.9). Detailed descriptions of the operations for primary breast cancer are outside the scope of this book. Following surgery the patient may receive radiotherapy in some centres or systemic adjuvant

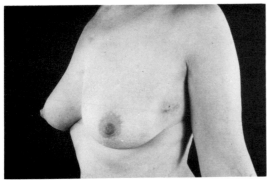

Figure 23.9 A woman who underwent subcutaneous mastectomy with subsequent prosthetic implant for breast cancer

hormone treatment for 2–4 years or a course of cytotoxic chemotherapy: these depend upon local protocols and upon the prognosis of the patient.

Locally advanced primary cancers

Tumours greater than 5 cm diameter may be assumed to have distant metastases and have a 20% survival at 5 years. They may prove difficult to control locally and are often inoperable without leaving tumour behind. Radiotherapy gives good

palliation in only around 50% of cases. In hormone responsive tumours, tamoxifen 10 mg b.d. results in local control lasting 1–7 years and also slows the growth of the occult metastases.

Advanced breast cancer with distant metastases

Once distant spread becomes symptomatic, the patient will die from her disease. Treatment is essentially by palliation.

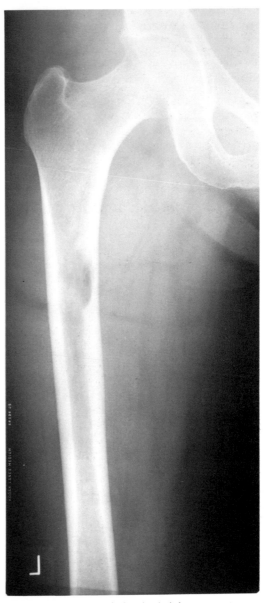

Figure 23.10 Radiograph showing lytic bony metastases

Secondaries may present almost anywhere, but the commonest sites are bone (Figure 23.10), liver, lung and pleura. The diagnosis is not always straightforward and any woman who has undergone treatment for primary breast cancer should have a new symptom such as back pain fully investigated, no matter how many years after the original surgery. Persistent bone pain requires a bone scan; dyspnoea or persistent dry cough probably indicate endo-bronchial spread, the chest radiograph of which is difficult to interpret – bronchoscopy and biopsy may be required. Pleural effusions do not often yield cells for cytological diagnosis and if confirmation of the cause is needed then lung biopsy has to be carried out. Pericardial effusion is unusual but gives severe discomfort. The very ill patient may be suffering from hypercalcaemia; abnormal liver function tests are usually enough to provide the diagnosis in a woman who is known to have had carcinoma of the breast. In wholly CNS metastases the opinion of a neurologist often saves the need for the CT scan.

The appearance of distant metastases means that systemic therapy must be implemented. However, specific therapies also play a part depending upon the sites of metastases.

Therapies for specific problems in advanced disease

Bone

Irradiation should be used freely for bone metas-tases. This is especially indicated for bone pain and for metastases in danger of collapse, e.g. vertebrae, the neck of the femur and the fermoral shaft. Impending or actual fracture of the femoral neck or shaft is treated by orthopaedic stabilization with postoperative radiotherapy.

Pleural effusion

A pleural effusion is emptied by a 28 gauge intercostal suction drain. This is described elsewhere (Chapter 17). Once the pleural cavity is empty pleurodesis is attempted by injecting 100 mg mepac-rine in 20 ml of water down the drain, leaving for 2 h and then re-applying suction for 2 days. This may be repeated if the effusion recurs.

Endobronchial spread

This gives severe dyspnoea which may be relieved to some extent by general measures: a broad-spectrum antibiotic to eliminate supra-added infection, sal-butamol and prednisolone to eliminate any broncho-spasm or oedema and oxygen. Cytotoxic chemo-therapy is used as the initial systemic therapy in this condition.

Brain metastases

Some help may be gained from systemic dexametha-sone in a dose of 4 mg 6-hourly. Persistent severe headache may be helped by irradiation.

Hypercalcaemia

The initial treatment is to rehydrate the patient over 24–48 h with normal saline. If this fails to restore the serum calcium to normal limits, then calcitonin or diphosphates can be used. The effects are best monitored using calcium excretion measurement.

Pain

A non-steriodal anti-inflammatory drug (e.g. ibu-profen, diclofenac sodium) and an analgesic (e.g. dihydrocodeine) give good pain control in a large number of patients. If pain persists, oral morphine may be required. Tricyclic antidepressants (e.g. dothiepin 75 mg nightly) can be used as a co-analgesic. Patients, particularly those with bone pain not controlled by analgesic medication, often require palliative radiotherapy.

Systemic therapy in advanced disease

Systemic therapy may be hormonal or by use of cytotoxic chemotherapy. On treatment the tumour deposits may apparently disappear altogether or get smaller (response) or stay static or progress. Side effects of many regimens of cytotoxic chemotherapy are unpleasant, while those of hormonal manipu-lation may be negligible. Therefore the initial systemic therapy used in most cases is endocrin-ological, although some units will rely upon oestrogen receptor measurements and other guides to likely response.

First-line hormone therapy

Premenopausal women until recently underwent oophorectomy whereas postmenopausal patients were given tamoxifen 20 mg twice daily. Tamoxifen acts by blocking the effect of circulating oestrogen on the cells and is a drug with very few side effects. Recently a new agent, goserelin (Zoladex) has been marketed. It blocks the action of the ovaries and surgical oophorectomy is now unnecessary. The premenopausal woman will probably receive both tamoxifen and goserelin in future. Side effects of goserelin are again few, apart from those of the menopause.

Those patients who respond to first-line endocrine therapy do so for an average of 18 months. They then progress again and therapy has to be changed.

Only those who responded to first-line endocrine therapy are given further endocrine treatment. One choice is megestrol acetate given in high dose (320 mg/day).

Cytotoxic chemotherapy

Cytotoxic therapy is often used after the failure of, or relapse from, endocrine therapy. Secondary breast cancer responds to combinations of chemotherapeutic drugs in 40–60% of cases. However, response is short-lived and the side effects may be distressing: hair loss, nausea, cystitis, sore mouth. Recently, less toxic drugs and regimens have been introduced, some using only a single agent; mitozantrone (Lederle) and epirubicin (Farmitalia) in low dose are currently being evaluated.

Cytotoxic therapy should be introduced as the first line along with endocrine therapy for the patient breathless due to lung metastases and for very aggressive tumours (short disease-free interval, secondary presentation with liver metastases, poor histological differentiation).

Breast cancer screening

Breast cancer screening by mammography every 3 years is being introduced in the UK, for women tween of ages of 50 and 65 years. Screening below the age of 50 has not been shown to be effective.

Mammographic screening gives rise to the discovery of palpable and impalpable lesions. These may be small breast cancers, radial scars (benign complex sclerosing lesions) which mimic the spiculate appearance of some cancers (Figure 23.11), fibroadenomas, fat necrosis or sclerosing adenosis.

When the radiologist sees an abnormality on a screening film he or she must decide whether it looks sufficiently dangerous to require open biopsy. The breast is palpated by a surgeon. If there is no palpable lump and yet the decision has been made that biopsy is required, stereotactic guided excision will be the procedure used. However, an attempt at preoperative diagnosis can be made by obtaining stereotactic cytology.

A number of devices have been manufactured which may be attached to mammogram machines. These work by taking two films centred on the lesion but with the machine swung through a 30° arc; the location and depth of the lesion are computed and the machine repositioned using controls of horizontal, lateral and vertical movement. A needle may then be placed down a guide channel exactly to the centre of the lesion.

Excision of a stereotactically located lesion

The operation depends upon the preoperative diagnostic cytology. If the cytology shows a cancer, the procedure will be therapeutic and probably wide excision will be carried out with lymph node biopsy or low axillary clearance. As stated earlier, the details of these procedures are outside the scope of this book. If no preoperative diagnosis has been obtained, a diagnostic operation is required with as little cosmetic damage as possible.

Diagnostic stereotactic biopsy is carried out after a marker wire has been placed in the breast. The marker equipment should be stout enough to be felt easily by the surgeon after incision within the breast tissue. The tip should engage firmly in the tissue. At present the ideal needle/wire combination has not been designed but one that combines these two necessities is the Nottingham needle (Nottingham Lesion Location Device, Mediplus Ltd). This needle places a flexible wire with a strong barb into the lesion through a needle which is then withdrawn. A cannula is replaced around the needle at operation allowing the point to be felt through the tissue. The position of the wire is checked by taking a lateral film.

The operation is carried out under general anaesthetic. A small circumferential incision (around 3 cm long) is made over the point of the needle, which is estimated by measuring from the skin entry and from the direction of the needle. Subcutaneous dissection is carried out for several centimetres around the incision and up as far as the needle shaft just under the skin. The breast tissue is cut directly down with the scalpel at 90° to the needle so that the shaft of the needle is again encountered 1–2 cm above the tip. The shaft is

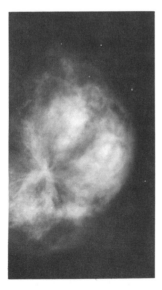

Figure 23.11 Spiculate lesion on a mammogram mimicking a carcinoma – in fact a benign radial scar

grasped with an artery forceps and the assistant holds the needle steady. The tip is now defined. Sometimes a clear lesion can then be felt and is removed. If not, the tissue around the needle tip is excised by cutting with the scalpel down parallel to the needle on both sides and across around 1 cm below it. The tissue including the needle tip is then pulled upwards with tissue forceps and sharp dissection frees it from behind. A piece around 1.5 cm square is removed. This is immediately radiographed (Figure 23.12) which is best carried

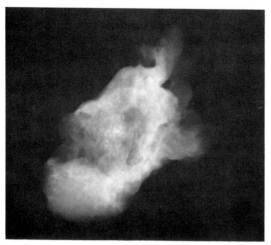

Figure 23.12 Specimen radiograph of an area of microcalcification removed by stereotactic marker biopsy. The piece of tissue (shown here magnified) should weigh less than 10 g when taken for diagnosis.

out in a machine designed for specimen radiographs (e.g. Faxitron, Vinten Intruments): a processor dedicated for mammography is not required for the films which can be developed in the routine radiography department if this is nearer to the operating theatre than the mammographic unit. The surgeon should mark the edges of the tissue with distinctive sutures for orientation.

Once the surgeon is satisfied that the biopsy taken is the lesion identified on the radiograph then the tissue is sent for histology. The skin is sutured with a suction drain left in the cavity. Frozen section is not advised for these lesions, which require care and time for correct interpretation. The pathologist later uses the specimen radiography machine to aid in the identification of the lesion by making serial slices and radiographing these.

Conclusion

The care of women with breast disease involves many procedures which are carried out by surgical junior staff. The trainee surgeon must be aware of the management lines for breast disease and be confident in diagnosis and in the necessary practical procedures. He should be able to tell the patient in simple language about the various therapeutic options that are available. He needs to be satisfied that any consent given is fully informed. The detailed counselling of the patient should be carried out by the senior surgeon. In acquiring knowledge and confidence there is no substitute for adequate patient experience.

24

Surgical oncology

R. D. Rosin

Most cancer patients will be, treated by general surgeons. However, there is a need for surgeons with a specific interest in oncology to coordinate cancer care, deal with the rarer malignant tumours and perform some of the standard oncological operations.

Malignancy probably accounts for one in three of the patients in most busy surgical wards. This chapter will deal with the more specialized tumours, particularly their investigation, treatment and the complications encountered as well as discussing oncological emergencies.

General concepts in the management of malignancy

In virtually every case, it is better for the patient to be aware of their diagnosis as they may have to face major surgery, radiotherapy or chemotherapy either singly or in combination. If active treatment is impossible, the patient needs to know or have some idea of the prognosis. If this is the position, it should be remembered that 'some hope is better than no hope, which in turn is better than despair'. The patient should never feel abandoned. If the family should request that the diagnosis be kept from their relative, then it must be remembered that the patient has a right to know if he wishes. However, occasionally it might be in the best interest for the patient not to be fully informed.

The management of advanced cancer, treatment of pain and care of the dying are covered in other chapters.

Decision making

Any decision must be based on the characteristics of both the host and the tumour (Table 24.1). The

Table 24.1 Host and tumour features

Tumour	Host
Anatomy and histology	Age
Stage or extent of disease	Performance status
Growth rate	Other morbid disease
Sensitivity or resistance to treatment	Distribution of metastases
	Functional reserve of system

important host characteristics include age, fitness and the presence or absence of concomitant serious disease. There are a number of tumour factors that critically influence treatment decisions. The site and histological type may influence therapy as well as the stage or extent of the disease. Its biological activity as reflected in its growth rate and the potential responsiveness to individual therapeutic modalities are also important. The question of when to treat and specifically what form of treatment to use, and whether it ought to be a single modality or combination, can be difficult to answer.

The question of therapy for patients with advanced metastatic disease is often even more difficult. If measurable lesions are present, they will permit precise monitoring of therapy and allow withdrawal of treatment that produces any morbidity without reducing the size of the tumour (Table 24.2).

Concepts of local, systemic and combined modality therapies

Malignant conditions have a local, regional and systemic phase – the length of each depends on the type and site of the malignancy. Cancer therapy can also be divided into local/regional and systemic.

343

Table 24.2 Objective response

Complete	100% reduction for minimum of 4 weeks without the appearance of new lesions
Partial	50% reduction in the measured size without increase in other lesions and a minimum duration of 4 weeks
Stable	<25% reduction in measurable disease without other lesions developing
No response	>25% increase in the size of the lesion or the development of new lesions
Improvement	20–50% reduction in size lasting at least 4 weeks

Local disease can be treated locally by either surgery or radiotherapy. In circumstances where local therapy is associated with a high recurrence rate, a combination of modalities may be effective, e.g. prophylactic postoperative radiotherapy following excision of an early breast carcinoma (Table 24.3).

Table 24.3 Effective combined modality therapies

Modalities	Tumour
Surgery and radiotherapy	Rectal cancer Sarcoma
Surgery and chemotherapy	Breast cancer Osteogenic sarcoma
Radiotherapy and chemotherapy	Brest cancer Sarcoma Pancreatic cancer

Systemic treatment includes that distributed not only to the local area, but also to other areas throughout the body, e.g. chemotherapy, hormone therapy or immunotherapy. Its use is based on the tendency for any primary malignant tumour to metastasize outside the local or regional area. The combination of local and systemic therapy is commonly called 'adjuvant therapy' which has resulted in improved local control and prolonged survival for some types of tumours.

For patients with advanced disease, combined modality therapy may be useful. The response to therapy must be carefully evaluated. The responsiveness may be determined in descending order of reliability and objectivity by survival, tumour regression and symptom response.

Diagnostic problems in cancer management

The diagnosis of cancer may be simple from the histology. For many tumours, however, the diag-

nosis depends on organ invasion since the lesion may be equivocal histologically.

A major diagnostic problem is that of a 'tumour of unknown origin'. Therapeutic management is rarely difficult, but the diagnostic implications are substantial in that a search for the primary is often arduous and expensive and even if identified may not justify therapy.

Therapeutic problems in cancer management

The first question to be asked could be 'when to treat cancer?'. Then, should one give sequential treatment or everything at the start? Sequential treatment has less morbidity but the potential for long-term control and perhaps for cure is limited and often even non-existent.

Whilst considering the when and how of therapy, it is also important to consider the duration, particularly of adjuvant or combined modality chemotherapy. This issue is not resolved, as adjuvant chemotherapy has not been definitely established as an important and absolute treatment for any tumour. However, it is becoming increasingly popular.

Effective treatment, i.e. treatment that induces regression, must not just *prolong* life, but must also be associated with an improved *quality* of life.

The complete management of the cancer patient

Staging

Clinical staging is vital prior to treatment plans being designed. A knowledge of the likely sites of metastases will lead to an appropriate but not excessive search for them and, if discovered, may limit an operation. The use of preoperative adjuvants such as radiotherapy or chemotherapy or the avoidance of an operation may be decided upon by the staging of the tumour. Sampling of suspicious tissues is vital prior to operation and the surgical oncologist clearly must have in mind preoperatively whether the planned procedure and treatment should be an attempt at cure or palliation. In the former instance, care must be taken to adhere to the principles of adequate local excision, not to enter the tumour bed, and to excise *en bloc* the regional lymph nodes if indicated.

Preoperative preparation

The patient must be in the best possible physical condition to withstand the surgery. Fluid balance, anaemia and nutritional dificiencies must be corrected. Immediate operation is usually not vital, and makes little sense considering cell kinetics; it is probably best to delay operation if necessary to improve the patient's status as this will ensure a smoother postoperative course. Particular attention must be paid to the timing of operation following radiotherapy to prevent postoperative necrosis or delayed healing. The usual preoperative measures such as informed consent and cross-matching of blood must not be forgotten.

Operation

If resection for cure is feasible, it should be performed without hestitation. More difficult situations arise if the cancer is not resectable due to invasion of vital structures. Should this occur, the first objective must be to determine precisely by frozen section examination whether or not it is truly unresectable. Involvement of neighbouring structures that can be excised does not preclude an attempt at cure. Reoperation on patients later often adds the difficulty of adhesions or infection. If the patient's life can be extended with reasonable quality, or if the patient may be made more comfortable by palliative surgery, it should be undertaken. Non-curative resection of massive cancers is acceptable if reducing the bulk of the tumour allows chemotherapy or other treatments which are effective with certain tumours, (e.g. ovarian cancers and lymphomas), an improved chance to act against fewer malignant cells.

Postoperative radiotherapy can be facilitated by marking the tumour bed with clips or the placement of tubes for postoperative after-loading local irradiation or implant chemotherapy. The placement of indwelling catheters for selective infusion should also be considered.

Only the surgeon performing the operation can be certain about the findings, and therefore must be responsible for writing and/or drawing the exact findings. The extent of disease, resection margins, involvement of lymph nodes, and whether or not resection was 'curative' must be recorded accurately.

Specific malignant tumours
Soft tissue sarcomas

These represent just less than 1% of all malignant neoplasms. They are often present as asymptomatic soft tissue swellings which are ubiquitous in their anatomical distribution. There are no reliable physical signs to distinguish between benign and malignant soft tissue swellings and therefore all that persist or grow should be biopsied and examined histologically. They have two serious properties in their natural history: the tendency to recur after excision and the risk of metastases.

The objective of treatment is survival with the least anatomical and functional loss. Soft tissue radiographs, ultrasound examination and occasionally arteriography are all useful, but the most important investigation in assessing the pattern of involvement of a primary lesion is, if available, NMR scanning and if not, a CT scan.

The diagnosis depends on histological examination and this should be performed on an incisional biopsy. The latter should be performed through a carefully placed incision (see Figure 24.1) so as not

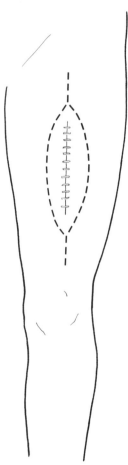

Figure 24.1 Biopsy incision placed in the longitudinal axis over quadriceps tumour

to compromise subsequent radical excision of the lesion. Aspiration cytology or needle biopsy should not be used except in rare situations as tissue cultures and electron microscopy are often necessary for accurate diagnosis and these require larger samples of tissue. Care must be taken to obtain excellent haemostasis as haematomas can lead to spread of the tumour far beyond the site of natural tumour invasion. Combined modality treatment is now usually employed with a wide excision of the tumour followed by postoperative radiotherapy and chemotherapy.

Lymphomas

These account for approximately 4% of all malignant diseases. Non-Hodgkin's lymphoma can occur at any age, but the incidence increases exponentially with advancing years. The average age at presentation is 50. Hodgkin's disease has a peak incidence in the third decade of life, but has a bimodal age distribution with another peak around 60 years.

Over the last two decades Hodgkin's disease has been transformed from an almost terminal disease to one in which an increasing number are being cured by radiotherapy and/or chemotherapy. Successful treatment is dependent on accurate knowledge of the extent of the disease. With the increasing sophistication of imaging techniques the surgeon's role in the overall management of Hodgkin's disease is minimal. If a laparotomy is performed and splenectomy carried out, it must be remembered that the patient will be more prone to pneumococcal pneumonia and therefore the procedure should be covered either by penicillin or a pneumococcal vaccine.

Cancer of the breast

The breast is the commonest site for cancer in women, and the chief cause of death in many countries. The incidence varies greatly with geography. Rare under the age of 25 years, breast cancer increases steadily in frequency with age and reaches a peak in old age with an incidence of 1200 per 100 000 women over the age of 80. The overall incidence in the UK is of the order of 25 per 100 000 whereas in Japan there are only 5 per 100 000 women.

Usually the diagnosis is obvious on clinical examination but no decision concerning treatment can be made without histological proof. With the advent of breast screening using mammography an increasing number of impalpable lesions are being discovered and histological confirmation can sometimes prove difficult (see p. 334).

With palpable lesions, fine needle aspiration should be performed provided the expertise is available to examine the specimen cytologically, If not, or if the cytology is equivocal, a needle biopsy can be performed under local anaesthetic.

The surgical management of primary breast cancer has changed dramatically in the last two decades. Whereas previously, mastectomy was almost always performed with or without regional node clearance, now breast conservation with postoperative radiotherapy is preferred if possible as the survival figures are the same.

It is best if the patient can be seen by both the radiotherapist and surgeon prior to any procedure so that treatment can be tailored to the patient. The size of the tumour, size of the breast and location of the tumour within the breast will all be important in deciding the best method of treating that patient. If a mastectomy is necessary, it must be remembered that the loss of a breast could have a tremendous impact psychologically on the patient, her husband and family. Counselling preoperatively is important and mention should be made of the possibility of breast reconstruction at a later date. Once carcinoma of the breast has been diagnosed, a search for metastases in the common sites should be undertaken. This would include an ultrasound of the liver and a bone scan. For the postmenopausal woman, the use of tamoxifen has been shown to be of benefit. There is still debate as to the value of adjuvant chemotherapy in the premenopausal woman, but unfortunately if metastases occur, then either radiotherapy and/or chemotherapy may be necessary.

Liver tumours

The incidence of primary cancer of the liver in industrialized countries is low. However, it is very common in Japan (17 per 100 000) and West Africa (58 per 100 000). Men are four times more commonly affected than women. Possible causative factors are hepatotoxins (e.g. aflatoxin), hepatitis B virus, malnutrition, alcohol, α-1 antitrypsin phenotypes and hormonal influence.

Metastatic carcinoma of the liver is 20 times more common than primary liver cancer, and usually secondary to cancer of the lung, gastrointestinal tract or breast. Of all patients dying of malignant disease subjected to post-mortem examination, 30–50% have liver metastases.

Most resectable liver tumours produce few symptoms when first seen, as compared with those liver tumours that are easily detected when they first present and are too far advanced to be surgically curable. Early symptoms are mild right upper quadrant discomfort with occasional shoulder-tip pain if the diaphragm is involved, epigastric pain and intermittent nausea. The diagnosis is usually made by ultrasonography, CT scans, hepatic arteriography and peritoneoscopy. The latter is a useful diagnostic procedure which allows biopsies to be taken under direct vision. The identification of alpha-fetoprotein is diagnostic and present in 60–90% of cases of hepatocellular carcinoma. It is also a good indicator of recurrence as it will disappear after successful resection of the tumour.

The only curative therapy available for primary liver cancer is surgical resection. For this to be possible, the tumour must be confined to one segment or lobe of the liver with no evidence of distant metastases. The patient must be fit enough to undergo such major surgery. The indications for hepatic resection for metastases are less well defined. Most resections for metastases have been for carcinoid, colorectal cancer and renal tumours. In those patients who have hepatic metastases from a colorectal primary, if surgical resection is feasible, there is a 40% 5-year survival. Multifocal bilobar involvement excludes surgical resection. As liver tumours receive their blood supply from the hepatic artery, it is logical to deliver chemotherapy agents directly into it for regional perfusion. This can be accomplished either by cannulating the hepatic artery, usually via the gastroduodenal artery at laparotomy or by the placement of a catheter percutaneously via the femoral artery. The advent of totally implantable pumps and ports have made direct hepatic perfusion more attractive. Regional perfusion should not be used unless the primary lesion has been removed and there is no evidence of extrahepatic metastases. The results of continuous hepatic infusion with 5-fluorodeoxyuridine for colorectal metastases are encouraging. Complications can arise either from the cannula or from the chemotherapy. The most common complication of the latter, especially if there is a large percentage of the liver replaced with tumour, is jaundice. Some patients with high-dose chemotherapy have developed sclerosing cholangitis. If an implantable pump is employed, it must be refilled according to its cycle and never allowed to run dry. If a port has been used, the hepatic artery cannula should be flushed through the port with heparinized saline at weekly intervals.

Testicular tumours

The vast majority of testicular tumours are malignant and account for between 1% and 2% of all malignant disease in men. It is the most common type of cancer in males aged between 20 and 35 years, and there has been an increase in incidence during the past 20 years. An increased risk is observed in men who have had a cryptorchid testicle. Diagnosis should be suspected clinically in any male with a scrotal mass. Staging is carried out with the use of CT scanning. Tumour markers (β-HCG) are useful in the non-seminoma tumour.

In men who have widespread disease from a seminoma or who have a teratoma, chemotherapy will probably be used and therefore before surgery sperm should be stored if a family is contemplated in the future. If the diagnosis is not clearcut, a frozen section of the testicle can be performed but an inguinal approach must be used with atraumatic cross-clamping of the spermatic cord prior to biopsy. If the diagnosis is still equivocal, it is better to remove a benign mass in preference to the possibility of leaving a malignant tumour behind.

If not performed preoperatively, lymphangiography and CT scan of the abdomen and pelvis are necessary investigations once the diagnosis is made. If an elevated tumour marker returns to normal following treatment, this is strong evidence that the disease has been eradicated. Similarly, a return to an elevated marker implies disease recurrence.

Cutaneous neoplasms

Skin cancer is the most common cancer in many countries where the population is predominantly white. In the USA, it accounts for 25% of all cancers and 50% in Australia. Prolonged and continuous exposure to sunlight in outdoor workers is the most common aetiological factor. Long-standing scars following burns, trauma and lupus may also be complicated by skin cancer (Marjolin's ulcer).

Among the many neoplasms that arise from skin, few require any form of major surgery. Most are treated by curettage, fulguration, radiotherapy or simply local excision. When surgery does become necessary, adequate excision with free margins of resection is usually curative.

Basal cell carcinomas are generally 4–5 times more frequent than squamous cell carcinomas. The majority of both types develop in the skin of the face, mainly around the nose, eyelids and cheeks. Basal cell carcinomas, also known as rodent ulcers, are very slow growing and can present in a nodular or ulcerative form which can be pigmented. Squamous cell carcinoma varies in presentation from a scaly and ulcerated lesion or elevated nodular mass to a punched-out infiltrating ulcer or a large fungating tumour.

In general the principles of diagnosis and staging of the various kinds of skin cancer are similar. The diagnosis is either strongly suspected clinically, or it is clinically atypical with the diagnosis unknown until biopsy results are available. As the incidence of metastatic disease from a basal cell carcinoma is so small, only physical examination is necessary unless some symptom or sign warrants further investigation. In the case of squamous cell carcinoma, it should be routine that a very careful lymph node examination is performed. While the cure rate for skin cancer exceeds 95%, the time, effort, expense and disfigurement are of more major proportion.

Excisional biopsy is always preferable as for the majority of cases it is curative. It also has the advantage of providing a pathologist with a complete specimen. The principal advantage of surgical excision and treatment is that it removes the lesion in one quick and usually unequivocal procedure. It also allows a definitive assessment of the extent of the neoplasm by examination of the margins of resection. Usually, these procedures are carried out under local anaesthetic as an outpatient. Occasionally, because of the anatomical site, a split skin graft may be necessary.

Malignant melanoma, especially if neglected, remains one of the more lethal forms of skin cancer. Although it is an infrequent tumour, much interest has been shown in it recently because of its rapidly increasing incidence, its wide variation in different ethnic groups, and its pathological and biological features. In most countries, the incidence has doubled or even trebled over the last 10–20 years. The highest mortality rates are recorded in Australasia (6 per 100 000). The explosion in incidence of malignant melanoma can be explained by the increased exposure to sun, especially in fair skinned people, and a decrease in the ozone layer allowing more dangerous light waves to pass through.

Over 60% of malignant melanomas arise in pre-existing benign pigmented lesions. As a rule, the diagnosis of malignant melanoma presents no difficulty to the practised eye. Reports that a pigmented area has suddenly altered its appearance, increased in size, changed colour, ulcerated or bled, must be viewed with great suspicion whilst itching can also be a symptom of change. Amelanotic melanomas (approx. 15%) can be difficult to diagnose. Excision biopsy should be performed with at least 1 cm clearance at each side, as this may prove adequate treatment for thin, good prognosis tumours. Prognosis depends on anatomical site, the presence of absence of ulceration, and histologically, the depth and thickness of the lesion as well as its mitotic rate.

Treatment depends on clinical staging and the estimated thickness of the lesion. It may be necessary after excisional biopsy to do a wider excision, the width depending on the histological features.

Isolated hyperthermic limb perfusion has been used for 30 years to treat recurrent disease, and recently it has been used as an adjunct to more conservative surgery for poor prognosis stage I limb melanomas. The lower limb can be perfused via the iliac vessels, and the limb isolated by buttock tourniquet, or via the femoral vessels when an upper thigh tourniquet is employed. The upper limb is perfused via the axillary vessels, utilizing a shoulder tourniquet. The leak rate should be monitored and the temperature then raised to at least 39°C.

Preoperatively the patient must be warned that there is a 10–15% chance of some postoperative oedema and that the limb will also become very red and hot. Blood should be cross-matched as the pump may need priming, and the clinical physics department warned that the leak rates during the operation will need to be monitored.

High systemic leak rates could be caused by poor application of the tourniquet, lack of control of anastomotic vessels or over-enthusiastic pumping with a high flow rate, leading to loss of fluid and drug to the patient. Overheating the blood (greater than 41°C) can lead to tissue necrosis. A high systemic leak rate will lead to nausea and vomiting and if very high, even to bone marrow depression.

When regional lymph nodes are clinically involved, therapeutic block dissection should be performed. Once again, the patient should be warned that there is a slight chance of postoperative oedema following the operation. This oedema can be lessened by the use of compression stockings.

Very extensive recurrences, not amenable to isolated limb perfusion or refractory to that treatment, can be treated with intralesional inoculation using BCG, or cryosurgery, local radiotherapy and/or by laser treatment.

Treatment of metastases and management of effusions

The treatment of metastatic disease represents the largest problem in clinical oncology as 60–70% of all patients with cancer will at some time develop distant metastases. Aggressive management of metastases on some occasions can contribute to long-term survival and, hopefully, a better quality of life. The risk of metastases is particularly high in certain specific organs because they are the initial capillary bed through which the blood is filtered after spreading from the primary site.

Although patients with generalized metastases may benefit from effective systemic chemotherapy because of its ability to reach most parts of the body, in many situations more localized treatment may add to the patient's survival and wellbeing. Some organs will contain a solitary metastasis or be the only site of metastases for a specific tumour. These may be suitable for surgery, radiotherapy or combined treatment.

Brain metastases

Carcinoma of the lung and breast have a predilection for spread to the brain. Malignant melanoma also tends to spread to this site. Improved management of patients with generalized metastases has led to longer survival and a greater incidence of spread to the brain. In general, radiotherapy would be the principal and often sole treatment.

Lung metastases

Almost one-third of patients with malignant disease have pulmonary metastases at some time during the clinical course of their illness. Current approaches to their management include chemotherapy for tumours sensitive to drugs, radiotherapy to augment chemotherapy and, very occasionally, pulmonary wedge excisions of focal discrete lesions.

Liver metastases

Most clinicians regard liver metastases as incurable. Most patients who develop metastases in the liver have them either at the time of diagnosis and resection of the primary tumour, or within 2 years of this event. The use of surgical resection, if possible, and regional perfusion have already been mentioned.

Bone metastases

Pain, pathological fracture and forced immobility caused by bone metastases significantly decrease the quality of life of the cancer patient. Over 80% of patients with bone metastases will have a breast, lung or prostatic primary. It is rarely life-threatening and occasionally patients live for years following the discovery of spread to their bones. They will require treatment to palliate the pain and prevent fracture in weight-bearing bones.

Localized radiation is highly effective and usually results in complete relief of the symptoms. Internal fixation before irradiation should be considered for lytic lesions in the weight-bearing bones to reduce the risk of pathological fracture.

Malignant pleural effusions

These are most commonly associated with carcinomas of the lung and breast, or with lymphomas. Patients commonly present with dyspnoea, cough or chest pain, though 20% can be asymptomatic. Their successful treatment may allow months or years of productive life. The diagnosis is made on chest radiograph and aspiration of the effusion with cytology. Pleural biopsy may be necessary if the cytology is negative.

Aspiration alone, even when the pleural space is completely emptied, does not prevent reaccumulation of fluid. Obliteration of the pleural space is necessary and thus any agent introduced should produce mesothelial fibrosis and pleural sclerosis rather than have a specific anti-malignant property. Surgical techniques are occasionally necessary and pleurectomy has been shown to be effective.

Malignant pericardial effusions

Their formation is usually gradual and the associated symptoms which include dyspnoea, cough, pain, orthopnoea, cyanosis, venous distention, leg oedema and cardiac enlargement may all be attributed to the overall systemic effects of carcinomatosis unless there are reasons to suspect pericardial involvement. Tumours that most commonly metastasize to the pericardium are lung and breast cancers, leukaemias, lymphomas and melanoma.

Malignant ascites

If tense malignant ascites develops and fails to respond to diuretics or aspiration and intraperitoneal cytotoxic drugs, peritoneovenous shunting can give good palliation. Two types of shunts are commonly used: the Denver which must be manually worked, and the Le Veen which has a valve. The shunt is tunnelled from the peritoneal cavity subcutaneously to the internal jugular vein. Postoperatively, a large diuresis usually occurs. Unfortunately the shunts are prone to clotting and can become infected.

Oncological emergencies

These are secondary complications of cancer that have either life-threatening potential or major irreversible morbidity if untreated. Untreated spinal cord compression may cause major morbidity including paraplegia and conditions requiring prolonged nursing care, but is not itself life-threatening.

The clinical management of oncological emergencies often involves immediate therapeutic intervention without specific organ diagnostic evaluation, e.g. brain metastases. All of the oncological emergencies are treatable so that one can often reverse the clinical syndrome with standard noninvasive and tolerable therapy. These emergencies may be effectively treated so that recurrence is prevented and prognosis determined by another site of disease.

Organ-related cancer complications

These complications of cancer do not represent emergencies in that they do not have life-threatening potential but do have major implications for morbidity. It may be remembered that in each visceral organ, benign processes may mimic the malignant disease so definitive diagnostic evaluations are necessary. Acquired infections, complications of therapy, incidental degenerative diseases or unrelated acute or chronic diseases are all potential problems that influence the therapeutic approach as well as confuse the diagnostic picture (Table 24.4). The patient with cancer is not immune to diabetes mellitus or coronary artery disease, and is just as susceptible as the non-cancer patient to incidental uncommon and rare diseases.

Table 24.4 Complications of cancer related to organs involved

Gastrointestinal tract	Infection, obstruction, organ failure, perforation, serositis, malabsorption
Genitourinary system	Obstruction, haemorrhage
Bone	Pathological fracture, infection
Lung	Infection, obstruction, serositis
Blood	Anaemia, haemorrhage, infection
Skin	Allergy, infection
Central nervous system	Seizures, neurological syndromes, cord compression, altered consciousness

Superior vena cava syndrome

The superior vena cava (SVC) syndrome develops as a consequence of a pathological process within the mediastinum and is considered an oncological emergency because of the acute cerebral syndrome that results from venous obstruction and increased intracerebral pressure. If left untreated, venous obstruction in the upper thorax can progress to stasis of blood flow and eventually to intravascular clotting with major secondary sequelae. It is almost invariably due to malignant disease (Table 24.5) and

Table 24.5 Non-malignant causes of the superior vena cava syndrome

Infectious	Syphilitic
Idiopathic	Sclerosing mediastinitis
Vascular	Catheter and pacemaker-induced phlebitis
Traumatic	Mediastinal haematoma
Degenerative	Goitre

is most commonly due to bronchogenic carcinoma, especially of the right lung. Lymph nodes in the mediastinum (Figure 24.2) encase the SVC and its thin wall and the low intravascular pressure within the venous system results in it being compressed relatively easily.

The increased venous pressure clinically manifests with venous distension of the neck and the upper thorax. Secondarily, oedema of the face, neck and

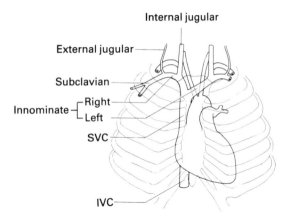

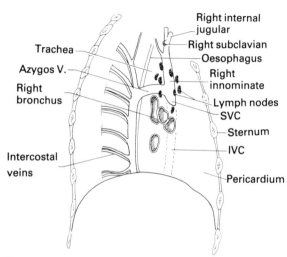

Figure 24.2 (*a*) Anterior view of thoracic cage and mediastinal vascular structures; (*b*) Mediastinal lymphadenopathy encasing the SVC

upper torso develops. This can lead to conjunctival oedema with visual disturbance and proptosis. Finally, symptoms of nervous dysfunction including headache, progressive dysarticulation and coma may occur. Concomitant obstruction of the trachea and oesophagus resulting in dysphagia, dysphonia and dyspnoea is possible.

The SVC syndrome diagnosis is made clinically and does not require radiological procedures for either confirmation or for establishing the site of obstruction. Chest radiography may demonstrate a large mass, but especially with metastatic lesions the mediastinal lesion may be quite small and detectable only by tomography. Venous access in the upper extremities must be avoided including venepuncture for any reason. Surgical manipulations in the neck, thorax, bronchi or oesophagus are likewise contraindicated.

The primary treatment is radiation, even without a histological diagnosis. After a relatively low dose, alleviation of the local oedema and venous obstruction may allow biopsy and further treatment. In children and young adults the syndrome is invariably due to lymphoma, and when this is thought to be the likely diagnosis, radiation should include the mantle field. In sensitive tumours, chemotherapy as a primary treatment may be effective and preclude the need for radiotherapy. It also plays a part in patients with the syndrome which is resistant to radiotherapy as well as being useful if maximum radiation has already been administered. Diuretics, anticoagulants and corticosteroids are of no proven efficacy. Surgical intervention is indicated as a secondary procedure only following resistance to other local and systemic modalities.

It is estimated that 10–20% of patients with the syndrome may survive longer than 2 years, justifying aggressive therapy.

Cardiac complications

Clinical cardiac complications are relatively uncommon, although heart metastases are present in 10% of post-mortems of patients with malignant neoplasms. The predominant clinical manifestation of cardiac metastases is the development of a malignant pericardial effusion. Because of the insidious clinical evolution of effusion, recognition of the life-threatening potential of cardiac tamponade is crucial. Effusions may be produced by either tumour implantations on the serosal surface with secondary exudations of fluid directly from the tumour, or by obstruction to the lymphatic flow emanating from the cardiac musculature as a consequence of mediastinal or hilar neoplastic infiltration with transudation of fluid within the pericardial sac.

Malignant pericardial effusion may be effectively treated for a long time by single pericardial aspiration. Radiotherapy may be used for patients with a radiosensitive tumour such as breast cancer. Equally, in chemotherapy-sensitive tumours such as lymphoma and the haematological malignancies, drugs may be superior to radiotherapy. Cardiac injury resulting from radiation or chemotherapy is a well recognized complication. Adriamycin (doxorubicin) in particular is associated with cardiomyopathy.

Spinal cord compression

This is one of the most devastating complications of cancer. Palliation for this complication is of paramount importance for survival is frequently prolonged and the paralytic effects of cord compression can be an overwhelming ordeal for both the patient and the family. Nursing care, physical therapy, rehabilitation and psychosocial attention are all part of the expanded health care needs of patients with residual neurological damage from spinal cord compression. The two critical determinants of succesful palliation are early clinical recognition of the syndrome and maximum combined modality therapy once the syndrome is diagnosed. The most common tumours with which spinal cord compression develops are lung and breast cancers, because of the high general incidence of these tumours. Prostatic cancer, renal cell carcinoma, lymphoma, myeloma and sarcoma are the next most frequent tumours in sequence. The incidence of spinal cord compression is increasing and the clinical consequences are devastating so that it represents a major clinical problem. Anatomically the two types of spinal cord compression are (Figure 24.3):

1. Extradural compression.
2. Intramedullary compression from metastases within the spinal cord proper.

The mechanism of tumour implantation is generally through haematogenous metastases, first to the vertebral body, from which point the tumour moves out to compress the dura, compressing the cord directly. Therefore, over 80% of patients with spinal cord compression from the extramedullary or extradural mechanism will have radiographic changes seen either with straight radiographs or nuclear scans. The second pathogenetic mechanism of spinal cord compression is retroneural growth from paraspinal areas through the intervertebral foramina with the development of secondary compression by direct impingement on the cord. In this instance, the tumour grows from the retroperitoneal or retrothoracic space in continuity with the paraspinal musculature, and along the nerves emanating from the spinal canal.

The primary symptom associated with spinal cord compression is pain which may develop as a preclinical symptom in up to 90% of patients. This pain may be insidious and is most often attributed to a low back pain syndrome or in patients with known bony lesions, a simple bone involvement with tumour. Paresis and paralysis evolve in sequence in the lower extremities. Sensory loss in the extremities develops after motor weakness; the last neurological insult is autonomic dysfunction with bladder and bowel incontinence.

Acute spinal cord compression occurs most typically in trauma with secondary haematoma of the cord or vertebral fracture and direct tumour compression. The development of acute spinal cord compression generally indicates a compromise in the arterial supply to the cord with secondary cord

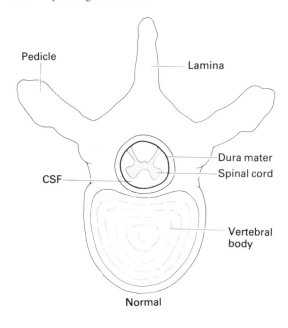

Normal

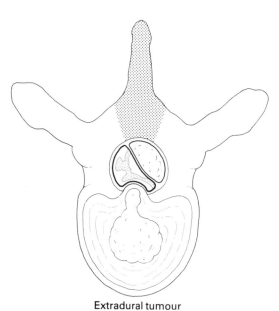

Extradural tumour

Figure 24.3 (*a*) Normal spinal cord and vertebral body; (*b*) Extradural spinal cord compression from metastases

infarction. If this develops, the prognosis is ominous. Alternatively, in rapidly growing tumours the clinical syndrome may appear over a short interval without vascular infarction.

Motor, sensory and sphincter symptoms may be observed independently without evolving in a chronological sequence. Autonomic dysfunction occurs most commonly with lesions below the third lumbar vertebra where the spinal cord ends.

When spinal cord compression occurs, the primary tumour is generally known. Multiple myeloma is the most common cause of spinal cord compression from an unrecognized primary tumour. Decompression laminectomy is contraindicated in this disease. Myelography is indicated in all patients with back pain and malignancy, even in the absence of neurological signs, and especially if bone lesions are undetected. Two primary tumour types associated with long survival after spinal cord compression are the soft tissue sarcomas and renal cell carcinoma. These tumours are often characterized by local growth and solitary metastasis. Renal cell carcinoma is almost invariably associated with bone lesions. Both these types of tumours are notoriously resistant to both radiation and systemic therapy and therefore surgical intervention is necessary as a primary approach. Prolonged survival in such patients necessitates early diagnosis because of the devastating effects of paraplegia.

The attitude towards spinal cord compression secondary to metastatic carcinoma is often nihilistic, particularly when considering surgery. Such a generalization is not tenable without a consideration of the total clinical picture. The traditional role for determining surgical intervention was based on the density and duration of the neurological deficit. The quantitative deficit, however, is only one component in the determination of therapy; other considerations include the primary tumour source, whether the tumour is radiosensitive or chemosensitive, extent of the tumour, and the presence of other morbid disease.

Surgical decompression is the first line of treatment for most tumours. This is accomplished by laminectomy or removal of the bony structures that encompass the cord posteriorly. This allows expansion of the oedematous cord, thus relieving the pressure on the nerves. In addition, the tumour mass may be wholly or partially excised. Often, laminectomy of multiple, contiguous vertebrae is necessary. Clips should be placed at the extreme ends of the laminectomy site to guide postoperative radiotherapy. Radiation is the treatment of choice for spinal cord compression secondary to radiosensitive tumours such as multiple myeloma and lymphoma. In these patients, laminectomy may be contraindicated as the tumour responds so rapidly and often completely to radiotherapy. Postoperative radiotherapy is always applied independent of the primary tumour source. Corticosteroids are used routinely as a prophylactic measure in patients receiving radiotherapy, although the necessity for these drugs has not been established in a controlled study. There is little evidence that systemic or intrathecal chemotherapy has any place in the management of spinal cord compression. It should be used to control systemic disease if the tumour is chemosensitive.

In summary, spinal cord compression is always reversible if detected prior to irreversible neurological changes. The improvement of occasional patients even in the presence of dense neurological deficits means that surgery should almost always be attempted. Contraindications are the disease type and the development of cord infarction from compression of the anterior spinal artery, but this is very rarely possible to diagnose clinically.

Hypercalcaemia of malignancy

Hypercalcaemia is frequent in cancer patients. It can occur at any point in the course of the disease and may be the first clue to the presence of cancer. It may not be clinically evident, but conversely, it can be the most debilitating aspect of the disease. Hypercalcaemia developing in association with malignancy may be directly related to the tumour due to the secretion of parathormone or to osseous metastases. It may, however, be unrelated to the malignancy and be due to another disease, e.g. primary hyperparathyroidism. Whatever the mechanism, hypercalcaemia may develop in as many as 10% of patients with advanced malignancy.

Hypercalcaemia, whether due to benign or malignant disease, can produce a number of different signs and symptoms. Anorexia, nausea, vomiting and constipation as well as vague abdominal pain can all occur. It must be remembered that hypercalcaemia is associated with an increased incidence of peptic ulcer. Polyuria, polydipsia and dehydration can also occur. The central nervous system manifestations include apathy, weakness, personality change and headaches.

The majority, i.e. over 90%, of patients with hypercalcaemia have bone metastases. As the bone is destroyed, calcium is released into the blood at a rate that exceeds maximal renal clearance.

Primary hyperparathyroidism, vitamin D intoxication, hypophosphatasia, Addison's disease, sarcoidosis, milk-alkali syndrome and immobilization must all be considered when hypercalcaemia is discovered.

Of the various treatment options for hypercalcaemia, the one most frequently used initially is to promote calcium excretion. This is accomplished by an infusion of large quantities of intravenous fluids containing sodium. Diuretics may be added to increase the rate of calcium excretion. However, thiazides are contraindicated because they can retard urinary excretion of calcium and aggravate the hypercalcaemia. Patients with diminshed cardiac or renal function will not tolerate aggressive chemotherapy with mithramycin C. In addition, patients undergoing this type of therapy are prone to losses of other electrolytes such as potassium and magnesium. Therefore, the serum levels of these electrolytes must be carefully monitored and appropriate replacements given. The adminstration of inorganic phosphate provides a rapid and dose-dependent decrease in serum calcium by promoting precipitation and deposition of calcium into bones. Phosphate therapy can be given intravenously, orally or rectally. Intravenous phosphate is reserved for acute hypercalcaemia and has now been superseded by agents such as mithramycin. However, oral phosphate is still useful for chronic outpatient therapy. Mithramycin was developed as a cytotoxic agent that has particular activity against certain testicular carcinomas, but was found directly to affect the skeleton where it inhibits bone resorption. Because of the site of action, the drug is useful in all cases of hypercalcaemia of cancer, regardless of the mechanism of the high serum calcium. Prostaglandin-blocking agents such as indomethacin and aspirin should not be used for patients with hypercalcaemia secondary to bone metastases, but should be used only when a hormone mediator is suspected.

Specific oncological operations and the insertion of central venous cannulae

Axillary block dissection

An incision within the axilla will give good exposure and excellent cosmetic results. The best exposure is probably gained by incision close behind and parallel to the pectoralis major muscle. The pectoralis minor muscle should be divided in its tendinous portion at the coracoid process. Dissection takes place above the course of the thoracodorsal nerve to the pectoralis major anteriorly, latissimus dorsi posteriorly and the axillary vein superiorly. All subcutaneous fat and lymphatic tissue up to the apex of the axilla is removed. Care must be taken to observe and preserve the long thoracic and thoracodorsal nerves if they are not involved with tumour. Suction catheters are used to close the dead space and remove lymphatic effusions. These catheters should be sutured in securely. Postoperative complications include the formation of a lymphocoele following removal of drains, lymphoedema of the arm, and nerve damage as detailed above.

Inguinal lymph node dissection

Inguinal block dissection can either be superficial which includes all the contents of the femoral triangle and lymphatic tissue below the inguinal ligament, or radical which encompasses the iliac and obturator nodes as well. A superficial inguinal block dissection removes the contents of the femoral triangle bordered by the sartorious muscle laterally, the adductor magnus muscle medially and the inguinal ligament superiorly. The long saphenous vein is divided at the apex of the femoral triangle and all the tissue including the deep fascia removed. The long saphenous vein is then ligated at its entry into the femoral vein. The tissue lying on the inguinal ligament is excised in continuity, and the lymphatics ligated in the femoral canal to lessen the chance of a lymphocoele forming. It is policy if the skin flaps are thin to excise the skin edges as their blood supply would be tenuous. Because of the potential contamination of the skin in this area, the origin of the sartorius can be divided and the muscle transposed to cover and protect the femoral vessels. Large suction drains should be inserted prior to skin closure.

Radical block dissection of the groin incorporates a retroperitoneal dissection above the inguinal ligament clearing the iliac vessels from the femoral canal to the bifurcation of the common iliacs. The peritoneum is peeled away medially and upwards. Lymphatic tissue which surrounds the external iliac vessels is dissected off while the obturator nodes are removed in continuity from the obturator fossa and by clearing the obturator nerve. A drain is not usually needed as the peritoneum and its contents obliterate the space. The femoral canal should be closed as for a femoral hernia repair.

Lymphoedema can occur in some patients following lymphatic clearance and can become a debilitating complication. Patients who develop lymphoedema may have had hypoplasia of the lymphatic channels preoperatively. It can lead to functional disability, skin ulceration, lymphangitis and verruca formation. The treatment of lymphoedema includes gravitational drainage, elastic support, intermittent compression and very occasionally surgery.

Central venous access

The advent of effective but sclerosant chemotherapy for certain tumours has given rise to problems of venous access when repeated courses of treatment are necessary. Inadequate peripheral veins due to thrombosis or sclerosis have made it necessary to use venous access catheters, usually located proximally in either the superior or inferior venae cavae, and with an externally situated injection port. These require great care by the patients and nursing staff in order to minimize the risk of damage or infection.

In 1973, Broviac introduced a cuffed Silastic catheter for parenteral hyperalimentation. The Hickman catheter then became the popular choice for bone marrow transplantation, prolonged in-

travenous feeding and for chemotherapy. The development of double-lumen and triple-lumen catheters has superseded the Hickman catheter when there is a need for giving chemotherapy and parenteral nutrition simultaneously.

Initially, catheters were placed in either the subclavian or internal jugular vein using a percutaneous approach. However, it has been shown that catheter insertion is probably safer using a cutdown technique and the complications are very much less. Catheter-related sepsis remains one of the most serious complications and may be reduced by employing strict aseptic techniques in insertion and management of the line with the use of catheter tunnelling and by ensuring the clinician is experienced in the insertion of these catheters.

The catheter can be inserted into the cephalic, external or internal jugular veins (Figure 24.4). The

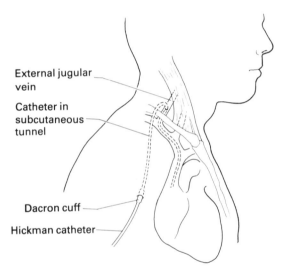

External jugular vein

Catheter in subcutaneous tunnel

Dacron cuff

Hickman catheter

Figure 24.4 Position of central venous catheter

extravascular part of the catheter is placed in a subcutaneous tunnel and the Dacron cuff should be placed halfway along the tunnel to act as an effective bacterial barrier. In every case, the catheter position must be checked and this is most easily performed using an image intensifier in the theatre. Ideally the tip of the catheter should be in the superior vena cava, just above the right atrium. If the Dacron cuff is placed just within the mouth of the subcutaneous tunnel, it seals the incision and soon becomes fixed. Subsequently, it is more easily extracted at the end of treatment by either simple traction or minimal dissection, whereas a cuff placed halfway along the tunnel will require incision and freeing.

A more recent development has been to use totally implantable systems with subcutaneously located injection reservoirs which are entered using a right-angled needle. The cannula is placed either into the external or internal jugular vein and the port, or chamber, is usually sited on the anterior chest wall.

Apart from the careful care of external catheters, especially the principles of 'junctional care', both externally placed catheters and implantable systems will need heparinization at regular intervals. The care of these catheters should be in the hands of experienced chemotherapy nurses or a nutritional team if that exists in the hospital.

Tumour of unknown origin

Primary cancer of unknown origin constitutes a substantial number of cases seen at referral centres. Most therapeutic decisions are based on the precise definition of the tissue of origin of the primary tumour. The problem is therefore important in clinical management.

The primary lesion may be too small to be capable of detection by routine clinical means; may be located in occult sites such as the retroperitoneum; or have undergone spontaneous regression becoming impossible to identify (e.g. malignant melanoma).

The diagnosis of a tumour of unknown origin is contingent on histopathological confirmation of malignancy and the exclusion of a primary tumour of that site. Therapy is determined primarily by considerations of the tumour most sensitive to treatment and secondarily by the most likely site of origin. Further biopsies to obtain the histopathological diagnosis or more sophisticated examinations such as electron microscopy may be necessary. Lymphoma is the most treatable 'undifferentiated' tumour, and may be definitively identified pathologically by T or B cell characteristics.

Tumour markers may be helpful, such as acid phosphatase for carcinoma of the prostate, parathormone levels if an oat cell carcinoma is suspected, as well as alpha-fetoprotein (AFP), carcinoma embryonic antigen (CEA) and human gonadotrophin (HCG).

Pulmonary lesions in the patient without previous cancer should undergo thoracotomy only after ascertaining that other sites of metastases do not exist. Bone lesions should be evaluated by establishing the number of lesions, taking a biopsy of the most accessible lesion and focusing on treatable tumours. Breast cancer can be occult, is a common tumour affecting bones or bone marrow, and is the most sensitive to treatment.

The patient presenting with a tumour of unknown origin may be subject to an extensive diagnostic search for the primary. While the diagnostic evaluation may overlap into a staging work-up, this is unwarranted and often unnecessary. One must first establish the histological diagnosis of malignancy which can be evaluated with special pathological studies. Then, one should assume that the primary tumour is maximally treatable, e.g. lymphoma if undifferentiated and adenocarcinoma of breast and ovary in women, and prostate in men. One should not over-investigate the patient.

Summary

Cancer treatment involves diagnostic and therapeutic decision-making that bridges many subspecialities of medicine. Palliation of secondary symptoms is often possible, and this may lead to an improved quality of life as well as prolonged survival. Combined modality therapies for patients with primary or regional disease, for whom the prognosis is limited, or the statistical likelihood of recurrence is high, has opened up new possibilities. The thrust of such treatments is the promotion of cure, or at the very least an alteration of the natural course of the disease. In patients with advanced cancer, the therapeutic goal is palliation and the choice and timing of therapy may prove difficult decisions. One must always remember that effective treatment must not simply prolong life, but also improve the quality of life.

25

Vascular disease

M. Horrocks

Diseases of the peripheral vascular system present with pain, swelling, ulceration or gangrene more commonly affecting the lower limb than the upper limb. This may be attributable to the three main systems – arterial, venous or lymphatic. Each system is dealt with below.

Arterial

Although disease of the arterial system is less common than disease of the venous system, it nevertheless accounts for more limb- and life-threatening conditions and may be conveniently divided into three areas: trauma, aneurysmal disease and occlusive disease.

Trauma

Peripheral arteries may be injured by either closed or open trauma and such injuries are being increasingly seen in areas of urban violence.

Closed injuries

These include pressure, e.g. too tight a tourniquet for too long, damage to the artery at the time of fracture, e.g. supracondylar fracture of the femur or humerus with a bone spicule causing damage directly to the artery wall.

Open injuries

Arteries may be damaged as part of a fracture from a knife or gunshot wound or accidentally during major surgery. Different types of injury are recognized which may give rise to different symptoms.

Spasm

This is a reversible narrowing of an artery caused by damage to the wall but reversible within a short time. Spasm is a dangerous diagnosis to make as in the early stages it may be indistinguishable from thrombosis. A diagnosis should only be made with caution and with good evidence, e.g. arteriographic appearance.

Thrombosis

This is a direct consequence of trauma to the artery and usually follows endothelial disruption. Very often at operation the outside of the artery may look normal or slightly narrowed at the site of injury.

Division of an artery

This may be complete or incomplete. Incomplete division may produce profound haemorrhage with fresh bleeding or massive haematoma. Complete division, particularly when caused by blunt trauma, often bleeds surprisingly little because the proximal vessel will occlude and thrombose in response to the injury.

Aneurysm

This may be true or false. True aneurysms are uncommon after trauma and occur many months or years after the injury because of weakness to the arterial wall. False aneurysms are more common and these develop secondary to a complete division of the artery.

Arteriovenous fistulae

These occur after open arterial injury when an abnormal communication is made between adjacent artery and vein and this matures into a permanent fistula.

Clinical features of arterial damage

In the event of an artery being damaged to the extent that thrombosis occurs, the features of acute ischaemia will ensue. These are the four 'P's: pain, pallor, pulselessness and paralysis. In the event of these symptoms time is very short to sort the problem out and irreversible ischaemia will ensue within 3–4 h of the injury. It is essential in this situation that the patient be investigated and treated as quickly as possible.

In the event of an open injury causing haemorrhage, the diagnosis is self-evident. The haemorrhage will be easy to control by direct pressure but symptoms of distal ischaemia must also be looked for and recognized quickly.

Aneurysm formation can occur any time following arterial injury – false aneurysms usually present in the first day or two following injury and present as a pulsatile mass at the site of injury. True aneurysms, however, may develop many months or years after the injury and should be investigated as outlined below.

Arteriovenous fistulae are relatively uncommon consequences of trauma and present either with local mechanical problems, a loud machinery murmur or the consequences of a high shunt, e.g. high output cardiac failure.

Investigation of vascular trauma

In addition to careful clinical examination, a simple Doppler velocimeter is helpful in diagnosing arterial injuries. The systolic pressure distal to the site of injury compared with systemic systolic pressure gives a good index of tissue perfusion distal to a suspected injury site. In normal healthy people with no evidence of chronic arterial disease the two pressures should be similar. Any significant reduction in perfusion pressure to an injured limb suggests an arterial injury and further investigation such as duplex scanning or angiography are indicated.

Duplex scanning is helpful particularly in the diagnosis of false aneurysm or narrowing of the vessel due to tissue distortion. Duplex scanners are becoming increasingly available but in the presence of acute ischaemia it is probably wise to proceed directly to an arteriogram. Arteriography is the principal technique for investigating arterial injuries (Figure 25.1). The technique can be performed under local anaesthetic and a catheter introduced

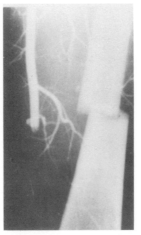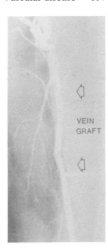

Figure 25.1 Arteriogram (Left) showing interruption of arterial flow beside a fracture; (Right) its restoration by a vein graft

via the femoral artery into the suspect area of trauma. It should be remembered in a case of crush injuries that the artery may be damaged in more than one place and care should be taken to see that the run-off is properly visualized before proceeding to surgery.

Treatment

There is really no place for conservative management of vascular trauma once the diagnosis is made. Bleeding should be controlled by local pressure as soon as possible and obvious bleeding wounds should be explored expeditiously and primary arterial repair carried out. In the presence of division of the artery, emergency arterial repair is indicated as soon as the diagnosis is made.

Principles of repair

Prior to exploring a damaged major artery, proximal control should be gained as soon as possible with a sling passed around the feeding artery. The area of damage should be carefully exposed so that 2 cm distally and proximally of the normal vessel are seen (Figures 25.2, 25.3 and 25.4). the patient should be systemically heparinized as soon as contol is achieved to prevent retrograde or pregrade intravascular thrombosis; 5000 units of heparin intravenously is sufficient for most situations.

In the presence of complex vascular injuries, temporary restoration of circulation can be achieved by the insertion of intravascular shunts into the proximal and distal ends of the artery. Simple Silastic catheters with heparinized blood are quite sufficient to preserve circulation for 1–2 h while complex repairs are undertaken. It should be remembered that damaged veins should also be

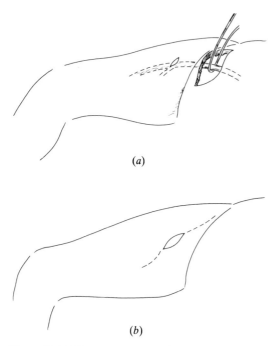

Figure 25.2 (*a*) Temporary contol of external iliac artery before exploring a stab wound of the groin. (*b*) The stab wound is extended along the line of the femoral artery before attempting to expose the lesion

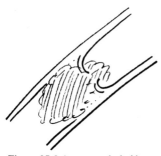

Figure 25.3 Artery occluded by contusion: curled up inner coat and platelet thrombus require surgical removal

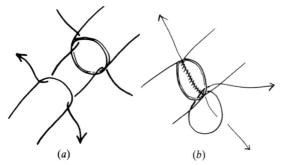

Figure 25.4 (*a*) End-to-end anastomosis – slinging sutures. (*b*) Continuous suture. For posterior layer either rotate the anastomosis or suture from within the lumen

repaired using a similar technique. It is often helpful to place the distal part of the limb into a transparent polythene bag following preparation so that the distal circulation can be assessed during the operative procedure.

Once the vessel has been opened then thrombus should be removed and the ends of the artery freshened up back to normal wall. Sometimes it is possible to do a primary repair of the artery at this stage but more usually a segment of interposition vein graft is required to obtain adequate length. Vein is better harvested from an unaffected limb and the long saphenous vein from the thigh is an ideal conduit in most cases. Completion angiography should be performed where there is any doubt as to functional result of the repair and the circulation can be checked using clinical examination, i.e. the return of pulses, simple Doppler pressure or an intraoperative flow meter. It is essential that the return of circulation is confirmed before the wound is closed.

Postoperative management

It is advisable to give antibiotics for 48 h following these repairs and low-dose heparin in the form of 5000 units subcutaneously twice daily for 5 days to prevent rethrombosis at the site of injury. If, however, there is extensive soft tissue damage with haematoma, heparin may be contraindicated.

Aneurysms

An aneurysm can be defined as an enlargement of an artery of more than twice the expected size and the following types are recognized:

1. A true aneurysm is where the wall of the artery itself becomes weakened and pressure from within causes an expansion of the wall with concomitant enlargement in the lumen.
2. A fusiform aneurysm is a true aneurysm in which there is diffuse dilatation of the artery and the abdominal aortic aneurysm would be a typical example of this type.
3. A saccular aneurysm is where only one wall of the artery becomes dilated and frequently the aneurysm communicates with the lumen of the artery by a small neck.
4. A dissecting aneurysm is where there has been a breach in the intima of the artery with blood dissecting into the wall of the vessel to produce a second channel. This may either rupture back into the artery lumen or may rupture externally with catastrophic results.
5. An arteriovenous aneurysm is where there is abnormal communication between an artery and a vein through a dilated channel.

6. A false aneurysm is following the seepage of blood through a damaged wall producing a cavity which contains blood and is lined by a clot and fibrous tissue and supported by the surrounding structures.

Aetiology of aneurysms

Congenital aneurysms are relatively uncommon in the peripheral arterial tree and the most common example is a berry aneurysm which occurs intra-cranially in the Circle of Willis.

Traumatic aneurysms follow damage by penetrating wound, often in association with a fracture. These may present many months or years after the injury and may present with symptoms of pressure.

Inflammatory or mycotic aneurysms may be seen following a subacute bacterial endocarditis or even as a manifestation of tertiary syphilis. More common now are inflammatory aneurysms secondary to intravenous drug abuse and many of these patients may have HIV or hepatitis infection.

Atherosclerotic aneurysms are by far the most common and account for the vast majority of peripheral vascular aneurysms. The commonest site is the abdominal aorta distal to the renal arteries, but more extensive thoraco-abdominal aneurysms are increasingly seen and other common sites are the femoral artery, the popliteal artery and internal iliac artery.

Clinical features

Many aneurysms present because of their size and pulsatile expansile nature or with one of the many complications. Abdominal aortic aneurysms, because of their site, are less difficult to detect clinically and only about 50% of patients presenting with abdominal aortic aneurysms have an easily palpable expansile mass. Abdominal aortic aneurysms have been found in approximately 2% of the elderly population in the western world and this incidence appears to be steadily increasing. The rate of discovery of aneurysms is more rapidly increasing because of chance findings during physical examination, radiographs or ultrasonic examination. Aneurysms of the abdominal aorta are not only the most common site for atherosclerotic aneurysm formation but also the most dangerous, with a high risk of rupture.

Clinical presentation of aortic aneurysms

Most abdominal aortic aneurysms are asymptomatic, being found on routine physical examination, plain radiograph performed for other reasons or discovered by the patient himself.

In a significant proportion the first symptom is that of leakage which can vary from catastrophic intraperitoneal leakage with rapid death to a warning pain, often in the back or lower abdomen, leading to urgent admission to hospital. More than 50% of ruptured abdominal aortic aneurysms die before admission to hospital is possible. Of those that survive to reach hospital, immediate surgery is mandatory.

Other presenting features

Of patients with expanding abdominal aortic aneurysms 10–20% will have quite severe back pain and may well present to other departments. It is not uncommon for such patients to have a history of persistent backache or loin pain which may be misdiagnosed as renal colic. Occasionally the thrombus material within the aneurysm may dislodge and embolize down in the leg presenting as acute leg ischaemia. Ureteral obstruction is an uncommon complication of aortic aneurysms, usually caused by direct pressure from the expanding wall or compression of the ureter by periaortic scarring in the so-called 'inflammatory' aneurysms.

Diagnosis

In patients of normal build aneurysms can usually be palpated but this becomes increasingly difficult with obese patients. It should be remembered that the aortic bifurcation lies at the level of the umbilicus and that the aneurysmal mass lies at or above the navel in the epigastrium. The lateral borders of the aneurysm can be felt to converge in the epigastrium so that if the upper border of the aneurysm is felt then almost certainly the aneurysm will be infra-renal. In those patients in whom the aneurysm obviously extends under the rib cage, the possibility of suprarenal extension should be considered. Further radiological evidence of size and situation should be confirmed before proceeding to surgery.

Plain radiograph

Although many aneurysms contain mural calcification which will show up on a plain radiograph, some 60% of aneurysms will not be visualized by such technique. Ultrasound (Figure 25.5) remains the simplest and easiest way to confirm the diagnosis, being both sensitive and specific. The presence of a large amount of bowel gas at the upper end of the aneurysm may not be visualized and no information is obtained about run-off. Computed tomography (CT) (Figure 25.6) and magnetic resonance imaging (MRI) have been advocated in the assessment of abdominal aortic aneurysms; both techniques give good information about the site and size of aneurysms, MRI giving more information about intravascular flow and assessment of the upper end. MRI appears to be more sensitive and

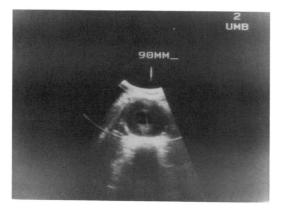

Figure 25.5 Ultrasound scan of abdominal aneurysm

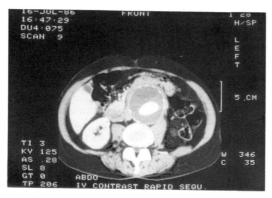

Figure 25.6 CT scan of aneurysm (with intravenous contrast)

specific for diagnosing the inflammatory version where the wall is often thickened and may involve the surrounding structures, e.g. ureter, duodenum and inferior vena cava. Many surgeons make routine use of angiography to assess aortic aneurysms although in many cases little additional information is obtained. It may be helpful to have an angiogram when the extent of the aneurysm is uncertain or when information about accessory renal vessels is very helpful. In those patients who also have occlusive disease with symptoms of claudication, an angiogram is essential to delineate the run-off and to allow planning of reconstructive surgery. Angiography for aneurysms should be done with great caution, with the catheter being introduced from some distal site in the arterial tree, e.g. the femoral artery, and care should be taken not to disrupt clot from the lumen of the aneurysm.

Treatment of abdominal aortic aneurysm

The decision to operate on an aortic aneurysm depends on the balance of the risk of the procedure against the risk of the natural history. The risk of rupture increases with the size, 6 cm aortic aneurysms having a 30% chance of rupture at 5 years. However, it is well known that aneurysms even smaller than 4 cm rupture and in younger fitter patients it can be justified to operate on aneurysms greater than this size. The risk of survival once ruptured varies enormously from hospital to hospital but is approximately 50%, being worst in those patients who have a free intraperitoneal haemorrhage. Overall risks of elective aneurysm surgery are approximately 5% mortality, with some specialized centres claiming figures as low as 2% mortality. Factors such as coexistent cardiac disease, decreased renal function and chronic obstructive airways disease tend to give a poorer chance of survival. Somewhat surprisingly, chronological age does not appear to be a risk factor for either elective or ruptured aneurysms up to the age of 85 years.

Operative technique

Choice of approach varies between a long midline incision or a transverse incision to go transperitoneally, or a left oblique abdominal incision and a retroperitoneal approach. The extent of the aneurysm should be assessed but care should be taken not to manipulate or disturb the aneurysm so as to prevent embolization of atherosclerotic material into the legs. The neck of the aneurysm should be exposed from the front by identifying the left renal vein and then dissecting behind it. It is not usually necessary to go round the neck of the aneurysm but just to define enough room on either side of the neck to place a clamp from the front. Similarly the iliac vessels, both external and internal, can be identified in the pelvis from a lateral approach but it is not necessary to dissect these vessels out thus reducing the risk of damaging the iliac veins. Once the vessels above and below the aneurysm have been dissected the patient can be heparinized systemically (approximately 4000 units is quite sufficient) and the aneurysm may be opened. Any lumbar vessels which are back-bleeding may be oversewn with an absorbable suture and the graft is then inlaid into the aneurysm as shown. It is rarely necessary to re-implant the inferior mesenteric artery but this can be done using a patch technique if the left colon appears ischaemic.

Following suturing of the graft, blood can be allowed initially down the internal iliac arteries before the external iliac arteries are released thus preventing atheroemboli and trash foot. Following successful revascularization of both legs the graft should be covered with the remains of the aneurysm sac. It is important to have full cooperation of the anaesthetist at the time of declamping so that the clamps are taken off the distal vessel slowly and any concurrent hypotension can be managed.

Ruptured aortic aneurysm

In a patient presenting with acute abdominal pain, if a diagnosis of ruptured aortic aneurysm is made the patient should be transferred to the operating theatre. There is rarely any benefit to be gained from any radiological investigation and in the vast majority of cases the diagnosis is obvious once it is thought of. The best place to resuscitate the patient is on the operating table rather than in the anaesthetic room. Patients should be wheeled into the operating theatre and placed on the operating table fully conscious, and while the anaesthetist is putting in venous and arterial lines the patient can be catheterized and prepared for surgery. The abdomen should be cleaned with warm chlorhexidine and spirit and draped leaving good access to both groins. Only once the patient is ready for the operation should the anaesthesia be induced. The surgeon should then proceed to repair the aneurysm without undue haste unless a free rupture has occurred. It is important in dissecting out the neck of the aneurysm not to damage any concomitant veins as venous bleeding in this situation is usually followed by death. In patients where the aneurysm cannot be controlled easily it is often possible to pass a balloon catheter into the aneurysm and up into the suprarenal aorta and stop haemorrhage by inflating the balloon. Once this is done the neck of the aneurysm can then be identified and a clamp placed in the appropriate place.

Successful outcome of surgery for ruptured aortic aneurysm depends on the general condition of the patient on arrival at the hospital, speed of diagnosis and the care and precision with which the patient is dealt with by both anaesthetist and surgeon. Once proximal control has been obtained, distal control can be achieved by opening the aneurysm and passing balloons from inside down the iliac arteries.

Popliteal aneurysms

It is estimated that over 90% of peripheral aneurysms occur in either the femoral or popliteal artery, the large majority being asymptomatic. By far the commonest cause is atherosclerosis although mycotic and anastomotic aneurysms are well described, particularly in the groin. There is a well known association between these distal aneurysms and abdominal aneurysms and approximately 25% of patients with popliteal aneurysms also have an abdominal aortic aneurysm. These more distal aneurysms tend to occur in the older age group and many of these patients exhibit other manifestations.

Hypertension, myocardial disease and peripheral vascular disease

Approximately 50% of popliteal aneurysms present as asymptomatic swellings behind the knee, often noted on routine examination. The most common complication is thrombotic, giving rise to thrombosis or emboli and consequent ischaemia of the lower limb. Sudden thrombosis of the aneurysm may give rise to acute ischaemia with a high risk of loss of limb. Popliteal aneurysms may rarely rupture. Diagnosis is made on the basis of careful clinical examination; if patent the aneurysm is felt as an expansile pulsatile mass in the popliteal fossa but following thrombosis all that will be felt will be a non-pulsatile mass. It is often easy to feel the popliteal aneurysm with the knee bent to 45°. Both ultrasound and CT scanning have been shown to be useful in the diagnosis of popliteal aneurysm but arteriography remains the investigation of choice. This not only shows the extent of the aneurysm but also the state of the run-off vessels before subsequent repair.

Treatment is best achieved by interposition graft with autologous vein being the conduit of choice when available. PTFE or Dacron interposition graft can also be employed but long-term results appear to be inferior.

The popliteal aneurysm can be approached either from the medial side or from the posterior aspect, the medial approach having the advantage of further exposure above and below the aneurysm and the ability to harvest as much vein as required. Operative angiography or intraoperative flow measurements should be taken to confirm patency and good functional result.

Femoral aneurysms

Femoral aneurysms have a similar natural history to popliteal aneurysms in that they tend to develop the complications of rupture, thrombosis and embolization. Diagnosis tends to be much more simple and treatment is by primary repair either with vein or with interposition Dacron. Anastomotic aneurysms in the groin can be approached in a similar way provided they are not infected, when an interposition of a further piece of Dacron graft is usually essential to prevent undue tension on the anastomosis.

Aneurysm at other sites, e.g. subclavian artery, brachial artery and carotid artery, should be treated along similar lines. In the case of cartoid artery aneurysms a temporary inlay shunt should be used to preserve cerebral circulation. In general smaller aneurysms are better treated by autologous vein interposition grafting rather than by repair with Dacron or PTFE.

Chronic ischaemia

This is defined as a slow progressive deterioration in arterial blood supply to a limb with concomitant loss of function. In the leg this may present initially as intermittent claudication which progresses to rest pain or frank gangrene. The commonest site of occlusive disease in the leg is in the femoropopliteal segment giving rise to calf muscle claudication. Patients with aortoiliac disease tend on the whole to be slightly younger and have more severe disease and their symptoms affect the whole leg.

Differential diagnosis

Approximately 15% of patients presenting with pain on walking relieved by rest have their symptoms due to another cause. The commonest causes are lumbosacral root irritation, arthritis of the hip or chronic venous insufficiency. In patients with true claudication their distal pulses should be diminshed or absent and the foot should become pale and pulseless after exercise.

In severe ischaemia with rest pain there may be muscle wastage with atrophic toes and thick coarse nails. The whole foot may show marked colour change on elevation and there may be pressure sores or ulcers on the toes.

Causes of chronic ischaemia

The vast majority of cases of chronic ischaemia are due to atherosclerosis of either the femoropopliteal or aortoiliac segment. Emboli from the heart or the abdominal aorta can give rise to chronic ischaemia and this may be complicated by thrombosis of the adjacent vessel. Buerger's disease is an uncommon condition affecting the small arteries in the hands and feet of young men who are heavy smokers.

Clinical examination

Careful examination should demonstrate the presence or absence of peripheral pulses throughout the body. The palpation of distal pulses in patients who are obese or have oedema can be extremely unrewarding and non-invasive studies are necessary.

Doppler ankle pressures

Using a simple Doppler velocimeter and a sphygmomanometer it is possible to assess the degree of vascularity of a limb. The ankle systolic pressure index is ankle pressure divided by the brachial pressure and is useful taken before and after exercise. In normal people the ankle pressure is the same as or greater than the brachial pressure before exercise and this ratio improves with walking. In patients with true intermittent claudication the resting ankle–brachial index will be low and this will fall further after exercise, taking several minutes to return to normal. The depth to which the ratio falls and the length of time of recovery are good indices of the severity of the disease and of the collateral circulation.

Duplex scanning

Duplex scanning is increasingly used to assess aortoiliac and femoropopliteal segments and with care and enthusiasm practically the whole of the peripheral arterial tree can be insonated and good images of the vessels obtained (Figure 25.7).

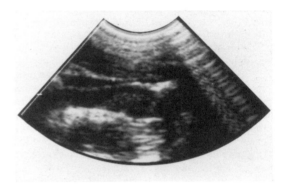

Figure 25.7 Duplex scanning of femoropopliteal segment

Arteriography

Arteriography remains the investigation of choice for deciding on treatment options once the decision to treat has been made. Angiography will not assess the severity of the disease and only gives an outline of which part of the arterial tree is active, thus enabling decision as to which treatment option is most appropriate.

Arteriography is best done using the Seldinger technique by introducing a catheter into the groin (Figure 25.8). The catheter is then passed up into the abdominal aorta so that good visualization of all vessels can be obtained. Intra-arterial digital subtraction angiography gives the most accurate information, particularly about run-off, but even this may underestimate the disease when the circulation is very poor (Figure 25.9).

Treatment

Most cases of intermittent claudication should be treated conservatively. The natural history of claudication is that two-thirds of the patients will

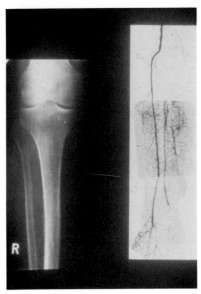

Figure 25.8 Arteriogram of femoropopliteal artery

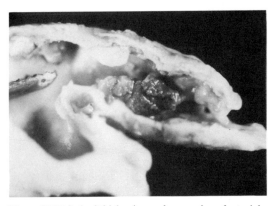

Figure 25.9 Marked thickening and narrowing of arterial wall, with clot formation

stay much the same or improve and only 20% of the claudicants will go on to develop rest pain or gangrene which will require surgical treatment. The mainstay of conservative treatment is to stop the patient smoking, encourage them to take exercise as much as possible and to keep their weight down. Attention should be drawn to any cases of hyperlipidaemia and any diabetics should be well controlled.

In those patients with worsening disease or who have onset of rest pain or gangrene, interventional treatment is indicated.

Angioplasty

Angioplasty is taking an increasing role in the management of patients with occlusive arterial disease (Figure 25.10). It is now possible to dilate occlusions of the iliac artery up to 5 cm in length and occlusions of the superficial femoral artery up to 15 cm in length by the passage of an angioplasty balloon. The role of laser and atherectomy devices has yet to be fully defined but enthusiastic groups have reported good results. Via the femoral artery it is possible to dilate the majority of isolated iliac and superficial femoral artery lesions with results similar to those of bypass surgery. In cases where angioplasty is not indicated or has failed, surgical treatment may be required. In certain areas of localized disease such as the carotid bifurcation, endarterectomy (which is removal of the atheromatous plaque) is possible with primary closure of the outer part of the remaining arterial wall. In those cases where there is more extensive occlusive disease, bypass surgery using Dacron or vein is the treatment of choice. It may be possible to revascularize the limb by extra-anatomical means such as an axillobifemoral or femorofemoral cross-over graft.

Lumbar sympathectomy has a fairly limited place in the management of chronic ischaemia. Increasingly the sympathectomy is done by a lumbar paravertebral block using an image intensifier to localize the tip of the injection needle. Lignocaine is infiltrated along the needle track and, provided there is warming of the affected lower limb and the needle is thought to be in the correct place, 5–10 ml of 5% phenol may be injected. This technique is often best done by experts in pain relief as severe complications can arise if the phenol in injected in the wrong place.

Sympathectomy tends to be used to relieve rest pain or aid the healing of skin ulcers in those patients who are either unstable or who have not responded fully to vascular reconstruction.

Reconstruction of the aortoiliac segment

In cases of severe bilateral iliac occlusion where lesser procedures are not possible, aortobifemoral grafting remains the treatment of choice. It should be remembered that elective aortic surgery carries considerable morbidity and mortality but excellent long-term results in terms of limb salvage. The operation is performed through a long abdominal incision and bilateral groin incisions in much the same way as an abdominal aortic aneurysm, and a prosthetic graft such as Dacron or PTFE may be sewn from the front of the abdominal aorta down to the common femoral or profunda femoris artery in each groin. Great care should be taken to prevent thromboembolic emboli occurring during the oper-

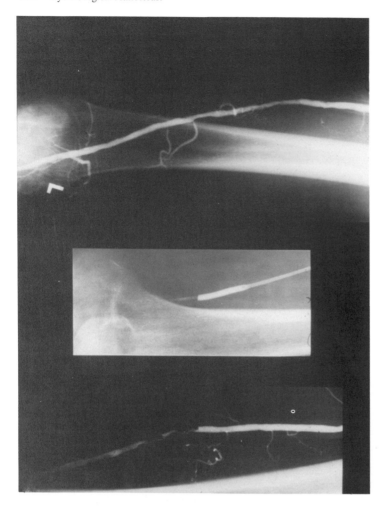

Figure 25.10 Dilating a narrowed femoral artery with an angioplasty balloon

ation and prophylactic antibiotics should be used in all cases. In the femoropopliteal segment autologous vein remains the conduit of choice with the vein being used either *in situ* or reversed. The vein can also be used from the arm or other leg and the short saphenous vein provides another source. Attention to detail is essential in this sort of surgery and often magnifying loupes or an operating microscope will help to ensure an accurate anastomosis.

Follow-up

It is increasingly apparent that results of femoro-popliteal vein grafting are complicated by the development of stenoses either within the graft or at and around the distal anastomosis. Various techniques of follow-up have been advocated including duplex scanning, regular arteriography and impedance analysis, all of which have been shown to improve patency rates when the stenoses have been corrected. If possible the patients should be followed closely for the first year following bypass surgery to try and prevent early occlusion.

Amputation

Amputation is one of the oldest surgical procedures, being first done for leprosy, ergotism and as a form of punishment. The widespread prevalence of occlusive vascular disease accounts for the vast majority of current amputations. Most surgeons are trained with a negative approach to amputation, feeling that preservation of the limb should be attempted; amputation is the very last resort. When amputation is the only outcome the operation is often relegated to the end of a list and delegated to relatively junior surgeons. As a result of this the results of amputation are far from ideal, with poor rates of healing and poorly planned rehabilitation.

The surgeon's responsibility does not end once the wound is healed but patients must be guided through the difficult period of rehabilitation and their return to the community. Properly planned amputation is a form of reconstruction which can return a patient to the community fully mobile in a relatively short period of time. Over the last 30 years, with the development of limb fitting units and the use of new materials it is possible to make prostheses to fit almost any stump, making it possible for surgeons to use all viable skin and tissue to the patient's best advantage.

Selection of level of amputation

Classic sites of election for amputations are less important now than previously because of the newer prostheses available. Figure 25.11 shows the various sites of amputation in the upper and lower limb. In patients with severe occlusive disease requiring major amputation, selection of the site of amputation is extremely difficult. Many non-invasive and invasive tests are available to determine the level but none has proved decisive. Skin temperature,

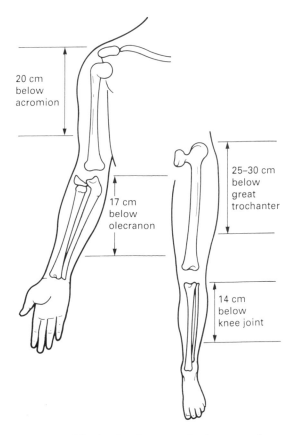

Figure 25.11 Elective sites for amputation in upper and lower limb

20 cm below acromion

17 cm below olecranon

25–30 cm below great trochanter

14 cm below knee joint

arteriography, transcutaneous Po_2, laser Doppler studies and many others have all been tried with variable results. It is clearly in the patient's interest to try and preserve the knee joint as this considerably improves the chance of subsequent rehabilitation.

Principles of surgery for amputation

There are two types of amputation to be considered: elective procedures in which there is freedom to fashion skin flaps and select the level according to blood supply and urgent amputation for fulminating infection or trauma where the viability of muscles and healthy skin are the most important factors. Urgent amputation for trauma or severe infection is best done by fashioning the flaps as for elective amputation but leaving the wound open with intention of delayed primary closure at approximately 5 days. When this technique is used flaps should be made more generously than otherwise as they can become slightly oedematous and more difficult to close later. In elective amputations the flaps are fashioned according to the level selected and skin and fascia divided at the same level. Underlying muscles should then be tapered down to the level of the bone with the intention of making a cylindrical stump for the prosthesis. The periosteum should be divided at the level at which the bone is to be sectioned and the bone should be cut cleanly and all rough edges smoothed down with a rasp.

Major blood vessels should be separately tied and ligated and major nerves pulled down and divided but not tied. Once bleeding has been controlled the muscles should be closed over the bone end by approximating the deep fascia on both sides. A suction drain should be inserted into the muscle area and brought out on the lateral side. The skin can then be closed, ideally with monofilament subcuticular suture, and this may be supported by dressings approximating the skin edges together. It is usual to remove the drain after 24–48 h (see p. 68).

Postoperative care

The use of early temporary prosthetic devices to encourage early mobilization has been enthusiastically supported in recent years though many elderly patients with arterial disease cannot cope in the first week or two following amputation. Amputation stumps should be dressed firmly in the early postoperative period to control oedema and possible haematoma. Dressings are best left undisturbed for the first 4–5 days following amputation unless there is good indication to take the dressing down. Once the wound has healed, patients can be mobilized on a temporary prosthesis. The use of the Panaid is particularly helpful in patients with below-knee amputations.

Amputations of the lower limb

Amputation of toes and forefoot

Amputation of one or more toes has a significant effect on walking, with loss of push-off power. Amputation is usually performed through a racquet-shaped incision and may be done at any part of the toe, the most common site being the metatarsal-phalangeal joint. Removal of the first or fifth toe is usually best done with removal of the head of the metatarsal, otherwise callus may be formed once walking is commenced. Transmetatarsal amputation limits push-off power even more but many elderly people can manage to walk quite adequately using hip and knee extensors. In transmetatarsal amputation it is important to suture the long tendons of flexion and extension together to preserve the power and integrity of the ankle joint. Symes' amputation was advocated for many years as an alternative to long below-knee amputation and when successful can produce a durable end-bearing stump. This level of amputation, however, requires a complex prosthesis and is rarely cosmetically acceptable. When a prosthesis is available a well formed below-knee amputation is usually preferable.

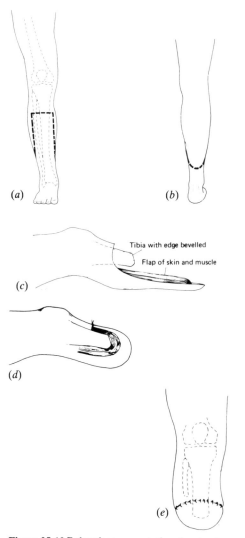

Figure 25.12 Below-knee amputation showing long posterior Burgess skin flap containing muscle, bevelling of tibial edge, and skin closure away from bone end

Below-knee amputation (Figure 25.12)

This amputation is the level of choice for patients with severe occlusive vascular disease, particularly for diabetics. It can be fitted with a satisfactory prosthesis and because of retention of the knee joint results in a high chance of walking again for the patient. The Burgess myoplastic technique is the most widely used with the long posterior flap being brought across the lower part of tibia and sutured anteriorly away from the weight-bearing centre. Prostheses fitted to the below-knee amputation stump are of the tendo-bearing type with a soft sponge-feel component to simulate movement of an ankle joint. The socket distributes weight over the surface of stump preventing pressure on the suture line itself.

Amputations through the knee

Once a popular site for amputation, through-knee amputations are less popular because of difficulties with fitting a prosthesis. This type of amputation is often favoured for elderly patients where major amputation is required for occlusive vascular disease in whom there is little hope of walking again. It provides them with a long lever with which to help get themselves around the bed and is preferred to an above-knee amputation.

Mid-thigh amputation (Figure 25.13)

In these opertions as much femur as possible should be retained as this provides more power and muscle balance for a subsequent prosthesis. In the amputation the anterior and posterior flaps are usually cut to equal lengths and the muscle sutured over the bone with care to ensure a good functional result postoperatively. A prosthesis fitted to an above-knee amputation is of a total contact type which is supported by a waist belt or by negative pressure in the socket. The socket is attached to a knee joint which provides control of knee movement to lock the limb straight if required.

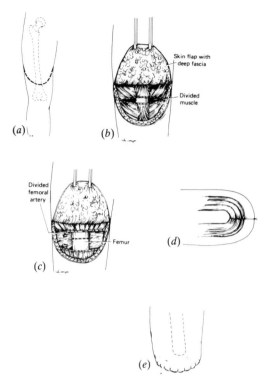

Figure 25.13 Mid-thigh amputation, preserving good length of femur

Hip disarticulation and hemipelvectomy

These high amputations are rarely performed and usually only for malignant disease or irreparable high thigh trauma. The lack of a thigh stump makes the fitting and control of a prosthesis even more difficult.

Amputation of the upper limb

Amputation of the upper limb is usually necessary for trauma, malignancy and rarely for peripheral vascular disease. The psychological impact of these amputations is much larger than for lower limb disease, particularly as patients are by and large younger. Amputations can be done at any site as modern prosthetic fitters can manufacture a suitable artifical limb for cosmetic purposes and to restore some function.

Venous disease

The price man has to pay for his upright posture is the liability to develop varicose veins and problems with the deep veins in the leg. Normal flow of blood in the lower limbs is from subcutaneous tissue and skin to the superficial veins and thence to the deep veins. These in turn drain into the femoral, iliac femoral veins and the inferior vena cava. The passage of blood up the veins is helped by the presence of valves which prevent reflux and help the muscle to pump blood up towards the heart. The valves are subjected to high pressures – the maximum is equal to a column of blood extending from the ground to the level of the heart, some $100\,cmH_2O$ in an average adult. Venous insufficiency is more common in women than men and may give rise to congestive pain, some localized tissue damage and unsightly varicose veins.

Varicose veins

The precise cause of this condition is not known although factors such as heredity trait, prolonged standing, child-bearing and previous deep vein thrombosis are all known to be aetiological factors. The commonest cause is due to incompetence of the valve at the sapheno-femoral junction, with reflux down the long saphenous vein. A similar pattern may occur at the short saphenous vein.

Clinical features

Varicose veins become extremely prominent and unsightly and patients may seek treatment because of the unpleasant appearance. As the veins become more marked there may be some interference with venous return and oedema of the ankle can occur towards the end of the day. As this swelling gets worse valves guarding the communication between deep and superficial veins become increasingly incompetent, giving rise to the appearance of subcutaneous venules and venous flares. By the time this happens the nutrition to the skin around the medial malleolus is often threatened and such patients are subject to varicose ulceration. The sapheno-femoral junction may be extremely incompetent and produce a blow out called a sapheno-varix which may be confused with a femoral hernia. This may be easily distinguished because the sapheno-varix will disappear when the patient lies down and a fluid thrill can be elicited over the sapheno-varix by tapping gently on the varicose veins lower down the thigh.

Clinical assessment

A cough impulse may be elicited down the main course of the long saphenous vein, which can be eliminated by compression at the groin. Fluid thrills can be transmitted up the vein by percussion confirming continuity of the main venous trunks.

Trendelenburg's test (Figure 25.14)

This is a simple clinical test to show the main site of incompetence in the leg. The leg is raised above body level to drain the varicose veins, then the suspected incompetent feeding proximal vein is compressed with a tourniquet and the patient then asked to stand up. If the site of leakage has been correctly identified the varices remain empty and if the tourniquet is then released these veins promptly fill. A simple directional Doppler may be used to demonstrate reflux in superficial varicose veins and is invaluable in indentifying the sites of incompetence in the superficial venous system.

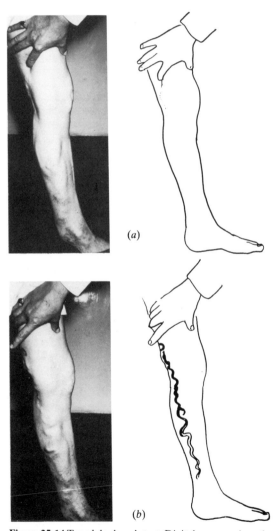

(a)

(b)

Figure 25.14 Trendelenburg's test. Digital compression of the main saphenous vein in the thigh, after elevation: (a), no early refilling, (b) release of compression allows incompetent downward filling. Compression site is marked with a circle before operation.

Treatment of varicose veins

Simple mild varicose veins in the elderly and the unfit can be treated with elastic support stockings, relieving the symptoms of pressure and preventing deterioration. Most younger patients, however, find this form of treatment unacceptable and prefer either injection sclerotherapy or surgery.

Injection sclerotherapy

This consists of injecting a sclerosant, e.g. ethanolamine into the lumen of the vein in order to thrombose the vein. It is important that as soon as the sclerosant is injected the vein is compressed and firmly bandaged for at least 7 days. Injection treatment does not, however, remove the source of incompetence of the superficial venous system and recurrence is more likely than after definitive surgery.

Surgical treatment

Once the long or short saphenous system has been identified as the source of incompetence, then that system is best divided and removed. For long saphenous incompetence a sapheno-femoral disconnection is essential and this is best done under a general anaesthetic. It is important to identify all the tributaries at the sapheno-femoral junction so that each one is ligated and divided. It is then preferable to strip the long saphenous vein down to the knee joint in order to remove any mid-thigh perforating veins. More obvious superficial varicose veins can then be removed through small incisions with the avulsion technique. It is rarely necessary to remove the lower half of the long saphenous vein as this is rarely diseased or incompetent.

Complications of varicose veins

Superficial thrombophlebitis

When a large varicose vein becomes thrombosed the vein becomes tender, raised, red and indurated along its course. It is often extremely painful and may give rise to some oedema and swelling of the leg. Treatment consists of compression with a firm elastic support, pain relief with analgesics and reduction of inflammation by non-steroidal anti-inflammatory agents for 7 days.

Bleeding

This is often due to minor trauma to a dilated vein giving rise to profuse bleeding perpetuated by high pressure within the vein and incompetence. Treatment is simple; the patient should be advised to lie down with the leg elevated and a pressure bandage applied to the area of bleeding. After a period of 5 min elevation, bleeding will usually have ceased.

Ulceration (Figure 25.15)

Ulceration may be due to varicose veins or to incompetent valves in the deep venous system. This is particularly common if there has been a previous deep vein thrombosis where the deep veins have recanalized but valves have suffered irreversible damage. A patient presenting with an ulcer round the ankle should be asked if there is any previous history of a venous thrombosis or if they had a painful swollen leg after trauma or immobilization in bed for medical or surgical reasons. If the valves of the deep veins are incompetent then pressure is transmitted back down the venous system to the gaiter area above the ankle.

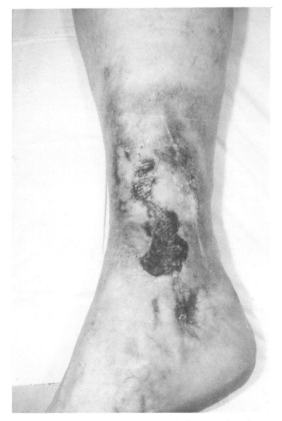

Figure 25.15 Varicose ulceration and pigmentation above the medial malleolus

If a deep venous damage is suspected then an ascending venogram or ambulatory venous pressures should be measured by direct cannulation of a vein.

Patients should be confined to bed with elevation of the foot so that the high venous pressure is abolished. Ulcers will usually then heal fairly quickly provided there is no evidence of any impairment of the arterial circulation. A swab should be taken for culture and antibiotics given as appropriate. By and large, local antibiotics are of little value and tend to induce sensitivity making the ulcer worse. In many cases a prolonged period of bed rest is inappropriate and in such cases healing can be obtained by compression elastic bandaging of the leg, thus emptying the dilated superficial veins and aiding the muscle pump to act efficiently. These bandages can be replaced at regular intervals until the ulcer heals (see p. 73).

Once the ulcer has healed the patient should be fitted with a firm graduated pressure stocking and it is unlikely that the ulcer will recur. Sometimes, however, large incompetent perforating veins are demonstrated on venography and these can be ligated and associated varicose veins treated by stripping.

Lymphatic system

Lymphoedema results from obstruction of lymphatic flow from the leg, either caused by a congenital abnormality of the lymphatic system or damage to the lymphatics by disease or surgery.

Congenital abnormality of the lymphatics in the lower limb produces oedema which can present either at birth or in adult life. Females are more commonly affected than males and there may well be a family history. The lymphatic system can be demonstrated either by isotope lymphography or by lymphangiography. In addition to congenital hypoplasia or absence of lymphatics, lymphoedema may follow an inflammatory process such as streptococcal cellulitis or filariasis and may occasionally follow radical surgery such as block dissection of the groin.

Lymphoedema of the arm is not uncommonly seen after carcinoma of the breast due to post-irradiation fibrosis, surgical damage to the lymphatics at radical mastectomy or because of recurrent tumour in the axilla.

Clinical features

Although it is frequently reported that lymphoedema can be differentiated from other forms of oedema on the simple physical sign of absence of pitting on pressure, this is an unreliable physical sign until the lymphoedema is long-standing and chronic. Diagnosis is made by excluding other obvious causes such as cardiac failure or renal disease and by demonstrating abnormalities of the lymphatics on isotope lymphography or lymphangiography.

Treatment

If the swelling is mild this can be reasonably well controlled with a well fitted graduated pressure stocking. If the swelling is prolonged and serious then prolonged elevation of the limb at night may help but very often these patients have to accept a chronically dilated limb. Many operations have been tried to improve the appearance of lymphoedema involving excision of the oedematous subcutaneous tissue down the the deep fascia, but very often the cosmetic result after surgery is little better than the original presenting symptoms. As yet there are no satisfactory operations for relieving long-standing lymphoedema.

26

Injuries and infections of the hand

G. Hooper

Injuries of the hand

Injuries of the hand as a result of domestic and industrial accidents are extremely common; it has been estimated that in an industrialized country such as Great Britain between one-quarter and one-third of all injured patients attending hospital will do so as a result of hand injuries.

Any hand injury, no matter how apparently trivial, has the potential to cause serious loss of function if inadequately assessed and treated. All doctors dealing with hand injuries in general practice, the workplace or the Accident and Emergency department must be constantly aware of this. Many such injuries are dealt with on an outpatient basis and a serious responsibility rests upon the junior staff who are required to undertake their initial treatment. In larger centres their work should be supervised by a surgeon particularly interested and experienced in this type of surgery but this is seldom possible in smaller hospitals. If the patient with a serious hand injury cannot be referred to an appropriate centre immediately it is important that early treatment should be directed to obtaining rapid healing of skin and preventing stiffness, thus leaving the hand in excellent condition for any later reconstructive surgery. In most cases it is this initial treatment that determines the final result.

General principles

Documentation

This is most important, especially as many industrial injuries will be the subject of later compensation claims. A note should be made of the patient's dominant hand, occupation and description of the accident. The site of the injury should be recorded on a simple diagram, together with any abnormal findings on clinical examination, such as deformities, loss of movement or sensation, and the results of radiographic examination.

To avoid confusion phalanges, digits and metacarpal bones should *never* be referred to by number, but always by name: a phrase such as 'the first phalanx of the second finger' is ambiguous. The phalanges are called proximal, intermediate and distal. Digits and their associated metacarpal bones are referred to by name: thumb, index, middle (or long), ring and little. The terms medial and lateral are not used in the hand: ulnar and radial are preferred. The surfaces of the hand are called palmar (or flexor) and dorsal (or extensor).

Facilities

Initial treatment of open wounds should not be carried out in an Accident and Emergency department unless a properly equipped operating theatre is available. Aseptic precautions are essential. Special instruments are needed for hand work, such as small-bladed knives, fine forceps, skin hooks, small artery forceps, fine scissors, needles and suture materials.

Anaesthesia

Full anaesthesia of the part is necessary. A general anaesthetic is often preferable, but brachial plexus block, Bier's block, wrist block or ring block of the finger may have a place, depending on circumstances (see Chapter 8). Local infiltration anaesthesia is usually unsatisfactory as it causes further swelling in the area of injury and obscures the local anatomy.

Digital nerve block (ring block) is useful for distal wounds and infections in the digits but it is best avoided if there has been a crushing injury and there is any doubt about circulation. After cleaning the skin, 1 ml of 2% lignocaine *without adrenaline* is injected around each digital nerve at the base of the finger, using a fine hypodermic needle. Anaesthesia is complete in 10 min.

Tourniquet

Operations on the injured hand should be done with a pneumatic tourniquet applied to the upper arm, so that a bloodless field is obtained and delicate tissues are spared the trauma of repeated swabbing. A tourniquet of rubber tubing should never be applied around the upper arm, because of the risk of nerve damage by uncontrolled local pressure. Except in infected cases, the limb is emptied of blood by applying an Esmarch bandage tightly from the

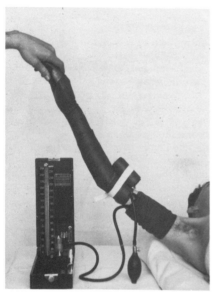

Figure 26.1 Method of obtaining a bloodless field in operations on the hand. Before the tourniquet is inflated, the limb is emptied of blood by means of an Esmarch bandage applied from the finger tips proximally

fingertips to just above the elbow with the arm elevated (Figure 26.1). The tourniquet is then inflated to a pressure of 20–30 mmHg above systolic pressure, after which the rubber bandage is removed. In a healthy person the tourniquet can be retained for a period of 60–90 min with safety.

Elevation of the limb for 2–3 min before inflating the tourniquet produces exsanguination that is nearly as good as that obtained with the Esmarch bandage. It is the method of choice when the hand is infected or the wound is very contaminated.

Preparation of the part

All wounds of the hand are potentially contaminated and thorough cleaning is essential, using soap and water initially. After checking that anaesthesia is complete the entire hand is placed in a basin and lathered energetically, using a handful of wool or gauze in preference to a nailbrush. When as much dirt as possible has been removed, the soap is washed away with sterile water. The skin around the wound may then be painted with an antiseptic agent, which should not be allowed to enter the wound.

A wire grid (Figure 26.2) or malleable lead hand are very effective in steadying the hand during operation.

Prevention of stiffness

Stiffness of the hand is a surgical catastrophe that is usually preventable. The mobility of the hand is dependent upon the interplay of many gliding structures within the tendon and joint systems. This gliding mechanism can be obstructed in three main ways, by infection, oedema and incorrect splintage.

Infection

Any infection of the hand is likely to cause swelling and fibrosis and hence stiffness. Major primary infections of the hand will be dealt with later in the

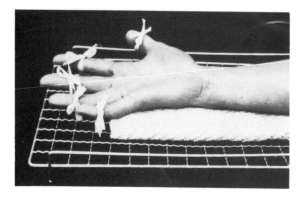

Figure 26.2 A wire grid, which is easily sterilized, makes an excellent support for the hand during operation. The digits are held in extension by separate tapes tied to the grid

chapter. They are relatively uncommon but infections resulting from neglected or inadequately treated minor wounds are not.

Oedema

Oedema of the hand is inevitable after crushing injuries, infections or prolonged operations. It must be anticipated and controlled by elevating the hand. The patient can be taught to hold the hand up or, in the case of an inpatient, the hand can be elevated by a support (Figure 26.3). *The common broad arm sling does not elevate the hand and it should not be used after hand injuries or operations*. If the underlying condition allows, active finger movements should be encouraged in order to 'pump away' oedema fluid, which is fibrin-rich and acts as a glue on the gliding structures in the hand. If the hand cannot be moved actively it should be splinted in the 'position of immobilization' while elevated.

Sometimes oedema develops days or weeks after injury or operations, usually because the hand has been held dependent and not actively used. This is an indication for admission to hospital so that the patient can be supervised in both elevation and active mobilization.

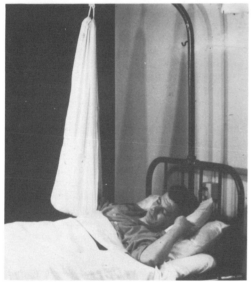

Figure 26.3 Elevation of the hand in a roller towel. The forearm is vertical and not constricted. The elbow is bent 90° and rests comfortably on a pillow

Incorrect splintage

Careless or inexpert application of splints, plaster or bandages is likely to hold the metacarpophalangeal joints in extension and the proximal interphalangeal joints in flexion. Irreversible stiffness is very liable to occur if a swollen hand is held in this position for more than 10–14 days.

It cannot be stressed too much or too often that the correct position for immobilization of the joints of the hand is with the metacarpophalangeal joints flexed, the interphalangeal joints extended and the first web space held open with the thumb abducted. This is known as the *safe position* or *position of immobilization*. In this position the capsular ligaments of all the joints are fully extended and the hand can be splinted for up to 3 weeks without the danger of iatrogenic stiffness due to secondary contractures. The boxing-glove dressing is a very satisfactory method of splinting the hand in the desired position (Figure 26.4).

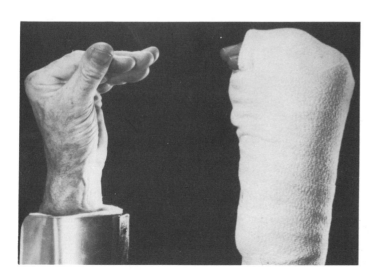

Figure 26.4 The 'position of immobilization' is as shown on the left, with the metacarpophalangeal joints flexed, the interphalangeal joints extended and the thumb abducted to prevent contracture of the thumb web. The wrist must be held in slight dorsiflexion. This position can be maintained by a boxing-glove dressing of fluffed gauze, orthopaedic wool roll and crêpe bandage. A plaster-of-Paris backslab will control the wrist and prevent the bandage from coming loose

Common examples of splintage techniques that violate this basic principle of safe positioning are the use of a straight wooden splint (Figure 26.5), or strapping the flexed fingers over a roll of bandage in the palm of the hand. They have no place in the management of hand injuries.

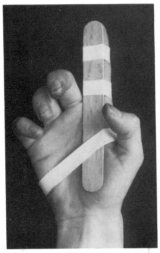

Figure 26.5 A straight splint holds the metacarpophalangeal joint in extension and impedes the movement of uninjured fingers. It has no place in the management of hand injuries

Rehabilitation

Careful supervision is essential after any hand injury. Even if major treatment is not necessary it is always advisable to recall the patient within a week of two to check that the hand is being used actively and not overprotected. The assistance of a hand therapist is often invaluable.

Wounds of the hand
General principles

All except the most superficial wounds must be explored carefully, in order to remove all foreign material and determine the full extent of the injury. Adequate facilities, anaesthesia and tourniquet control are essential.

Except in clean-cut wounds, debridement is necessary. Great care is needed after crushing injuries in assessing the viability of the skin. Haemorrhage is controlled by careful use of the bipolar minicoagulator. Nothing but harm can result from blind plunging of forceps into a bleeding wound of the hand. Primary suture of the skin is

permissible only in the circumstances detailed below.

Primary repair of deeper structures such as cut nerves and tendons should only be contemplated by a surgeon skilled in the management of such injuries. The junior doctor must remember that no harm will come to the hand if primary care is concentrated on wound healing and prevention of stiffness; reconstructive procedures can always be carried out later by a more experienced surgeon.

Wound excision

The first aim of treatment is to avoid infection, which is particularly disastrous since it may spread to tendon sheaths or deep fascial spaces. Even if confined to the skin, infection may cause permanent disability due to the formation of an indurated scar. The most common type of hand infection seen now is in a minor wound that has become infected due to inadequate wound excision and a misplaced reliance on the efficacy of antibiotics given in inadequate dosage.

Formal excision of the wound is rarely practicable or necessary in the hand. Any ragged, devitalized or grossly contaminated skin edges are excised so as to leave the wound margins as healthy as possible. It is always better to accept a slight deficiency of skin than to leave skin that is likely to become necrotic and infected. Subcutaneous fatty tissue often prolapses through skin wounds on the palmar aspect of the hand; if bruised or contaminated it should be excised.

Thorough exploration ensures the removal of any foreign material and devitalized tissue and will allow any damage to deeper structures to be identified. It may be necessary to extend the wound but any incisions used for wider exposure should be made with care and forethought. No hand incision should cross a major crease at right angles, otherwise a contracted keloid scar may result. Incisions should lie either in or parallel to a crease, or be placed where creases are absent (Figure 26.6). Zig-zag incisions which approach the crease at 45° and then turn through 90° at the crease are also acceptable. A transverse wound on the flexor aspect of the hand can be extended by making a distal longitudinal incision at one end and a proximal one at the other; in the fingers these longitudinal incisions should lie in the midlateral line, dorsal to the flexion creases.

Primary skin closure

Primary suture is permissible only when: (1) the wound is recent, (2) contamination is minimal, and (3) the skin edges can be brought together without tension.

Fine non-absorbent material on a cutting needle should be used: 4/0 nylon is very suitable. The

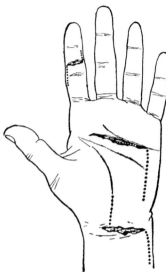

Figure 26.6 Incisions that are permissible for extending wounds of the hand. Incisions should be made in, or parallel to, skin creases or in areas where skin creases are absent

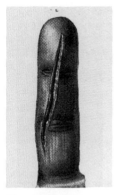

Figure 26.7 A clean-cut superficial linear wound on the palmar aspect of a finger does not gape, because of the attachment of skin to deep fascia. Stitches are therefore unnecessary

minimum number of sutures are inserted and tied without tension. The thick superficial horny layer of the palmar skin does not heal by first intention and often desquamates, giving a gaping appearance to the wound after removal of of sutures.

When conditions are not suitable the skin should not be sutured. Adequate apposition may be obtained by the pressure of dressings alone; if not, the wound must be left open and allowed to heal by granulation or, preferably, covered by skin graft. With such treatment healing will occur without suppuration and with a supple scar – a result far superior to that obtained when primary suture has been followed by even a mild degree of infection.

Superficial linear cuts and lacerations

The wound should be explored carefully but, if it is a relatively clean cut, debridement is not necessary. On the palmar surface of the hand wounds do not gape, unless there is tension in the subcutaneous tissues, so that stitches are unnecessary (Figure 26.7).

Wounds with raised skin flaps

It is important to assess the viability of the skin by its colour and the presence of bleeding at the free edge, and this can only be done by letting down the tourniquet after debridement of the wound. If the edges appear ischaemic the flap is trimmed until it bleeds. Subcutaneous fat is trimmed as it has poor vitality, then the flap is laid back in position and secured with the minimum number of fine stitches and a compression dressing. There must be no tension on the flap, or sloughing will occur; it is far better to leave a defect to which a skin graft can be applied.

Distally based flaps are usually ischaemic and unlikely to survive. A common mistake of the inexperienced is to replace such a flap, which inevitably becomes necrotic and infected, putting the function of the hand at risk. If it is likely that the entire flap may be non-viable, it should be excised and replaced with an appropriate skin graft or flap which will almost certainly require the skills of a specialist hand or plastic surgeon if the defect is large.

Wounds with loss of skin

All lost skin should be replaced as soon as possible; this not only hastens healing but by preventing infection limits fibrosis and contracture. Skin may be replaced by grafting, local or distant flaps. When there has been severe crushing of the hand it is wise to delay grafting for 48–72 h until oedema has been controlled by elevation. In the meantime the hand is splinted in a boxing-glove dressing.

Skin grafts

Partial-thickness grafts are readily available and take successfully in a large proportion of cases, even in the presence of mild sepsis. A suitable donor site with hand injuries is the upper inner aspect of the forearm. Owing to poor wearing qualities these grafts are less satisfactory on the palmar than on the dorsal surface, but as a temporary expedient they are excellent.

Full-thickness grafts are better on the palmar surface of the hand, but are less certain to take than split-thickness skin in conditions where complete asepsis cannot be assured. They may be taken from the groin, cubital fossa, forearm or post-auricular area and usually the donor site can be closed without difficulty. The skin is cut accurately to the shape required, subcutaneous fat removed and the graft stitched under normal tension and held with a tie-over dressing.

Local flaps

Small defects on the palmar or dorsal surface of a finger can be covered by rotating a flap from its lateral aspect (Figure 26.8a). The donor area is then covered with a split-thickness graft. Alternative methods of obtaining local flap cover include the cross-finger and thenar flaps (Figure 28.8b, c) but these techniques are definitely not recommended for the inexperienced because of the very real risks

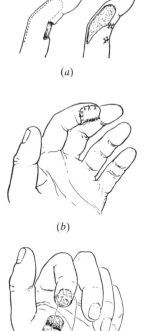

(a)

(b)

(c)

Figure 26.8 Methods of replacing skin loss in the fingers by local flaps: (*a*) rotational flap from side of finger to palmar surface; (*b*) a cross-finger flap; (*c*) a thenar flap

of flap failure, or contractures since the hand must be splinted in an undesirable position. A split-skin graft applied as a temporary expedient, with later reconstruction by an expert, is much to be preferred.

Pedicle flaps from distant sites

Local flaps are seldom sufficient when large areas of skin have been lost, although sometimes it is possible to use the skin from an injured digit which requires amputation as a flap, after filleting out the bones and removing the nail.

Large flaps to replace skin on the hand may be raised from the abdominal wall, groin or pectoral area. There are considerable advantages in using an axial pattern flap based on constant blood vessels as the flap can be quite long in proportion to its width, without compromising survival. Often the defect caused by raising the flap can be closed by direct suture.

An additional advantage of the pectoral flap is that the hand is elevated and oedema is less likely, but the scar in the donor area may be unacceptable, particularly to a female patient. In these circumstances the groin flap based on the superficial circumflex femoral artery may be preferable.

Wounds with division of nerves

The median and ulnar nerves are most often severed in transverse wounds across the front of the wrist (Figure 26.9). Late lesions of these nerves can be detected by appropriate muscle wasting, motor weakness (Figures 26.10–26.13) and loss of sensation to light touch. These tests are difficult to apply in young children but absence of sweating may be apparent and the denervated skin will fail to wrinkle after prolonged immersion in warm water.

It is very difficult to identify loss of nerve function after a recent injury when a patient is distressed, in pain and usually unable to cooperate with standard testing. The golden rule is that if there is a wound overlying a nerve, then the nerve must be presumed to be damaged and examined carefully during surgical treatment of the wound.

A severed median or ulnar nerve should be sutured primarily provided that conditions are ideal, i.e. the wound is recent and clean-cut and the operator has the experience and necessary facilities. The method of choice is epineurial repair using magnification and 8/0 or 10/0 non-absorbable suture.

Secondary suture is preferable if initial conditions are not ideal. At the first operation the nerve ends should be approximated with a couple of non-absorbable sutures; the site of injury should be

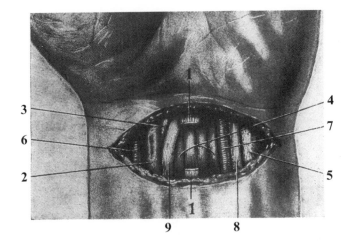

Figure 26.9 Anatomy of nerves and tendons at a level just above the wrist joint – a common site of injury. In this case the tendon of palmaris longus has been severed. 1, Palmaris longus; 2, flexor carpi radialis; 3, flexor pollicis longus; 4, flexor digitorum superficialis; 5, flexor carpi ulnaris; 6, radial artery; 7, ulnar artery; 8, ulnar nerve; 9, median nerve

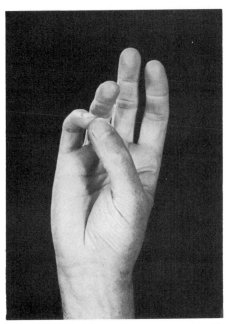

Figure 26.10 Test for median nerve function. The thumb is opposed to the little finger by the action of the thenar muscles

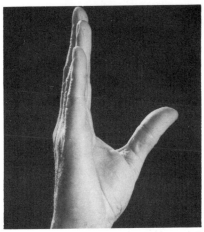

Figure 26.11 Another test of median nerve function. Abduction of the thumb from the plane of the palm by the action of abductor pollicis brevis

neuroma. The nerves are quite large and their repair is not as difficult as might be supposed. Since they are pure sensory nerves, the results of suture can be excellent but are directly proportional to the care and accuracy of repair.

Wounds with division of tendons

Tendons are often divided in incised wounds of the wrist, hand and fingers. Tendon function should therefore be tested carefully in patients with such wounds. When the hand is relaxed the fingers lie in a fairly constant posture, with increasing flexion in the more ulnar digits. This is determined by the tone in the flexor and extensor muscle masses. Sometimes a glance is enough to lead one to suspect a severed tendon because it is obvious that the posture of one or more fingers is altered (Figure 26.14).

isolated from adjacent structures by silicone-rubber tubing, if available. This allows a much easier secondary repair when the nerve is re-explored 3–5 weeks after injury, as tissue reaction around the nerve is minimized and the thickened epineurium is easily identified as a separate layer when placing sutures.

Digital nerves are often divided in wounds involving the sides of the fingers. They should be repaired as this decreases the residual anaesthesia of the finger and the chance of developing a tender

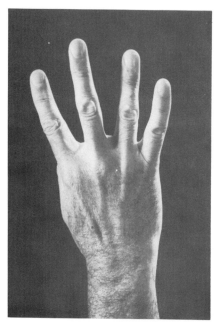

Figure 26.12 Test for ulnar nerve function. Abduction of the fingers in the plane of the palm. Contraction of the first dorsal interosseous muscle and the abductor digiti minimi can be palpated

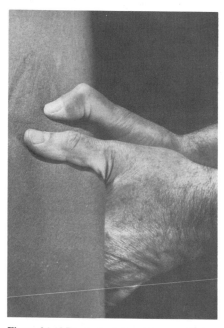

Figure 26.13 Paralysis of the adductor pollicis causes Froment's sign in ulnar nerve lesions: when gripping a thin board the affected thumb is bent at the interphalangeal joint by the action of the flexor pollicis longus (innervated by the median nerve)

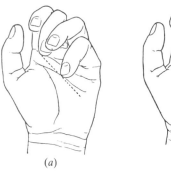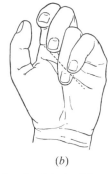

(a)	(b)

Figure 26.14 'Spot' diagnosis of tendon injuries. The abnormal position of the ring finger in (a) suggests a severed flexor tendon; that in (b) a severed extensor tendon

The results of tendon repair are likely to be disappointing owing to the developement of adhesions between the tendon and surrounding structures at the point of suture, commonly and inevitably the result of a clumsy repair with the wrong suture material. As with nerve injuries, the primary treatment of tendon injuries depends on the condition of the wound and the experience of the surgeon dealing with the injury. In contaminated wounds or severe crushing injuries primary repair is not recommended.

Flexor tendons

Between the metacarpophalangeal joints and the middle phalanx the flexor tendons are enclosed within a firm, fibrous sheath. Absolute fixation of the tendons with loss of digital function will result if dense adhesions form in this area. When both tendons are severed in the fibrous flexor sheath the inexperienced surgeon should suture the skin wound only in the first instance and refer the patient for later reconstruction by an expert. At a secondary procedure the cut tendons can be replaced by a free tendon graft, usually of palmaris longus tendon. This ensures that the points of tendon suture are outside the flexor sheath, where surrounding tissues are more elastic and adhesions are less important.

Excellent results can be obtained when primary repair is carried out by an experienced surgeon using delicate instruments, magnification and the correct suture technique. The ends of the tendons must be accurately coapted with non-absorbable sutures of wire or nylon inserted by a technique that ensures the tendon is strongly held without crushing, kinking or fraying. Elastic traction is applied to the injured finger and over-extension is prevented by a back splint (Figure 26.15). This arrangement allows controlled passive movement of the tendon which will limit the tethering effect of any adhesions that

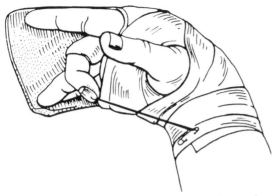

Figure 26.15 Elastic traction after primary tendon repair

form after repair. Close supervision by an experienced hand therapist is necessary.

Flexor tendons in the palm or at the wrist are surrounded by loose synovium or paratenon. Primary repair usually gives better results than in the digital sheaths as adhesions are less restrictive. Primary repair is recommended when the flexor pollicis longus tendon is divided distally, but results of primary repair in the thenar area or at the level of the metacarpophalangeal joints may be poor and the inexperienced surgeon is best advised to close the skin wound and refer the patient for later tendon grafting.

Extensor tendons

Primary repair of extensor tendons using fine, non-absorbable sutures is recommended if conditions are suitable. Extensor tendons are generally believed to be easier to repair than flexor tendons, but the results do not always support this view. Extensor tendons do not lie in a rigid sheath (except under the extensor retinaculum) and, since their excursion is less than flexor tendons, the effect of adhesions is less severe. However, because extensor tendons are flat it is difficult to obtain accurate end-to-end apposition without bunching or overlapping. Furthermore, an extensor tendon is frequently divided where it forms the posterior expansion over a joint; the joint is usually opened and movement may be impaired by adhesion.

On the dorsum of the proximal interphalangeal joint the injury is often confined to the central slip which inserts into the base of the middle phalanx. No immediate disability is apparent and the injury is likely to be missed, unless the wound is properly explored. As the severed ends separate the lateral bands of the extensor expansion slide anterior to the axis of the proximal interphalangeal joint, causing flexion of this joint and hyperextension of the distal interphalangeal joint. The occurrence of this 'boutonnière deformity' can be prevented by early repair of the tendon followed by splintage of the finger with the interphalangeal joints in extension.

Wounds with division of vessels

Revascularization

Major blood vessels such as the radial or ulnar artery should be repaired using 9/0 nylon and magnification. It is possible to repair smaller vessels down to a diameter of 1 mm or less, using the operating microscope and 10/0 sutures, thus revascularizing parts of the hand that might otherwise have become ischaemic. These procedures are very time-consuming and place great demands on theatre facilities, but it is essential that they are available in major accident centres.

Replantation

Consideration must be given to replantation using microvascular techniques if a part has been completely severed. There is no doubt that replantation after major loss of the hand, several digits or the thumb can benefit function immensely, but a good case has not been made for replanatation of a single digit other than the thumb. Replantation is usually very successful when the part has been cleanly severed with a minimum of crushing but success is less likely if there is a severe crushing element or the part has been avulsed.

The severed part should be placed in a sterile plastic bag containing no ice, preservatives or fluid and then placed on (not in) ordinary ice in an insulated container. The nearest specialist replantation centre must be notified *before* transferring the patient and care should be taken that the amputated part is sent with the patient.

Special types of wound

Wounds with foreign bodies

Unless these can be easily palpated, their removal can be difficult and great damage can result from digging around the wound in their pursuit. Radiographs in two planes should be taken immediately before operation, if the object is thought to be radio-opaque. Various devices, for example a paper-clip taped to the skin, can be used to assist localization by radiography and then a corresponding mark is made on the skin before preparation. An incision should be made across the axis of a long object such as a needle. Wooden foreign bodies are always contaminated and the wound should not be sutured after their removal.

Grease-gun and paint-spray injuries

Typically these affect the index finger of the non-dominant hand. In a moment of carelessness, the nozzle of a blocked high-pressure gun is held against the finger to test it; if the nozzle suddenly clears a fine jet of grease or paint may penetrate the tissues for a considerable distance. The entrance point may appear to be no more than an innocent puncture wound, but distension of the tissue planes with the material causes ischaemia and amputation is almost inevitable if treatment is delayed. Immediate exploration is indicated with removal of as much of the foreign material as possible. The digit should be widely explored through incisions that extend into the palm if necessary. The wound should be left open.

Bites and allied injuries

All wounds sustained from contact with teeth are potentially serious, owing to the risks of infection, and the risks are greatest with human bites. Any wound of the knuckles sustained from contact with an adversary's teeth should be treated with great respect. Exploration and debridement should be particularly thorough and carried out with adequate anaesthesia. If the joint has been involved it should be thoroughly irrigated with saline and left widely open. The hand is then splinted in the position of rest. Intensive antibiotic treatment must include a drug effective against anaerobic organisms (see Hand infections below).

Burst finger

This is the result of severe crushing. The skin literally bursts open and the tendons, bones and joints may be exposed (Figure 26.16). It is usually impossible to close the wound without tension

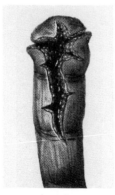

Figure 26.16 Burst finger. The gaping is due mainly to swelling and the wound cannot be closed without tension. Stitches are therefore dangerous

because of swelling of subcutaneous tissues. Stitches should therefore be avoided as far as possible although a few loose sutures may be necessary to secure a covering for exposed tendons and bones. After careful debridement, the wound edges are approximated by the pressure of dressings alone.

Injuries of the fingertip

The pulp of the finger is a most important functional part of the hand. Injuries that damage the pulp can be very troublesome and result in severe impairment of function unless dealt with competently from the earliest stage.

Amputation

A severed fingertip may sometimes be sutured back successfully in young children, but in adults this is not recommended because necrosis is common and healing by secondary intention is very slow.

The aim of treatment is to achieve rapid healing without hypersensitivity of the fingertip. This usually requires some trimming of the terminal phalanx to allow direct closure of the skin. One should not hesitate to sacrifice some length of a finger to obtain primary closure with well-padded skin on the pulp; failure to do this results in tight, adherent, hypersensitive skin and the finger will not be used. Before closing the skin the digital nerves are identified, cut back well away from the site of the scar and sealed with *bipolar* diathermy. The digital vessels are also sealed.

Skin grafts, either partial or full-thickness, are very liable to become adherent to underlying bone and are rarely necessary after partial amputation of the fingertip, although they have a place when there is loss of skin alone. Distant skin flaps have the disadvantage that they are relatively insensitive. Local V–Y advancement flaps overcome this problem, but are not recommended for the occasional operator.

Subungual haematoma

A painful collection of blood under the nail is usually the result of a crushing injury, and is often associated with a fracture of the terminal phalanx. It can be evacuated by drilling a hole in the nail with a sharp scalpel or needle, under ring block if necessary (Figure 26.17).

Splinter below the nail

Infection may follow if the splinter is left. It may be difficult to remove unless a wedge of nail overlying the splinter is excised under digital block anaesthesia (Figure 26.18).

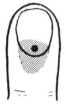

Figure 26.17 Trephining the nail to evacuate a subungual haematoma

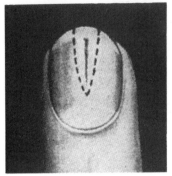

Figure 26.18 A wedge-shaped piece of nail should be removed to give access to a foreign body beneath it

Mallet finger

This is due to avulsion of the insertion of the extensor tendon from the terminal phalanx (Figure 26.19) and may be caused by a trivial incident, such as catching the finger when bed-making. The distal interphalangeal joint should be held in extension using a small plastic splint which must be worn continuously except when washing the hand. There is no need to immobilize the proximal interphalangeal joint (Figure 26.20). It may be necessary to use the splint for 6–8 weeks.

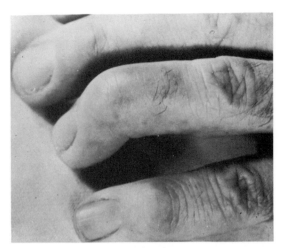

Figure 26.19 Mallet finger deformity

Fractures of the hand

These are very common. They may be isolated or, less often, part of a complicated injury involving skin loss and other soft tissue damage.

A radiographic examination, with films taken in two planes at right angles to each other, is mandatory if a fracture is suspected, both to confirm the diagnosis and guide treatment. On the basis of the clinical examination and radiograph a decision should be made on the following points:

1. Is the fracture *stable* or *unstable*? A stable fracture is one that is undisplaced and is not likely to displace or, if already displaced, is in an acceptable position.
2. Is *reduction* necessary? Fractures with unacceptable displacement or deformity that will hinder function in the future should be reduced.

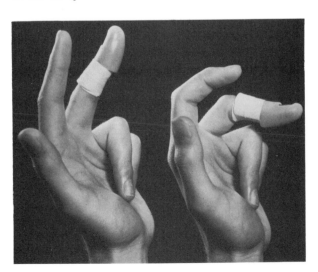

Figure 26.20 A simple plastic splint for a mallet finger. Easily applied, maintained and cleaned. Note that the proximal interphalangeal joint should not be immobilized

3. Is *splintage* needed and, if so, what type should be used?
5. Is the fracture one that may require *internal fixation*?

Stable fracture

The majority of isolated fractures of the metacarpals and phalanges are stable and require no reduction or immobilization. Common examples are linear fractures of the metacarpal shafts, fractures of the neck of the little finger metacarpal bone without malrotation of the finger and the simpler undisplaced fractures of the phalanges. The finger can be protected by splinting it to an adjacent digit using 'buddy strapping' or a simple removable splint (Figure 26.21) and early active movement must be encouraged. Much harm can be done by unecessary and prolonged immobilization in a splint or plaster, which can lead to irreversible joint stiffness.

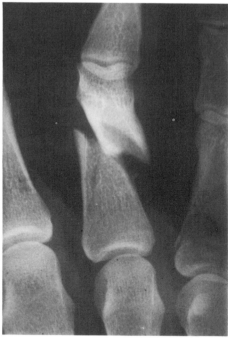

Figure 26.22 A typical unstable fracture of the proximal phalanx

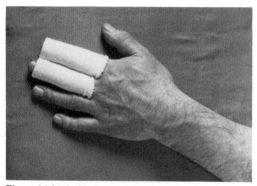

Figure 26.21 A simple splint for stable fractures of the phalanges

Unstable fractures

Oblique and transverse fractures of the proximal phalanx are intrinsically unstable and will often displace because of the pull of attached tendons (Figure 26.22). They should be reduced with appropriate anaesthesia and then splinted. A most satisfactory form of external immobilization is provided by a strong strip of aluminium padded with foam sponge and applied to the volar aspect of the digit (Figure 26.23). As always, the injured digit is

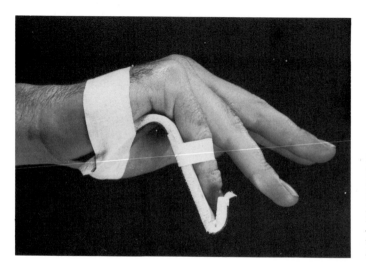

Figure 26.23 A light metal splint, padded with foam rubber, used to immobilize a phalangeal fracture. Note that the metacarpophalangeal joint is flexed and the interphalangeal joints are extended – the 'position of immobilization' in which the joints are least likely to develop fixed contractures

splinted in the 'position of immobilization' with the metacarpophalangeal joint at 90° and the interphalangeal joint in not more than 15° of flexion. There is no need for the splint to extend proximal to the wrist. It is a general principle that uninvolved digits should not be splinted if at all possible. For this reason plaster splinting is seldom required and can be positively harmful by impeding the use of the uninjured part of the hand.

There is no place for traction in the management of unstable fractures of the hand.

Internal fixation

Most fractures can be managed satisfactorily with the methods described above, but internal fixation may be required for (1) unstable fractures that cannot be controlled by splintage; (2) displaced fractures entering joints; and (3) multiple fractures, especially if there is associated soft tissue damage.

Fine Kirschner wires, intraosseous wiring or small screws are adequate to stabilize most fractures in the hand (Figure 26.24). Compression plating has little place and is virtually contraindicated for phalangeal fractures as the soft tissue dissection required is only too likely to cause adherence of adjacent soft tissues.

Open fractures

Careful debridement is necessary. Completely detached fragments of bone are removed and bone ends that are grossly contaminated must be cleaned by trimming. The care of the skin wound follows the principles given previously.

If the fracture is stable a boxing-glove bandage will provide a satisfactory support and dressing. It is often necessary to treat unstable fractures by internal fixation, particularly if there are multiple fractures, difficult skin problems or circulatory embarrassment. In these circumstances Kirschner wires should be used as for closed fractures, provided there has been adequate excision of the wound.

Injuries of joints

Ligamentous injuries

Sprains are quite common and will settle down without specific treatment, although occasional discomfort may persist for some months.

There are two ligamentous injuries that are easily missed and cause prolonged disability. If rupture of the ulnar collateral ligament of the metacarpophalangeal joint of the thumb is undetected at the time of injury, the thumb will remain weak and unstable when gripping. The ligament will not heal

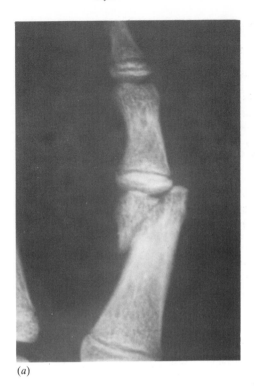

(*a*)

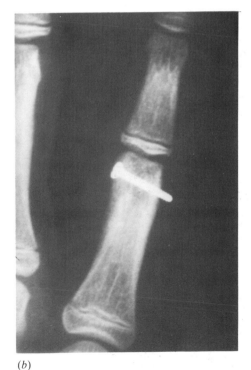

(*b*)

Figure 26.24 (*a*) An unstable intra-articular fracture; (*b*) internal fixation with a small screw

satisfactorily by immobilization alone, as it is usually avulsed from the base of the proximal phalanx and comes to lie superficial to the adductor aponeurosis which separates it from its attachment. An operation is necessary to reattach the ligament. Similar prolonged disability can result from a rupture of one of the collateral ligaments of the proximal interphalangeal joint of a finger. If instability can be demonstrated on stress examination the ligament should be repaired surgically as this will result in a quicker recovery of joint function.

Dislocations

Dislocations of the interphalangeal joints can usually be reduced easily under ring block anaesthesia. The temptation to 'pop back' an obviously dislocated joint should be resisted until a radiographic film has been taken to exclude an associated fracture. Another film should be taken to confirm reduction and the collateral ligaments must be examined.

Dislocations of the metacarpophalangeal joints may be difficult or impossible to reduce by closed means because of soft tissue interposition. Force should never be used and an open reduction should be performed if there is any difficulty.

Fractures involving joints

Internal fixation may be necessary to restore the articular surface and allow early mobilization.

Acute infections of the hand
General principles

The classic surgical infections of the hand are now relatively uncommon. Lack of experience may result in inadequate treatment with unnecessary prolongation of disability and sometimes even serious loss of function.

The general principles of management of hand infections are, however, straightforward:

1. Rest is required in the diffuse stage of infection.
2. Elevation is required to reduce swelling.
3. Diffuse, spreading infections are controlled by antibiotics. Surgical drainage is not helpful.
4. Surgical drainage, not antibiotic treatment, is indicated when localized pus has formed. Abscesses must be drained by small incisions sited to provide direct drainage without risking damage to important structures. *There are no standard incisions in the surgery of the infected hand.*

In the diffuse stage of infection

During the stage of cellulitis before an abscess has formed the aim of treatment is to abort the infection if it is early, or to localize it if it is more advanced. Fomentations, 'hot soaks' and 'drawing' ointments are unnecessary. The mainstays of treatment are rest, elevation and antibiotic therapy.

Rest

The hand is splinted in the position of immobilization with a volar plaster-of-Paris slab or a boxing-glove dressing.

Elevation

This is necessary to reduce oedema and prevent stiffness. Most patients with hand infections require admission to hospital where it is possible to maintain elevation by suspending the arm from an overhead support.

Antibiotic therapy

This may abort some early infections completely. It is essential for the control of spreading cellulitis, lymphangitis and bacteraemia. Most suitable antibiotics are effective by mouth but in a severe infection they should be given by injection to ensure rapid onset of action. At this early stage of infection antibiotics must be given on an empirical basis. Flucloxacillin (500 mg orally every 6 h for adults) is the most frequently used antibiotic, since most hand infections are caused by penicillinase-producing staphylococci or, in the case of spreading infections, penicillin-sensitive streptococci). Before it is given enquiry should be made for previous sensitivity to any variety of penicillin. Tetracycline (250–500 mg orally every 6 h for adults) or clindamycin (150–300 mg every 6 h before meals) are suitable alternatives if such a history is obtained. The possibility of infection by mixed organisms should be borne in mind and the antibiotic regime altered appropriately. Infections due to *Bacteroides* are common in bite wounds and metronidazole (400 mg orally every 8 h) is usually effective.

In the stage of localization

No operation should be done unless there is definite evidence of localized pus, which may be present when the patient is first seen or after some days of conservative treatment. Recognition of abscess formation is therefore all-important. It is suggested if a diffuse ache is replaced by a severe throbbing pain that keeps the patient awake. Confirmatory signs are: (1) visible subcuticular pus; (2) well-localized tenderness found by pressing gently on the suspected area with the closed points of a pair of forceps; and (3) the appearance of a dusky cyanotic spot in the centre of a reddened area of cellulitis.

Anaesthesia

No incision should be made without complete anaesthesia. 'Freezing' with an ethyl chloride spray is useless. General anaesthesia is usually preferable and should give full relaxation; there is no place for a 'whiff of gas', which so often results in a struggling patient and does not permit the careful, unhurried technique that is essential for success.

The operation

It is essential that the operation be carried out in a bloodless field with tourniquet control in order to obtain a clear view into the depths of an abscess cavity. The arm is exsanguinated by elevation before inflating the tourniquet.

The skin of the affected area is cleaned with a solution of 0.5% chlorhexidine in spirit and the incision is made. The aim is to provide drainage by the most direct route by an incision which will heal with the least possible scarring. The site of the incision is chosen before anaesthetizing the part and is usually at the position of maximum tenderness. If possible it should lie parallel to flexor creases and not cross them.

Subcuticular pus may represent the superficial component of a collar-stud abscess (Figure 26.25).

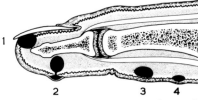

Figure 26.25 Diagram of finger to show various types of abscess: 1, apical abscess; 2, pulp abscess with collar-stud extension; 3, subcutaneous abscess; 4, intracutaneous abscess

The operation is commenced by uncapping the superficial abscess and then a deep connection is sought. If present, it is gently probed to determine its extent and then enlarged by an incision through the dermis to permit inspection of the walls of the deeper cavity. The edges of the incision are parted and pus is mopped out with a pledget of cotton-wool. Any loose slough is picked out with fine forceps and obviously dead subcutaneous fat is cut away, care being taken not to remove any healthy tissue. During the removal of dead tissue the depths of the cavity are inspected frequently to make sure

that important adjacent structures, such as tendon sheaths or digital nerves, are not damaged.

If subcuticular pus is not visible the abscess is opened by an incision 0.5 cm in length placed immediately over it. After pus is located the wound is enlarged as necessary to allow free drainage and exploration as described above.

Irrespective as to whether the abscess is superficial or deep the edges of the skin are cut back with fine pointed scissors to form a narrow, diamond-shaped opening. No drains are used and the wound should never be plugged with a gauze wick. A dry gauze dressing is applied and held in place with a boxing-glove dressing or, in the fingers, a tubegauze dressing (see p. 69). The tourniquet is then removed and the arm elevated.

After-care

The dressing must be kept dry. A dressing change is carried out the day after operation with appropriate sedation or anaesthesia; as a rule the dressing can be removed easily, but may need soaking off in a 1% solution of cetrimide. The wound edges should be separated gently and the abscess cavity inspected carefully to make sure that drainage remains adequate; there is any doubt about this the abscess cavity must be further explored under anaesthesia. A fresh dressing is then applied. Subsequent dressing changes are carried out at intervals of 1–3 days until healing is complete.

Antibiotics are not usually required after the first 24 h unless: (1) the abscess is very large, (2) there are signs of bone infection, or (3) there is evidence of continuing spreading infection.

It may be necessary to continue splintage and elevation for several days if there is much oedema or surrounding cellulitis. Active mobilization should, however, be encouraged as soon as the infection is under control.

Specific types of infection
Paronychia

Acute infection of the nail fold is very common. It begins as a cellulitis but pus rapidly forms and localizes at the sides of the nail or superficial to its base. Without treatment pus may discharge spontaneously by separation of the cuticle from the surface of the nail, but more often the pus continues to extend beneath the nail which eventually floats on a pool of pus.

Antibiotic therapy is used only if the infection is seen at a very early stage and there is a prospect of it being aborted completely. If pus has formed, operation is required, not antibiotics. Pus is released by stripping back the cuticle and lateral nail folds from the surface of the nail, using the closed points of fine dissecting forceps (Figure 26.26). No cutting is needed, except to trim away any loose portions of cuticle. Drains are not used, nor is it necessary to tuck gauze between the nail fold and the nail. A portion of the base of the nail should be resected if it is undermined by pus, to allow free drainage (Figure 26.27). The nail will be obviously loose and lacking its normal lustre. Care should be taken that no small fragments of dead nail remain.

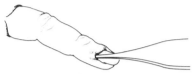

Figure 26.26 Elevation of nail fold to drain a paronychia

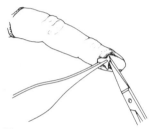

Figure 26.27 Resection of base of nail if there is pus beneath it

Pulp abscess

Infection of the terminal pulp is relatively common and potentially serious. Pus may not be localized when the patient is first seen and it is a bad mistake to incise too early.

Before localization, pulp infections are treated conservatively with rest and antibiotics but operation is required forthwith if there is clear evidence of localized pus. The old 'hockey-stick' (Figure 26.28a) and 'fish-mouth' incisions should not be used. The incision should be made directly over the abscess, as indicated by the point of maximum tenderness (Figure 26.28b). Collar-stud abscesses are common in the pulp and failure to recognize the

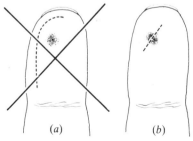

Figure 26.28 Incision for pulp abscess: (*a*) wrong; (*b*) correct

deep extension to the pocket is the commonest mistake made in the treatment of this condition. Pulp abscesses are often complicated by bone infection or sloughing of soft tissue if treatment has been delayed. Early osteitis may resolve with drainage of the pulp abscess and antibiotic therapy but in more severe cases there may be sequestration of much of the distal part of the terminal phalanx. The wound will not heal until the sequestrum has separated, which may take several weeks, with consequent prolonged disability, a course of events that underlines the importance of dealing with pulp space infections by adequate drainage at the right time.

Apical abscess

This is a variety of pulp space infection, but is not so serious because the main pulp space is not involved and bone infection is rare. The abscess points under the free edge of the nail; it is drained by a transverse incision at the tip of the finger (Figure 26.29a) and a V-shaped wedge of nail is removed (Figure 26.29b).

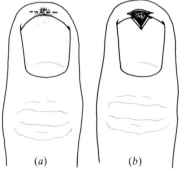

Figure 26.29 Apical abscess: (*a*) site of initial incision; (*b*) excision of V-wedge of nail

Subcutaneous abscess

This is similar in many respects to a pulp abscess, but occurs in the more proximal parts of the finger or the palm (Figure 26.25). It is treated along the same lines as a pulp abscess. Care must be taken when draining an abscess on the flexor aspect of the finger that the flexor tendon sheath is not opened. *Intradermal abscesses* are not common. They are small but very painful. Treatment is by drainage.

Carbuncle

A carbuncle is a result of infection of a hair follicle and therefore occurs on the dorsum of the hand. Treatment is conservative; antibiotics will encourage the infection to localize and after a few days a core of slough will separate, leaving a suprisingly large hole which heals rapidly.

Web-space abscess

This is commonly the result of minor trauma of the palmar skin, particularly if there has been blistering. Dorsal oedema may be marked, particularly in the early stages, and it may be difficult to decide where the pus lies. Later there is a characteristic separation of the fingers adjacent to the affected web.

Unless pus is obviously pointing, 24 h of conservative treatment is often worthwhile. The hand is splinted, elevated and spreading infection is controlled by antibiotics. When swelling has been reduced, the abscess is opened by a transverse incision on the palmar aspect, opposite the interdigital space and about 1 cm proximal to the free edge of the web. Initially the skin only is incised, to avoid damage to adjacent digital nerves. The abscess cavity is entered by blunt probing, and its extent is determined. Subcutaneous tissue is incised carefully to unroof the abscess and provide free drainage (Figure 26.30); a dorsal counter incision is not usually necessary. A vertical web-splitting incision must be avoided as it will produce a contracting scar.

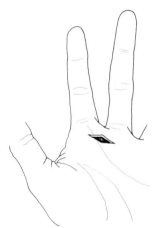

Figure 26.30 Site of incision for drainage of web-space abscess. Edges are cut back to form a diamond-shaped opening

Palmar abscesses

These uncommon abscesses may occur in the following sites:

1. Subaponeurotic. The abscess is deep to the palmar fascia and may follow a penetrating injury. Pus often extends along the line of penetration, causing a collar-stud abscess (Figure 26.31).
2. Mid-palmar space. Pus lies deep to the flexor tendons in the palm.
3. Thenar space. The abscess lies between the thenar muscles and adductor pollicis.

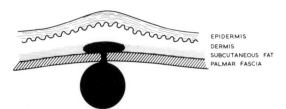

Figure 26.31 Subfascial abscess of the palm with a superficial collar-stud extension

Swelling of the dorsum of the hand is marked, because the skin is not bound down firmly to the underlying fascia as it is in the palm. The concavity of the palm is, however, obliterated in the region of the abscess and there is severe pain on local pressure in the palm.

A short period of conservative treatment is often needed to limit the spread of infection and to reduce oedema, but the abscess should be opened as soon as it has localized. A subaponeurotic abscess is opened by an incision in, or parallel to, a palmar crease but the fascia should be incised vertically to minimize the risk of damage to digital nerves and vessels. A mid-palmar abscess can be drained by an incision directly over the abscess; an alternative is to open the space via one of the lumbrical canals which can be entered by an incision in one of the interdigital web spaces. Whichever route is chosen very great care should be taken not to damage digital nerves and vessels. The thenar space may be drained by similar techniques; the entrance to the appropriate lumbrical canal lies on the radial side of the index finger in the first web space.

Tendon sheath infection

This infection usually follows a penetrating injury, particularly at the level of one of the flexor creases in a digit. The finger may be only slightly swollen, but is exquisitely painful and the pain is made worse by passive movements. Untreated, the infection can result in sloughing of the flexor tendon. The tendon sheath of the affected digit should be drained by two incisions, a transverse one in the distal palmar crease and a mid-lateral one in the distal part of the digit. A fine catheter is threaded up the sheath from the proximal incision and the sheath is irrigated with isotonic saline. The catheter is left *in situ* to allow further irrigation over the next 24 h, the hand is splinted in a boxing-glove dressing and systemic antibiotics are given in full dosage.

Septic arthritis

This common infection almost invariably follows a misplaced punch which strikes the mouth, causing a tooth to pentrate a metacarpophalangeal joint when the first is clenched; when the hand is relaxed the puncture wound is sealed and free drainage of infected material is prevented. Treatment consists of opening the joint, irrigating it with isotonic saline and giving antibiotics, which must be effective against the anaerobic organisms that are found in the human mouth flora. The joint is left open and the hand is splinted.

Erysipeloid

Infection with *Erysipelothrix rhusiopathiae* follows minor scatches from fish scales or meat bones. It is therefore most often seen in fishmongers, butchers and housewives. Ths finger is dusky red and swollen but not painful, although it may be itchy. The course of the infection is shortened by treatment with penicillin.

Herpetic whitlow

This is due to infection with the herpes simplex virus and is seen most commonly in nurses, doctors and dentists who come in contact with patients with infected orotracheal secretions. It is an acutely painful condition of the fingertip that may be confused with pulp abscess or paronychia, but the appearance of little vesicles around a central lesion is characteristic. Treatment is essentially symptomatic and the initial attack usually resolves in 7–10 days, although recurrence may occur. Painting the skin with a 5% solution of idoxouridine in dimethyl sulphoxide will sometimes relieve the acute pain if treatment is started early.

27

Paediatric surgery

L. Spitz and D. F. M. Thomas

Paediatric surgery is best organized in such a way as to concentrate specialized surgery, such as the correction of major congenital anomalies, in regional centres. Less complex problems, e.g. hernia, undescended testis, emergency surgery (intussusception, appendicitis, etc.) and trauma are generally shared with general surgeons who have had some training in paediatric surgery. The non-operative aspects of surgical management demand an understanding of the physiological and psychological differences between children and adults. Of equal importance to the general surgeon is the ability to recognize those conditions which should prompt referral to a specialist centre. The purpose of this chapter is to provide detailed practical guidance for surgeons involved in the care of children.

Definitions

Neonate

The neonatal period is defined as the first 28 days of extrauterine life. This standard definition can be modified to take account of the increasing survival of premature babies. In this modified definition gestational age is considered in addition to the duration of postnatal life. A neonate is an individual in whom the sum of gestational age and postnatal life is less than 44 weeks.

Infant

This imprecise term is generally understood to relate to the first year of life.

Child

Childhood ends with puberty. Since the onset and duration of puberty vary, an upper age limit of 14 years is usually applied.

The child as a surgical patient

Physiology

A full-term newborn baby weighs, on average, 3.5 kg and has a surface area of $0.19\,m^2$. The ratio of surface area to weight is twice that of an adult and imposes a very genuine risk of hypothermia or excessive insensible fluid loss. The neonatal kidney is unsophisticated and can function only within a limited homeostatic range. During the first four weeks of life the diuretic response to water load is poor and injudicious infusion of intravenous fluids can rapidly result in circulatory overload and oedema. Fluid restriction is generally better tolerated. Many hepatic enzyme systems are immature with the result that drugs and anaesthetic agents are only slowly detoxified. Drug dosages should be calculated individually on a weight basis with careful reference to the manufacturer's data or a paediatric prescribing compendium. Finally, a combination of low immunoglobulin levels and reduced leucocyte activity lower the child's resistance to infection, particularly in the newborn period.

Anatomy

Body size in itself does not present insurmountable problems. The results of surgery in very low birth weight babies are determined more by the medical complications of prematurity than by the technical limitations of surgery. In recent years the technology of paediatric care has improved considerably and a wide range of cannulae, infusion sets, catheters and drains are now available in appropriate sizes. An anatomical consideration of great importance, however, is the fact that congenital anomalies are frequently multiple. The discovery of one abnormality should always prompt a careful search for others. For example, exomphalos is frequently associated with severe congenital heart disease. Imperforate anus is a clearly visible anomaly but failure to diagnose a possible coexistent oesophageal atresia could result in fatal inhalation pneumonia.

Psychology

It is now widely accepted that admission to hospital may have harmful psychological sequelae and these are largely related to the child's age, the site and extent of the surgical procedure, the degree of associated discomfort and the duration and circumstances of hospital admission. It seems that children are most vulnerable between the ages of 1 and 4 years and whenever possible elective surgery should be performed outside this period or carried out on a day-case basis. General anaesthesia is preferable for all but the most minor surgical procedures. Questions are best answered honestly. A child who has been misled (albeit from good intention) that a procedure such as venepuncture will be painless will soon learn that the contrary is true and may harbour a continuing mistrust of doctors. On the other hand, there is no need to invoke unnecessary apprehension by an over-detailed account. Explanations and answers are best confined to immediate problems and procedures.

The benefits of unrestricted parental visiting far outweigh any minor irritations to the medical and nursing staff. The comforting presence of a parent is often very helpful in ensuring that vital infusions, catheters and drains remain in position for the time intended. We feel that every effort should be made to enable mothers of small children to be resident. Mothers who are breast feeding require encouragement and practical support to ensure that lactation is sustained during the period their child is taking 'nil by mouth'. Flexibility and a considerate approach will promote an atmosphere in which parents, medical and nursing staff can work together for the child's benefit.

Day-case surgery

Day-case surgery has proven benefits for the child and the family. Efficient routine is the key to its success.

1. Careful patient selection should be performed at the initial outpatient visit. Potential anaesthetic risks should be identified and investigated, e.g. sickle-cell screening tests for non-Caucasian children.
2. Clear, written instructions will be required by the parents. The time and place where they should report for admission should be clearly stated as

must be the instruction to give nothing by mouth for 6 h before admission. (For infants a period of 4 h is sufficient.)
3. If possible, day-case operations should be grouped together as a separate operating list. If this is not feasible, day-case procedures should be performed sufficiently early in the day to permit time for recovery. An experienced anaesthetist must decide whether children who have required endotracheal intubation can be allowed home on the same day but difficulty with extubation is an indication for overnight observation. Low grade fever (less than 38.5°C) is a common physiological response to surgery and, in the absence of other symptoms, does not justify extending hospitalization.
4. Subcuticular skin closure with absorbable suture material such as Dexon (polyglycolic acid) has obvious advantages in this group of patients.
5. Effective non-opiate postoperative analgesia is important. The use of intraoperative infiltration or nerve block with bupivacaine (Marcaine) is a valuable adjunct to conventional postoperative analgesia; 0.25% bupivacaine is injected towards the end of the operative procedure in a dosage up to 1 ml/kg. Clearly this form of analgesia is only appropriate for open procedures.

The following procedures are commonly performed on a day-case basis: herniotomy; circumcision; orchidopexy; endoscopy, e.g. cystoscopy, gastroscopy; minor orthopaedic procedures, e.g. change of plaster, manipulations; and minor ENT procedures, e.g. insertion of grommets.

Diagnostic procedures
Collection of blood
Venepuncture

The veins of the antecubital fossa are the most rewarding, followed by those of the dorsum of the hand, the scalp and the foot. Puncture of the internal jugular or femoral vein is rarely justified. In the case of the latter, there is a well-documented risk of resultant septic arthritis in the underlying hip joint. A tourniquet (such as a broad elastic band) is always useful, since it frees a hand to immobilize the child's arm or leg. Identify a suitable vein by inspection and palpation (very useful in chubby infants) and clean the venepuncture site with an antiseptic swab. A 21 G or 23 G needle is attached to the appropriate size of syringe and venepuncture is made with the bevel surface of the needle facing upwards. The aim is to enter rather than transfix the vein. Gentle suction is applied to the syringe – which should be allowed to fill slowly.

The use of a winged infusion needle is of particular value when large quantities of blood for serological investigations are required.

Heel prick

In the first few months of life this technique will invariably yield 1 or 2 ml of capillary blood. It is important to ensure that the foot is warm and well perfused. With the left hand, grasp the foot in such a way as to dorsiflex the ankle and encircle the heel with the thumb and forefinger. After cleaning with an antiseptic swab, make a stab with a disposable sterile lancet to a depth of about 2 mm. Blood should be collected by allowing it to drip into the container, not by scraping the lip of the container against the skin as this results in haemolysis. To promote the formation of discrete drops of blood, it may be helpful to apply a very thin film of sterile petroleum jelly to the skin of the heel at the start of the procedure.

Arterial sampling

Pulse oximetry and other forms of non-invasive oxygen monitoring have become widely available in recent years. The main purpose of this equipment is to provide continuous monitoring. It does not obviate the need for intermittent formal blood gas analysis, particularly in susceptible preterm infants. Arterial puncture remains, therefore, a valuable skill. The radial artery is the most appropriate for sampling in small children, but the temporal and brachial arteries can also be used. The technique of radial artery sampling is as follows: a 23 G or 25 G needle is fixed firmly to a 1–2 ml syringe (the syringe size being determined by preference for ease of handling rather than sample volume). Heparin is drawn into the syringe to prime the dead space of the hub and needle. The child's wrist should be in the neutral position, palm uppermost. It is often too difficult to locate the precise position of the artery by palpation but in small babies the radial artery may be visible as a blue line on the flexor aspect of the wrist. Otherwise, its surface marking is taken as the midpoint of the radial third of the wrist (just lateral to the tendon of flexor carpi radialis). With the bevel upwards the needle is advanced until bone is reached. Very gentle suction is applied to the syringe as the needle is very slowly withdrawn. If the artery has been successfully transfixed, blood will flow into the syringe. If the first attempt has been unsuccessful it may be repeated. Following sampling, it is important that firm local pressure is applied for at least 5 min to prevent haematoma formation. It must be noted that air bubbles or delay in analysis of the sample will invalidate the results. Samples which cannot be analysed within 10 min should be kept in ice.

Collection of urine

0–2 years of age (or until continent)

The perineum is first cleaned with soap and water and then dried with sterile cotton wool. Several self-adhesive urine collecting bags are commercially available; the most useful are those which incorporate a one-way device to prevent loss of the sample if the bag becomes detached. When a suitable volume (2–10 ml) has been collected the bag is removed and the urine drained into a sterile specimen container by removing the sealing strip (when provided) or by cutting a corner of the bag.

2–7 years of age (continent but unable to cooperate in the midstream collection manoeuvre)

A clean, ideally sterile, bowl is placed within a potty and after cleaning of the perineum as above the child is encouraged to void normally into the bowl.

7 years and over (or whenever the child can comprehend and perform the midstream manoeuvre)

Instructions are given to begin voiding, stop the flow in midstream and then void into a clean or sterile container. When the sample has been obtained, the child proceeds to complete bladder emptying.

Suprapubic puncture

This procedure is less popular than previously and its main value is to clarify repeatedly equivocal results obtained by other methods. Urethral abnormalities such as diverticula or the remnant of a recto-urethral fistula may produce persistent bacteriuria which is not representative of urine in the bladder and upper urinary tract. A full bladder is essential if this procedure is to be performed safely. The nursing staff are asked to note the time of voiding in order that puncture may be performed after an interval of at least one hour. The child is maintained in a supine position with the legs in abduction. The presence of a full bladder should be confirmed by percussion or palpation. After careful cleaning of the lower abdominal wall with antiseptic, the bladder is punctured by a vertical stab with a 21 G needle mounted on a 20 ml syringe. The point of puncture should be in the midline, 1–2 cm above the symphysis pubis. Depth of puncture depends on age, but is normally between 0.5 and 1.5 cm. When the sample has been collected the needle should be removed from the syringe before urine is transferred to a sterile container.

Urinary catheters

Whenever a urinary catheter is passed a specimen of urine should be obtained and sent for microscopy and culture. In addition, indwelling catheters should be sampled two or three times a week to screen for catheter-related urinary sepsis. The diagnosis must also be considered in any child with a catheter *in situ* who develops fever or unexplained symptoms.

Cerebrospinal fluid (CSF)

Meningitis features prominently in the differential diagnosis of unexplained clinical deterioration in children. For this reason it is fortunate that lumbar puncture is a relatively simple procedure in this age group. The conventional lumbar puncture needle has the benefit of a stilette to prevent blockage with tissue during insertion. However, if a suitable size needle is not available for smaller children, a 21 G needle or a winged infusion needle of the same calibre may also be used. Local anaesthetic is not used for lumbar puncture in neonates but it should certainly be used in infants. If drugs are to be instilled into the CSF (e.g. antileukaemic agents) it is wise to consider the use of a brief general anaesthetic. The child is positioned in the lateral position with the spine fully flexed. As with adults, it is of great importance to ensure that the plane between the iliac crests is strictly vertical and that the trunk is not allowed to roll over. The L4/L5 interspace is preferred in children and lies on, or caudal to, a line drawn between the superior posterior iliac spines. When the skin has been adequately prepared (e.g. with povidone-iodine solution) the needle is introduced strictly in the midline of the interspace and advanced slowly in the horizontal plane. The ligamentum flavum may offer little resistance and it is wise to remove the stilette frequently to check for the drainage of CSF. Ideally, manometry should be performed but in a sick, surgical baby the prime aim is to obtain adequate CSF for laboratory investigations with the minimum upset to the baby from prolonged handling. Common sense is required. A bloody tap is not infrequent, and if it occurs three numbered containers should be used to collect the CSF in order that microscopy may distinguish between the uniform blood staining associated with intracranial haemorrhage and the decreasing concentration of red cells which should characterize a bloody tap. The techniques of ventricular puncture and cisternal puncture are not described since we feel they should be performed only by experienced operators.

Intravenous fluids in paediatric surgery
Techniques and sites for intravenous infusion

Peripherally-sited cannulae should be used wherever possible. In the neonate, the use of umbilical, arterial or venous catheters may appear a tempting alternative but the complications such as lower limb ischaemia and necrotizing enterocolitis should limit their use to sampling and the administration of drugs for resuscitation.

Peripheral veins

Winged needles (e.g. Butterfly (Abbot))

These needles have the advantage of being easy to introduce by percutaneous puncture but unless they are well fixed the sharp tip tends to cut out of the vein, resulting in extravasation. Scalp veins are the most appropriate site since good fixation can be achieved. Shave the scalp in the parietal or temporal region and invoke the assistance of a nurse to immobilize the baby and place a finger over the proximal course of the selected vein. (Alternatively, an elastic band encircling the occipitofrontal circumference may be used as a scalp tourniquet.) The proposed puncture site is cleaned with, for example, isopropyl alcohol or chlorhexidine. The needle is advanced with the bevel upwards in the line of the vein until it has been successfully entered. Blood will be seen flowing back in the plastic tubing. *N.B.* It is easy to mistake the superficial temporal artery for a vein – in this case bright arterial blood will flow briskly into the tubing. The needle should be removed and firm local pressure applied. When the winged needle has been successfully introduced into a vein, a small volume of normal saline should be injected slowly to check that there is no extravasation. Strips of micropore or plaster-of-Paris are most effective in immobilizing the needle and this should be performed before attaching the infusion giving set. An inverted gallipot or similar container may be taped over the infusion site as additional protection against dislodgement of the needle.

Cannulae (Figure 27.1)

With practice, it is possible to introduce a 20 G or 22 G cannula into almost any visible peripheral vein. The skin of neonates and infants is relatively tough whereas their veins are fragile. Thus, in order to control the advance of the cannula through the subcutaneous tissues and guide its entry into the vein, it is necessary first to puncture the skin with a lancet. The veins on the dorsum of the hand are the most reliable sites in neonates and small infants

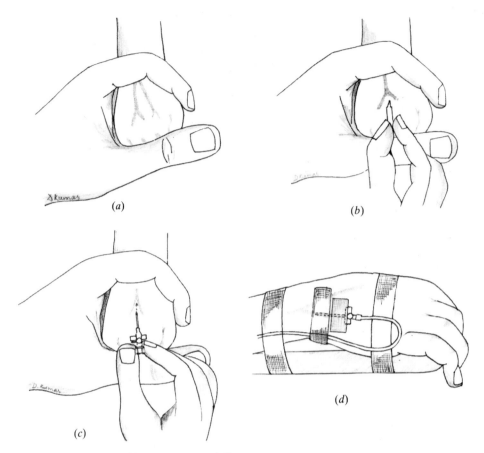

Figure 27.1 Technique of intravenous cannulation

(Figure 27.1a). A broad elastic band is a useful tourniquet which permits the assisting nurse the use of both hands to immobilize the child. Secure fixation and splintage of the infusion site is essential (Figure 27.1d). Umbilical catheters should *not* be used for the reasons already outlined.

Cannulating a dorsal vein of the hand (neonate or infant)

1. Use the left hand to grip and palmar flex the child's hand thus stretching and fixing the veins on the dorsum.
2. Clean the skin thoroughly with an antiseptic solution. With a lancet make a puncture site a few millimetres distal to a venous confluence or the proposed site of entry.
3. With the right hand introduce the cannula (bevel upwards) through the lancet puncture site and advance slowly until the vein has been entered. Remove the stilette and push the cannula gently up the vein using a rotating action if resistance is encountered.

4. Inject 1 ml of normal saline and observe for evidence of extravasation. If the saline flows easily and no swelling develops around the cannulation site, attach the infusion giving set and fix it in such a way as to prevent direct traction on the cannula. Splint the wrist in about 20° of palmar flexion.

Cutdown (Figure 27.2)

The advent of new paediatric cannulae has very much reduced the indication for this procedure. The antecubital veins may be employed but in an emergency the long saphenous vein at the ankle has the advantage of being the most consistent site anatomically. It should be noted, however, that the long saphenous route is unsuitable for major abdominal surgery or trauma since compression of or damage to the inferior vena cava may interfere with entry of infusion fluid into the circulation.

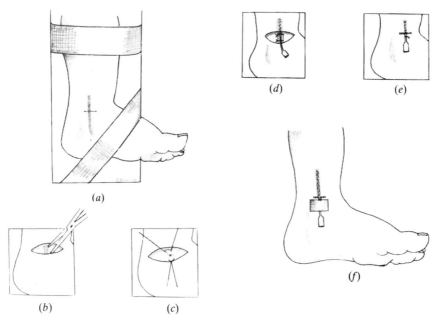

Figure 27.2 Technique of cutdown (long saphenous vein at the ankle)

Technique of cutdown on the long saphenous vein at the ankle points

Since this is a surgical procedure, full aseptic technique should be employed. A good light is essential. Before commencing the cutdown, immobilize the ankle by taping it firmly to a splint applied to its lateral aspect.

1. After cleaning and 'towelling up' the medial aspect of the ankle, infiltrate an area above and anterior to the medial malleolus with local anaesthetic, e.g. lignocaine 1%.
2. With a scalpel, make a transverse skin incision just above and anterior to the medial malleolus (the precise relationship and extent of the incision will depend on the child's age, but should rarely exceed 0.5–1.0 cm). Artery forceps should then be used to open up the subcutaneous tissues by blunt dissection until the long saphenous vein is evident lying on the tibia.
3. Mobilize the vein from surrounding fascia, taking particular care to separate it from the saphenous nerve which lies anteriorly. Pass two stay ligatures (e.g. Dexon 3/0) under the vein and by traction on the distal stay, lift the vein up into the incision. Incise about one-third of the vein's circumference and introduce the desired cannula or Silastic catheter. If a tourniquet has been used, the 'non-sterile' assistant should be asked to remove it at this stage.
4. The proximal stay ligature is tied around the vein to secure the cannula within it. Venous oozing from the distal direction is usually sufficient to require ligation of the distal stay to occlude the vein below the venotomy site.
5. The incision is closed with one or two sutures and covered with a sterile dressing.

Central veins

The indications for central venous catheterization include:

1. Major surgery or resuscitation.
2. Central venous pressure monitoring.
3. Long-term parenteral nutrition.

Percutaneous puncture, e.g. the internal jugular vein or subclavian vein

These techniques are valuable but not without complications, such as pneumothorax, haemothorax and damage to major vessels or the thoracic duct. For these reasons this route is not recommended for the occasional operator.

It may be possible to introduce a Silastic catheter at a peripheral site and thread it into a central position. The basilic antecubital vein and scalp veins have been used for this purpose. Venepuncture is performed with a large-calibre winged needle (the attached plastic tubing having first been removed) and Silastic tubing is fed through the needle to reach a central site. It is important to note that, in the event of failure, the catheter should not be withdrawn through the needle because of the real risk of cutting across it with the point of the needle. Both the catheter and needle should be removed together as a single manoeuvre.

Surgically placed central venous catheters, e.g. internal jugular vein, external jugular vein, subclavian vein, femoral vein

General anaesthesia is mandatory. After surgical exposure of the selected vein, a Silastic catheter is introduced and advanced into the right atrium. Radiological confirmation of the catheter position is essential. By creating a subcutaneous tunnel and bringing the catheter out at a distant site, rather than through the surgical incision, it is possible to minimize infection. With careful nursing, these catheters may remain in position for several weeks or months.

Fluids for infusion
Maintenance and postoperative fluids

1. Neonates: dextrose 10% saline 0.18%.
   N.B. If this combination is not available an approximation (dextrose 8% saline 0.18%) can be made up by the addition of 20 ml of normal saline to 80 ml of Dextrose 10% in a paediatric infusion burette.
2. Infants and children: dextrose 4% saline 0.18%.

Resuscitation

Plasma (plasma protein fraction) is the volume expander of choice.

Intravenous nutrition

See section on intravenous feeding, p. 395.

Intravenous fluid requirements
Maintenance fluids

The fluid requirements before operation and on the fourth and subsequent postoperative days are shown in Table 27.1

Examples

A 7.5 kg infant will require 7.5 × 100, i.e. 750 ml/day.

A 16.0 kg child would receive 1000 ml plus 6 x 50 ml, i.e. total 1300 ml/day.

A 28.0 kg child would receive 1500 ml plus 8 x 25 ml, i.e. total 1700 ml/day.

Table 27.1 Maintenance intravenous fluid requirements

Weight	Daily requirements
Neonates	
1500 g	180 ml/kg/24 h
1500–2500 g	150 ml/kg/24 h
2500 g	120 ml/kg/24 h
Infants and children	
10 kg or less	100 ml/kg/day
10–20 kg	1000 ml/day plus 50 ml/kg/day for each kg above 10 kg
Above 20 kg	1500 ml/day plus 25 ml/kg/day for each kg above 20 kg

Postoperative intravenous fluids
Neonates

First 48 h after operation: one-third of maintenance requirements. Third and fourth days after operation: two-thirds of maintenance requirements. Fifth and subsequent days: full volume maintenance requirements.

Infants and children

First 24 h after operation: half of maintenance requirements. Second and third days after operation: two-thirds of maintenance requirements. Fourth and subsequent days: full volume maintenance requirements.

Fluid balance – abnormal losses

The volumes of nasogastric aspirate, enteric fistula output and other extracellular fluid losses should be carefully recorded and replaced volume for volume with normal (0.9%) saline with the addition of 10 mmol potassium chloride/500 ml of saline solution.

Urinary output – normal and abnormal water loss

By the end of the first week of life, the normal urinary output has risen to 100–120 ml/kg/day. Following surgery the minimal acceptable output is 40 ml/kg/day (roughly 2 ml/kg/h). In older children insensible loss is relatively unimportant but is far more significant in neonates, particularly premature babies. The use of an overhead radiant heater or phototherapy for jaundice may increase fluid intake requirements by between 50 and 200%. Additional intravenous fluids should be given and careful monitoring of urinary output and serum electrolytes is essential.

Electrolyte replacement

Sodium (normal requirement 3 mmol/kg/day)

Provided abnormal losses are accurately replaced (see above), it is not normally necessary to calculate sodium balance on a formal basis. Nevertheless, one must be aware of the salt-losing potential of the neonatal kidney and plasma electrolytes should be checked daily. A plasma value of less than 130 mmol/l requires correction.

A suitable formula for replacement is:

Sodium requirement (mmol) = sodium deficit (mmol/l) x body weight (kg) x 0.6

(*N.B.* Normal saline 0.9% contains 154 mmol of sodium/l).

Potassium – (normal requirement 2 mmol/kg/day)

When 24 h have elapsed since operation and provided urine output has been re-established (at least 40 ml/kg/day), potassium replacement should be added to the infusion. A maintenance concentration is 20 mmol/l. Since potassium is an intracellular ion, plasma levels are an insensitive reflection of total body potassium status. Nevertheless, a value of under 3.5 mmol/l usually requires correction. The following rules are applied:

1. The deficit should be corrected with an infusion containing 20–40 mmol/l of potassium chloride.
2. The total input of potassium should not exceed 5 mmol/kg/day.
3. Urinary output should be adequate.
4. Plasma levels (and possibly ECG) should be checked every 12–24 h depending on the rate of replacement.

Correction of other metabolic deficits

Metabolic acidosis

It is difficult to give a precise value of base deficit beyond which correction is required. The indications for corrections depend on the clinical context. In practice, in a sick neonate or infant, a deficit of between 5 and 10 mmol/l justifies correction.

A suitable formula is:

Sodium bicarbonate required (mmol or ml of an 8.4% solution) – base deficit (mmol/l) $\times$ body weight (kg) $\times$ 0.3.

Hypoglycaemia

Irreversible cerebral damage can result from undetected or inadequately treated hypoglycaemia. The risk is much greater in children than in adult surgical patients. 'Small for dates' babies are at particular risk.

1. Correct any blood sugar level of less than 2.2 mmol/l (40 mg/100 ml) with an infusion of dextrose 10% (75–100 ml/kg/day).
2. Correct symptomatic hypoglycaemia immediately with an intravenous injection of dextrose 50% (1–2 ml/kg) as a stat dose, repeated as necessary and followed by dextrose 10% infusion.

Hypocalcaemia

A plasma value (total calcium) of less than 1.5 mmol/l merits correction with calcium gluconate 10% 1–2 ml/kg i.v. as a stat dose followed by an infusion containing calcium gluconate 10% 5 ml/100 ml of infusion solution. (*N.B.* calcium solutions interact with sodium bicarbonate.)

Resuscitation: correction of hypovolaemia

Plasma (PPF) is administered at an initial 'push' rate of 20/kg/h for infants under 10 kg in weight and 10–15/kg/h for older children. The infusion rate should be reviewed at or before 1 h. Visible or suspected concealed haemorrhage should be countered by transfusion with whole blood as soon as it becomes available. Two points are of importance:

1. Infection is an extremely common cause of unexplained collapse in the paediatric surgical patient. Empirical broad-spectrum antibiotic treatment should be started more readily than in adults.
2. Sick surgical neonates and infants are often glycogen depleted and exposed to the risk of hypoglycaemia during periods of stress. When calorie-free solutions are being used for resuscitation it is necessary to perform frequent, e.g. half-hourly, Dextrostix estimations of blood sugar. If necessary, infusions of plasma or blood should be alternated with dextrose 10% or, ideally, a second infusion set up to provide a continuous infusion of dextrose.

Intravenous nutrition

The last decade has witnessed a revolution in the postoperative management of children undergoing major gastrointestinal surgery. In contrast to adult patients, children have additional nutritional requirements for growth. In particular, consideration of brain growth dictates the much earlier use of intravenous feeding in this age group. There are also qualitative differences in children, for example, histidine is an essential amino acid and there are also requirements for other amino acids regarded as 'non-essential' in adults. A scaled-down adult regimen is inadequate – paediatric regimens must be tailored to their specific requirements. In many hospitals the solutions for parenteral nutrition, tailored to the individual requirements of each patient, are now dispensed from a central aseptic preparation area. This obviates the need for time consuming preparation of parental nutrition on the paediatric wards and reduces the risk of infection. If such a central service is not available, parenteral nutrition can be made up and administered according to the regimen detailed below.

Technique

Peripheral cannulae are used initially and by electively resiting infusion sites at 24-hourly intervals it is possible to forestall thrombosis and preserve peripheral venous access for several weeks. After a period of 3–4 weeks it is usually necessary to resort to the use of a central venous catheter. The arrangement of infusion pumps is shown in Figure 27.3. Dextrose and Vamin Glucose are infused alternately but Intralipid is given by continuous infusion apart from a 4 h period in the morning to

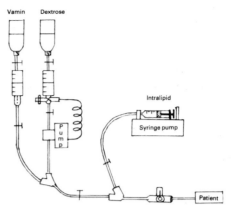

Figure 27.3 Diagram of method of administration of parenteral nutrition

permit clearing of blood lipids before samples are taken for laboratory investigations. A comprehensive regimen for prolonged total parenteral nutrition (TPN) is illustrated in Table 27.2. It is important to note that this applies only for infants under 10 kg in weight. Volumes and constituents should be modified accordingly for older children.

Precautions

Parenteral feeding regimens take no account of abnormal losses – these should be replaced volume for volume with the appropriate physiological

Table 27.2 Infusion rates and additives for introduction of parenteral nutrition and subsequent total parenteral nutrition (TPN) in infants up to 10 kg body weight

	Duration (hours/ day)	Infusion rates (ml/kg/h)			
		Day 1	Days 2 and 3	Days 4 and 5	Days 6 and TPN
Intralipid 20 plus Vitlipid Infant*	20	0.3	0.6	0.8	1.0
Vamin glucose plus Ped-El†	8§	2.5	4.0	5.0	6.0
Dextrose 10% (plus to each 500 ml: K_2HPO_4 17.42%: 4.0 ml NaCl 30%: 1.6 ml) plus Solivito‡	16§	6.0	–	–	–
Dextrose 10%‖ (plus to each 500 ml: K_2HPO_4 17.42%: 4.0 ml NaCl 30%: 1.0 ml) plus Solivito‡	16§	–	–	5.0	–
Dextrose 10%‖ (plus to each 500 ml: K_2HPO_4 17.42%: 35 ml NaCl 30%: 0.6 ml) plus Solivito‡	16§	–	–	5.0	–
Dextrose 10%‖ (plus to 500 ml: 16§ K_2HPO_4 17.42%: 3 ml) plus Solivito‡	16§	–	–	–	5.0

* Vitlipid Infant: 1 ml/kg to a maximum of 4 ml added to Intralipid syringe daily.
† Ped-El: 5 ml/kg to a maximum of 100 ml added to burette daily.
‡ Solivito: 1 ml/kg to a maximum of 4 ml added to burette daily (5 ml per vial).
§ Order of infusion: Vamin → Glucose → Glucose → Vamin, etc.
‖ Dextrose 15% may be given by central line but not by peripheral vein. (Reproduced from the *British Journal of Intravenous Therapy*.)

solution (normally 0.9% normal saline). Close biochemical monitoring is mandatory. During the first week of TPN the following investigations are required:

Blood urea ⎫
Blood electrolytes ⎬ daily
Blood glucose ⎪
Urinary glucose ⎭

Full blood count ⎫
Blood calcium/magnesium ⎬ twice weekly
Liver function tests ⎭

After the first week of TPN the frequency of these investigations is halved, i.e. urea, etc. on alternate days, full blood count, etc. weekly.

Sepsis is by far the most frequent complication of TPN and should be suspected as the probable cause of any fever or unexplained clinical deterioration. Treatment of this complication consists of removal of the central line or catheter and the cessation of TPN. Dextrose saline should be administered through a re-sited peripheral infusion – plasma may be required initially if there is hypovolaemic septic shock. Blood culture and culture of the catheter tip are required but broad-spectrum antibiotic treatment should be started immediately.

Blood transfusion

Viscous fluids such as packed red cells, platelet concentrate or even whole blood do not flow easily through the fine cannulae used in neonates. In particular, Silastic central venous catheters block so readily as to preclude their use. A peripherally sited cannula or needle is preferred. If blood will not drip through the infusion system under gravity several alternatives are possible.

1. Increase the 'hydrostatic' head of pressure by raising the height of the bag or bottle of blood above the patient.
2. Attach a three-way tap and syringe to the giving set, draw up and slowly inject a calculated volume of blood through the cannula every hour or half an hour (more frequently if the aim is to replace active blood loss).
3. Use a syringe pump to infuse under pressure at the appropriate rate. *N.B.* Blood should not be transfused by means of a peristaltic pump (e.g. IVAC). Haemolysis may result from this form of pumping action.

If a choice of blood preparations is available, whole blood is appropriate for:

1. Replacement of acute blood loss.
2. Volume expansion in septicaemia with or without disordered coagulation.

The freshest available whole blood or fresh frozen plasma should be used to supplement low levels of clotting factors in neonates and in septic states. Freshly packed red cells are appropriate for correction of anaemia due to chronic blood loss or impaired erythropoeisis. Platelet concentrate may be required for the specific correction of thrombocytopenia. Haematological advice should be sought.

Rate of transfusion
Acute blood loss

Peroperative loss is estimated by weighing swabs and measuring the contents of sucker bottles. Replacement is given volume for volume with whole blood. Other acute losses, e.g. gastrointestinal haemorrhage, must be replaced initially at an empirical rate determined by clinical judgement and the vital signs. An initial rate of 20 ml/kg/h would be modified in the light of clinical response, pulse and blood pressure readings (plus CVP values, if available).

Anaemia and subacute blood loss

As an approximate guide, 7 ml of whole blood/kg of body weight will raise the Hb by 1 g/dl.

Accurate replacement is calculated as follows:

Blood volume in infancy: 80 ml/kg body weight.
Whole blood for transfusion usually contains around 12 g/Hb/dl.
A 3000 g infant has a Hb of 7.0 g/dl.
Total blood volume: 3000 x 80 240 ml.
Total body Hb content: $240 \times 7/100 = 16.8$ g.
Ideal Hb concentration is 12.0 g.
Ideal total body Hb content $= 240 \times 12/100 = 28.8$ g.
Patient's Hb deficit = 12.0 g.
Hb of transfused blood: 12 g/dl.

Therefore, volume of transfused blood required is 100 ml.

N.B. When top-up transfusion is required, the total volume transfused during any 24 h period should not exceed 20 ml/kg. In the example above 60 ml of whole blood would be given on the first day followed by the balance of 40 ml on the following day.

Bowel preparation

The aim of preparation is to empty the bowel of any faecal residue, thus minimizing the risk of gross

Table 27.3 Bowel preparation

	Diet	Washouts
Two days before operation	Nourishing fluids	Twice
Day before operation	Clear fluids	Twice
Day of operation	Nil by mouth	None

peritoneal soiling and facilitating the surgery (Table 27.3). Since anaerobic bacteria appear to play a particular role in the genesis of postoperative infection, an endeavour is made to reduce their numbers and to ensure adequate tissue levels of antimicrobials at the time of surgery. Metronidazole is instilled into the rectum following preparatory large bowel washouts and systemic broad-spectrum antibiotic cover (e.g. gentamicin or mezlocillin) may be given during induction of anaesthesia.

Washout technique

0–6 months

A nasogastric tube is passed into the rectum and a 20 ml syringe attached. Saline is gently injected, then permitted to drain. The procedure is repeated until a total volume of about 200 ml has been used.

6–12 months

As above except that a Jacques or similar catheter is employed. The syringe volume is 50 ml and total washout volume 500 ml.

Over 12 months

A conventional washout set (funnel and tubing) is suitable. Depending on the age of the child, colonic capacity and faecal consistency, up to 2–3 litres may be necessary.

General care during operation

The prime considerations are prevention of hypothermia and accurate replacement of blood or other extracellular fluid loss. Insensible heat loss is a major threat to neonates.

1. Induction of anaesthesia is best performed under the thermal protection of an overhead radiant heater.

2. The ambient temperature of the operating theatre should be as high as is consistent with the comfort of the theatre staff – 25°C is ideal.
3. Body parts (e.g. limbs, head) not relevant to the operative procedure should be insulated by wrapping in aluminium foil.
4. An electric heating pad should be prewarmed and placed on the operating table.
5. Although it is not always feasible to pass infusion solutions through heating coils, some attempt must be made to warm those packs or bottles which have been stored under refrigeration.

Blood transfusion becomes necessary when 10% of the circulating volume has been lost (total blood volume = 80–85 ml/kg).

Measured losses are calculated from the weights of small batches of used swabs weighed frequently throughout the operation. Experience is required to make accurate estimates of additional losses from other sources (e.g. fluid absorption by surgical drapes and evaporative loss from exposed intestine). As a general guide, intravenous fluid is administered during surgery in a volume of 4–6 ml/kg/h.

Premedication

It is the responsibility of the anaesthetist to see the patient before operation and prescribe the appropriate premedication.

Routine premedication

(For dosage details see below)

Infants under 1 year of age: atropine only.
Small children (10–15 kg): atropine plus sedation, e.g. trimeprazine, pethidine injection.
Older children (over 15 kg): oral benzodiazepine premedication or papaveretum and hyoscine.

Much of the distress associated with induction of anaesthesia in children can be alleviated by the use of local anaesthetic cream under an occlusive dressing applied to the proposed site of venepuncture 1 h before operation, e.g. EMLA cream.

Neurosurgery (including head injuries)

Atropine only – avoid sedatives or CNS depressant.

Potential or actual upper airway obstruction

Atropine only. Preoperative sedation can seriously jeopardize the upper airway.

Dosage

Atropine

Up to 2.5 kg body weight: 0.15 mg
2.5–8 kg: 0.2 mg
8–15 kg: 0.3 mg i.m. 45 min before operation
15–20 kg: 0.4 mg
Over 20 kg: 0.5 mg

Papaveretum and hyoscine

Papaveretum 0.4 mg/kg
Hyoscine 0.008 mg/kg i.m. 1.5 h before operation.

N.B. Maximum dose of papaveretum 15 mg.

Trimeprazine (Vallergan)

Oral route only: 2–4 mg/kg 2 h before operation.

Injection Pethidine Compound (Inj. Peth. Co.)

Dose 0.06–0.08 ml/kg 1 h before operation.
(Pethidine content = 1.5–2.0 mg/kg)
Preparation: Pethidine 25 mg
            Promethazine 6.25 m in 1 ml
            Chlorpromazine 6.25 mg in 1 ml

Postoperative analgesia

Neonates

The use of opiates for neonatal analgesia carries a real risk of respiratory depression. The use of opiates in this age group requires specialist supervision and for the time being is probably best limited to specialist neonatal surgical centres.

Infants and older children

Continuous morphine infusion for children has been introduced recently. Its main use is in the management of postoperative pain following major surgery.

The technique is not applicable to children under 1 year of age. A suitable regimen is as follows:

Morphine 0.5 mg/kg is added to 50 ml of normal saline and the solution is then infused continuously at a rate of 1–3 ml/h. The rate is adjusted according to the analgesic response. Careful nursing supervision is required to detect possible respiratory depression and malfunction of the infusion pump.

Papaveretum   0.2–0.3 mg/kg i.m.
Pethidine   1 mg/kg i.m.
Morphine   0.1 mg–0.2 mg/kg i.m.
Paracetamol Elixir to 1 year 120 mg
                   1–5 years 240 mg
(Preparation 120 mg in 5 ml)
Metoclopramide (Maxolon)
    1–5 years 2.5 mg } i.m. or orally 2–3 times/day
    5–10 years 5 mg }
(Maximum total daily dose 0.5 mg/kg).

Neonatal surgery

Surgery during the neonatal period comprises largely the treatment of congenital anomalies. The specialized knowledge and expertise required when undertaking neonatal surgery necessitates the concentration of facilities, including the sophisticated support services of anaesthesia, pathology (histological and chemical), radiology and nursing care, within large centres serving widely dispersed populations. As will be shown later, infants can be safely transported over long distances provided adequate precautions are taken.

Diagnosis of congenital malformations

1. Antenatal detection of an anomaly.
2. Postnatal diagnosis:
    (a) External deformities;
    (b) Concealed anomalies:
        (i)   Respiratory distress
        (ii) Bilious vomiting
        (iii) Delayed passage of meconium
        (iv) Delayed micturition
        (v)   Passage of blood in the stools
        (vi) Abdominal masses

Antenatal detection of an anomaly

Certain social and physical conditions should alert the physician to the possibility of a fetal anomaly.

These include extremes of maternal age, primigravida and high multiparous mothers, low socio-economic status, single mothers and those who smoke during pregnancy, poor nutrition, diabetes and hypertension. Polyhydramnios in the mother may be indicative of a high intestinal obstruction, such as oesophageal atresia, duodenal or high jejunal atresia. Oligohydramnios should lead one to suspect the presence of renal agenesis, infantile polycystic disease or urinary obstruction.

Antenatal ultrasound is capable of detecting a wide range of fetal abnormalities during pregnancy. These include central nervous system disorders such as anencephaly, hydrocephalus, microcephaly, encephalocele and myelomeningocele, urinary tract anomalies, e.g. hydronephrosis, dysplasia, posterior urethral valves and tumours, and gastrointestinal problems. Typical examples of gastrointestinal malformations amenable to prenatal ultrasound detection include intestinal atresias (particularly duodenal atresia), diaphragmatic hernia, anterior abdominal wall defects (exomphalos and gastroschisis), and meconium ileus. Sacrococcygeal teratoma and cystic hygroma are examples of other lesions which can be detected. Fetal echocardiography can provide detailed information of congenital cardiac malformations which may be vitally important in determining the likely prognosis for the infant.

Increased maternal serum levels of alpha-fetoprotein (AFP) confirmed by high levels of AFP in the amniotic fluid may indicate the presence of a myelomeningocele although gastroschisis and multiple pregnancies also produce high levels. Amniocentesis is also helpful in the diagnosis of sex-related congenital malformations such as Duchenne muscular dystrophy and haemophilia and in enzymatic deficiency diseases. Chromosome analysis is helpful in detecting conditions such as Down's syndrome, Turner's syndrome, Klinefelter's syndrome, trisomy 13 and cri-du-chat syndrome (detection of short arm of fifth chromosome).

Postnatal diagnosis

External/surface deformities

Routine physical examination soon after birth will reveal externally obvious malformations such as cleft lip, myelomeningocele, exomphalos, gastroschisis, imperforate anus, ectopia vesicae, etc. Brief notes on these and other congenital anomalies will follow later in this section.

Concealed anomalies

The recognition of the significance of certain clinical features should alert the physician to suspect an abnormality of one of the internal viscera.

Respiratory distress

In the neonate respiratory distress is defined by the following features:

(a) Tachycardia (heart rate > 160/min).
(b) Tachypnoea (respiratory rate > 60/min).
(c) Expiratory grunting.
(d) Sternal and intercostal recession.
(e) Cyanosis.
(f) Apnoeic episodes.

Although idiopathic respiratory distress syndrome (IRDS), meconium aspiration and cardiac failure account for the majority of causes of respiratory distress, surgical conditions may be responsible and a radiograph of the chest and abdomen is mandatory in all cases. The surgical causes of respiratory distress include diaphragmatic hernia, oesophageal atresia with or without tracheo-oesophageal fistula, congenital lobar emphysema, tension pneumothorax and obstructive lesions involving the upper airways such as choanal atresia, Pierre Robin syndrome, cystic hygroma, etc.

Bilious vomiting

The presence of green bile in the vomitus is indicative of mechanical intestinal obstruction unless an alternative diagnosis, such as necrotizing enterocolitis or septicaemia, can be positively established. Non-bilious vomiting which is persistent may be due to gastro-oesophageal reflux, pyloric stenosis or a high duodenal obstruction.

Additional features of intestinal obstruction include abdominal distension (Figure 27.4), failure to pass meconium and hyperactive bowel sounds. The degree of abdominal distension is directly related to the level of the intestinal lesion. Distension is confined to the upper abdomen in duodenal and high jejunal obstruction, while in lower obstructions massive distension occurs, occasionally severe enough to cause respirator embarrassment. Small amounts of meconium may be passed even in complete intestinal atresias but the amount and colour of the meconium in these circumstances is not normal. Erythema and/or oedema of the anterior abdominal wall (Figure 27.5 is indicative of peritonitis or ischaemic intestine.

The causes of neonatal intestinal obstruction are:

1. Intraluminal – e.g. meconium ileus, milk inspissation, meconium plug syndrome.
2. Intramural – e.g. atresias and stenoses, Hirschsprung's disease, anorectal malformations
3. Extrinsic – e.g. malrotation ± volvulus, irreducible inguinal hernia, intussusception, duplication cysts.

Plain abdominal radiographs in the erect and supine positions are essential in the diagnostic

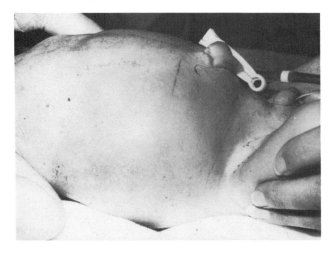

Figure 27.4 Abdominal distension due to Hirschsprung's disease in a neonate

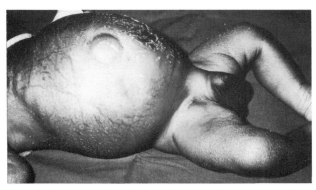

Figure 27.5 Oedema of the anterior abdominal wall indicates the presence of peritonitis – the circular depression is due to pressure from the bell of a stethoscope

work-up, while contrast studies are necessary for selected cases.

Delayed passage of meconium

Ninety-eight per cent of full-term infants and over 90% of premature infants will evacuate meconium spontaneously within the first 24 h of life. Failure to do so should alert the clinician to the possibility of Hirschsprung's disease. A suction rectal biopsy for ganglion cells should be performed in infants whose symptoms fail to resolve spontaneously. Infants with the other causes of mechanical intestinal obstruction will fail to pass meconium for mechanical reasons.

Failure to micturate

Normally the infant should pass urine within the first 24 h of life. The state of hydration of the infant who fails to micturate during this period should be assessed. If hydration is adequate, further investigation of the kidneys and urinary system should be undertaken with specific reference to posterior urethral valves and other causes of bladder outlet obstruction.

Rectal bleeding

In the neonatal period the passage of blood and mucus in the stool, especially when accompanied by abdominal distension and bile-tinged vomiting, is highly suspicious of necrotizing enterocolitis (NEC). Pneumatosis intestinalis on plain abdominal radiograph is diagnostic of NEC. Other causes of rectal bleeding in infancy include malrotation with volvulus, duplications, Meckel's diverticulum, intussusception and anal fissures. In the majority of cases, especially when there are merely small streaks of fresh blood on or in the stool, no cause can be found and the source is usually attributed to superficial ulceration in the anal canal or lower rectum.

Abdominal masses

The most common abdominal masses in infancy are benign conditions of the kidney (hydronephrosis, multicystic disease). Tumours, such as neuroblastoma and nephroblastoma, are rarely diagnosed in the neonatal period, with the exception of mesoblastic nephroma, a tumour closely related to Wilms' tumour but following a more benign course. Other benign cystic conditions such as mesenteric or duplication cysts may either be found on routine physical examination or may present with symptoms of intestinal obstruction due to compression of the adjacent intestine.

Transport of the surgical neonate

The newborn infant can be transported safely over a long distance provided adequate precautions are taken to maintain body temperature, monitoring facilities are available if required, and the accompanying staff are experienced and adequately equipped to deal with any cardiorespiratory emergency. When resuscitation is required for shock, hypothermia, respiratory insufficiency, disturbances of fluid, electrolytes or acid–base homeostasis, it is essential that therapeutic measures commence at the base hospital. Transfer may be delayed until the condition of the infant has stabilized. Where urgent surgery is essential, e.g. intestinal volvulus, gastrointestinal perforation or profuse haemorrhage, resuscitation measures should be continued during transfer by the transportation team.

The following requirements are necessary for the safe transfer of a surgical neonate:

1. Transport incubator ideally equipped with facilities for monitoring of heart rate, body temperature, inspired oxygen concentration and with an inbuilt mechanical ventilator (Figure 27.6).
2. Equipment necessary for cardiorespiratory resuscitation including laryngoscopes, endotracheal tubes, suction apparatus, chest drainage tubes and a variety of inotropic and respiratory stimulant drugs.
3. All surgical neonates, irrespective of whether there is evidence of intestinal obstruction, should have a nasogastric tube in position on free drainage with regular aspiration to ensure that the stomach is empty. This will prevent vomiting and aspiration during transfer.
4. A specimen of maternal blood (10 ml). This minimizes the amount of blood required from the infant for compatibility studies. Blood for transfusion should be available during all neonatal surgical procedures.
5. A valid consent form for surgery. The mother, having recently given birth, will not be able to accompany the infant to the referral centre and the father may have other commitments to care for siblings at home.
6. Copies of all records regarding the pregnancy, delivery and perinatal period including biochemical investigations, radiographs, etc. should be made available to the referral centre.
7. Special precautions:
   (a) Oesophageal atresia: the blind upper pouch must be kept empty during transfer to prevent aspiration of saliva. This is best achieved by continuous or frequent intermittent suction by an indwelling tube (the double-lumen Replogle tube is best suited for this purpose). Reflux of gastric content into the distal tracheo-oesophageal fistula and aspiration pneumonia is prevented by positioning the infant in the upright prone position.

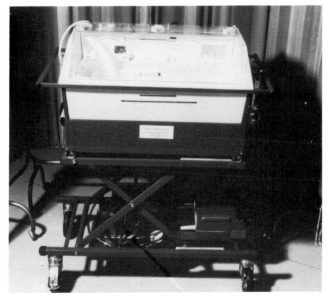

Figure 27.6 An example of a transport incubator

(b) Diaphragmatic hernia: infants presenting after the first 12–24 h can usually be managed in a high oxygen atmosphere. If this is inadequate and especially for infants presenting with acute respiratory distress soon after birth, an endotracheal tube and gentle mechanical ventilation are required. Ventilation by means of a face mask is strictly contraindicated as this forces air into the intestines which further compromises respiration. In all cases a large *patent* nasogastric tube should be passed and left on free drainage in order to limit the volume of gas entering the intestines. Any sudden deterioration during resuscitation or transfer should lead one to suspect the presence of a tension pneumothorax. This is best treated in the acute situation by inserting a hypodermic needle into the pleural space via the second intercostal space anteriorly on one or both sides and aspirating the free air. Formal insertion of an underwater chest drain can then be performed.

(c) Exomphalos and gastroschisis: the chief risk to these infants is loss of large quantities of fluid and heat through the exposed intestine or thin covering membrane. These losses are best restricted by wrapping the intestine or intact exomphalos sac in plastic film. Moist saline swabs rapidly become cold and dry out and should be avoided.

Preoperative preparation

1. Cross-match 1 unit of fresh whole blood.
2. Vitamin K (phytomenadione, 1 mg i.m.) is administered if not previously given in the immediate postnatal period.
3. Check Dextrostix preoperatively and if necessary give 50% glucose intravenously to prevent hypoglycaemia.
4. The infant should be normothermic.
5. Correct any acid–base and fluid or electrolyte imbalance.

Specific neonatal problems

In this section it is intended to discuss briefly the clinical presentation and diagnostic evaluation of some of the common neonatal surgical conditions. The emphasis is on early diagnosis and prompt referral to specialized centres.

Congenital diaphragmatic hernia

Herniation of abdominal viscera into the affected hemithorax occurs through the foramen of Boch-

dalek (an embryonic remnant of the pleuroperitoneal canal) in the posterolateral part of the diaphragm. The left side is affected ten times more frequently than the right. Compression on the developing lung during intrauterine life results in pulmonary hypoplasia. The greater the severity of pulmonary hypoplasia, the earlier the infant presents with respiratory distress and the worse the ultimate prognosis.

Clinical features

Respiratory distress (for clinical criteria see above), apparent dextrocardia (i.e. in left side defects), audible borborygmi in the left hemithorax and a scaphoid abdomen.

Confirmation of the diagnosis

Straight radiograph of the chest and upper abdomen will reveal bowel shadows in the pleural cavity with shift of the mediastinum to the contralateral side. There is usually a paucity of gas shadows within the abdomen (Figure 27.7).

Treatment

Treatment consists of immediate resuscitation including mechanical ventilation and the use of cardiorespiratory supportive drugs. The operative

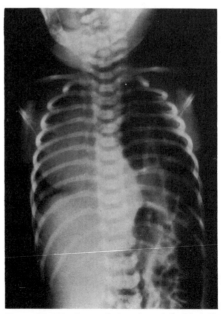

Figure 27.7 Radiograph showing a left-sided diaphragmatic hernia with the heart displaced into the right hemithorax. There is continuity between the intra-abdominal and left thoracic gas shadows

repair was, until recently, regarded as an emergency but it is now common practice to allow the infant's condition to stabilize for a variable period before submitting it to surgery. The operative repair consists of transabdominal reduction of the hernial content, closure of the diaphragmatic defect and correction of an associated intestinal malrotation.

Oesophageal atresia

In 90% of cases of oesophageal atresia there is an associated distal tracheo-oesophageal fistula (Figure 27.8). The presence of polyhydramnios in the mother during pregnancy should alert the clinician to the possibility of an oesophageal atresia or high intestinal obstruction.

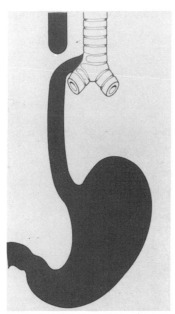

Figure 27.8 Diagram of the commonest type of oesophageal atresia with the associated distal tracheo-oesophageal fistula

Clinical features

Because the infant is unable to swallow saliva, repeated oropharangeal suction is required to maintain a patent airway. This 'excess' mucus is the first sign of oesophageal atresia and the diagnosis should be established at this stage and not when the infant is offered a feed, when coughing, dyspnoea and cyanosis will occur.

Confirmation of the diagnosis

A large calibre (No. 10–12 Fr.) radio-opaque catheter should be passed into the oesophagus. In oesophageal atresia the progress of the catheter is arrested approximately 10 cm from the mouth or nose. A straight radiograph of the chest and abdomen (without radio-opaque contrast material) will confirm the level of the obstruction. Gas within the stomach is an indication of the presence of a distal tracheo-oesophageal fistula (Figure 27.9).

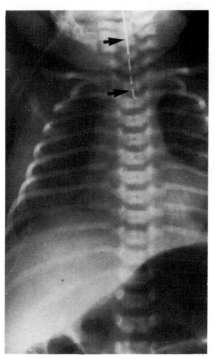

Figure 27.9 Radiograph showing the radio-opaque tube in the upper oesophagus in an infant with oesophageal atresia. Gas in the stomach indicates the presence of a distal tracheo-oesophageal fistula

Treatment

The tracheo-oesophageal fistula is ligated and divided and a primary end-to-end oesophago-oesophageal anastomosis constructed via a right extrapleural thoractomy.

Gastro-oesophageal reflux

The lower oesophageal sphincter is relatively underdeveloped in infancy and reflux of gastric content is a common phenomenon. The majority of infants respond to conservative treatment with small thickened feeds, and the maintenance of an upright posture with or without the addition of antacids.

Clinical features

Early symptoms include persistent vomiting with or without haematemesis, failure to thrive, constipation and frequent respiratory infections. A recently recognized complication of gastro-oesophageal reflux in early infancy is episodes of apnoea and cyanosis due to aspiration (near-miss sudden infant death syndrome – SIDS).

Confirmation of the diagnosis

This is by barium oesophagogram (including evaluation of gastric outlet), oesophagoscopy, prolonged pH monitoring, oesophageal manometry and 'milk scan' using ⁹⁹Tc sulphur colloid to assess pulmonary aspiration. pH monitoring is the most accurate investigation. Barium studies provide anatomical data while endoscopy provides information on the oesophageal mucosa.

The indications for surgical intervention include failure of conservative treatment, a peptic oesophageal stricture (Figure 27.10), refractory ulcerative oesophagitis and near-miss SIDS where the cause of the apnoeic attacks has been demonstrated to be aspiration of refluxed gastric content.

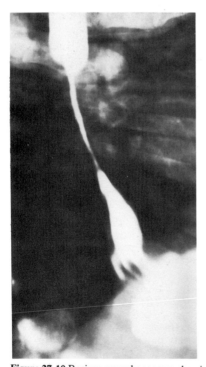

Figure 27.10 Barium oesophagogram showing a long midoesophageal stricture and a distal hiatus hernia with gastric rugae extending above the diaphragm

Pyloric stenosis

Hypertrophic pyloric stenosis is one of the commonest causes of vomiting in the infant beyond the immediate neonatal period. It occurs more frequently in boys than girls in the ratio of 4:1. Symptoms usually commence between the ages of 2 and 4 weeks.

Clinical features

Symptoms consist of projectile non-bilious vomiting within 20–30 min of a feed, failure to thrive and constipation. On physical examination there may be evidence of dehydration, gastric peristaltic waves may be visible across the left upper quadrant of the abdomen and a pyloric 'tumour' may be palpated in the right hypochondrium. The 'tumour' is best felt soon after a vomit or in the early stage of a 'test feed'. In experienced hands, a tumour is palpable in over 90% of cases.

Confirmation of the diagnosis

Palpation of the pyloric 'tumour' is sufficient clinical evidence for confirmation of the diagnosis. In cases where a tumour cannot be felt, barium studies or, more recently, ultrasonography will establish the diagnosis (Figure 27.11).

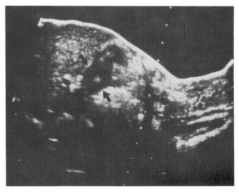

Figure 27.11 Ultrasound scan showing the pyloric mass with a centrally placed pyloric canal

Treatment

Surgery is the only acceptable form of treatment for infantile hypertrophic pyloric stenosis. Preoperative preparation of the infant includes correction of fluid and electrolyte imbalances with particular emphasis on restoring depleted potassium, sodium and chloride ions. The surgery is never an emergency and should be delayed until the infant's condition is optimal.

The operative procedure consists of a pyloromyotomy which involves splitting the hypertrophied muscle of the pyloric canal longitudinally down to, but not including, the mucosa. The myotomy should extend from the gastroduodenal junction through the hypertrophied pyloric muscle onto the antrum of the stomach.

Oral fluids are best omitted for at least 12 h postoperatively to avoid postoperative vomiting. Thereafter feeds may be rapidly reintroduced. The postoperative stay in hospital should rarely extend beyond 48–72 h.

Intestinal atresia

Atresias of the intestine develop as a consequence of an intrauterine mesenteric vascular or intestinal catastrophe, such as mesenteric arterial thrombosis or embolus, intestinal volvulus, intussusception, or strangulation. These are usually isolated anomalies in contrast to duodenal atresias which are frequently associated with other congenital malformations, such as Down's syndrome, congenital cardiac defects, oesophageal and anorectal anomalies.

Clinical features

Bile-stained vomiting is the only absolute sign of neonatal intestinal obstruction. Abdominal distension is dependent on the level of the obstruction, being virtually absent in high small bowel obstructions and increasing progressively the further distal the obstructive lesion is in the intestinal tract. Meconium already present in the distal intestine when the atresia developed may be passed, but more often only mucus plugs are evacuated per rectum.

Confirmation of the diagnosis

An erect and supine abdominal radiograph will reveal the presence of dilated loops of proximal intestine with air–fluid levels. The rest of the abdomen, particularly the pelvis, is opaque except in low intestinal obstructive lesions (Figure 27.12). *N.B.* Small intestine cannot be differentiated from large intestine on plain radiograph in the infant under 6 months of age.

Malrotation with or without volvulus

During early fetal differentiation, part of the development and elongation of the intestinal tract

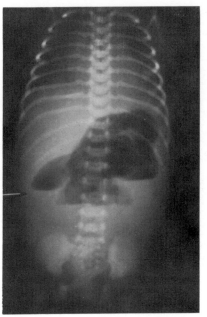

Figure 27.12 Erect abdominal radiograph in an infant with midjejunal atresia showing dilated loops of intestine with air–fluid levels in the upper abdomen

takes place in the physiological umbilical hernia. Re-entry into the peritoneal cavity is completed around the twelfth week of intrauterine life. During this process of re-entry a definite sequence of events is followed whereby the caecoiliac loop undergoes an anticlockwise rotation of 270° before becoming fixed in the right iliac fossa. A similar rotation affects the duodenal loop. Failure to complete the normal rotational process results in the midgut loop being suspended from the posterior peritoneum on a narrow base which is prone to undergo volvulus. In addition, abnormal bands (Ladd's bands) overlie and compress the duodenum causing intermittent obstruction (Figure 27.13).

Clinical features

Uncomplicated malrotation presents with intermittent episodes of bile-tinged vomiting. There may be little or no abdominal distension. When volvulus occurs the entire midgut loop (from the duodenojejunal flexure to the mid transverse colon) becomes ischaemic due to vascular compression. These infants pass dark blood per rectum and rapidly become shocked and acidotic.

Confirmation of the diagnosis

A plain abdominal radiograph may show a 'double-bubble' appearance of air–fluid levels in the stomach and duodenum but when a volvulus has

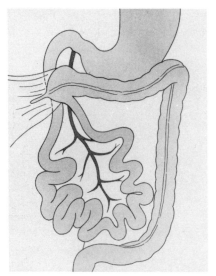

Figure 27.13 Diagrammatic appearance of the common variety of midgut malrotation. The caecum is subhepatic in position and Ladd's bands extend across the duodenum to the posterior abdominal wall

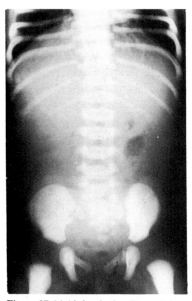

Figure 27.14 Abdominal radiograph in an infant with malrotation and volvulus. The 'gasless abdomen' is an ominous sign

occurred the plain radiograph appears 'gasless' (Figure 27.14). If the infant's condition permits, a contrast study should be performed to confirm the diagnosis. The upper gastrointestinal series which demonstrates the configuration of the C-loop of the duodenum is generally preferred to the barium enema which only defines the position of the caecum.

The presence of intestinal malrotation should be regarded as a surgical emergency. A few hours of intensive resuscitation should be followed by urgent laparotomy.

Treatment

The volvulus is untwisted and any frankly gangrenous bowel resected. Congested bowel rapidly recovers following reduction of the volvulus. Operative correction consists of widening the base of the mesentery and placing the bowel in the non-rotated position, i.e. small intestine on the right and large intestine on the left of the peritoneal cavity. An incidental appendicectomy should be carried out to avoid delay in diagnosis of a subsequent appendicitis due to its abnormal position.

Meconium ileus

This is the earliest and most frequent gastrointestinal manifestation of cystic fibrosis or mucoviscidosis. Caucasians are more frequently affected than coloured races. The obstruction is caused by thick tenacious meconium impacted within the lumen of the small intestine.

Clinical features

All three cardinal features of intestinal obstruction are present. Abdominal distension is usually evident at birth and may be prominent. Bile-stained vomiting occurs early and the infant usually fails to pass meconium of any description. Distended loops of intestine packed with meconium may be palpable on abdominal examination. A positive family history of cystic fibrosis is a further helpful diagnostic feature.

Confirmation of the diagnosis

The plain abdominal radiograph shows distended loops of intestine of varying calibre, a paucity or absence of air–fluid levels and a bubbly appearance within the meconium mass (Figure 27.15). A contrast enema will show the small 'unused' microcolon containing inspissated mucus plugs. Final confirmation of the diagnosis is obtained on a sweat test where the sodium and chloride contents are grossly elevated (in excess of 70 mol/l).

For the uncomplicated case of meconium ileus, gastrografin enema may be therapeutic as well as diagnostic. Indications for operative treatment include the presence of a mechanical intestinal obstruction (e.g. atresia), peritonitis and the failure of gastrografin enema to relieve the obstruction.

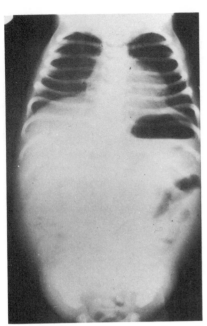

Figure 27.15 Abdominal radiograph revealing a 'soap-bubble' appearance in the right lower quadrant in an infant with uncomplicated meconium ileus

Hirschsprung's disease

The aganglionic segment always involves the rectum to a greater or lesser extent and progresses proximally for a variable distance. In 90% of cases the abnormality is confined to the rectosigmoid region. Total colonic aganglionosis affects 5% of patients with Hirschsprung's disease.

Clinical features

Delayed passage of meconium beyond the first 24 h of life is the single most constant presenting feature of Hirschsprung's disease. There is usually associated abdominal distension and bile-stained vomiting. Colonic hyperperistalsis may be visible on abdominal inspection. The degree of obstruction may be total, particularly in long-segment disease, or intermittent. Meconium plug syndrome, i.e. abdominal distension relieved by the passage of a large plug of meconium, should be regarded as indicative of Hirschsprung's disease until the diagnosis has been positively excluded. Enterocolitis of Hirschsprung's disease, which presents with profuse diarrhoea in addition to subacute intestinal obstruction and which may rapidly lead to dehydration and shock, is responsible for most of the mortality and morbidity associated with this condition. Enteroco-

litis develops as a consequence of delayed diagnosis and is rarely seen before 2 weeks of age.

Confirmation of the diagnosis

Barium enema may show a typical 'cone' in the distal rectum (Figure 27.16) but this is unusual in the neonatal period. Retention of barium for longer than 24 h is the main diagnostic criterion on the barium study at this age. The only absolute method of confirming or refuting the diagnosis is by rectal biopsy. An experienced histopathologist should be able to identify ganglion cells in a suction rectal biopsy containing an adequate amount of submucosa (Meissner's plexus). In selected cases, a full-thickness biopsy for evaluation of the myenteric plexus (Auerbach) may be required.

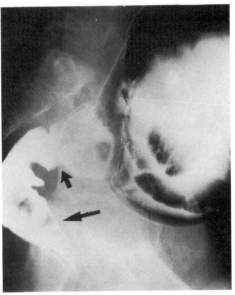

Figure 27.16 Barium enema in Hirschsprung's disease showing an irregular contracted aganglionic lower rectum with coning into the dilated ganglionic proximal intestine

Treatment

The initial treatment consists of a colostomy performed in ganglionic intestine. This requires frozen section confirmation of ganglion cells at the level of the proposed colostomy. In infants with severe enterocolitis, a period of resuscitation, consisting of rehydration and bowel decompression with gentle rectal saline washouts, will allow the patient to withstand surgery more safely. The definitive procedure is delayed until the child is at least 3 months of age.

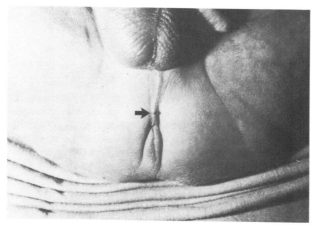

Figure 27.17 Covered anus with a spot of meconium in the midline raphe indicating the 'low' nature of the lesion

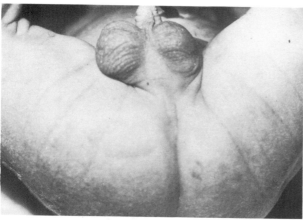

Figure 27.18 'High' (supralevator) anorectal agenesis showing a partially split scrotum. The presence of meconium in the urine in this infant was diagnostic of a recto-urethral fistula

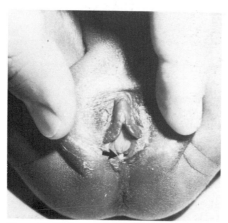

Figure 27.19 Anovestibular fistula in a female infant with a 'low' anorectal malformation

Anorectal malformations

The clear differentiation between supralevator (high) and infralevator (low) lesions is vitally important to the future anorectal continence of the child (Figures 27.17, 27.18 and 27.19).

Clinical features

An absent or malformed anus should be detected soon after birth. A diagnostic scheme for anorectal anomalies is outlined in Figure 27.20.

Confirmation of the diagnosis

A clinical diagnosis is sufficient in the majority of cases. Where doubt exists an inverted lateral radiograph (normally after the first 24 h of life) may be helpful in defining the level of the agenesis.

Treatment

Treatment consists of a colostomy followed some 3–6 months later by a 'pull-through' procedure for high lesions, while low lesions are treated immediately by a local anoplasty procedure.

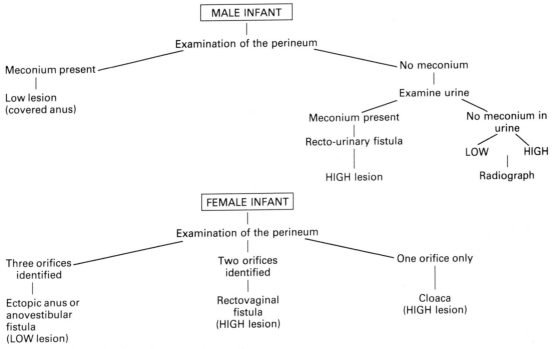

Figure 27.20 Diagnostic scheme for anorectal anomalies

Necrotizing enterocolitis

Although only recently recognized as a distinct entity, necrotizing enterocolitis (NEC) has assumed major significance in neonatology as well as in paediatric surgery. The aetiology is unknown but mesenteric circulatory disturbance consequent upon perinatal stress is generally accepted as providing the final common pathway in the pathogenesis of the condition. The role of infective agents, particularly clostridial infection, remains to be proven.

Clinical features

The first sign of NEC is reluctance of the baby to feed. The presence of blood and mucus in the stool, abdominal distension and bile-tinged vomiting soon follow. If untreated, the disease may progress to full-thickness necrosis of the intestine with perforation. Even following successful conservative treatment, approximately 5–10% of patients develop strictures of the involved intestine.

Confirmation of the diagnosis

A plain abdominal radiograph showing air bubbles within the wall of the intestine (pneumatosis intestinalis) is diagnostic of NEC (Figure 27.21). Pneumoperitoneum denotes an intestinal perforation.

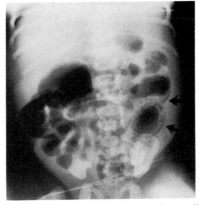

Figure 27.21 Abdominal radiograph revealing intramural gas (pneumatosis intestinalis) in the left colon

Treatment

In the early stages of the disease process, conservative treatment is usually successful. This comprises nasogastric decompression, parenteral broad-spectrum antibiotics (penicillin, metronidazole and gentamicin) and withholding oral feeds for 14 days during which time parenteral nutrition is provided. The indications for surgical intervention include intestinal perforation, the failure of conservative measures and stricture formation.

Inguinal hernia

Inguinal herniotomy is the most common surgical procedure undertaken in the neonatal period (excluding circumcision). With a few exceptions the hernia is of the indirect variety entering the processus vaginalis which has failed to obliterate.

Clinical features

The mother notices a lump in the groin which appears intermittently when the baby cries (Figure 27.22). The incidence of irreducibility is high in early infancy and this may be the very first sign of the presence of a hernia.

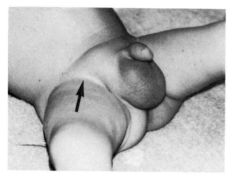

Figure 27.22 Right indirect inguinal hernia in a male infant

Confirmation of the diagnosis

Frequently the clinician will not be able to detect a hernia during consultation. In these cases, the history from the mother or family practitioner is sufficient for the surgeon to proceed with an exploration of the groin.

Treatment

The operation consists of a simple herniotomy, which is undertaken as a day-case. The operation should be scheduled as soon as possible. The majority of incarcerated hernias can be successfully reduced once the infant has been adequately sedated. Herniotomy should then be carried out within 48–72 h. Irreducibility exposes the intestine to ischaemic necrosis and the blood supply to the ipsilateral testis may also be compressed with resultant testicular atrophy.

Exomphalos and gastroschisis

Failure of complete regression of the physiological umbilical hernia results in the formation of an exomphalos of major (defect greater than 5 cm in diameter) (Figure 27.23) or minor extent. Antenatal rupture of a minor exomphalos results in eviscer-ation of intestine which becomes thickened and oedematous due to exposure to amniotic fluid. The defect is usually to the right of a normally formed umbilical cord (gastroschisis).

Clinical features

The exomphalos sac consists of amniotic membrane externally and peritoneum internally with the two layers separated by Wharton's jelly. The thin sac which is relatively avascular is liable to rupture if left untreated. A high percentage of major exomphalos are associated with other congenital anomalies, e.g. congenital heart defects, while minor lesions and gastroschisis are usually isolated abnormalities.

Spina bifida

Failure of closure of the neural arches results in a widely dispersed spectrum of lesions. Antenatal diagnosis is possible by detection of high maternal serum or amniotic alpha-fetoprotein levels. The diagnosis may also be suspected on antenatal ultrasound scan.

Clinical features

A spina bifida occulta may be suspected by the presence of an overlying tuft of hair, a haeman-gioma, lipoma, dermoid or sinus, usually in the sacral region of the spine. A meningocoele consists of a sac containing cerebrospinal fluid without neural tissue, and may either be membrane- or, uncommonly, skin-covered. A myelomeningocoele is characterized by the presence of exposed neural tissue or the spinal lesion, below which there is paralysis of the lower limbs, and anal and urinary sphincter dysfunction to a greater or lesser extent.

Treatment

Except for the severest cases where surgical closure of the defect would be technically impossible, operative closure of the myelomeningocele should be carried out within the first 24 h of life in order to prevent deterioration of neurological function and bacterial infection. Assessment of the suitability of patients for surgical treatment should only be made by experienced medical practitioners

Cystic hygroma

The abnormal lymphatic tissue (lymphangioma) is most commonly located in the neck. It may be evident in the newborn period or only become visible after the first few weeks of life. Sudden

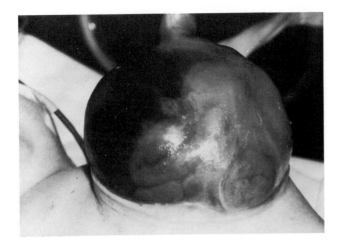

Figure 27.23 Major exomphalos. The liver is visible through the transparent amniotic membrane in the upper part with the intestine in the lower part of the exomphalos sac

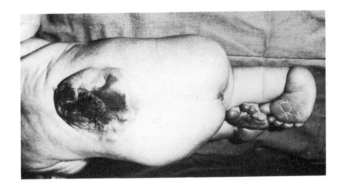

Figure 27.24 Lumbar myelomeningocele. Neural tissue is evident in the central plaque. Note the deformity of the lower limbs and the patulous anus

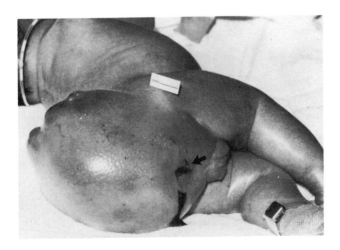

Figure 27.25 Massive sacrococcygeal teratoma displacing the anal orifice anteriorly. Radiograph commonly shows areas of calcification

enlargement due to infection or haemorrhage may result in tracheal compression. For this reason, early surgical excision is recommended, even if only partial resection can be achieved.

Sacrococcygeal teratoma

This is the most common tumour recognized at birth. It arises from the coccyx (notochord remnant) and is usually benign at birth. The incidence of malignant degeneration increases exponentially by a factor of 10% for each month after birth.

Clinical features

A large mass on the buttocks is easily identified but occasionally the lesion is entirely intrapelvic and may only be diagnosed on abdominal or rectal examination (Figure 27.25).

Treatment

Early complete excision, including the coccyx, in the neonatal period is indicated to avoid possible complications and malignant transformation. The long-term prognosis in these circumstances is excellent, although anorectal and urinary function may have been affected.

28

Treatment of snake bite

D. A. Warrell

Venomous snakes belong to five families of which two, Elapidae and Viperidae, contain all the species of major medical importance. These species have a pair of fangs – enlarged teeth bearing a groove or channel, usually with adjacent replacement fangs, in their upper jaws. The venom glands, situated behind and below the eye, are surrounded by compressor muscles which squeeze the venom along the venom ducts which connect with the venom channels at the base of the fangs.

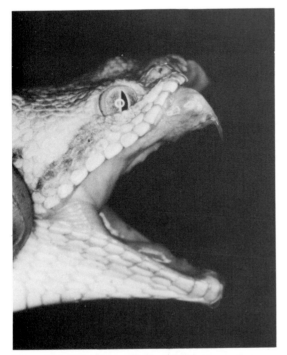

Figure 28.1 Hinged fang with sheath of the saw-scaled or carpet viper (*Echis carinatus*) (Family Viperidae)

Types of snakes

Viperidae

The Viperidae have the most highly evolved venom apparatus. The curved fangs which may reach a length of 50 mm in the gaboon viper (*Bitis gabonica*) are hinged so that they can be folded away in a membrane sheath when not in use (Figure 28.1). There are two sub-families, the viperinae, old world vipers and adders including the European adder (*Vipera berus*); and the Crotalinae, pit vipers, which include rattlesnakes, moccasins and lance-headed vipers of the Americas and the Asian pit vipers. The Crotalinae possess heat-sensitive pit organs between the eye and the nostril which enables them to detect their warm-blooded prey (Figure 28.2). The name 'viper' implies production of live young (ovovivi-parity), but some species lay eggs and the term is not strictly applied. The Viperidae are usually relatively short, thick snakes with broad heads and a definite neck. Many have keeled scales and most have a repeated dorsal pattern which may be striking or brightly coloured.

Elapidae

These include cobras, kraits, mambas and coral snakes. They have short, permanently erect fangs (Figure 28.3). Spitting cobras of Africa and Asia are able forcibly to eject venom from their fangs for a distance of several metres towards the eyes of an aggressor. This is a purely defensive device. The venom channel makes a right-angled turn forward just before its exit from the front of the fang. Australasian terrestrial venomous snakes such as the taipan, tiger snake, death adder and brown snakes are usually classified with the Elapidae, but have been grouped with the sea snakes by some taxonomists.

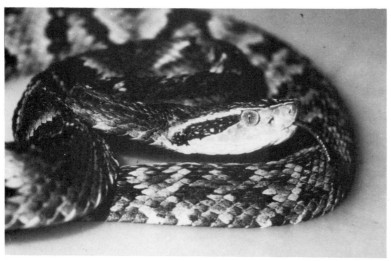

Figure 28.2 The jararaca (*Bothrops jararaca*), the most important cause of snake bites in Sao Paulo State, Brazil. It has a heat-sensitive pit organ between the eye and the nostril

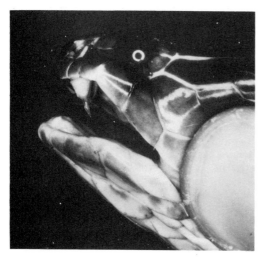

Figure 28.3 Short permanently erect fang of the Sri Lankan cobra (*Naja naja naja*) (Family Elapidae)

Hydrophiidae (sea snakes)

These are adapted to marine life by having flattened, paddle-like tails, reduction or loss of the large ventral scales used for traction by terrestrial snakes, an elongated single lung which allows prolonged dives and a salt-excreting gland in the floor of the mouth.

Atractaspididae (burrowing asps or burrowing or mole vipers or adders)

This is a small family confined to Africa and the Middle East. They have very long fangs which are used one at a time with a side-swiping action to impale their prey which consists of other burrow-dwelling reptiles and amphibians.

Colubridae

A large family of snakes generally regarded as harmless and including the British grass snake and smooth snake. However, bites by 40 or more species of Colubridae can cause local and even systemic effects in humans. Members of the sub-family Boiginae (back-fanged snakes) have grooved fangs at the backs of their mouths which can inoculate venom. Other species, with enlarged but solid maxillary teeth lacking any groove or channel, can by a sustained chewing action introduce enough venomous saliva to cause envenoming. The African boomslang (*Dispholidus typus*) and bird, twig or vine snakes (*Thelotornis* sp.) have on rare occasions killed herpetologists who handled them carelessly and allowed a sustained bite. Two species of Asian keel-backed snakes (genus *Rhabdophis*) have also caused severe envenoming. The message is clear; all colubrid snakes should be treated with caution.

Distribution of venomous snakes

Venomous snakes are abundant, especially in tropical countries, in all types of terrain including deserts, jungles, marshes, lakes and rivers, up to altitudes of 5000 m. The range of the adder (*Vipera berus*) enters the Arctic Circle. However, there are no venomous snakes in the Antarctic, on most islands of the western Mediterranean, Atlantic,

Caribbean and Pacific (except the western Pacific) and in Madagascar, Chile, New Zealand, Ireland and Iceland. Sea snakes abound in the Indian and Pacific Oceans, in estuaries, for distances of several hundred miles up some rivers, and in freshwater lakes in the Philippines, Cambodia and the Solomon Islands.

Table 28.1 lists the species responsible for most deaths and morbidity in different parts of the world. Some famous species, such as the king cobra (*Ophiophagus hannah*), bushmaster (*Lachesis muta*) and gaboon viper (*Bitis gabonica*) are not included because, despite their great size, potent venom and notoriety, they bite humans very rarely. Bites by sea snakes, once an important hazard to fisherman in parts of Asia, now appear to be rare, possibly because hand operated shore nets have been replaced by mechanical methods in many areas.

Epidemiology of snake bite

Snake bite reaches its highest incidence in rural areas of the tropics where it is an occupational risk of agricultural workers and hunters. In most countries the true incidence is underestimated by official statistics, but the problem has also been exaggerated. In some countries, such as Brazil and Thailand, mortality has declined sharply over the last few decades as locally produced antivenom has become widely available.

The incidence of snake bite may show marked seasonal fluctuations with peaks coinciding with the planting and harvesting of rice (e.g. Russell's viper bite in South East Asia) or with increased farming activity before the start of the annual rains (e.g. saw-scaled or carpet viper bites in the West African savanna region). There may also be diurnal variations in incidence; rubber plantation workers in

Table 28.1 Snakes responsible for most deaths and morbidity

Area	Scientific name	English name
North America	*Crotalus adamanteus* *Crotalus atrox* *Crotalus viridis* subspecies	Eastern diamond-back rattlesnake Western diamond-back rattlesnake Western rattlesnakes
Central America	*Crotalus durissus durissus* *Bothrops asper*	Central American rattlesnake Terciopelo, caissaca
South America	*Bothrops atrox* *Bothrops jararaca* *Crotalus durissus terrificus*	Fer de lance, barba amarilla Jararaca South American rattlesnake
Europe	*Vipera berus* *Vipera ammodytes*	Viper, adder Long-nosed viper
Africa	*Echis carinatus* *Bitis arietans* *Naja nigricollis* *Naja haje* *Dendroaspis* species	Saw-scaled or carpet viper Puff adder Black-necked spitting cobra Egyptian cobra Mambas
Asia, Middle East	*Echis carinatus* *Vipera lebetina* *Vipera palaestinae*	Saw-scaled or carpet viper Levantine viper Palestine viper
Indian subcontinent and South East Asia	*Naja naja, N. kaouthia, N. sumatrana* etc. *Bungarus caeruleus* *Vipera russelli* *Calloselasma (Agkistrodon) rhodostoma* *Trimeresurus albolabris* etc. *Echis carinatus*	Asian cobras Indian krait Russell's viper Malayan pit viper Green arboreal pit vipers Saw-scaled or carpet viper
Far East	*Naja naja* *Trimeresurus flavoviridis* *Trimeresurus mucrosquamatus* *Agkistrodon halys, A. blomhoffi, A. caliginosus*	Asian cobra Habu Chinese habu Mamushi
Australasia	*Acanthophis antarcticus* *Notechis scutatus* *Oxyuranus scutellatus* *Pseudonaja textilis*	Death adder Tiger snake Taipan Eastern brown snake

South East Asia are frequently bitten by Malayan pit vipers before dawn as they make their rounds of the rubber trees. Bites by spitting cobras in Africa, and by kraits in India, Sri Lanka and South East Asia often occur while the victims are asleep in their huts at night. Flooding, the movement of large numbers of people into areas infested by venomous snakes and unexplained increases in the population of venomous snakes have been associated with epidemics of snake bite.

Regional snake bite problems

UK and Europe

The mortality from snake bite is very low. The adder (*Vipera berus*) bites about 100 people each year in the UK and 200 in Finland, and in the UK there have been only 14 deaths during the last 100 years and in Finland 21 deaths in 25 years. In France, where the principal species is *V. aspis*, there have been 23 deaths in the past 7 years. The most dangerous European species are probably the long-nosed viper (*V. ammodytes*) and Levantine viper (*V. lebetina*).

North America

In the United States there are approximately 7000 venomous snake bites each year with 9–14 deaths attributable to rattlesnakes (Western and Eastern diamond-back, Mojave, Pacific and timber rattlesnakes, etc., genus *Crotalus*). Copperhead moccasins (*Agkistrodon contortrix*) are responsible for most venomous bites. Handling snakes for bravado or religious rituals results in some severe and fatal bites. In Mexico there are probably about 30000 bites per year with 100–200 deaths. The dangerous species include rattlesnakes (*Crotalus durissus*) and pit vipers (*Bothrops asper* and *Agkistrodon bilineatus*).

Central and South America

Medically-important species include rattlesnakes (*Crotalus durissus* subspecies) and many species of the ubiquitous and abundant genus *Bothrops* (lance-headed pit vipers). In Brazil there were an estimated 4800 deaths in 1929 and 2000 in 1949. The incidence of bites is now about 20 per 100000 per year with few deaths. In Costa Rica, hospital admissions for snake bite have been estimated at 22.4/100000 population/year, with five deaths per 100000, mostly attributable to *Bothrops asper*. In French Guyana, the incidence of snake bites is about 75/100000 population/year of which 7.2% are severe or fatal. Snake bite is also reported to be an important medical problem in Colombia, Bolivia, Venezuela and Ecuador.

Africa

The saw-scaled or carpet viper (*Echis carinatus*) is the commonest cause of snake bite morbidity and mortality throughout the savanna region of the northern part of Africa. In the Benue Valley of north eastern Nigeria, the incidence of bites by this species was almost 500/100000 population/year with a mortality of 12%. Other medically important species are the puff adder (*Bitis arietans*) and spitting cobras which occur throughout Africa, except in the rain forest areas; and in East and southern Africa, black and green mambas (*Dendroaspis polylepis* and *D. angusticeps*). Night adders (genus *Causus*) are responsible for large numbers of bites throughout Africa, but envenoming is usually mild. In the desert and mountainous regions of North Africa, *Vipera lebetina*, *V. latastei* and *Cerastes cerastes* are responsible for some bites.

Middle East

Small numbers of snake bites have been reported from Israel, Jordan, Saudi Arabia, Iran and Iraq. Medically important species include *Echis carinatus* and *E. coloratus*, *Vipera palaestinae*, *V. lebetina* and the burrowing asp (*Atractaspis engaddensis*).

Indian subcontinent and South East Asia

An estimated 15–30000 people die each year of snake bite in Pakistan and India, where the principal species are cobras (*Naja naja*), krait (*Bungarus caeruleus*), saw-scaled viper (*Echis carinatus*) and Russell's viper (*Daboia russellii*). In Sri Lanka there are more than 60000 bites and almost 1000 deaths per year (6/100000 population per year) attributable to *D. russellii*, *B. caeruleus* and *Naja naja*. Throughout most of South East Asia, arboreal green pit vipers (genus *Trimeresurus*) are responsible for most venomous bites, but most deaths are caused by Malayan pit viper (*Calloselasma rhodostoma*), cobras, Malayan krait (*Bungarus candidus*) and in Thailand and Burma, Russell's viper. In Burma, where Russell's vipers are responsible for more than 70% of all bites and deaths, snake bite has been as high as the fifth major cause of all deaths in the country. There are still more than 1000 deaths a year and in some areas the mortality has been as high as 38/100000 population per year. In Peninsular Malaysia, there are more than 5000 bites per year (50/100000 population) but with a very low mortality. Most bites are caused by Malayan pit vipers and cobras. In the past, sea snake bite was a common cause of death among fishermen along the coasts of India, Peninsular Malaysia, Thailand and Vietnam. The beaked sea snake *Enhydrina schistosa*, which lives inshore and in estuaries, is the most important cause.

East Asia

In China and Taiwan, snake bite does not appear to be very common. Important species include cobras, Chinese krait (*Bungarus multicinctus*) and various species of mamushi (genus *Agkistrodon*), the sharp-nosed viper or 'hundred pacer' (*Deinagkistrodon acutus*) and Chinese habu (*Trimeresurus mucrosquamatus*). Most venomous bites are caused by arboreal green pit vipers; *Trimeresurus stejnegeri* in Taiwan and *T. albolabris* in Hong Kong. In Taiwan, the mortality from *T. stejnegeri* bites was 2%, and from *T. mucrosquamatus* (116 bites per year) was 7.3%. The highest case mortality followed bites by *D. acutus*, *Bungarus multicinctus* (18% mortality) and *Naja naja*. In the Amami, Ryuku and Okinawa islands of Japan, the habu (*Trimeresurus flavoviridis*) inflicted an average of 610 bites with six deaths per year during the 1960s.

Australasia

In Australia there were more than 200 bites per year with an average of 4.5 deaths per year during the 30 years up to 1977, but recently the average mortality has fallen to one. There are a large number of highly dangerous genera including *Notechis* (tiger snakes), *Pseudonaja* (brown snakes), *Austrelaps* (copperhead), *Pseudechis* (black snakes), *Acanthophis* (death adders), *Oxyuranus* (taipans) and *Tropidechis* (rough-scaled snake). In New Guinea, there is a high incidence of snake bites and mortality caused by taipan, death adder and possibly small eyed snake (*Micropechis ikaheka*). Sea snakes (*Enhydrina schistosa*) cause some bites in rivers many miles up from the sea.

Venom composition

Snake venoms are the most complex poisons, containing 20 or more components including enzymes, non-enzymatic polypeptide toxins, non-toxic proteins, carbohydrates, metals, lipids, free amino acids, nucleotides, biogenic amines and other compounds. Venoms of Elapidae, Australasian terrestrial snakes and Hydrophiidae are notable for their polypeptide and phospholipase A_2 neurotoxins, which block neuromuscular transmission by preventing release of acetylcholine at the nerve terminals or blocking receptors post-synaptically. Viperidae venoms are rich in proteases and procoagulant enzymes. However, some elapid venoms show marked proteolytic and procoagulant activity, while some Viperidae venoms contain neurotoxic phospholipase A_2.

Clinical features of snake bite

One-third to one-half of patients bitten by venomous snakes, and bearing fang marks indicating that the skin has been punctured, develop no evidence of envenoming. When symptoms and signs do appear they may be attributable to snake venom, to fear and to first-aid and other pre-hospital treatment. Many patients anticipate a rapid and painful death and so the clinical picture may be dominated by physiological manifestations of anxiety, such as hyperventilation, or even frank hysteria. First-aid and traditional treatments, which are often the first resort, before the patient sees a doctor, may produce dramatic, damaging and clinically misleading effects; bleeding from local incisions, congestion or ischaemia from tight tourniquets, and vomiting from emetic herbal remedies. Heavy-lidded and drowsy patients suspected of having neurotoxic envenoming may in fact be physically exhausted and sleepy after a long and hurried journey to the hospital.

Early symptoms

Immediate pain from the mechanical trauma of the bite is the rule followed, in the case of most Viperidae and some elapid bites, by increasing throbbing pain over minutes or hours caused by the injected venom. However bites by sea snakes, kraits and coral snakes are virtually painless apart from the initial pricking or stinging sensation. Sea snake bites may pass unnoticed by wading fishermen and krait bites may not wake the slumbering victim. Persistent bleeding from the fang marks suggests a haemostatic abnormality. Local swelling, sometimes noticeable within minutes of the bite and usually within 2 h is typical of envenoming by Viperidae and some Elapidae, particularly the spitting cobras of Africa and most Asian cobras. Bites by sea snakes, kraits, coral snakes and some species of African and Asian cobra and Australasian elapids cause virtually no local signs. Severe systemic envenoming by tropical rattlesnakes (*Crotalus durissus terrificus*) and Russell's vipers may be associated with negligible local envenoming. Early syncope, vomiting, colic, diarrhoea, angio-oedema and wheezing may occur after bites by some Viperidae (including the European adder) and Australasian elapids. Nausea and vomiting are common early features of severe envenoming by many species of snakes.

Local envenoming

Massive local swelling, which progresses for several days to involve the entire bitten limb and adjacent areas of the trunk, may follow bites by Viperidae.

As the venom is taken up by the lymphatics, linear erythema or bruising may appear along the course of superficial lymphatics (for example, on the medial surface of the calf and thigh) and over enlarged, tender regional lymph nodes. Blisters containing serous or serosanguinous fluid are first seen in the first few hours at the site of the bite and, with severe

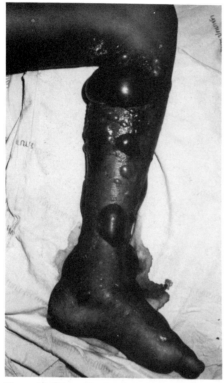

Figure 28.4 Extensive local swelling, bruising, blistering and early tissue necrosis 48 h after a bite on the calf by a Malayan pit viper (*Calloselasma rhodostoma*) in Thailand

envenoming, extend up the bitten limb (Figure 28.4). These changes result from increased vascular permeability caused by venom proteases, phospholipases, hyaluronidase, endogenous autacoids released by the venom (e.g. histamine, serotonin and kinins) and venom haemorrhagins which damage vascular endothelium. A third of the circulating blood volume may be extravasated into a swollen limb. Myotoxic and cytolytic factors present in some venoms can cause tissue necrosis which may also be a complication of thrombosis, external compression by a tourniquet, raised tissue pressure within a tight fascial compartment and infection. There is a high risk of local necrosis after bites on the digits because of the high concentration of venom and pressure within a relatively indistensible compartment. Early signs of necrosis include demarcation of an area of anaesthetic skin with altered pigmentation, fluctuance and a putrid smell. Venom spreads in fascial planes, undermining apparently normal skin and producing 'skip lesions' extending up the affected limb (Figure 28.5). Viperidae notorious for the production of severe local swelling, blistering and necrosis include African puff adder (*Bitis arietans*), Palestine viper (*Vipera palaestinae*), Malayan pit viper (*Calloselasma rhodostoma*), Japanese habu (*Trimeresurus* sp.), South American *Bothrops* sp. and bushmaster (*Lachesis muta*) and North American rattlesnakes. Venoms of some elapid snakes can also cause severe local effects (e.g. Asian cobras and African spitting cobras).

Hypotension and shock

A common cause is hypovolaemia resulting from extravasation into a bitten limb or massive gastrointestinal haemorrhage. Viperidae venoms may cause vasodilatation by a direct action on blood vessels or by releasing endogenous vasodilators. The

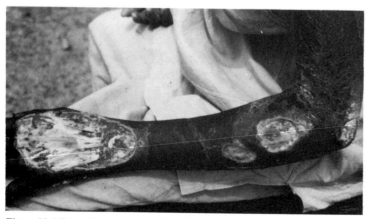

Figure 28.5 Extensive tissue necrosis with 'skip lesions' in a patient who presented 8 weeks after being bitten on the dorsum of the hand by a puff adder (*Bitis arietans*) in Nigeria

autopharmacological syndrome is exemplified by early recurrent syncope, angio-edema, colic, diarrhoea and other autonomic symptoms after bites by European vipers and Palestine vipers. Viperidae venoms can also affect the myocardium directly causing arrhythmias and other electrocardiographic abnormalities. Snake bite may stimulate psychogenic vasovagal shock in some patients.

Bleeding and clotting disturbances

Snake bite is by far the most important cause of 'defibrination syndrome' and non-clotting blood in tropical countries. Venoms of many Viperidae, Australasian elapids and Colubridae contain procoagulant enzymes which cause consumption coagulopathy. There is excessive bleeding from wounds and venepucture sites. The combination of defibrination, platelet dysfunction and haemorrhagin-induced damage to blood vessel walls can produce severe spontaneous systemic bleeding into the gastrointestinal tract, brain and other tissues.

Renal failure

This may occur as a complication of severe systemic envenoming caused by almost any species, but is particularly common after bites by Russell's vipers, tropical rattlesnakes, *Bothrops* species, Australasian elapids and sea snakes. Mechanisms may be 'pre-renal' (renal ischaemia resulting from shock, obstruction by fibrin thrombi or vasoconstriction) or damage to the kidney by interstitial haemorrhage and the direct nephrotoxic action of the venom, products of intravascular haemolysis and rhabdomyolysis and immunological complications of antivenom treatment. In parts of India, Sri Lanka and Burma, Russell's viper bite is the commonest cause of acute renal failure.

Paralysis

A characteristic evolution of neuroparalytic signs, reminiscent of myasthenia gravis and botulinum intoxication follows envenoming by Elapidae (kraits, coral snakes, mambas and some cobras), Australasian elapids, sea snakes and a few species of Viperidae (tropical rattlesnake, south Indian and Sri Lankan Russell's viper, southern African berg adder *Bitis atropos* and east Asian Pallas' pit viper). Premonitory symptoms include blurring of vision, a feeling of heaviness of the eyelids and buccal paraesthesia. There is progression from loss of upward gaze and ptosis to total external ophthalmoplegia, facial paralysis, inability to open the mouth, protrude the tongue, swallow and speak and further

to generalized flaccid paralysis and death from respiratory paralysis (Figure 28.6). Exceptionally, as in the case of some bites by black mambas (*Dendroaspis polylepis*) and other large elapids, respiratory paralysis may develop within 15–30 min after the bite. However, this progression usually takes several hours and in some cases the appearance of paralytic signs may be delayed for more than 10 h.

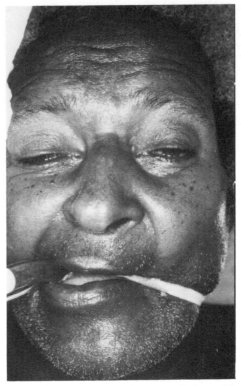

Figure 28.6 Ptosis and respiratory paralysis requiring mechanical ventilation in a patient bitten by a Taipan (*Oxyuranus scutellatus canni*) in Papua New Guinea

Generalized skeletal muscle breakdown (rhabdomyolysis)

Phospholipase A_2 in venoms of sea snakes, Australasian elapids, tropical and timber rattlesnakes and Indian and Sri Lankan Russell's vipers damage skeletal muscle and release myoglobin, muscle enzymes and potassium into the circulation. In the case of sea snake bites clinical symptoms begin within 0.5–3.5 h of the bite. They include generalized muscle aches, pains, stiffness, tenderness and resistance to passive stretching, trismus and loss of tendon reflexes. Some 3–8 h after the bite the urine becomes 'mahogany' or 'Coca-Cola' coloured (myoglobinuria). Products of rhabdomyolysis may cause renal failure. Deaths are attributable to respiratory paralysis, acute cardiac effects of hyperkalaemia and renal failure. Myoglobin in urine produces a positive 'stix' test for haemoglobin/blood.

Treatment
First-aid

This can only be carried out by the victim, or people who happen to be around at the time, using materials which are readily to hand. Many traditional and newly fashionable methods do more harm than good because they are damaging or delay transfer to medical care.

Recommended first-aid measures

1. Reassure the patient.
2. Immobilize the bitten limb with a splint or sling. Firm binding of the splint with a broad crêpe bandage is effective. The aim is to prevent muscular contraction which will enhance absorption and spread of venom.
3. Move the patient to a dispensary or hospital as quickly, comfortably and passively as possible. Take the snake responsible for the bite, provided it can be killed or secured without risking further bites.
4. Avoid harmful and time-wasting procedures such as incisions, excisions, cauterizations, amputations, instillation of chemicals, application of ice packs, electric shocks, and ingestion or application of herbal remedies.
5. Avoid the use of tourniquets, constricting bands, bandages or pressure pads unless the snake was

an identified dangerously neurotoxic elapid or sea snake. In these cases alone, where there is a risk of respiratory paralysis before the patient reaches hospital, a tight (arterial) tourniquet should be applied around the upper part of the limb. This should be released for 1 min every 30 min and applied for not longer than 2 h in total. If the materials are available, a less uncomfortable method is to splint the limb and firmly bind it with a crêpe bandage. The aim is to delay life-threatening neurotoxicity until the patient can be brought to a place where he can be intubated and artificially ventilated.

Medical treatment

Snake bite is a medical emergency which should be assessed and treated by medically trained staff in a dispensary or hospital. Because of uncertainties about the species responsible and the amount of venom injected, and the variable speed of evolution of signs and symptoms and envenoming, most patients bitten by snakes should be observed for at least 24 h. Exceptions are those cases where the snake can be identified reliably as non-venomous. The history must establish the time and circumstances of the bite, identification of the snake (ideally from examination of the dead specimen, otherwise from a description) and the progression of symptoms. The patient is examined for evidence of local and systemic envenoming. Fang marks, extent of local swelling and tenderness, and tender enlargement of local lymph nodes should be recorded. Gingival sulci, nose, skin and other sites should be examined for evidence of spontaneous bleeding (Figure 28.7). The earliest sign of paralysis

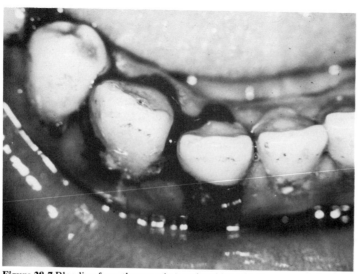

Figure 28.7 Bleeding from the gums in a patient bitten by the saw-scaled or carpet viper (*Echis carinatus*) in Nigeria

is ptosis (failure of lid retraction causing hooding of the pupil when the patient is asked to look upwards). Signs of respiratory muscle paralysis include dyspnoea, exaggerated abdominal respiration, contraction of intercostal muscles and cyanosis. Muscle tenderness and stiffness suggests rhabdomyolysis. Cardiovascular assessment includes measurement of blood pressure and pulse rate, assessment of skin temperature, level of consciousness and urine output.

A few ml of venous blood should be placed in a clean, dry glass test tube and left for 20 min at ambient temperature. Failure of the blood to clot indicates defibrination. Other useful simple laboratory measurements include peripheral leucocyte count, haematocrit, urine microscopy and stix testing and electrocardiogram.

Monitoring of snake bite victims should include frequent assessment of new symptoms and signs, level of consciousness, ptosis, pulse rate and rhythm, blood pressure, respiratory rate and progression of local envenoming. In patients with paralytic envenoming, the ventilatory capacity (peak expiratory flow, or vital capacity) or expiratory pressure should be measured.

Antivenom

Antivenom, which is hyperimmune animal (usually horse) serum, is the only specific treatment for envenoming. Antivenoms are expensive, are often in short supply and can cause life-threatening reactions. For these reasons they must be used only when indicated (Table 28.2) and should be administered only by medically trained staff able to use the optimal route (slow intravenous injection or infusion) and to detect and treat serious reactions. Antivenoms are effective only against the specific venoms stated on the ampoule or package insert.

Table 28.2 Indications for antivenom treatment

Systemic envenoming:
  Hypotension, shock, other signs of cardiovascular
    toxicity
  Neurotoxicity
  Rhabdomyolysis
  Impaired consciousness
  Spontaneous systemic bleeding
  Non-clotting blood
  (WBC > 20 000 μl, elevated serum enzymes)
  Acidosis

Local envenoming:
  Known necrotic venom
  Swelling involving more than half of the bitten limb
  Rapid progression of swelling
  Bites on digits and into other tight fascial compartments

Polyspecific or polyvalent antivenoms are produced to cover all the important venomous species in a particular geographical area. These are invaluable when the species of snake is unknown. When the species diagnosis is certain, the optimal treatment is with a monospecific antivenom. The initial dose of antivenom varies with the particular manufacturer, but in most cases is not less than five 10 ml ampoules. *N.B. Children need the same dose as adults.*

Skin and conjunctival sensitivity tests are of no predictive value and should not be used. The effectiveness of the initial dose of antivenom is judged by the clinical response. If life-threatening signs such as respiratory paralysis and shock persist, the dose should be repeated within 1 h. In the case of procoagulant venoms, the initial dose is repeated every 6 h until blood coagulability is restored. Coagulability is assessed by the simple whole blood clotting test described above. Late recurrence of envenoming caused by continuing absorption of venom from the injected 'depot' of venom can occur, and so severely envenomed patients should be observed in hospital for several days.

Antivenom reactions

Early (anaphylactic) reactions present with itching, urticaria, tachycardia, fever, coughing and vomiting within 10 min to 2 h of starting antivenom treatment. Immediate treatment with 0.1% (1 in 1000, 1 mg/ml) adrenaline is effective. The adult dose is between 0.5 and 1.0 ml and for children 0.01 ml/kg, given by subcutaneous, or in more urgent cases intramuscular, or even *very slow* intravenous injection. This should be followed by an antihistamine such as chlorpheniramine maleate (adult dose 10 mg, children 0.2 mg/kg) by slow intravenous injection. Life-threatening anaphylaxis (shock, bronchospasm, angio-oedema) can be prevented and reversed by adrenaline. Pyrogenic reactions start later and should be treated by cooling the patient and giving antipyretic drugs. Late (serum sickness type) reactions develop 5–24 days after treatment. They are characterized by recurrent itching, urticaria, fever, lymphadenopathy, arthralgias, periarticular swelling and albuminuria. Mild cases should be treated with an oral antihistamine. Prednisolone (5 mg four times a day for 5 days in adults, 0.7 mg/kg/day in divided doses for 5 days for children) is effective in more severe cases.

Supportive treatment

Artificial ventilation (manual or mechanical) is life-saving in patients with respiratory paralysis. Antivenom, even in adequate doses, may act too slowly to prevent respiratory arrest. Endotracheal intubation with a cuffed tube is usually adequate unless the patient requires prolonged ventilatory support.

Anticholinesterases

Anticholinesterases, e.g. neostigmine, may produce a dramatic improvement in neuromuscular transmission in patients envenomed by some neurotoxic species, especially Asian cobras. All patients with neurotoxic envenoming should be given a 'Tensilon test' as in cases of suspected myasthenia gravis. After an initial intravenous injection of atropine sulphate (adults 0.6 mg, children 50 μg/kg) to block unpleasant side effects of acetylcholine, edrophonium chloride (Tensilon) is given by slow intravenous injection (adults 10 mg, children 0.25 mg/kg). Patients who show definite improvement in respiratory muscle strength can be maintained on neostigmine and atropine.

Hypotension and shock

These may be reversed by antivenom alone or by correcting hypovolaemia. A plasma expander, preferably whole fresh blood or fresh frozen plasma, is infused. Refractory cases may respond to dopamine infused into a central vein (2.5–5 μg/kg/min).

Renal failure

In oliguric patients, urine flow may increase following cautious rehydration, diuretics and dopamine. Peritoneal or haemodialysis may be required in patients who do not respond to conservative treatment and develop signs of uraemia.

Surgical aspects of snake bite treatment

An aggressive surgical approach to the management of snake bite has been advocated especially by surgeons in Texas who treat bites by the western diamond-back rattlesnake (*Crotalus adamanteus*). This involves surgical exploration and excision of the bite site (to remove the venom depot) and extensive fasciotomies to prevent compartmental syndromes, and irrigation of tendon sheaths and joint cavities to remove venom. However, surgery may be dangerous in acutely envenomed patients, especially if their blood is incoagulable and they are hypotensive and shocked. The results of fasciotomy may be disfiguring and even crippling. There is continuing argument between those who believe that early use of adequate amounts of antivenom is sufficient to prevent tissue destruction, and those

who believe that elective surgery is needed in addition to antivenom.

There is little evidence in favour of early surgical treatment of the bite site. Local infection should be prevented by the use of prophylactic antimicrobials such as penicillin or erythromycin, and a booster dose of tetanus toxoid should be given. If the wound has already been tampered with (for example, incised with unsterile instruments) the spectrum of antimicrobial activity should be broadened by addition of gentamicin or cefuroxime. Fluctuant collections of pus at the site of bites by *Bothrops jararaca* are unusually common in Brazil. Bacteria, typical of the oral flora of these snakes, have been isolated indicating that the infection is introduced by the snakes' fangs. These abscesses should be aspirated or opened by incision and the patient treated with a suitable broad-spectrum antimicrobial agent. Blisters and bullae are best left alone unless they become large and threaten to rupture. In this case they should be aspirated to dryness with a fine needle. The bitten limb should be nursed in the most comfortable position; this will often involve elevation in a sling. It is best to avoid occlusive dressings which conceal the evolution of envenoming and may become soaked with exudates and blood. Flies may be a nuisance in hot climates. Spraying the area with insect repellant (containing diethyltoluamide) or putting the patient under a mosquito net may help.

Surgical debridement is indicated at the earliest signs of necrosis. Local, spinal or general anaesthesia will be required to allow a thorough exploration, as tissue damage may be far more extensive than suggested by the superficial appearances. Immediate split skin grafting is recommended. Large skin defects are likely to persist as chronic ulcers in tropical countries and may suffer malignant change after 8 years or more (Figure 28.8). Keloid formation is an added problem associated with the healing of large denuded areas (Figure 28.9). Amputation is greatly feared in many parts of the tropics and discourages many patients from coming to hospitals. Every effort should be made to preserve a limb. A farmer crippled by amputation will probably have to make his living by begging.

Complications of snake bite

Intracompartmental syndromes

Bites by snakes with necrotic venoms such as rattlesnakes, Malayan pit viper, habu, puff adder and South American *Bothrops* sp. can cause swelling and necrosis of muscles within tight fascial compartments such as the anterior tibial compartment (Figure 28.10).

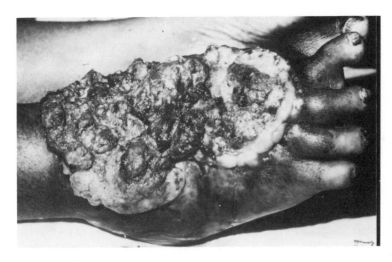

Figure 28.8 Squamous cell carcinoma developing at the site of a chronic ulcer and osteomyelitis caused by snake bite (*Calloselasma rhodostoma*) 8 years previously

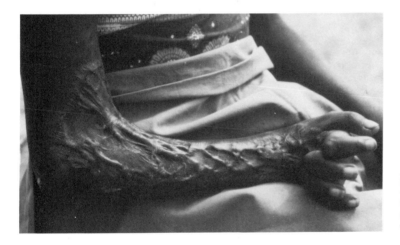

Figure 28.9 Keloid formation in a Nigerian girl who was bitten on the elbow by a spitting cobra (*Naja nigricollis*) 1 year previously, with extensive skin necrosis

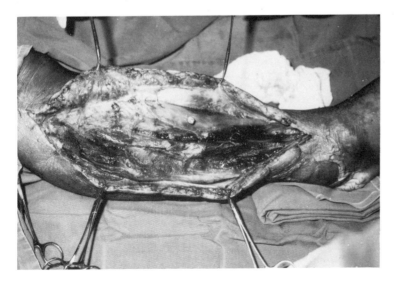

Figure 28.10 Necrosis of muscles in the anterior tibial compartment following a bite on the calf by a 'fer de lance' (*Bothrops atrox*) in Para State, Brazil

Swelling of soft tissues may increase the tissue pressure to such an extent that perfusion is impaired and ischaemic damage is added to the effects of the venom. Signs of intracompartmental syndrome are excessive pain, weakness of the compartmental muscles and pain when they are passively stretched, hyperaesthesia of areas of skin supplied by nerves running through the compartment and obvious tenseness of the compartment. Detection of peripheral arterial pulses by palpation or by Doppler ultrasound does not exclude intracompartmental hypertension. Accident surgeons have found that intracompartmental pressures of more than 45 mmHg are associated with a high risk of ischaemic necrosis. Surgical decompression (fasciotomy) is indicated in these circumstances, but in the case of venom-induced intracompartmental syndromes, there is good evidence from animal experiments that fasciotomy will not prevent necrosis of envenomed muscle. Clinical signs of intracompartmental syndrome in an envenomed limb are not reliable, but measurement of intracompartmental pressure by a simple system (for example, a teflon cannula introduced perpendicularly into the compartment and connected by fine tubing to a saline manometer and infusion pump) provides an objective indication for the procedure. Fasciotomy must not be performed before blood coagulability has been restored by antivenom. This can be accelerated by giving fresh whole blood and concentrates of platelets and clotting factors.

Necrosis

Local necrosis, resulting in the loss of a terminal phalanx or whole digit, is frequent after bites on the fingers or toes. Early adequate treatment with antivenom is essential, but the problem of preventing necrosis and serious functional impairment has not been solved. Expert surgical intervention may be required.

Snake venom ophthalmia

If venom is 'spat' into the eyes, urgent generous irrigation with water or any other available bland fluid is essential as is the case with other chemical irritants. Unless a corneal abrasion can be excluded by fluorescein staining or slit lamp examination, topical antimicrobials such as tetracycline or chloramphenicol should be instilled and the eye closed with a dressing pad.

Prevention of snake bite

Travellers to snake-infested areas can reduce the risk of snake bite. Unfortunately, the measures described below are impracticable for the farmers and hunters resident in these areas, who have to walk and work barefooted and barehanded in fields, plantations and jungles. Snakes should never be approached, disturbed, cornered, attacked or handled even if they are thought to be harmless species, are in the possession of snake charmers, or appear to be dead. Even a severed snake head can bite. Venomous species should not be kept as pets or performing animals. Protective clothing such as boots, long socks and trousers should be worn when walks in undergrowth or deep sand are unavoidable. A light should be carried at night. Particularly risky activities are collecting firewood, moving logs, boulders, boxes or debris likely to conceal snakes, climbing rocks and trees covered with dense foliage, or swimming in overgrown lakes or rivers. Wading in the sea or estuaries, especially in sand or near coral reefs, should be avoided in sea snake-infested areas. Campers should try to sleep off the ground or use sewn-in groundsheets to prevent nocturnal intrusions by snakes.

Organizers of expeditions to remote snake-infested areas should find out in advance about the likely range of venomous species and about the location of hospitals, dispensaries and the availability of antivenom in the neighbourhood. Although the risk of snake bite is low it may be justified to take a supply of an appropriate antivenom, as local hospitals may be out of stock. Medically untrained people should not give antivenom except in an extreme emergency when it could be given by multiple deep intramuscular injections into the anterior and lateral thighs.

29

Care of the dying

James Kyle

While the advice given in this chapter is particularly applicable to the management of patients in the terminal stages of neoplastic disease, it is also relevant in the case of those who are dying from non-neoplastic conditions. For both groups of patients the aims of the doctor and the supporting hospital team must be to ensure that the patient is as active and interested as possible in the most appropriate surroundings, and also to allay his fears and doubts and to build up trust. Once mutual trust and understanding have been established, often medication becomes much simpler.

In the management of malignant disease the time comes when the doctor must cease in his attempts to prolong life – 'the good doctor is aware of the distinction between prolonging life and prolonging the act of dying' (Lord Horder). This must be an active decision taken by a senior doctor after very careful assessment of the patient's condition. In practice, frequently there is an overlap between active treatment of the underlying disease and the palliative treatment. Combined therapy at times may be appropriate and always there must be a willingness to review both the diagnosis and prognosis. However, when it is clear that the end is in sight the doctor should prepare the patient and his relatives for that final stage. Relatives most commonly prefer that patients spend their few remaining weeks or months in familiar surroundings and this aspect of care falls most frequently on the family doctor. However, they may be admitted to hospital or to a special hospice for 'terminal care', particularly if symptoms are severe.

It is not within our terms of reference as doctors to hasten death. Nevertheless, when in advanced malignant disease death is inevitable, it is not justifiable to employ artificial methods of supporting or replacing vital body systems when the patient's comfort does not call for such measures.

A doctor must not take any step whose prime intention is to end the patient's life. However, it is permissible to prescribe therapy which may shorten the patient's life so long as the clear aim and object is to relieve pain and suffering.

The latest antibiotics are not needed for a terminal bronchopneumonia. Artificial stomas should be avoided if possible. In his dying hours, the paramount consideration is the patient's comfort. Consequently it is the doctor's responsibility to relieve physical and mental distress and to prepare the patient for the end. It is shirking this responsibility to leave the care of the dying patient to others. The consultant must play a leading role, and on ward rounds he should always talk to any dying patient. The tact and patience of a considerate doctor can do much to allay the patient's fears and comfort the relatives. A simple honest approach and a willingness to listen are important in establishing trust between patient and doctor.

Some patients at first may not want to know the truth; their wishes must be respected. Later on their attitude of denial may change as trust and confidence are built up. Again a patient may request that only selected information be given to relatives. Not infrequently relatives will endeavour to instruct the doctor how much he should tell the patient, but the doctor must always remember that the overriding consideration must be that patient's best interest.

Each patient must be treated as an individual. A patient care plan should be drawn up by the medical, nursing and other supporting staff; the plan will need to be regularly reviewed and modified in the light of experience with that particular individual. All staff must be constantly aware that the patient must never feel isolated or deserted.

Relief of pain

Before starting analgesic therapy, it is necessary to make as accurate a diagnosis as possible of the cause of the pain. A full history is taken, including the patient's own description of the pain, and of any aggravating or relieving factors. A careful neurological examination is made, for example, for loss of sensation, and some radiographs may be necessary. As a person's reaction to pain can be markedly influenced by psychological factors, e.g. depression or loneliness, the psychological state of patients (and of relatives) needs to be assessed.

Pain in malignant disease tends to be constant, and constant control is required. This implies the prescription of a regular schedule of pain-relieving drugs which should be designed to anticipate rather than to treat pain. Under no circumstances should a patient ever be in the position of 'watching the clock' for his next dose of analgesic; nor should he feel the need to justify it by first experiencing pain.

Not all pain is the direct result of extension of the lethal disease itself. Pain may be caused by swelling, infection or by non-fatal coexistent conditions, such as haemorrhoids. Simple remedies, for example, elevation, tapping of effusions and appropriate suppositories may afford relief. Furthermore discussion and explanation of each symptom enables the patient to relax, thereby reducing the drug dosage required. If desired by the patient, alcohol has a sedative effect and induces mild euphoria. In terminal care units there should be no unnecessary restrictions on the administration of alcohol, and it may be given regularly. Other luxuries not normally available in hospital, e.g. honey, should be provided for a patient who wants them.

The drugs available for the relief of pain are the analgesics and the narcotics. These can be potentiated by the phenothiazines, which will also control nausea and vomiting, or by sedatives, which will ensure adequate sleep. Most of these drugs are effective orally and injections may not be required.

Mild pain

It is important to start analgesic therapy early, at the first sign of pain. Aspirin (600 mg) and paracetamol (1 g) are useful analgesics for the control of mild pain and can be given 4–6 hourly (Table 29.1). Dihydrocodeine bitartrate (DF 118) causes troublesome constipation; if given it should not be repeated regularly.

It is always better to try simpler analgesics first and only to increase the potency and dosage of the analgesic drug chosen when it is necessary in order to produce adequate relief from pain. If the patient is vomiting the analgesic must be given by injection.

Table 29.1 The commonly used analgesics

1. Oral

Aspirin	600 mg	} 1–2 tablets 4-hourly for
Paracetamol	1000 mg	mild to moderate pain
Buprenorphine (Temgesic)	0.4 mg	1–2 tablets sublingually
Morphine	5–120 mg	4-hourly for moderate to severe pain

2. Parenteral

Diamorphine	2.5–4.5 mg	4-hourly (s.c. or i.m.)
Buprenorphine (Temgesic) in presence of pain from increased intracranial pressure	0.3–0.6 mg	8-hourly (s.c. or i.m.)

3. Rectal

Oxycodone pectinate (Prolodone)
Suppositories – useful when oral and parenteral routes difficult

1. Bone pain		
Soluble aspirin	600 mg	1–3 tablets 4–6 hourly
Flurbiprofen (Froben)	50 mg	1–2 tablets 6–8 hourly
2. Raised intracranial pressure		
Soft tissue infiltration		
Nerve compression pain		
Dexamethasone (Corticosteroids)	2–4 mg	6-hourly
Prednisolone	5–10 mg	t.d.s.

As the effect of the tablets or injection wears off in 4–6 h, the return of pain should be foreseen and regular repeat medication be ordered and given before pain is felt again.

If aspirin is used, it should be given 4-hourly and in soluble (calcium aspirin) buffered (without acid) form. Paracetamol (Panadol), the active metabolite of phenacetin, is used increasingly. Distalgesic, combining paracetamol 325 mg with dextropropoxyphene hydrochloride, is effective in a dose of 2 tablets q.d.s. Distalgesic is a most useful preparation. Buprenorphine (Temgesic) is effective when given sublingually – 1 or 2 tablets (0.4 mg) placed under the tongue 6- or 8-hourly. If and when these drugs begin to fail, it is better to move directly to the morphine group of drugs.

It is common to give, as an adjuvant to these mild pain-relievers, promazine (Sparine) or chlorpromazine (Largactil), 25–75 mg 6-hourly, and diazepam. They help to relieve the patient's anxiety.

Moderate and severe pain

When pain is more severe, the narcotics morphine or diamorphine (heroin) are unquestionably the best drugs available. Oral medication may be tried first, using morphine sustained release tablets (MST) 10 mg every 8 h.

Nausea can be controlled by syrup of prochlorperazine maleate, 5–10 mg, and additional sedation by syrup of chlorpromazine, 25–50 mg. Chlorpromazine suppositories, 100 mg, may be used instead.

Once pain is severe parenteral therapy will be required. It is usual to start with 10 mg morphine sulphate or 5 mg diamorphine hydrochloride subcutaneously and to increase the dose as necessary. The drugs can be given as an intramuscular injection. In some cases morphine may with advantage be administered subcutaneously, using a constant infusion pump or similar device. An intravenous bolus is rarely justifiable. The longer acting opioid oxycodone may be given rectally, one 30 mg suppository every 8 h. The use of diamorphine is banned in many countries. In solution it is rather unstable, but a fresh preparation may be given subcutaneously in the terminal stages. The amount of morphine mostly has to be gradually increased, and in a few cases may reach a maximum of 2000 mg/24 h. However, this is not always so, and if fears and doubts are removed, occasionally the dosage can be reduced. Somewhat smaller dosage may be advisable in patients over 70 years of age. When prescribing narcotics in dosages above those normally employed, it is advisable for the house-surgeon to have the order countersigned by a more senior medical colleague.

Side effects of morphine

Morphine and its derivatives may cause nausea, vomiting, depression of the cough reflex and constipation. Diamorphine has the advantage that it does not cause vomiting or constipation. Nausea can be prevented by haloperidol (Serenace) 1.5 mg at night or prochlorperazine (Stemetil) 5 mg t.d.s., and respiratory depression by nalorphine hydrobromide (Lethidrone) or naloxone hydrochloride (Narcan) 0.4 mg i.v. Addiction, drug tolerance and withdrawal symptoms are not problems in terminal care.

Other analgesics

Pethidine, 50 mg, is a short-acting analgesic. Both methadone (Physeptone) 5 mg and levorphanol (Dromoran) 1.5 mg may accumulate in the body, while dipipanone (Diconal) has a tendency to cause marked sedation. In severe stabbing pain sodium valproate (Epilim) 200 mg b.d. can be tried.

Alcohol itself may prove a useful adjuvant, and there is much to be said for a bottle of whisky or brandy at the bedside.

Local therapy

Although hope of cure has been discontinued it may be worth considering local radiotherapy to ease pain, e.g. from a metastasis in a long bone. Radiotherapy can be given with benefit when vaginal bleeding is a problem, for haemoptysis and when mediastinal metastases are obstructing the bronchus, superior vena cava or oesophagus. A single treatment of 8 Gy may suffice.

Interruption of pain pathways

If severe pain of nerve or spinal origin is present, an anaesthetist or neurosurgeon should be consulted about nerve blocks, or even cordotomy. Recently, methods of interrupting pain pathways in the medulla by the percutaneous insertion of electro-coagulating electrodes have been under trial and may prove more applicable in patients with malignant disease.

Alternatively, the posterior nerve roots corresponding to the segmental distribution of the pain can be blocked by intrathecal injection. Coeliac axis may be tried for upper abdominal pain and paravertebral blocks for chest wall pain. Epidural injections of steroids are sometimes helpful.

For bone pain some of the non-steroidal anti-inflammatory drugs will give worthwhile relief, e.g. flurbiprofen (Froben) 50–100 mg 6-hourly. Local radiotherapy may help.

Other adjuvant drugs

Anti-inflammatory drugs such as aspirin, flurbi-profen, 200 mg per day in divided doses or Naproxen, 0.5–1 g per day, give some relief when pain is caused by metastases in bone, liver or in the pelvis. The headache resulting from raised intracranial tension may be eased by steroids, e.g. dexamethasone, 10–20 mg per day; they may also be exhibited when there is spinal cord compression.

Other symptoms of advanced cancer

Pain is not the only symptom of advanced malignancy, and vomiting, dysphagia, cough, dyspnoea, ulceration or fungation may cause distress. The following are brief guides to management (Table 29.2).

Nausea (see Table 29.2)

This may be drug-induced or result from hypercalcaemia, uraemia, or raised intracranial pressure. In most cases a chlorpromazine suppository given first thing in the morning frequently provides an effective antidote. The food offered to the patient should be interesting, and be varied by a sympathetic nursing staff according to the patient's whims and wishes.

Vomiting

If not caused by mechanical obstruction, drug toxicity should be suspected. The vomiting may be psychological and reassurance, careful diet, iced

Table 29.2 Other drugs used in terminal care

Nausea and vomiting		*Night sedation*	
Prochlorperazine (Stemetil)		Nitrazepam (Mogadon)	5–10 mg
Tablets	5 mg	Flurazepam (Dalmane)	15–30 mg
Syrup	5 mg in 5 ml	Chlormethiazole (Heminevrin)	10 ml syrup. 2 tablets
Suppositories	5 mg or 25 mg		or caps
Injections	125 mg i.m.	Temazepam (Normison)	10–20 mg
Metoclopramide (Maxolon)		*Diarrhoea*	
Tablets	10 mg	Codeine phosphate	15–60 mg t.d.s.
Syrup	5 mg in 5 ml	Diphenoxylate hydrochloride 2.5 mg	2 tablets, 6-hourly
Injections	10 mg in 2 ml	(Lomotil)	
Tranquillizers		Atropine sulphate 0.025 mg	
Diazepam (Valium)		Loperamide hydrochloride 2 mg	1 tablet, 8-hourly
Tablets	2, 5, 10 mg	(Imodium)	
Syrup	2 mg in 5 ml		
Injections	5 mg/ml	*Hiccough*	
(*Note:* Valium is more quickly absorbed orally than parenterally)		Chlorpromazine (Largactil)	25 mg oral or i.m. 100 mg as suppository
Chlorpromazine (Largactil)		Metoclopramide (Maxolon)	10 mg oral or i.m.
Tablets	10, 25, 50, 100 mg		
Syrup	25 mg in 5 ml	*Oral candidiasis*	
Suppositories	100 mg	Nystatin (Nystan)	1–2 tablets or 5 ml 6-hourly
Injections	10 mg/ml, 25 mg/ml		
Haloperidol (Serenace)		Amphotericin (Fungilin)	Lozenges
Tablets	1.5, 5, 10, 20 mg		
Liquid	2 mg/ml	Gentian violet	
Injections	5 mg/ml, 10 mg/ml	Ketoconazole (Nizoral)	20–400 mg daily
(Useful when agitation is prominent)		*Urinary frequency*	
Antidepressants		Emepronium bromide (Cetiprin)	100 mg 2 tablets t.d.s.
Amitriptyline (Tryptizol)	10 mg t.d.s.		
Maprotiline hydrochloride (Ludiomil) Begin with small doses Effects may be slow to appear	10 mg t.d.s.		

water, sedatives and antiemetics may help. Those used most frequently are prochlorperazine maleate (Stemetil) 5 mg t.d.s.; cyclizine (BP) 50 mg (oral or i.m.) or metoclopramide monohydrochloride (Maxolon) 10 mg t.d.s.

Dysphagia

If mechanical obstruction is present consider giving relief by insertion of a Moussin-Barbin or similar tube. An endoscopist may be able to clear the lumen with a laser beam. Inability to swallow saliva is distressing and frequent mouthwashes may help. Gastrostomy and jejunostomy may only prolong suffering and are now seldom used.

Mouth cancer

Advanced cancer in the mouth may be very painful but frequent antiseptic washes and local anaesthetic sprays can help. Salivation may be a problem and it is difficult to control dribbling. Conversely, a dry mouth leads to cracked tongue and lips and episodes of fungus infection – lip ointments, boiled sweets and fungicides (nystatin) may help. A painful red tongue may respond to tablets of nicotinamide.

Cough

This is best controlled by linctus codeine or diamorphine.

Dyspnoea

This can be very distressing but bronchial relaxants (ephedrine, aminophylline and atropine) and sedatives (e.g. chlordiazepoxide, 5–10 mg t.d.s.) can help. An open window may give relief.

Fungating growth

Frequent dressings with liquid paraffin, hypochlorite solutions or proflavine emulsion may control discomfort and odour. Fortunately, the patients themselves are rarely troubled by the unpleasant smell, but isolation with aerosols or 'smoke bombs' may be required for the sake of relatives and nursing staff. Exhaust ventilation in the patient's room helps.

Depression

This is commoner in younger subjects. The tricyclic antidepressants are of benefit, but tend to produce confusion and oversedation when given to patients receiving narcotics. Small doses are advisable initially, e.g. amitriptyline (Tryptizol) 10 mg t.d.s. or maprotiline hydrochloride (Ludiomil) 10 mg t.d.s.

It is worth remembering that 25–30% of patients in a terminal care unit will be able to return to their own homes (at least for a time) once their more demanding symptoms have been relieved.

General care
Constipation

When needed, a regular and effective laxative should be given. Magnesium hydroxide plus liquid paraffin emulsion, 20 ml b.d., along with senna tablets 2 b.d. is useful. Lactulose, 20 ml is now popular.

Faecal impaction

This is best prevented by twice-weekly enemas or suppositories. Aperients should be used only in small doses, particularly if the patient is bedridden. As narcotics constipate, the patient should be assured that lack of a daily bowel movement is not harmful.

A patient who has become impacted should be sedated and then *two* manual evacuations performed at intervals of some hours to ensure that the rectum and lower colon are properly emptied.

Incontinence

Incontinence of urine and faeces may be troublesome: the former indicates the insertion of an indwelling catheter of Silastic or Gibbon type. Appropriate antibiotic should be given if necessary.

Bedsores

Frequent attention to the skin or the provision of a sheepskin rug or ripple mattress helps to prevent bedsores in the bedridden patient. Hammock-type beds and the Koro tilting bed have proved useful, and help to reduce the physical burden on the nursing staff.

Sleep

Adequate restful sleep should be achieved by sedation, preferably with nitrazepam (Mogadon) 10–20 mg orally. In the elderly, temazepam (Normison) 10–30 mg is generally effective. Chlormethiazole (Heminevrin), 2 capsules (384 mg base), is also useful.

The dying

Death is the inevitable end of all human beings – the only certainty in life is death. There is need for education of the population to accept death as the natural, if final, part of human experience.

Death from malignant disease is usually a gradual process of withdrawal and thus the sympathetic doctor can do much to help the patient and his relatives. The patient should be encouraged to talk and his questions be answered frankly and simply. While it is not our duty to tell a patient he is about to die, it is equally not in his interests to deny him the truth should he choose to know it. The tendency now is to tell the patient the truth. Young doctors may at first find this a difficult and unpleasant task, but gradually gaining a patient's trust and confidence is a very rewarding exercise. It is important to consider the emotional make-up of the patient. The blunt truth, put across in an uncaring manner, can be harmful. Fortunately unpleasant facts can usually be couched in and softened by kind words. Admittedly patients may take from the words just the parts that they want to. Elderly patients tend to accept their fate philosophically. Young patients may be resentful that they are going to die, and considerable patience, tact and sympathy are required in dealing with them. Hearing the truth helps to reduce fear of the unknown.

All humans have responsibilities and worries and many will die happier if they first have the opportunity to leave their affairs in good order. For this reason frank discussion should not be avoided until the patient is moribund, by which time it is frequently too late. A talk with a social worker or financial adviser may give peace of mind to the patient. Discussion renders it easier for the one who is dying to die and for those who are left to mourn.

Dying patients require constant encouragement and must never be passed by on the ward round. At no time should the patient ever feel abandoned. The doctor should spend a little time every day talking and listening to him. If desired the hospital chaplain should be informed about a dying patient as soon as possible so that he can establish a relationship of trust and help the patient overcome his fears. Religious faith can help a man bear his trials with strength and expectation, and a doctor, whatever his own beliefs, must never say anything to destroy hope for a new and better life.

Relatives also require encouragement and help. Frequently they are reluctant to accept the truth and the house surgeon may have to repeat, many times, the reasons for the patient's condition if misunderstanding is later to be avoided. Above all, he must do his utmost to allay the inevitable sense of guilt which relatives feel by his assurance that everything possible has been done. Under no circumstances must he indicate that something more might have been done or that the patient or his relatives were at fault in not seeking medical care at an earlier date. Relatives should be told not to discuss the patient's condition when with him and not to whisper at the foot of his bed. Acuity of hearing is often preserved until the end. They should be encouraged to help to show their love for the patient by performing little tasks for his comfort, preferably in the privacy of a single room. Some patients and some relatives find it difficult to talk about approaching death. For them little acts of kindness may speak louder than words, settling quarrels, smoothing out differences and setting the final seal on the bonds of friendship which have united them throughout life.

As death approaches it should be remembered that the peripheral circulation will fail and subcutaneous injections of narcotics may cease to be effective. Drinks of iced water, cool spongeing and an electric fan help to keep the patient cool. There is no need for the patient to spend his last hours on his back and by turning him on his side choking can be prevented. The 'death rattle' is due to retained bronchial secretions and may be reduced by suction. A timely injection of hyoscine 600 µg may help.

Has death occurred?

It is not always easy to be certain that a patient is dead. This is particularly true when the patient has had brain metastases, has been artificially cooled down or is being maintained on a ventilator. The embarrassment of the young doctor is increased when there are relatives present, anxiously awaiting his verdict. With advanced malignant disease there is no place for resuscitative measures and a little time can be taken to make certain that death has occurred.

The usual method of determining the presence of death is by auscultation with a stethoscope over the apex of the heart for sounds of circulatory activity and over the trachea and bronchi for any respiratory sounds. Silence in the room or ward is essential as the sounds may be very feeble. At least 2 min (by the clock) must be spent on auscultation. If there is any doubt it is advisable to come back after 5 min and again listen; in the meantime the relatives are told that life is not yet extinct.

Fragmentation of the blood columns in the retinal vessels as seen through the ophthalmoscope is another test of death that is sometimes employed. The most rapid and certain confirmation is that provided by a monitoring electrocardiograph, the complexes flickering to a steady line on the screen of the oscilloscope.

In a patient who is being maintained on a ventilator, fixed dilated pupils are a sign of irreversible cerebral damage. There is no need to request electroencephalography tracings. In the presence of these signs it is justifiable to disconnect the ventilator and observe whether spontaneous respiration returns within 1 min. If it does, the patient is not dead and the ventilator should be reconnected. The difficult subject of brain death is considered on p. 454.

Death and transplantation

When there is any possibility of the organs of a dying patient being used for transplantation, then two senior attending doctors must make the decision that the patient is dead and that his vital body systems are no longer capable of independent activity. The decision must never be made by a member of the transplantation team.

When it seems probable that a dying/dead patient's organs would be suitable for transplantation, a tactful approach should be made to the relatives in order to obtain their consent for organ removal. Patients with carcinomatosis are not suitable as donors.

Bereavement

A good hospital doctor dealing with the relatives of a patient who has died needs to have some understanding of the emotional disturbances which they are experiencing, sometimes for the first time. The word 'bereavement' is derived from 'bereft' which means robbed – the relatives feel robbed of a loved one. The mourning reaction is usually immediate, may be delayed and can become pathological, leading to melancholia and depression which require psychiatric treatment. The nature and depth of the reaction depend on many factors including the age and degree of kinship and of dependence of the relative, previous experience and geographic proximity to the former home of the deceased. The pathological form may be the result of guilt feelings.

Normal mourning has a clear beginning and end and passes through four stages:

Stage 1: Shock, disbelief, anger, loss. Normally this stage ends with the funeral.
Stage 2: Idealization, extolling the virtues of the departed – *de mortuis nil nisi bonum*.
Stage 3: Ambivalent stage, when there is a more rational balancing of the profit/loss account.
Stage 4: Disengagement. The relative starts to prepare for a new way of life in the changed circumstances. It may occur at different times depending on age.

The duration of each stage can vary; one or more stages may be omitted.

In abnormal mourning the bereaved person becomes stuck in one of the four stages, or passes through them in the wrong order. Abnormal anger may take the form of unjustified complaints against the doctor. The house surgeon should inform the family doctor of the death of a patient in hospital. The family doctor can then call once or twice at the home of immediate relatives to make sure that the mourning reaction is proceeding normally and is not becoming pathological.

30

Major civil accidents

A. B. Matheson

At any time, a major civil accident or natural disaster may occur which results in so great a number of casualties that the ordinary emergency services are overwhelmed. To cope with such an event the emergency agencies such as the police, fire service, ambulance service and the health authority prepare in advance contingency plans and publish them to their staff. The Accident and Emergency (A and E) department will be the fulcrum of any hospital plan and the Junior Casualty Officer should at an early date familiarize himself with the proposed arrangements and know what his duties and responsibilities would be in such an event.

Overall planning

It is impossible to foresee in exact detail every conceivable disaster which might occur, but the capabilities of the emergency services to respond routinely to a given number of casualties should be known and a figure arrived at where the emergency plan has to be adopted. Consideration should be given to particular risk areas within the hospital's catchment, such as airports, mines, motorways, factories or oil installations. Geographical regions at risk from natural disaster such as hurricane, flooding or earthquake which could result in widespread devastation and the loss of even the most basic of services require state contingency plans to provide aid to the surviving population. These plans may very well involve the military authorities and the provision of health services will be but a part.

The aims of the emergency services when faced with a more localized disaster will be to rescue the victims and transport them to hospital, there to be treated as quickly and efficiently as possible. If suitably located, a group of hospitals may respond to a single incident, and in these circumstances planning should encompass the numbers and types of casualties which each institution could accept. A more isolated but major hospital might very well have to cope entirely on its own, in the initial stages at least, but calling on its distant neighbours for specialized assistance if the need arose and became apparent. The police, ambulance and rescue services will have formed their own contingency plan but all these agencies, along with the hospital, must knit together closely and for this to happen good communications and liaison are essential.

The hospital plan and response

The hospital plan is simple in concept – it is to cease all unnecessary work of the hospital, so releasing staff and facilities for the treatment of the disaster victims. A capability of handling other emergencies must, of course, be maintained. The hospital response, on the other hand, must be flexible. The numbers and type of staff called in should relate to the number and type of casualties received or expected. The response must also be capable of being varied as clearer details of the disaster emerge. Again, for this to happen smoothly good communications are necessary.

Communications

The first intimation of a disaster is likely to be from the police through the hospital telephone exchange. The telephone operator should have clear written instructions as to who to contact in this event. It is likely to be a Senior Medical Adminstrator or the Senior Casualty Officer or both. Regrettably nowadays it is necessary to have some sort of check mechanism to ensure that the information is genuine and so prevent the work of the hospital being disrupted unnecessarily in response to a hoax call.

The decision having been taken to implement the hospital major civil accident plan, key personnel are then informed. A list of these people annotated by the posts they hold, and with their telephone numbers, should be kept at the telephone exchange.

The Medical Administrator should set up a control point, ideally near or within the A and E department where he can liaise closely with the A and E staff and be in contact with other departments in the hospital by telephone. He should also be in contact with the disaster site, either by telephone or by radio over the police or ambulance communications network. All information regarding casualties is fed to this point, and from it wards and other departments are advised of what to expect.

Additionally, it is useful to set up a Casualty Information Bureau within the A and E department, ideally manned by police officers and provided with information regarding patients by the A and E and other hospital staff. The bureau should have a direct telephone line to police headquarters and other separate outside telephone lines, as it is important that the hospital exchange lines remain free for essential calls.

The police should broadcast through television and radio an emergency telephone number where anxious friends and relatives can obtain information regarding casualties. This number should put them in contact with an information bureau at the local police headquarters. Enquiries from the news media should be handled by the hospital administration through a designated Press Officer.

Personnel

Key personnel within the A and E department at this stage are the Senior Casualty Officer, the Senior Nursing Officer and the Senior Medical Administrator, who has assumed the role of Hospital Medical Controller. The last will require the assistance of a lay administrator.

Arrangements are put in hand for casualties to be received in the A and E department and the Senior Casualty Officer and the Senior Nurse, acting on such information as is available to them, arrange for additional staff to be called in as necessary. It is important that staff are allocated, as far as possible, tasks with which they will be familiar, and frequently junior members of staff who have recent experience of the working of the A and E department may be more useful than senior staff to whom the A and E department is foreign.

Depending on the circumstances of the incident it may be worthwhile designating a Site Medical Officer. This should be a senior doctor experienced in handling casualties who goes immediately to the scene of the disaster to report back an accurate assessment of the number of casualties and their types, again using the police or ambulance radio networks as necessary.

The Hospital Medical Controller

The Senior Medical Administrator is in a position to take a broad view of the hospital response to the incident. He is situated in or near the A and E department and in close liaison with its staff. He is in contact with the police, ambulance service and the Site Medical Officer should there be one. He is therefore well placed to advise wards, theatres and departments, such as the radiographic department and the Blood Transfusion Service, as to what will be required of them. He may be supported in his tasks by other medical administrators and will certainly require the assistance of a lay administrator.

Lay Administrator

His duties are logistic. He will be required to provide portering and other staff for the movement of patients and materials about the hospital; initially, for example, clearing wards for the receipt of casualties, and later transporting patients from the A and E department to the theatres and wards. He will also be responsible for ensuring that all departments have sufficient supplies to perform their work.

Site Medical Officer

This should be the most senior member of medical staff who is familiar with the handling of casualties and who can be spared from the hospital. He is designated to go to the scene of the incident and report back. His primary duties there will *not* be clinical but he should liaise closely with the police and the rescue services in making an accurate assessment of the number and type of casualties. He may find it useful to set up a casualty clearing point where rescued victims are gathered and sorted or triaged. There he can discuss with the Senior Ambulance Officer the order and means of their transfer to hospital. He will also be in the best position to decide if a mobile surgical team is necessary and can request one through the Hospital Medical Controller. He will direct the activities of the team when it arrives.

Mobile surgical team

Disaster victims should receive their treatment in hospital, but in some instances rescue may be delayed for some time, for example, when casualties are trapped, and it is then that a mobile surgical team can do useful and even lifesaving work. The team should be small, possibly consisting of two doctors and a nurse. It is better to have two or three such teams working individually, but under the direction of the Site Medical Officer, than one large team. The personnel should be experienced in dealing with casualties, but need not be very senior. People who are to go out as part of the team should be designated according to the posts they hold in the hospital plan and a team leader identified before leaving.

Protective clothing, preferably in conspicuous colouring carrying some form of identification, should be worn. They should take with them all the necessary instruments, fluids and drugs in pre-packed hampers prepared in advance for this purpose. On arrival at the site they should report to the Site Medical Officer or to the Senior Police Officer. The assessment that is made of a casualty, including the perceived urgency of the case and any treatment given, should be recorded on a suitable casualty label and securely attached to the victim's clothing. Members of the team should be careful not to inhibit the activities of the rescue workers.

Receipt of casualties at the A and E department

If it can be so arranged, it simplifies matters if all casualties are admitted through one entrance to the A and E department. Clear instructions can then be given to the ambulance drivers, and at this entrance there should be a Senior Ambulance Officer with a supply of blankets and stretchers taken from the emergency stores so that ambulances can be re-equipped and turned round with as little delay as possible.

Inside the entrance there should be stationed a senior member of medical staff performing triage. His function is sorting, not treating. It is a responsible task. The surgeon who undertakes it needs courage; he must display the ability to make difficult decisions and to take command. He divides the casualties as they arrive into three categories:

1. Critically injured – those in immediate danger of death, principally severe injuries to the head, chest, abdomen and extensive burns.
2. Less urgent cases who nevertheless require admission.
3. Injured, but possibly not requiring admission – the 'walking wounded'. Many will have skin cuts caused by flying glass, some are dazed, many are frightened and most are covered in dust and debris.

The critically injured go at once to a resuscitation area where there is a team of junior doctors supervised by a senior anaesthetist. It is essential

that each patient has a clear airway established and an intravenous line set up. The less seriously injured who still require admission present a problem if they arrive in large numbers. It is advantageous to have a large ward or area cleared for their reception. There a senior surgeon takes charge and decides the order in which the patients will receive treatment. A third area will be necessary to accommodate the 'walking wounded'. Although their definitive treatment may have to be delayed for some time they should be made as comfortable as possible by dressing and splintage and should be reassessed at an early stage to ensure that no deterioration is occurring or serious injury has been overlooked.

Documentation

It is likely that the standard methods of documentation will have to be abandoned during a major civil incident. A documentation team of clerical staff should be assembled and positioned near the entrance door. Every arriving casualty should have several copies of a self-duplicating casualty form filled out with as much information as is available. It is esential that one copy accompanies the patient wherever he goes and another is sent to the police information bureau. It may not be possible to discover the names of all victims initally and a simple means of identifying unknown patients should be devised, such as giving them consecutive letters of the alphabet, or a number.

Mortuary

If many fatilities occur the usual mortuary facilities of the hospital may prove inadequate and an area which will serve as a temporary mortuary should be designated. It should, of course, be at a discreet distance from the parts of the hospital accessible to the public, and it should be staffed by the police.

Stand-down

As the A and E department is the first to respond to a major disaster, so it is likely to be the first department of the hospital to resume normal working. As patients are transferred to the theatres and wards of the hospital for definitive treatment and the incoming flow of victims reduces to a trickle or ceases, so the memebers of the A and E staff can be stood down. Fresh staff who had been rested for a period during the emergency may then go on duty and the department revert to its regular routine. It may be of advantage to maintain the hospital contol point for two or three hours after the last victim has been admitted and the police information bureau may require to remain open for several days following the incident until all victims have been accounted for and all relatives informed. Eventually the time will be reached where the Hospital Medical Controller in consultation with colleagues can decide that the emergency is passed and a general stand-down will be declared, and the hospital will gradually return to the usual routine.

Wider considerations

Modern information gathering and braodcasting techniques mean that news of a disaster is very quickly disseminated and indeed the hospital may get its first inkling of an incident from these sources. The hospital soon becomes the focus of attention, both for anxious friends and relatives requiring information about their loved ones and the national or even international news media seeking to report the story. If no arrangements are put in hand to cater for the particular and legitimate needs of these groups, they could unwittingly impede the clinical work of the department. It is important therefore to have contingency arrangements which will anticipate that problem.

As soon as a major emergency is declared the hospital should be made secure against unauthorized entry and police assistance will almost certainly be necessary to achieve this. As few entrances as is compatible with the functioning of the hospital should remain open, but manned by both hospital staff and the police to allow authorized entry. Off-duty hospital staff should carry identification passes to permit entry.

Legitimate enquirers such as friends and relatives should be admitted to some part of the hospital and accommodated separately from, but in reasonable proximity to, the clinical areas. There they can be offered comfort and support by the clergy and social workers. They should be provided with as much information regarding events as it is humane to release. If at all possible, separate areas away from the common gaze should be organized for the reunion of families and the grieving of the bereaved.

Particular attention should be paid to press relations and the Press Officer should regularaly update them. The issuing of casualty and survivor lists, however, should remain a matter for the police. Regular press conferences can be useful, and requests for photographs and interviews with patients may, if appropriate, be accommodated by operating the so-called rota system where three or four reporters are allowed such access on the understanding that they will share their material with all of their colleagues.

Surprisingly soon after a major incident the hospital may find itself the centre of public and press attention because of visits by VIPs, so adding to security problems, and once more potentially compromising its clinical activities. Visits may be made by the presidents or chairmen of the companies involved, ministers and civil servants from the government department or departments in whose sphere of influence the incident occurs, politicians, and heads of state or their representatives. Those VIPs whose interest extends to the investigation and initiation of enquiry into the incident should be accommodated at the earliest possible date, but in a quiet and discreet manner. Other VIPs will wish to visit to offer comfort and support to the victims, the survivors and their relatives, and to thank the emergency services. These visits will unavoidably create enormous media interest and security problems, and while they are invaluable in terms of maintaining the morale of all concerned, if at all possible the hospital authorities should most tactfully suggest that they be delayed for at least 48 h following stand-down of the emergency.

The physical injuries suffered by victims of a disaster are often readily identifiable, but the psychological hurts can be more insidious and difficult to perceive. These traumas can affect survivors as well as victims and relatives and indeed extend to members of the emergency sevices as well. Even members of the caring professions may not be immune. Social workers, clergy and members of the psychiatric staff should have early involvement with all of these groups so that problems can quickly be identified and the work of alleviation begun forthwith.

31

Postoperative chest complications and artificial ventilation in surgical patients

J. M. Imray and D. C. White

Some disturbance of lung function is an almost inevitable occurrence during the postoperative period and there are many potential causes for this. In most cases this disturbance manifests itself as a period of arterial hypoxaemia whose duration and intensity depend on the site and duration of the operation, the age of the patient, the preoperative state of the lungs, the anaesthetic technique and the postoperative sedation.

In addition to this period of arterial desaturation, the causes of which will be discussed below, a minority of patients develop definite pulmonary pathology which may be classified as:

1. Atelectasis (the commonest).
2. Bronchopneumonia and bronchitis.
3. Lobar pneumonia.
4. Aspiration pneumonitis.
5. Lung abscess.
6. Pulmonary oedema.
7. Pulmonary embolus.
8. Fat embolus.
9. Pneumothorax.

Factors affecting the incidence of complications

Chest complications are here defined as the development of a productive cough, pyrexia and the appearance in the chest of physical signs which were absent preoperatively. If radiological criteria are used then the incidence of complications may be notably higher. Their incidence has changed little in 40 years. Possibly improvements in prevention and treatment have just kept pace with more adventurous surgery in poor-risk patients.

Site of operation

This is the single most important factor:

Upper abdominal operations: 20–25% incidence
Lower abdominal operations: 5–10% incidence
Non-abdominal operations: less than 1% incidence

Open vesical or prostatic surgery, however, carries a risk comparable to upper abdominal surgery. This compares unfavourably with trans-urethral prostatic surgery in which the incidence is 1–2%.

Duration of surgery

The longer the surgery, the greater the risk. One series reports an incidence of 3% for procedures lasting under 1 h to 58% in operations prolonged over 4 h.

Pre-existing lung pathology

Patients with chronic bronchitis are three times as likely to develop a bad chest after operation and in these patients the complication is likely to be an acute exacerbation of their existing condition.

Emergency surgery

An increased incidence of most complications is found following emergency surgery and chest complications are no exception. Causes are: (1) inadequate preoperative assessment and treatment of any pulmonary conditions; (2) the frequency of vomiting with its attendant risk of inhalation; and (3) the frequent poor condition of the patient before surgery.

438

Age

These complications are commoner after the age of 70 because of the increase in chronic lung disease with age.

Sex

The increased incidence in men is related only to their increased incidence of smoking, but the difference grows less as more women take up the habit.

Smoking

This causes an increase in secretions of the bronchial glands and at least doubles the risk of chest complications.

Obesity

The work of breathing is greatly increased and all indices of respiratory efficiency are impaired.

Dental sepsis

Pulmonary abscess may occur in patients with bad teeth and gums.

Anaesthesia

There is no significant difference in the incidence of chest complications following either local or general anaesthesia, nor for that matter between agents used. Errors in technique, such as failure to adequately reverse muscle relaxants and prolonged unconsciousness, are both conducive to complications.

Causes of chest complications

Some causes have been given above but it has long been recognized that inability to breathe deeply and to cough and so expel secretions from the lungs are the most important factors. This inability results from the pain felt in the wound and from muscular spasm and this is why the incidence of chest complications is so much greater after upper abdominal (and thoracic) operations in which the mechanics of breathing are affected.

Additional important factors are impairment of diaphragmatic movement by the presence of a pneumoperitoneum and, after thoracic surgery, the reduced chest wall movement.

It has been shown that on the first day after upper abdominal surgery the vital capacity, peak flow rate (PFR) and forced expiratory volume in 1 s (FEV_1) are all reduced to less than 50% of normal and a gradual return takes place, reaching above 80% on the tenth day.

Another mechanism tending to cause accumulation of bronchial secretions is the paralysis of the bronchial cilia by inhaled anaesthetic agents. These cilia normally propel secretions up the bronchial tree. Furthermore the secretions themselves may be thickened and made harder to remove by the drying action of unhumidified gases and by drugs such as atropine which tend to dry up secretions. Dehydration may produce a similar effect.

Bronchospasm may also prevent the removal of secretions; fortunately asthmatics do not usually develop attacks in the postoperative period.

Recently it has been shown that after anaesthesia and regardless of the site of operation there is a reduction in the functional residual capacity (FRC) of the lungs. This is the volume of gas in the lungs at the end of a normal expiration. The cause of this reduction in FRC is not clear but it has the effect that closure of small airways occurs earlier during expiration than would otherwise be the case. With increasing age and in the presence of lung pathology this closure may take place, or may even be permanent, within the normal tidal volume range. There will then be unventilated alveoli in which pulmonary blood is not being oxygenated (shunting) and this will result in the postoperative arterial desaturation already referred to. This condition may continue for as long as 6 days after operation. In addition, airway closure, even if only intermittent, will predispose to atelectasis.

Another factor possibly involved in the production of lung complications is the filtration by the lungs of debris of white cells, platelets and fibrin such as accumulate in stored blood. During large blood transfusions if no filter is used this debris will be trapped in the pulmonary capillaries and may lead to impaired function and alveolar collapse.

Decreased cardiac output and pulmonary oedema are also factors which may be involved in the postoperative period and will affect pulmonary function.

Preoperative assessment

From what has already been said it should be possible to identify those patients in whom there is a high risk of pulmonary complications developing. Provided the surgery is elective in nature a good deal can be done to improve the situation and thereby reduce the risk of pulmonary complications developing in the postoperative period.

Existing pulmonary pathology must be assessed. In addition to routine chest radiography, simple respiratory function tests such as vital capacity, FEV or PFR can be performed and by comparison with normal values the degree of disability can be estimated. Performance of the last two tests before and after the administration of a bronchodilator makes it possible to determine how much airway obstruction is due to bronchospasm and so potentially reversible.

If purulent sputum is present this can be treated by appropriate antibiotics after sputum culture and also by physiotherapy. Elective surgery during acute respiratory infections should be avoided.

Dental sepsis may lead to lung abscess postoperatively so carious teeth should be removed 3 weeks before surgery to allow the gums to heal.

Smokers should refrain from smoking for 3 weeks before operation to give time for the reduction in bronchial hypersecretion. This ideal is rarely achieved in practice.

Obese patients must be encouraged to diet and lose weight before elective surgery.

The patient should meet the physiotherapist and receive explanations and practice in the breathing exercises which will be employed postoperatively.

Blood-gas measurements are not normally required. If clinically the patient's pulmonary condition is so bad that these measurements are abnormal at rest then he may require mechanical ventilation in an intensive care unit postoperatively.

Postoperative management

At the end of the operation it is important to ensure that muscle relaxants have been fully reversed and that the upper air passages have been sucked clear of secretions. Oxygen should be given routinely after major surgery. It should be given at a concentration high enough to counteract the arterial desaturation.

As soon as the patient is sufficiently awake he should be encouraged to breathe deeply and cough and also to move about in bed. These exhortations should be made every hour at least (the 'stir up' regime).

Analgesia

Coughing and deep breathing are best done after a dose of analgesic with the nurse, physiotherapist or doctor supporting the abdominal wound. Judgement is needed in prescribing doses of narcotics postoperatively. If too much is given the patient will lie immobile and with respiratory depression but if too little is given pain will prevent coughing.

There are wide variations in the practice of prescribing narcotics postoperatively, but it seems probable that there is a general tendency not to prescribe enough. Better results would be obtained by more analgesia accompanied by more frequent encouragement to cough and breathe deeply. Intermittent inhalations of Entonox (50% nitrous oxide in oxygen) may also be used to provide analgesia for physiotherapy and can be very effective.

Other methods of securing more complete analgesia include:

1. Intravenous infusion of an opiate, either continuously at a predetermined dose rate, or intermittently on patient demand.
2. The injection of the local anaesthetic, bupivacaine, into the epidural space via a catheter inserted at the appropriate level.
3. The injection of an opiate, e.g. morphine sulphate 5–10 mg diluted to 10 ml with saline again into the epidural space. A single injection gives excellent pain relief for 12–24 h.
4. A combination of both opiate and local anaesthetic.

These methods demand the continuous presence of skilled nursing staff because of the danger of possible hypotension associated with epidural bupivacaine and that of apnoea induced by morphine, so that the patient is best nursed in the intensive care unit.

Reduced incidence of chest complications can be achieved, without sacrificing analgesia, by the use of the respiratory stimulant, doxapram, given either as a single dose at the end of anaesthesia or by intermittent intramuscular injection in the early postoperative period.

Position

So far as the lungs are concerned neither the supine nor the sitting position is particularly advantageous as in both these positions parts of the lung are permanently dependent. Probably the semiprone position with the patient turned regularly from side to side is the best as this does permit drainage of the upper lung.

Signs, symptoms and treatment of chest complications

Atelectasis

This is commonly present to some degree after upper abdominal surgery and may be demonstrable radiologically without any symptoms but if any appreciable degree of infection, bronchial obstruction or shunting of blood through unoxygenated lung occurs then signs and symptoms will be present.

The condition occurs typically within 48 h of operation and is usually basal in origin and unilateral. The area involved may vary from a segment to a massive collapse of a whole lung. Characteristically, tachypnoea is present (30–60 respirations/min) with dilatation and movement of the alae nasi accompanied by slight cyanosis. The heart rate is rapid and movement of the affected side of the chest is reduced. Decreased breath sounds, rhonchi and dullness to percussion may be present over the affected area. In the absence of pleural involvement there is no pain on inspiration.

Radiological findings

Radiologically segmental areas of homogeneous density are seen and since there is a reduction of lung volume the mediastinum may be drawn over to the affected side. Note that a temporary paralysis of one half of the diaphragm is not uncommon after upper abdominal surgery and this tends to promote collapse of the adjacent lower lobe. Some of these features are seen in Figure 31.1.

Treatment

This consists of measures directed to removing the secretions blocking the airways. These include encouragement to cough, postural drainage accompanied by percussion and compression of the chest wall synchronized with the respiratory movements. If bronchospasm is present bronchodilators such as isoprenaline, salbutamol or aminophylline may help.

Various measures to soften or liquefy secretions have been advocated. The best is the inhalation of steam or nebulized water.

The most effective way of removing secretions is direct suction by means of a catheter inserted down the bronchus. This may be done by passing the catheter down a previously inserted endotracheal tube or by bronchoscopy. Care must be taken not to promote pulmonary collapse by too much suction. If a cuffed endotracheal tube is used it is sometimes possible to reinflate a collapsed portion of lung using positive pressure from an Ambu bag.

Bronchopneumonia and bronchitis

These infective conditions may occur following atelectasis but more commonly they are acute exacerbations of pre-existing conditions. Signs and symptoms are similar to those of atelectasis but with a major infective element present, purulent sputum which may be copious, is found together with extensive rales and rhonchi. A specimen of sputum is sent for culture and sensitivity tests. Pleural effusions may occur (Figure 13.2).

Treatment

As for atelectasis, together with appropriate antibiotics according to the results of sputum culture and sensitivity tests. If pleural effusions are sufficiently large drainage may be required.

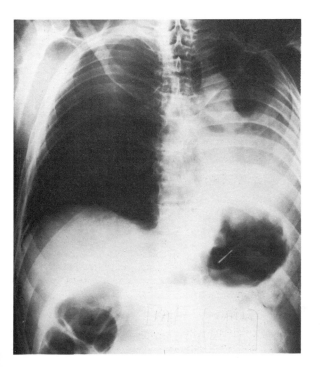

Figure 31.1 Postoperative atelectasis of left lower lobe. The trachea is drawn to the left. Free air is seen under the right hemidiaphragm. The gastric distension should be reduced by the nasogastric tube. Bronchoscopy required

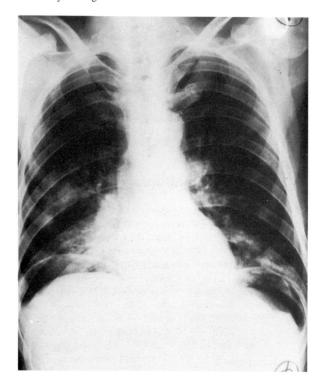

Figure 31.2 Bilateral basal bronchopneumonia after a laparotomy. There is a large postoperative pneumoperitoneum

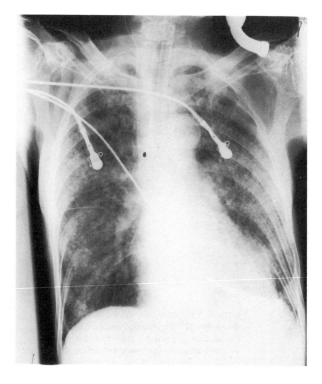

Figure 31.3 Aspiration penumonitis following inhalation of acid gastric contents. The patient is being ventilated; the endotracheal tube and chest ECG leads are seen

Aspiration pneumonitis

Symptoms begin shortly after the aspiration of gastric contents and this complication has a high mortality if the inhaled material has a pH below 2.5. The principal feature is increasing cyanosis unrelieved by oxygen. Tachypnoea, tachycardia and hypotension are present and expiratory bronchospasm usually occurs. The radiological appearance is of irregular mottled densities throughout the lung fields (Figure 31.3). In severe cases death may result quickly from pulmonary oedema or more slowly from progressive hypoxia.

Treatment

Repeated tracheal suction through an endotracheal tube or tracheostomy is performed. Oxygen administration (high concentrations) is advisable. Bronchoscopy is undertaken to remove solid pieces of food if necessary. Cardiac failure may require digitalization. Bronchodilators and antibiotics should be used. Steroids have often been given in the treatment of this condition but the results are uncertain. Mechanical ventilation may be required.

The presence of a subphrenic abscess is frequently associated with atelectasis and infection in the adjacent lung (Figure 31.4).

Lung abscess

This results from the inhalation of infected material. A non-productive cough, pyrexia and leucocytosis are accompanied by a patch of consolidation in which a fluid level may be seen. The abscess may rupture into a bronchus or into the pleura producing an empyema and bronchopleural fistula.

Treatment

This is by antibiotics and by drainage of the abscess (see p. 223).

Pulmonary embolus

This usually arises from thrombosis in veins of the legs or pelvis and typically presents with the sudden onset of pain in the chest. It may occur at any time postoperatively but is commonest from the second to the fourteenth day. As well as the chest pain there is fainting, dyspnoea, tachycardia, hypotension and cyanosis. Venous pressure is raised. Haemoptysis is an important sign and radiographs may show enlargement of the right side of the heart with a shadow in the infarcted area of the lung. An isotope lung scan is valuable. ECG changes of right heart strain may be present. If the embolus is large, shock may be profound.

Prophylactic measures such as injection of subcutaneous heparin, 5000 units i.v. 8-hourly for 5 days, intraoperative followed by daily infusion of high molecular weight dextran or intraoperative intermittent pneumatic compression of the calves significantly reduces this danger (see also p. 259).

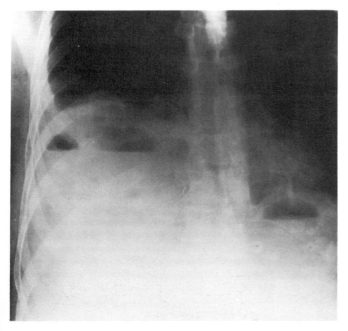

Figure 31.4 Large right subphrenic abscess, with fluid level. There is atelectasis in the lower lobe of the right lung

Treatment

This is by anticoagulants, together with oxygen and sedation. If repeated embolization is occurring, tying off the source of the emboli may be considered. A lung scan is advisable; a vascular expert should be consulted and venography may be advisable.

Fat embolus (see p. 147)

This is seen after multiple injuries, particularly those involving the lower limbs. It is due to the appearance in the circulation of multiple droplets of fat. Symptoms may not develop until 2 or 3 days after the injury and are due to the lodging of fat droplets in the brain, skin, kidneys, lungs, etc. Dyspnoea, cyanosis and frothy sputum are produced. Fat droplets may be identified in the sputum.

Radiological appearance is of widespread mottling throughout the lung field to which the term 'snowstorm' has been applied.

Fat embolism can be the cause of sudden collapse during surgery in a small number of patients undergoing hip replacement due to the forceful impaction of the prosthesis into the femoral neck, driving marrow fat into the circulation.

Treatment

Treatment of the pulmonary condition is directed to maintaining arterial oxygenation; oxygen is given, frequent tracheal suction is necessary and mechanical ventilation may be required. Provided adequate oxygenation can be maintained the prognosis is good, even after long periods of unconsciousness.

Shock lung (see p. 273)

Pneumothorax

This can occur at any stage in the postoperative period. It should not be missed and should always be considered in differential diagnosis when the patient develops acute respiratory distress. It is due to the rupture of an emphysematous bulla or bullae, which can be very small, into the pleural cavity. This may be initiated by positive-pressure ventilation during anaesthesia and occurs more commonly in patients with pre-existing lung disease.

Diagnosis

When small, this can be difficult, and may only be obvious on chest radiographs. As the airspace enlarges, signs of reduced movement on the affected side, hyperresonance, diminished breath sounds, bronchial in character, and then deviation of mediastinum and trachea to the opposite side with or without the presence of subcutaneous emphysema, make the diagnosis clear. It can be readily confirmed by aspirating air from the affected side through a fine bore needle inserted into the second intercostal space 2 cm from the internal edge, or if time allows, by chest radiographs.

Treatment

A small pneumothorax discovered incidentally on routine radiography (Figure 31.5) needs no treatment since air in the space will slowly be absorbed. A large pneumothorax needs under-water drainage and suction via an intercostal drain (see pp. 220–222). A life-threatening tension pneumothorax may initially be decompressed by the insertion of a large cannula (14 G Medicut) mounted on a three-way tap. In spite of continuous drainage occasionally an air leak into the pleural cavity persists. Thoracotomy with decortication of pleura may then be necessary.

Postoperative arterial desaturation and oxygen therapy

It should be remembered that a degree of hypoxaemia, due to the shunting of blood past non-aerated alveoli, is a constant feature of the early postoperative period. It is more marked in the elderly since the Pao_2 naturally declines with advancing years. This hypoxia can be readily reversed by increasing the concentration of oxygen in the inspired air, for example by giving 2–3 litres of oxygen/min through a simple mask. Patients who have pre-existing chronic bronchitis or emphysema with raised $Paco_2$ should be given oxygen in a more controlled manner. Such patients depend on a degree of hypoxia for respiratory drive. Too high an inspired concentration of oxygen would lead to further depression of their respiratory centres, with a rise in $Paco_2$ to dangerous levels. For this purpose, a variety of masks based on the Venturi principle and delivering precise concentrations of oxygen (25, 28, 35%) have been designed. In such a group of patients the use of doxapram, a respiratory stimulant, given by continuous infusion, may allow a necessary increase in the inspired oxygen concentration to achieve a satisfactory Pao_2 without associated respiratory depression. If, however, it is not possible to relieve hypoxia without provoking excessive increases in $Paco_2$ then artificial ventilation becomes necessary.

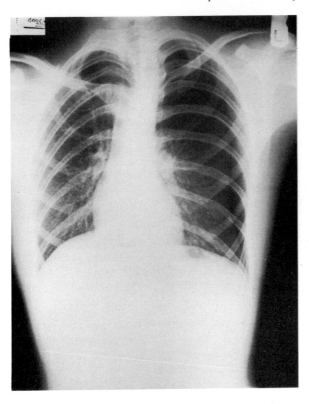

Figure 31.5 Left pneumothorax

Artificial ventilation in surgical patients

Artificial ventilation in the postoperative period can make it possible to operate successfully on patients who would otherwise be rejected for surgery or who, if operated on, would have little chance of survival. It is important that the technique be regarded as preventive of respiratory failure whenever the risk of this is high. Much better results are obtained if this approach is adopted rather than using the technique as a last resort in a patient who is already in advanced respiratory failure. This implies careful preoperative assessment of respiratory disabilities and close monitoring of respiratory function postoperatively in those patients in whom a high risk has been identified.

Patients receiving artificial ventilation should be nursed in an intensive care unit by nurses trained in this work and where medical supervision is experienced and continuous. It is inappropriate that this be undertaken in the general surgical ward since the consequences of quite small mishaps can be rapidly fatal when the staff are inexperienced with this form of therapy.

Indications for artificial ventilation

Surgical patients may require ventilation for a number of reasons: (1) The patient's preoperative respiratory function may be so poor that it may be possible to predict that the additional temporary impairment of respiration which always follows anaesthesia and surgery (particularly upper abdominal and thoracic) will be enough to push him into respiratory failure. In such a patient a planned period of ventilation may be carried out postoperatively and, in a properly organized unit, the risks of such a procedure are small. (2) Postoperative respiratory complications may become so severe as to necessitate ventilation. In practice, this most commonly occurs following upper abdominal or thoracic surgery in patients who had some degree of respiratory dysfunction preoperatively. Such people may appear to develop 'acute' respiratory failure but studies of respiratory function performed at the first sign of complications developing and subsequently would have shown insidious depreciation which could have been successfully averted by early ventilation. Unfortunately, the measures which are necessary when severe respiratory failure has developed, such as high oxygen concentrations, airway pressures and tidal volumes, may themselves produce further lung damage and make the situation irrecoverable. (3) The nature of the surgery may be such as to require the patient to be relieved of the work of respiration and to require accurate control of the composition and volumes of inspired gases, e.g. after cardiopulmonary bypass. (4) Diseases may be present preoperatively causing muscle weakness, such as myasthenia gravis or other muscular dystrophies. These conditions may be exacerbated postoperatively, necessitating ventilation. Ascending polyneuritis and acute porphyria are two conditions which may occur postoperatively and require ventilation. (5) Rarely a patient may become so weakened by surgical complications, such as multiple bowel fistulae accompanied perhaps by gross electrolyte abnormalities, as to make ventilation necessary. (6) Sepsis in the abdominal or thoracic cavity may be associated with shock leading to multiorgan failure, including the lungs – the so-called 'shock lung syndrome'. This condition is associated with a very high mortality, survival depending on an aggressive approach to the eradication of infection, circulatory support and ventilation until the lung pathology, essentially that of toxic damage to the pulmonary capillaries associated with alveolar exudates, resolves. (7) Raised intracranial pressure and cerebral oedema, resulting from head injury or following a period of cerebral hypoxia, for example after resuscitation from cardiac arrest, can be effectively reduced by mechanical *hyper*ventilation. Here a reduction in $Paco_2$ is is associated with a parallel reduction in cerebral blood flow.

Leaving aside those cases in categories (1) and (3) for whom a period of artificial ventilation has been planned preoperatively, the decision to begin ventilation of any patient is not always a straightforward one. There must be a reasonable chance that the pathological changes which have necessitated artificial ventilation will be reversible. The possibility of having a patient who cannot be weaned off a ventilator is not a pleasant one. The effects of anaesthesia and surgery on respiratory function in a fit patient are reversible. Under normal circumstances respiratory function, as measured by arterial oxygen tension (Pao_2), vital capacity (VC), peak flow rate (PFR) and forced expiratory volume in 1 s (FEV_1), returns to normal or nearly so by the third day after an abdominal operation. This means that if a patient gets into respiratory difficulties soon after surgery and requires ventilation the situation is a relatively favourable one in that that part of the respiratory dysfunction which is due to the operation should steadily improve throughout the postoperative period. The dysfunction referred to is caused by inability to cough and breathe deeply due to pain from the wound and also the postoperative arterial oxygen desaturation associated with a fall in functional residual capacity (FRC).

The decision to begin artificial ventilation

This is based on clinical observation of respiratory distress, inability to clear secretions from the lungs, together with deteriorating blood-gas figures. Signs and symptoms of respiratory distress are: (1) tachypnoea; (2) tachycardia; (3) cyanosis; (4) orthopnoea; (5) bronchospasm; (6) use of accessory muscles of respiration; (7) indrawing of chest wall on inspiration; (8) sweating; (9) mental confusion and drowsiness.

When the decision to ventilate has been made, the patient should then be transferred to the intensive care unit and intubated with an orotracheal tube. Once safely established on the ventilator, with hypoxia relieved, then a decision can be made whether to proceed to nasotracheal intubation (standard practice), whether to retain the orotracheal tube (short-term ventilation, i.e. 24–48 h) or to proceed to tracheostomy.

Tracheostomy versus intubation

Disadvantages of tracheostomy are:

1. It is an open wound and is particularly liable to infection.
2. Surgical complications, such as haemorrhage, emphysema and pneumothorax and also aspiration of blood, may occur.

Advantages of tracheostomy are:

1. Suction and clearing of secretions are easier.
2. Large tubes can be used, having low resistance to gas flow.
3. Patients are more comfortable.
4. It can be continued indefinitely.
5. Weaning is easier with a tracheostomy.

In general, if it is considered that ventilation will have to be continued for more than 2 weeks, then a tracheostomy should be considered although, particularly in young children, ventilation via a nasotracheal tube may be carried out safely and without complications for months. Permanent damage to the vocal cords is surprisingly rare.

Oral versus nasal intubation

1. Oral intubation is easier to perform.
2. A larger tube can be passed orally (size 8, 9 or 10) and this makes suction easier.
3. To tolerate prolonged oral intubation quite heavy sedation is usually required. This is quite feasible in the immediate postoperative period but cannot be continued indefinitely.
4. Oral tubes can be obstructed by the patient biting and precautions must be taken against this. Also it is possible for oral tubes to be extruded by use of the tongue and lips.

5. Nasal tubes sometimes cause epistaxis. This can be prevented and passage of the tube facilitated by instilling 1% ephedrine drops.
6. Distortions of the nasal anatomy, such as deviation of the septum or presence of polyps, may make passage of an adequate size of tube impossible. Tube sizes are given in millimetres of internal diameter. The minimum feasible size for prolonged nasal intubation in the adult is 6.

In view of these considerations, oral intubation is really only suitable for short-term ventilation such as for 24–48 h postoperatively. For this purpose, it is convenient to leave in the tube used for anaesthesia (provided this is plastic) and not reverse the muscle relaxant.

Complications of endotracheal intubation

The important complications are: (1) intubation of either bronchus; (2) obstruction; (3) tracheal dilatation; (4) tracheal stenosis.

Intubation of either bronchus

Usually the right, leading to collapse of the non-aerated lung (Figure 31.6). This is more likely to occur after emergency intubation and particularly in children. It is avoided by being aware of the possibility and is easily rectified by withdrawing the tube above the level of the carina.

Obstruction

This may occur because of simple kinking or because of blockage by secretions. If acute, it is a life-threatening situation and is only resolved by rapid reintubation. The accumulation of secretions results from faulty suctioning technique or inadequate humidification.

Tracheal dilatation

This is generally due to the cuff on the tube being overdistended over a long period in association with local infection. It may lead to breakdown of the trachea with erosion into surrounding structures, for example, the innominate vein.

Tracheal stenosis

This can occur at the level of the cuff or at the tip of the tube. Again infection and physical damage by an overdistended cuff or one which distends unevenly to displace the tip against the tracheal wall can be incriminated. It is more likely to occur after prolonged intubation and although usually diagnosed during the weaning period it may appear as a late sequela.

The cuffed tube

Improvements in tube and cuff design over the years have brought about a reduction in complications. Tubes used today are manufactured from soft, inert plastic and cuffs are so constructed that a gas-tight

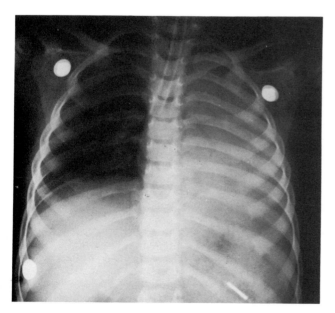

Figure 31.6 Endotracheal tube in right main bronchus. The left lung is unaerated

seal in the trachea is achieved under low pressure with a broad area of cuff applied to the tracheal mucosa, the so-called 'high-volume, low-pressure cuff'. If the blood supply to the tracheal mucosa at cuff level is to be maintained and necrosis avoided, then the pressure in the cuff must remain below capillary perfusion pressure. Once the cuff is inflated to produce a gas-tight seal it should remain inflated since intermittent deflation and inflation may damage the trachea and produce tracheal stenosis.

Damage is further reduced by avoiding the practice, once time honoured, of intermittent cuff deflation and inflation. This was done hopefully to lessen the risk of pressure necrosis of the tracheal mucosa. It is now generally accepted that once the cuff is inflated to a gas-tight seal it should remain so inflated.

Humidification

Under normal conditions, air reaching the main bronchi has attained body temperature and is saturated with water vapour at that temperature (air at 37°C can hold much more water vapour than at room temperature). This process of humidification and warming is carried out by the very large moist area of the nasal mucosa and to a lesser extent by the pharynx. If an endotracheal or tracheostomy tube is in place, the humidifying surfaces have been bypassed. Dry gases cause the trachea and bronchi to secrete a copious fibrinous exudate which dries, forming thick crusts which become detached and can cause serious obstruction. For this reason it is necessary to humidify the inspired gases.

Hot water humidifier

The hot water humidifier is the most satisfactory type of humidifier for routine use with ventilators. It consists of a tank of water maintained at a fixed temperature by an electric element and a thermostat (Figure 31.7). Gas from the ventilator going to the patient passes across the surface of the water, becoming saturated as it does so.

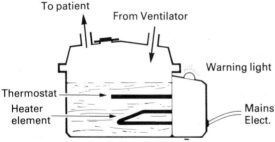

Figure 31.7 Simple humidifier for a ventilator.

The water should be kept at 60°C as this prevents the growth of organisms. There must be a sufficient length of flexible wide-bore tubing between the humidifier and the patient to allow the temperature of the humidified gas to fall to slightly below body temperature before it enters the patient's lungs and a thermometer may be placed at the patient's end of the airway to verify this point. Water will condense out in the tubing because of the temperature drop and some way of draining this should be provided. The humidifier must be placed lower than the patient so that there is no danger of water being accidentally spilled into the airway.

Nebulizer

Various forms of nebulizer are available which blow a mist of fine droplets into the airway. The most efficient is the ultrasonic nebulizer in which the water is broken up by dripping on to a plate vibrating at ultrasonic frequency. Nebulizers deliver a variety of sizes of droplets; if they are too large, they precipitate out before getting into the lungs. Ultrasonic nebulizers are so efficient that they may deliver too much water. This is absorbed into the circulation and at least in small children may produce *fluid overloading*. The water from nebulizers may also affect the compliance of the lungs so care is required in their use.

Condenser humidifier

The condenser humidifier is a device primarily intended to provide partial humidification when attached directly to a tracheostomy or endotracheal tube. It consists of a disc or brass gauze or concentrically rolled metal foil sheets having a low resistance to the passage of gas. The device is warmed by the heat of the patient's expiration (37°C) which is cooled by contracting the metal and water condenses out from the fully humidified expired air. The inspired air, which is at room temperature, is warmed by contact with the metal and then picks up some water vapour from the condensed water on the metal. These devices are only about 50% efficient. They must be mounted as close to the patient as possible and care must be taken that they do not get blocked by coughed-up secretions.

Ventilators

Very many types of ventilators are now in use, working on many different principles. Descriptions and discussion of the classification of ventilators are beyond the scope of this chapter. The most important considerations are: (1) the reliability of the machine; (2) the familiarity of the staff with its controls; (3) ease of sterilization – preferably by autoclave; (4) the ability to deliver accurately a known volume of gas to the patient; (5) a precisely controllable O_2 concentration of the inspired gases; (6) a safe and efficient means of humidification; (7) built-in alarms indicating disconnection, obstruction and gas leak.

The modern ventilator fulfils all the above criteria.

Intrathoracic pressure

During normal spontaneous respiration the intrathoracic pressure is always subatmosheric ('negative'). This keeps the lungs from collapsing and assists the return of blood to the heart. During intermittent positive-pressure ventilation (IPPV) the mean intrathoracic pressure is always above atmospheric and this tends to impede the venous return to the heart. To keep the mean intrathoracic pressure low and to minimize this undesirable effect, care has been taken in the design of ventilators to ensure that peak inspiratory pressure is quickly reached and that expiration then takes place as rapidly as possible. The expiratory rate depends on the elasticity of the patient's lungs and the resistance of the tubes, valves and ports through which he expires.

In addition, the combined length of the inspiratory and expiratory phases is arranged to take not more than one-third of the time available for each breath, i.e. there is an expiratory pause. These measures keep the intrathoracic pressure low and normally the effect on cardiac function is negligible.

Positive end-expiratory pressure (PEEP)

Recently it has been found that in lungs having pathological changes tending to cause collapse of airways they can be kept open, hence improving Pao_2, by maintaining some residual positive pressure at the end of expiration. This technique was first used in the treatment of respiratory distress syndrome of the newborn but has been found to improve lung function in atelectasis, emphysema, pulmonary oedema, aspiration pneumonitis and other conditions. Despite what was said previously, it has been found that in most cases a positive pressure of 10–12 cmH$_2$O can be tolerated by a patient with a normal cardiovascular system and this may greatly improve oxygenation in conditions of atelectasis. Such positive end-expiratory pressures can be produced by spring-loaded or weighted expiratory valves or by placing the expiratory port at the required depth in a tank of water.

Use of the ventilator

The following steps are taken by the doctor managing the ventilator:

1. Familiarization with the controls is the first step.
2. Selection of the correct ventilation rate – 12–16/min in the adult.
3. Selection of the correct tidal volume. Various nomograms are available which afford some guide. An approximate figure is 110 ml/kg body weight. Tidal volumes are most accurately read by placing the measuring device (Wright's respirometer or some other form of spirometer) so that it measures the gas actually expired from the patient's lungs and not on the inspiratory side where large errors may be introduced by compliance of tubing, cuff leakage, etc. In practice, the ventilator will initially be set by inspection of the movements of the chest wall during inspiration. IPPV is less efficient than spontaneous breathing and the chest movements should look greater than those of normal spontaneous breathing.
4. Selection of the correct oxygen concentration (FIO$_2$) Given a patient with normal lungs it should be possible to ventilate with air (21% oxygen) but in practice patients on IPPV always require some oxygen enrichment. It is important to limit this to what is necessary to maintain a Pao_2 in the region of 10–12 kPa. The reason for this is that oxygen at high concentrations is toxic to the lungs. An inspired oxygen concentration of above 50% for any great length of time is undesirable since it may produce signs of *oxygen toxicity*. Also if obstruction develops in the lungs at high oxygen concentrations pulmonary collapse occurs as the oxygen is completely absorbed. Unabsorbed nitrogen helps to keep the lungs expanded – the 'nitrogen scaffold'.

For these reasons, the FIO$_2$ must be carefully controlled in the light of blood-gas figures. Of course, in some cases, such as severe aspiration pneumonitis, it is essential to give 100% oxygen to prevent hypoxia. If so the prognosis is bad as clearly the lungs are extensively damaged. It is not always easy to control accurately the FIO$_2$ and an oxygen-measuring instrument may be needed.

Adequate ventilation is shown by the absence of cyanosis and cardiovascular stability. The settings of the ventilator and the FIO$_2$ are determined by the blood-gas measurements and these must be done as often as necessary until a stable state is attained. If many arterial samples are needed, then an indwelling arterial cannula should be considered.

The introduction of pulse oximetry is a major advance. It provides non-invasive measurement of oxygen saturation on a continuous basis, allowing accurate titration of inspired oxygen concentration, thus obviating the need for repeated blood samples.

Sedation or paralysis

In order to prevent the patient 'fighting' the ventilator it is necessary either to paralyse the respiratory (and other) muscles with curare or a similar drug or, alternatively, to give large enough doses of narcotics such as morphine. In the postoperative period the latter method is usually the one of choice since good postoperative analgesia is produced. Large doses of narcotics are often required and should be given freely.

Physiotherapy

Patients being ventilated require regular tracheal suction, with a frequency dependent on the amount of secretions being produced. This is done using a sterile non-touch technique. Dangerous hypoxia may result if the patient is disconnected from the ventilator for too long so that it is important that this process be completed within 10 s.

To permit drainage of secretions, the patient must be regularly turned from side to side and physiotherapy given as often as necessary to clear secretions from the chest and re-expand any areas of collapse which may be detected on the daily chest X-ray. The physiotherapy consists of posturing the patient to permit drainage of secretions accompanied by squeezing and percussion of the chest wall and 'bagging' – this consists of hyperinflation of the lungs with an Ambu type bag, followed by a rapid expiration to emulate a cough and so expel secretions.

These procedures are essential to keep the chest clear of secretions and prevent atelectasis. They may need to be done frequently but they may upset patients considerably. Care must be taken to avoid hypoxia and to be no more enthusiastic than is necessary.

Safeguards

When a patient is being ventilated an Ambu or similar self-inflating bag must be kept at hand and all staff must be familiar with disconnection of the patient from the ventilator and maintenance of ventilation with the bag. Modern ventilators are fitted with alarm systems giving warning of any major changes or of mechanical breakdown. Should such occur, it is essential that all personnel looking after these patients are competent to continue ventilation manually. Close supervision by nursing and medical staff is essential at all times, especially during weaning.

Weaning of the ventilator

Before artificial ventilation can be withdrawn, certain criteria must be met: a minimum vital capacity of 10–15 ml/kg body weight, a $PAo_2 - Pao_2$ difference of less than 40 kPa and a near-normal Pao_2 with an FIO_2 no more than 50% (except in those with pre-existing lung disease). These are figures which can serve as guidelines.

Before attempting to wean off the ventilator the blood-gas figures should be as near normal as possible. If the patient normally has a chronic compensatory metabolic alkalosis secondary to a respiratory acidosis then his blood-gas measurements should be adjusted to what is normal for him. Any sedative or muscle relaxant is allowed to wear off or is reversed. Everything that is being done is explained to the patient who is sat up in the bed as this is the best position for breathing. The morning is the best time to begin an attempt at weaning.

After disconnecting the ventilator the endotracheal or tracheostomy tube is attached to a T-piece system through which is blown humidified air using a hot-water humidifier (see Figure 31.7) with a fan blower incorporated. Oxygen enrichment is at a slightly better level than that required to produce a normal Pao_2 when the patient was being ventilated. If necessary, PEEP can be continued during the weaning period.

During weaning, the patient must be continuously observed and blood gases measured at intervals. It is often necessary to put patients back on the ventilator overnight during the weaning period. Endotracheal tubes may not be tolerated without a good deal of sedation which is not conducive to weaning so that such tubes sometimes have to be taken out before it is certain that weaning has been accomplished. They may then have to be replaced. In the case of a tracheostomy, a longer period of trial is possible. A fenestrated tracheostomy tube having a large window cut in the outer radius of the curved part of the tube is inserted. This permits the patient to breathe through the larynx and speak in a normal way. A cork can be put in the external end of the tracheostomy but the ability to suck out the trachea is retained as long as the tube remains in place.

Intermittent mandatory ventilation

This technique facilitates weaning and makes it a simple and safe process. The patient breathes spontaneously from a T-piece side circuit with humidication, oxygen enrichment and PEEP, if required, while the ventilator delivers, at given intervals, 'mandatory' inspiration, the frequency of which is gradually reduced to zero as weaning progresses.

After the patient has been weaned from artificial ventilation supplementary oxygen will continue to be required until he is able to maintain a Pao_2 above 9 kPa while breathing room air. This may take several days.

Withdrawal of ventilatory support

There will always be a small number of patients for whom it is inappropriate to continue ventilatory support. This is either because the nature of their illness is clearly incompatible with survival or because they have suffered irreparable brain damage leading to brain death.

The diagnosis of brain death and the withdrawal of life-support systems constitute an important issue and is dealt with separately in the subsequent section.

Brain death

The concept of brain death occurring in patients has developed in parallel with advancing techniques of resuscitation and intensive care and, in particular, the ability to maintain the vital function of breathing by a mechanical ventilator, even though there is permanent functional death of the brain stem.

When brain death occurs and ventilation is continued, death in the traditional sense – the cessation of heart beat – is always inevitable and follows within hours or days or, less commonly, weeks. There is therefore no justification in continuing any form of active treatment once this diagnosis has been made since this would needlessly prolong the distress of relatives, demoralize intensive care staff and waste a limited resource – the intensive care bed.

The decision to withdraw life-support measures has nothing to do with transplant surgery but is strictly clinical. If, however, relatives give permission for organ donation, then withdrawal can be made at a time appropriate to the needs of the transplantation team.

It is most important that there should be no confusion within the medical profession as to the circumstances in which the diagnosis of brain death should be considered and how it should be made, and that society recognizes that such a diagnosis is made with complete certainty. To this end, a code of practice with specific criteria has been formulated over the years in the UK by the Royal Colleges and their Faculties in consultation with Health Departments and others, including doctors, nurses, lawyers, coroners and administrators, with Health Councils and with major religious bodies.

Similar codes exist in other countries, e.g. the Harvard Code in the USA.

It is recommended that the following guidelines taken from this code are followed in every case. These guidelines were reaffirmed by the Royal Colleges in 1981.

Conditions for considering diagnosis of brain death

All of the following should coexist:

The patient is deeply comatose

1. There should be no suspicion that this state is due to depressant drugs. Narcotics, hypnotics and tranquillizers may have prolonged duration of action, particularly when some hypothermia exists. The benzodiazepines act cumulatively, their effects persist and they are commonly used as anticonvulsants or to assist synchronization with mechanical ventilators. It is therefore recommended that the drug history should be carefully reviewed and adequate intervals allowed for the persistence of drug effects to be excluded. This is of particular importance in patients whose primary cause of coma lies in the toxic effects of drugs followed by anoxic cerebral damage.
2. Primary hypothermia should have been excluded.
3. Metabolic and endocrine disturbances that can cause or contribute to coma should have been excluded. There should be no profound abnormality of serum electrolytes, acid–base status or blood glucose concentrations.

The patient is being maintained on a ventilator because spontaneous respiration had previously become inadequate or had ceased altogether

Relaxants and other drugs should have been excluded as a cause of respiratory inadequacy or failure. Immobility, unresponsiveness and lack of spontaneous respiration may be due to neuromuscular blocking drugs and the persistence of their effects should be excluded by eliciting spinal reflexes (flexion or stretch) or by showing adequate neuromuscular conduction with a conventional nerve stimulator. Equally, persistent effects of hypnotics and narcotics should be excluded as a cause of respiratory failure.

There should be no doubt that the patient's condition is due to irremediable structural brain damage. The diagnosis of a disorder which can lead to brain death should have been fully established

It may be obvious within hours of a primary intracranial event, such as severe head injury, spontaneous intracranial haemorrhage, or after neurosurgery, that the condition is irremediable. But when a patient has suffered primarily from cardiac arrest, hypoxia, or severe circulatory insufficiency with an indefinite period of cerebral anoxia, or is suspected of having cerebral air or fat embolism, then it may take much longer to establish the diagnosis and to be confident of the prognosis. In some patients the primary condition may be a matter of doubt and a confident diagnosis may be reached only by continuous clinical observation and investigation.

Tests for confirming brain death

All brain-stem reflexes should be absent (Figure 31.8)

1. The pupils are fixed in diameter and do not respond to sharp changes in the intensity of incident light.
2. There is no corneal reflex.
3. The vestibulo-ocular reflexes are absent. These are absent when no eye movement occurs during or after the slow injection of 20 ml of ice-cold water into each external auditory meatus in turn, clear access to the tympanic membrane having been established by direct inspection. This test may be contraindicated on one or other side by local trauma.
4. No motor responses within the cranial nerve distribution can be elicited by adequate stimulation of any somatic area.
5. There is no gag reflex or reflex response to bronchial stimulation by a suction catheter passed down the trachea.
6. No respiratory movements occur when the patient is disconnected from the mechanical ventilator for long enough to ensure that the arterial carbon dioxide tension rises above the threshold for stimulating respiration, i.e. the $Paco_2$ must normally reach 6.7 kPa (50 mmHg). This is best achieved by measuring the blood gases; if this facility is available the patient should be disconnected when the $Paco_2$ reaches 5.3–6.0 kPa (40–50 mmHg) after administration of 5% carbon dioxide in oxygen through the ventilator. This starting level has been chosen because patients may be moderately hypothermic (35°C), flaccid and with a depressed metabolic

Table 31.1 Check list of respiration and temperature observations, blood-gas analyses, brain stem reflexes, and drug and endocrine status that has to be completed by two doctors before diagnosing brain death (Royal Devon and Exeter Hospital)

Royal Devon and Exeter Hospital

Diagnosis of Brain Death

Patient's name ....

Cause of Structural Brain Damage ....

....

Doctor 1 ....

Doctor 2 ....

Questions   Answers
1. Respiration
   (a) If arterial blood gas analysis has been performed:
       (i)   Was the $Paco_2$ below 45 mmHg before the ventilator was disconnected?
       (ii) Is there any spontaneous ventilation within 5 min of disconnecting the ventilator?
       (iii) If arterial blood gas analysis has not been performed: Is there any spontaneous ventilation within 10 min of disconnecting the ventilator?

2. Brain stem reflexes
   (a) Do the pupils react to light?
   (b) Is nystagmus present when each ear in turn is investigated with ice cold water for 1 minute?
   (c) Does any response occur when each cornea in turn is touched?
   (d) Is any movement present in the head and neck, either spontaneously or in response to any stimulus?
   (e) Is there a gag reflex or reflex response following bronchial stimulation by a suction catheter passed down the trachea?

3. Body Temperature
   (a) Is the rectal temperature below 35°C?
   (b) If it is, has the patient got primary hypothermia?

4. Drugs
   (a) Have any neuromuscular blocking drugs been administered during the preceding 12 h?
   (b) If they have does any neuromuscular blockade remain?
   (c) Have any other drugs which may affect ventilation or the level of consciousness been administered during the preceding 12 h?

5. Is the coma due to a metabolic or endocrine cause?

Signed

Doctor 1 .... Doctor 1 ....

1st Test: 2nd Test:
Doctor 2 .... Doctor 2 ....

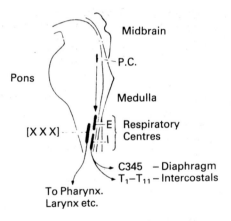

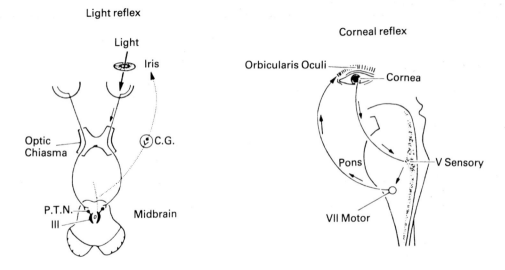

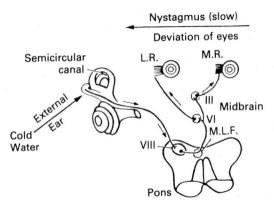

Figure 31.8 Neural pathways involved in brain-stem reflexes

rate, so that the Pa_{CO_2} rises only slowly in apnoea (about 0.27 kPa/min (2 mmHg/min)).

Hypoxia during disconnection should be prevented by delivering oxygen at 6 litre/min through a catheter placed in the lower trachea.

If blood-gas analysis is not available to measure Pa_{CO_2} and Pa_{O_2}, the alternative procedure is to supply the ventilator with pure oxygen for 5 min and to disconnect the ventilator for 10 min while delivering 5% carbon dioxide in oxygen at 6 litre/min by catheter in the trachea. This establishes diffusion oxygenation and ensures that during apnoea hypoxia will not occur.

Those patients with pre-existing chronic respiratory insufficiency, who may be unresponsive to raised levels of carbon dioxide and who normally exist on a hypoxic drive, are special cases and should be expertly investigated with careful blood-gas monitoring.

Other recommendations

1. The diagnosis of brain death must be made by two medical practitioners who have expertise in this field. One should be a consultant, the other being a consultant or senior registrar who should assure himself or herself that the preconditions have been met before testing is carried out. The length of time required before the preconditions can be satisfied varies according to circumstances and although occasionally it might be less than 24 h it may extend to days.

2. The two doctors may carry out the tests separately or together. If the tests confirm brain death, *they should nevertheless be repeated.* It is for the two doctors to decide how long the interval between the tests should be, but the time should be adequate for the reassurance of all directly concerned.

3. There may be circumstances in which it is impossible or inappropriate to carry out every one of the tests. The criteria are guidelines, not rigid rules, and it is for the doctors at the bedside to decide when the patient is dead.

4. It is suggested that the profession, in association with the Health Departments, design a check list which would be completed in all cases and form part of the hospital case record. Table 31.1 is an example of such a record used in the Royal Devon and Exeter Hospital.

5. There is now conclusive evidence that there is no need to pursue any form of extra confirmatory investigation, such as EEG recording or cerebral angiography.

6. Finally, should consent for organ donation be obtained, it is important that neither doctor making the diagnosis of brain death be a member of the transplant team.

The relatives of the patient should be kept informed, in a compassionate manner and using clear but simple language.

Appendix 1

Conversion tables

Temperature: centrigrade to fahrenheit

°C	°F	°C	°F	°C	°F	°C	°F
33	= 91.4	36	= 96.8	39	= 102.2	42	= 107.6
34	= 93.2	37	= 98.6	40	= 104.0	43	= 109.4
35	= 95.0	38	= 100.4	41	= 105.8	44	= 111.2

Temperature: fahrenheit to centigrade

°F	°C	°F	°C	°F	°C	°F	°C
91	= 32.8	96	= 35.6	101	= 38.3	106	= 41.1
92	= 33.3	97	= 36.1	102	= 38.9	107	= 41.7
93	= 33.9	98	= 36.7	103	= 39.4	108	= 42.2
94	= 34.4	99	= 37.2	104	= 40.0	109	= 42.8
95	= 35.0	100	= 37.8	105	= 40.6	110	= 43.3

Weights: metric to apothecaries'

1 kg	= 2 1b 3¼ oz
500 g	= 1 lb 1⅝ oz
100 g	= 3½ oz
25 g	= ⅞ oz
10 g	= ⅓ oz
1 g	= 15.43 grains
<1/2 or 500 mg	= 7.7 grains

Weights: apothecaries' to metric

¼ grain	= 15 mg
½ grain	= 30 g
15 grains	= 1 g
½ oz (avoir.)	= 15 g
1 lb	= 454 g

Measures: metric to imperial (liquid)

1 ml	= 17 minims
1 litre	= 1 pint 15 fl oz approx.

Measures: imperial to metric (liquid)

15 minims	= 1 ml
1 fl oz	= 30 ml
1 pint	= 568 ml

Measures of length

1 mm	= approx. 0.04 in
1 in	= approx. 2.5 cm

Appendix 2

SI units

The International System of Units (SI) was adopted by the Conference Générale des Poids et Mesures in 1960 as a coherent system based on the units: metre, kilogram, second, ampere, kelvin and candela. The mole was added in 1971. It is already adopted by some thirty countries as their only legally accepted system.

The following table of definitions and conversion factors lists some commonly used units:

Physical quantity	Unit	Symbol	SI definition
Length	Inch	in	2.54×10^{-2} m
Volume	Litre	l	10^{-3} m^3
Force	Newton	N	kg m s^{-2}
Force	Dyne	dyn	10^{-5}
Energy	Joule	J	kg m^{2}s^{-2}
Energy	Calorie (thermochemical)	Cal	4.184 J
Pressure	Pascal	Pa	kg m^{-1}s^{-1} = Nm^{-2}
Pressure	Conventional millimetre of mercury	mmHg	$13\,332.24 \times 10^{-2}$ Pa
Radiation dose	Rad	rad	10^{-2} 2J kg^{-1} l

Names and symbols for basic SI units

Physical quantity	Name of SI unit	Symbol for SI unit
Length	Metre	m
Mass	Kilogram	kg
Time	Second	s
Electric current	Ampere	A
Thermodynamic temperature	Kelvin	K
Luminous intensity	Candela	cd
Amount of substance	Mole	mol

SI units: range of normal blood values

'Normal range' means that values found in 95% of healthy adult subjects can be expected to fall within this range. The ranges quoted are locally derived, for the analytical methods used in one chemical pathology department, and alterations in these ranges may be notified from time to time. Significantly different ranges may apply in other laboratories using different analytical techniques. Consult the localbiochemist.

'Analytical precision' is indicated, where available, and is the expected standard deviation resulting from repeated analyses of the same sample. It may be useful to keep this inevitable source of variation in mind when assessing the significance of reported values falling outside the normal range, or of apparent day-to-day fluctuations in reported values in the same patient.

Blood

Analysis	Normal range	Analytical precision (S.D.)	Stability	Specimen (ml of blood for a single request)
Acid phosphatase	Up to 0.4 U/l	0.1	Poor (medium if serum separated)	2
Alkaline phosphatase	28–114 U/l	11	Poor (medium if serum separated)	5
Amylase	70–300 U/l	40	Good	2
Aspartate aminotransferase	6–14 U/l	2	Medium (invalidated by haemolysis)	5
Bilirubin	Up to 26 µmol/l	3	Medium (keep in dark)	5
Calcium	2.30–2.70 mmol/l	0.05	Good	5
Cholesterol M and F <40 years M and F >40 years	 3.4–7.3 mmol/l 3.4–8.8 mmol/l	0.2	Good	5
Cortisol M F M and F	 190–770 nmol/l 9 a.m. 110–690 nmol/l 9 a.m. <170 nmol/l midnight	50	Good (heparinized plasma required)	5
Creatinine	60–110 µmol/l	10	Good	5
Electrolytes Sodium Potassium Bicarbonate	 137–146 mmol/l 3.5–4.8 mmol/l 20–30 mmol/l	 1.2 0.1 1.0	Good if serum separated (otherwise very poor)	
Urea <40 years >40 years	 2.3–6.6 mmol/l 2.8–7.3 mmol/l	0.3	Good	
Gamma-glutamyl transferase (γ-GT) M F	 4–28 U/l 4–18 U/l	2.0	Medium	5
Iron	18–27 µmol/l	3	Good	10
Magnesium	0.75–1.00 mmol/l	–	Medium (invalidated by haemolysis)	2
Protein bound iodine	320–630 nmol/1	25	Good	10
Thyroxin (T4)	70–150 nmol/l			10
Albumin	30–47 g/l	1		
Total protein	59–83 g/l	2	Good	5
Phosphate	0.9–1.5 mmol/l	0.1	Poor (invalidated by haemolysis)	5
'Blood sugar' (fasting) M <40 years F <40 years M and F >40 years	 3.3–5.2 mmol/l 3.1–4.7 mmol/1 3.3–6.3 mmol/l	0.3	Medium. Oxalate/fluoride tube essential	2

Blood gas analysis

Normal ranges	Blood pH	7.35–7.42
	$Pa\text{co}_2$	4.5–6.0 kPa
	$Pa\text{o}_2$	10.6–13.3 kPa
	Standard bicarbonate	21–25 mmol/l
	Actual bicarbonate	21–25 mmol/l
	Base excess or deficit	0 ± 3 mmol/l
	Buffer base	38.48 mmol/l

Index